Handbook of Behavior Problems of the Dog and Cat

SECOND EDITION

G. Landsberg BSc DVM Dip ACVB
Doncaster Animal Clinic, Thornhill, Ontario, Canada

W. Hunthausen BA DVM
Animal Behavior Consultations, Westwood, Kansas, USA

L. Ackerman DVM DACVD MBA MPA
Westborough, MA, USA

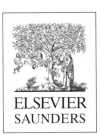

ELSEVIER
SAUNDERS

EDINBURGH LONDON NEW YORK OXFORD PHILADELPHIA ST LOUIS SYDNEY TORONTO 2003

SAUNDERS
An imprint of Elsevier Limited

First edition 1997
Second edition 2003
    Reprinted 2003, 2004 (twice), 2005, 2006, 2007, 2008 (twice)

ISBN: 978 0 7020 2710 9

British Library Cataloguing in Publication Data
A catalogue record for this book is available from the British Library

Library of Congress Cataloguing in Publication Data
A catalogue record for this book is available from the Library of Congress

Note
Medical knowledge is constantly changing. Standard safety precautions must
be followed, but as new research and clinical experience broaden our
knowledge, changes in treatment and drug therapy may become necessary or
appropriate. Readers are advised to check the most current product
information provided by the manufacturer of each drug to be administered to
verify there commended dose, the method and duration of administration,
and contraindications. It is the responsibility of the practitioner, relying on
experience and knowledge of the patient, to determine dosages and the best
treatment for each individual patient. Neither the Publisher nor the authors
assumes any liability for any injury and/or damage to persons or property
arising from this publication.

                                                            The Publisher

Note
The publisher has made every effort to obtain permission to reproduce all
illustrations used in this book.

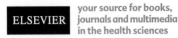

www.elsevierhealth.com

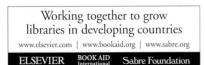

The
publisher's
policy is to use
paper manufactured
from sustainable forests

Printed in China
N/09

Handbook of Behavior Problems of the Dog and Cat

Dedications

To my wife Susan, my children Nadia, Rebecca, and David, and our Golden Retriever Marilyn
Lowell Ackerman

To my wife Susan, my children Joanna, Mitchell, and Jordan, my veterinary partner
Dr Stephen Waisglass, and our new playmate Buffy
Gary Landsberg

To my wife Jan Kyle and my buddies Ralphie, Beau, and Peugeot
Wayne Hunthausen

For Saunders:

Commissioning Editor: Joyce Rodenhuis
Senior Development Editor: Zoë A. Youd
Project Manager: Joannah Duncan
Design: Andrew Chapman

Contents

Preface

Not that long ago, animal behavior was considered an interesting diversion for veterinarians, but little emphasis was placed on this discipline in veterinary school curricula or continuing education for practitioners. Now, there seems to be a general 'awakening' in the veterinary profession as practitioners realize the importance of this subject to their clients, the well-being of their patients, and the success of their practices. Attention to behavioral signs and behavioral problems is an essential part of veterinary medicine since behavioral signs and behavioral changes are often the first or only signs of underlying health problems. But behavior also plays a critical role in the relationship between the pet and its owners. The behavior, or anticipated behavior, of the pet is often the most important consideration influencing its adoption, while the pet's behavior can also lead to the dissolution of the bond between it and the family. Unacceptable behavior is one of the more common reasons for abandonment and euthanasia of dogs and cats. North American statistics suggest that more pets are euthanized for behavioral reasons than for all medical reasons combined. This should be enough of an incentive for veterinarians to incorporate behavioral evaluations and counseling into everyday practice.

This book is designed to provide the veterinarian in general practice with the tools to help owners with concerns they might have about their pets' behavior. Most importantly, it helps veterinarians incorporate behavior consultation into their practices in a very meaningful way, and utilizes hospital paraprofessional staff to their optimum. Not only does the book introduce topics such as learning theory and behavior modification techniques, but it also covers the diagnostic and therapeutic options for the successful management of behavior problems. In this edition, we not only address neuropharmacology and psychoactive drug activity, but also examine important training techniques, nutritional intervention, and explore alternative forms of therapy. Throughout the text we have included cases to illustrate real-life clinical situations. To best illustrate the principles and because of veterinary–client confidentiality, our case examples are composite representatives of our caseload rather than actual clinical cases. To be successful in managing behavior problems, veterinarians must be more than animal trainers. The proper approach to behavioral problems does not differ significantly from any other medical discipline. One needs to carefully evaluate patient history, perform a thorough physical examination, formulate differential diagnoses, conduct diagnostic testing, initiate treatment options, and monitor the patient's responses. Proper diagnosis of the problem and selection of reasonable treatment modalities are solely in the realm of veterinary medicine; let this book serve as your guide.

We have also included in this book a number of the forms and handouts that we utilize in our consultations with clients. These forms and handouts, as well as our resource list and drug dosing table, have been reproduced on the accompanying CD so that they can be printed off for use in your practice. We hope that you find them valuable support aids for offering behavioral services.

To all of those who took the time to share with us their thoughts, ideas, and observations on behavior, we wholeheartedly thank you. Thanks to Dr RK Anderson for his kind words in the next preface of this book. Dr Anderson's development of the Gentle Leader™ head halter has provided us with an invaluable tool for humanely and effectively communicating with our pets. He has been a mentor and counselor for many of us who work in this field and we very much appreciate his support and guidance.

Thanks also to Dr Patrick Pageat for his additions to this book, which we hope will begin to clarify some of the additional diagnostic considerations and therapeutic modalities utilized by the 'French' school of veterinary behavior. And a very special thank you to our families who saw less of us, to our pets who received less attention and fewer walks, and to our partners and associates in practice who covered for us. You have no idea how much we appreciate your patience and value the support that you gave us while we worked on this project.

Lowell Ackerman
Gary Landsberg
Wayne Hunthausen
2003

Preface

The first edition of this book was a valuable and practical resource to help guide veterinary medical practitioners through the diagnosis and treatment of common behavior problems in dogs and cats. Readers of this second edition benefit even more from new knowledge in the field and the continuing educational expertise of the authors as lead speakers at national and international meetings on clinically important behaviors of our companion animals. The authors also have provided greater background information about the development of natural canine and feline behavior and have particularly emphasized new knowledge on the effects of disease and aging on behavior.

As an important new feature of this new edition, they have provided a number of extremely useful forms and handouts to help guide practitioners through the consulting process. These forms and handouts help to make this a book that every practitioner should have to improve behavioral services for companion animals in every practice. This is also the first text that looks at the French approach to behavior problems (in English) in an attempt to help understand some of the differences and similarities in the way behavioral problems are approached in different countries.

An increasing number of veterinary practitioners are making a concerted effort to provide behavior services. This not only helps to reduce the number and severity of behavior problems but also goes a long way to strengthening the bond between owner and pet and greatly reducing the possibility of relinquishment.

Practitioners can further their skills in this fast growing field by keeping abreast of the latest in continuing education and utilizing resources such as texts, videos, and handouts that help to educate themselves and their clients. No longer do we use punishment and dominance challenges to gain control of our pets. Understanding natural behavior, learning principles, behavior modification techniques, and the needs of our pets are the keys to success. This new edition will help veterinarians learn and use those keys.

Robert K Anderson DVM, MPH, DACVPM, DACVB, Professor Emeritus Director, Center to Study Human/Animal Relationships, CENSHARE College of Veterinary Medicine and School of Public Health, University of Minnesota 2003

Preface

The veterinary approach to the behavioral disorders of pets has always been very exciting to me. Understanding the origin of unacceptable and abnormal behavior is an interesting purpose. Being first trained in ethology by studying the behavior of insects, I am particularly interested in the structure of the sequence of the behaviors. But, because I am also first and foremost a veterinarian, my approach to veterinary behavior includes not only ethology but also physiology, psychopharmacology, and medicine. I approach behavioral disorders from both a medical and ethological angle, seeking to highlight the level of disorganization in behavioral function.

For 16 years, I have worked on shaping a theoretical and clinical body of work, in order to develop a set of diagnoses and therapeutic procedures. Using a very large number of cases and clinical trials, I have constructed a system of approach. Many clinical files (11 052) have helped support all the observations and conclusions which were offered in the first edition of my French textbook, and with the help of the authors of this book I have attempted to translate and summarize some of this information in this text. Much of this data was the result of clinical experimentation with psychotropic drugs. My collaboration with pharmaceutical laboratories has helped me to gain access to some unique drugs and to some in-depth pharmacological data. And now, my interest has become focused on the development of pheromone therapy. By studying chemical communication in the dog and cat and through the development of synthetic pheromone analogs, it has been possible to create a new therapeutic approach for some behavior disorders. I hope these new tools will be of great help to pets, pet owners, and veterinarians.

I am hopeful that the information that I provided for this text will lead to a better understanding of the French approach to the diagnosis and treatment of behavior problems in pets.

Patrick Pageat DVM, PhD
Behaviorist Diplomate of the French National
Veterinary Schools
Research and Development Director,
Pherosynthese s.n.c.
Le Rieu Neuf, F84490 Saint Saturnin D'Apt, France
2003

About the authors

Gary Landsberg

Dr Gary Landsberg received his DVM in 1976 from the Ontario Veterinary College. He is a partner in two companion animal practices, Doncaster Animal Clinic and Steeles Veterinary Service in Thornhill, Ontario, where he is in general practice as well as a behavior referral practice. Dr Landsberg is a diplomate of the American College of Veterinary Behaviorists and is the president-elect (2002–2004). He appears regularly in the media and has hosted his own radio and TV pet shows. He is on the advisory board for a number of veterinary journals and VIN (Veterinary Information Network). Dr Landsberg is a frequent speaker at veterinary conferences around the world and was the recipient of the American Animal Hospital Association's companion animal behavior award in 2000. He and his wife Susan have raised three great kids, Joanna, Mitchell, and Jordan, as well as their Bichon Frise, Buffy (prominently displayed throughout this book).

Wayne Hunthausen

Dr Wayne Hunthausen is the director of Animal Behavior Consultations in the Kansas City metropolitan area, which provides behavior consultations and training services for pet owners and a behavior externship program for veterinary students. He received his BA (zoology) and DVM (1979) degrees from the University of Missouri, and has been working in the area of applied animal behavior since 1982. Dr Hunthausen is an internationally renowned lecturer and author on the topic of pet behavior. He writes for a variety of veterinary and pet publications, and is co-author of the book *The Practitioner's Guide to Pet Behavior Problems* and co-editor of the books *Dog Behavior and Training: Veterinary Advice for Owners* and *Cat Behavior and Training: Veterinary Advice for Owners*, and he helped to develop and appeared in the child safety video *Dogs, Cats & Kids: Learning to be Safe with Animals*. Dr Hunthausen currently serves on the advisory board for the Society of Veterinary Behavior Technicians, and the boards of a number of veterinary journals. In 1996, he helped found the Interdisciplinary Forum for Applied Animal Behavior and serves on its executive committee. He has served as the president and executive board member of the American Veterinary Society of Animal Behavior. In 2002, Dr Hunthausen received the American Animal Hospital Association's PetCare Award for outstanding contributions to small animal behavior medicine. In his spare time, he is an avid photographer and enjoys skiing, cycling, movies and traveling with his wife, Jan, as well as hiking with their dogs Ralphie, Beau, and Peugeot.

Lowell Ackerman

Dr Lowell Ackerman is a board-certified veterinary dermatologist, an award-winning author, an international lecturer, and a consultant in veterinary practice management. He is a graduate of the Ontario Veterinary College and a diplomate of the American College of Veterinary Dermatology. In addition to his veterinary training, he also has an MBA from the University of Phoenix and an MPA from Harvard University. Dr Ackerman splits his time between clinical practice and consulting. He is a clinical assistant professor in the dermatology service of the Tufts University School of Veterinary Medicine. In addition to veterinary specialty practice, Dr Ackerman is a management consultant with Veterinary Healthcare Consultants, dealing specifically with issues such as veterinary fee structures, staff education, promotion, marketing,

governance, and the development of in-hospital profit centers.

Dr Ackerman is the author of 74 books, including *Business Basics for Veterinarians*, and over 150 book chapters and journal articles. He lectures extensively, on an international basis. Dr Ackerman is a member of the American Animal Hospital Association, the American Veterinary Medical Association, the American Society of Journalists and Authors, the Association of Veterinary Communicators, and the Association of Veterinary Practice Management Consultants and Advisors.

1

Behavior counseling and the veterinary practitioner

PET RELINQUISHMENT AND THE NEED FOR COUNSELING SERVICES

Despite the fact that the origins of pet domestication have been lost in history, the significance of pets in our lives today cannot be overemphasized. While the original association between pet and owner was probably utilitarian, by the latter half of the 20th century, many households considered pets as family members. It is apparent that pets in these loving environments live long, healthy lives and veterinarians contribute greatly to this longevity. However, those animals that fail to create a lifelong family bond with their adopted families often suffer a much different fate.

Clearly, pets are valued by our society, and roughly one in three North American households have pets. Nutritious and affordable diets are available for pets, vaccination is available for many debilitating diseases (e.g., rabies, distemper, panleukopenia, parvovirus, leptospirosis), and a variety of amenities are available for those that can afford them (day care centers, pet bakeries, summer camp for pets, etc.). Pet owners seem to be making a commitment to invest in the health of their pets by seeking preventive and corrective veterinary services, as needed. And yet millions of animals are abandoned each year, or euthanized for non-medical reasons.

There are a myriad of reasons why people acquire a dog or cat and then decide it just

1

doesn't fit their lifestyle. Empirical evidence suggests that this is not a rare occurrence. Statistics released by the National Council on Pet Population Study and Policy (NCPPSP) revealed that only 16% of dogs entering member shelters were ever reclaimed by their owners; over 25% were adopted out to other families and over 56% were euthanized. The results were even worse for cats. This suggests that many dogs and cats that appeared in shelters were not lost with owners searching diligently for them – they were abandoned. It is thus very important to determine the causes of relinquishment in these cases, since abandonment appears to represent a significant part of the problem.

Preliminary evidence suggests that education and counseling before and after acquisition of a pet may help reduce relinquishment. It seems that when people get pets for the wrong reasons, or the pets are not properly trained, or the new owners are not prepared for the responsibilities involved, these pets become like foster children, shuffled from home to home until they either find loving families or become the ward of some institution. When dogs end up in institutions such as shelters, few leave alive. Presumably, if owners can be effectively counseled on responsible pet ownership, relinquishment should be less of a problem.

Since more dogs and cats are euthanized for behavioral reasons than for all medical causes combined, effective behavioral counseling is also an important part of the equation. Some of the more critical behaviors for which owners seek counseling (and may choose to abandon their pets) include aggression, inappropriate elimination, and destruction of personal property. Many of these problems are the result of animals being adopted and then left at home alone while all family members are working or at school. The same problems that have resulted in latchkey children with uninvolved parents have also contributed to pets being left at home without supervision. Problem behaviors are to be anticipated in this scenario. Veterinary practitioners can be effective partners in correcting these problems, by increasing their knowledge and offering relevant services or directing clients to appropriate resources.

THE IMPORTANCE OF PROVIDING COUNSELING SERVICES

Pet behavior problems all too often result in the demise of the pet due to euthanasia or abandonment. The veterinary profession must be a leader in reversing this trend. Although many veterinarians routinely counsel owners (by some estimates accounting for 20% of a veterinarian's time), a comprehensive and standardized approach is sorely needed. It is our intention to provide the foundations for this approach within the pages of this book.

There are many reasons why veterinarians should be enthusiastic about behavior counseling. In addition to the altruistic reason of bettering the lives of pets and owners, there are also solid economic reasons for embracing these concepts. With preventive behavioral counseling and early intervention as problems arise, fewer pets will be rejected, abandoned, or destroyed. The benefits are obvious to all; by saving the pet's life and improving the bond between owner and pet, the owner's commitment to, and level of pet care, should be greatly enhanced. Veterinarians are in the unique position of having repeated contact with most owners during the early, formative months of the pet's life, when important information about preventive health and behavioral management must be disseminated. Getting a complete behavioral history is also an essential part of veterinary care, since the first sign of many medical problems is a change in the behavior of the pet.

Recent estimates indicate that between 6 and 15 million dogs and cats are euthanized each year in the United States at shelters alone, with less than 5% due to medical reasons. In one study, behavior problems were the third most common reason for shelter surrender in cats, after moving and owner allergies, and the most common reason for shelter surrender in dogs. In one Canadian study it was estimated that 11.5% of cats and 13% of dogs euthanized at veterinary clinics may be due to behavioral reasons.

Similarly, in a recent US study, veterinarians indicated that 10 to 15% of their euthanasia cases, or about 224 000 pets each year, are euthanized for behavioral reasons. In general, veterinarians in North America report that they do not routinely inquire about animal behavior and are not confident in their skills to treat behavioral problems. It is clear that with timely and accurate behavioral advice, fewer pets will meet premature and untimely deaths, and a significant cause of client loss can be eliminated.

To this end the American Veterinary Medical Association (AVMA) has recognized veterinary behavior as a board-certified specialty area (i.e., specialists are granted diplomate status in the American College of Veterinary Behaviorists). Other countries also have or are considering similar certification programs. However, it is also clear that efforts are needed to increase the number of veterinarians who incorporate behavioral inquiries and advice into their routine clinical practice. For existing practitioners this will require a concerted effort to include behavior as an integral part of continuing education. In addition, veterinary colleges must increase the behavioral content at the undergraduate level to ensure basic knowledge of: (a) normal species-typical behavior and the client behavioral advice needed to insure normal development; (b) learning and training principles; (c) animal restraint and husbandry; (d) abnormal behavior and its causes; (e) diagnostic considerations for animals with behavioral signs; and (f) the medical and surgical intervention that might be utilized to treat behavioral problems. It would also be valuable for veterinary students to learn about behavior counseling, from history taking to treatment, but this level of expertise might be an optional rotation or achieved through postgraduate continuing education.

PROVIDING BEHAVIORAL SERVICES IN PRACTICE

Providing behavioral services should be an important facet of every veterinary practice. There are several different roles a veterinarian

and veterinary clinic can take in this regard. These are highlighted in Figure 1.1. Each has the effect of promoting healthy behaviors in pets and reinforces the notion that the veterinary practice is a complete health care provider.

A recent study by the American Animal Hospital Association revealed that 78% of pet owners consider their veterinarian to be the first person to contact when seeking help for behavior problems. As many as 90% of dog owners noted one or more behavior problems that they would like to improve. All veterinarians should therefore have enough knowledge of normal and abnormal behavior to know when and how to give advice, and when and where to refer. However, the veterinarian with a medical background is in the unique position of being able to offer the broadest possible range of behavioral services throughout the life of the pet, including medical diagnostics, surgical intervention, and drug therapy. In fact, the first step in any behavioral case is to rule out underlying illness, since most behavioral changes and behavioral problems could have a medical cause. Also, if cases are then referred to a behavior consultant who is not a veterinarian, the referring veterinarian must take an active role in the diagnostic workup, as well as any medical, pharmacological, or surgical therapy that might be indicated.

The veterinarian who wants to provide complete behavioral counseling services must have a good understanding of animal learning, normal behavior, and behavior modification. Know your limitations and attempt to master one problem area at a time, such as feline housesoiling or canine destructive behaviors. Add additional behavioral problems only after you have mastered your approach to previous ones. For dogs, practitioners could begin by offering behavior counseling on topics such as puppy training, jumping up, coprophagia, digging, barking, begging, garbage raiding, chewing, play biting, and housetraining. Common feline behavioral topics might include litterbox training, plant chewing, jumping on counters, climbing, scratching, and nocturnal activity.

Approach	Considerations
Pre-selection consultation	• Consult with prospective pet owners to help them select an appropriate pet for their circumstances. Advise the owner about the health, behavior, and nutritional requirements of their new pet so that the home and family can be prepared in advance.
Preventive counseling	• Counsel owners how to raise their pet in order to minimize behavioral problems. Use handouts, pamphlets, books, and videos. Take full advantage of puppy and kitten vaccination visits to educate the family.
Puppy parties/training	• Encourage owners to participate in puppy programs to enhance early socialization and provide training advice. If you have the space and expertise, consider offering classes in the clinic.
Behavior management products	• Recommend and supply appropriate training devices (leashes, halters, chew-toys, motion-activated alarms, etc.) to prevent or correct undesirable behaviors. If you do not recommend the right products, the owners may make improper decisions.
Surgery	• Preventive: neutering can prevent estrous cycles in females and may reduce behavior problems associated with the effects of androgens such as sexual attraction to females, roaming, marking, masturbation, mounting and some forms of aggression.
• Early-spay neuter: many animal shelters in North America now spay puppies and kittens prior to adoption before 9 weeks of age, primarily as a form of population control. To date, numerous studies have found that there are no long-term adverse behavioral or medical effects associated with this surgery. In clinical practice, spaying and neutering might also be considered at an early age, but there seems little justification or advantage to admitting puppies and kittens into the hospital for surgery until all vaccinations and deworming have been completed.
• Surgery can also be a therapeutic option for the treatment of behavior problems such as those influenced by androgens (as discussed above) and those influenced by female hormones (e.g., estrous behavior, pseudopregnancy). Declawing (except in countries where the procedure is illegal or considered unethical) and teeth extraction or dental disarming might be alternatives to consider when euthanasia or relinquishment are likely.
Basic behavior counseling	• As puppies and kittens mature, undesirable behaviors may develop. Intervene early and dedicate sufficient time to counseling for each specific behavior problem. If managed unsuccessfully, consider referral before the behavior becomes even more ingrained and the family becomes more frustrated.
Behavioral screening	• Diseases of any organ system can cause or contribute to changes in behavior. Therefore screening for behavior problems and any behavioral changes is an important component of each health care visit and can aid in the early identification and diagnosis of medical conditions.
Medical history and diagnostics	• Practice good-quality medicine and complete medical assessment on all patients routinely. Perform a medical workup on every patient that requires a behavioral assessment. Run appropriate diagnostics to rule out all possible medical problems for the presenting behavioral signs.
Behavioral history and diagnostics	• Once medical problems for behavioral signs have been ruled out (or resolved), the behavioral diagnosis requires some knowledge and expertise in history taking and familiarity with the differential diagnoses for the presenting signs. A videotape, interactive discussion with the owner, observation of the pet and owner, and a written history might all be utilized.
Advanced behavioral consultations	• Make sure you feel competent in performing behavior counseling for advanced problems, such as aggression or phobic behaviors. If in doubt, contact a behavior referral center for advice or refer the case. Inappropriate counseling benefits neither the patient nor the veterinary practice.
Pharmacological management	• Drug therapy (as well as alternative therapies such as nutritional management and supplements) can be an important component or even a necessity for the successful resolution of many behavior problems. This might be the case if there are medical conditions causing or contributing to the signs (e.g., pain management, interstitial cystitis, seizure focus). Psychotropic drugs may be a useful therapeutic option or an integral part of the treatment program for some problems.

Figure 1.1 Types of behavioral service offered by the veterinary practice.

Behavior cases that are seen by referral practitioners have a somewhat different distribution. In general terms these problems are less common, require a great deal of time and commitment on behalf of the owner, and may have a poor prognosis. Cases seen at referral behavior clinics are usually those that require time and expertise for the diagnosis, assessment, and advice; cases that may have been refractory to previous attempts at treatment; or are disruptive or actually dangerous to people, other pets, or the pet itself. Depending on the problem, these cases may be beyond the expertise or interest of most practitioners and referral may indeed be the best option for all. On the other hand, the availability of competent behavioral counselors may be limited in a particular area, so that the veterinary clinic may be the best resource available to the client, even if the practitioner has limited behavioral counseling expertise. In these cases, the use of a variety of resources from the literature, such as that contained in this and other texts, client handouts, online consulting services (such as www.VIN.com), and phone or fax support from behaviorists (such as Telephone Behavior Consultations for Veterinarians – Hunthausen and Landsberg), may be the most practical option.

Although there is a great deal of variability between studies, Figures 1.2 and 1.3 provide an idea of the type of cases that might be most common in general practice (i.e., nuisance and training issues) as compared to referral practices (i.e., more dangerous or disruptive problems), as well as what problems might be sufficiently problematic for the owners to consider relinquishment or euthanasia. At behavior referral practices, aggression, inappropriate elimination, and destructive behaviors are the most common cases in dogs, while elimination has traditionally been the most common reason for referral in cats, followed by aggression (Fig. 1.3). However, a recent trend noted by some behaviorists is that aggression surpassed elimination as the most common reason for referral in cats. Although this may be a function of lifestyle changes and owner expectations, one explanation for this change in distribution is that practitioners are now more willing and able to treat elimination cases and that there are more therapeutic options available (drugs, pheromones).

The economics of providing behavioral services

All veterinarians should be performing some behavioral services or they are truly not providing complete client care, and they are economically disadvantaging themselves as well. While there are many humanitarian and ethical reasons to help clients celebrate the human–animal bond, this particular section of the book will deal

Most common problems according to owners[i]	Most common problems seen at referral practices[ii]	Problems leading to increased risk for relinquishment[iii]	Problems leading to shelter surrender[iv]
1. Jumping up 2. Barking 3. Begging for food 4. Jumping on furniture 5. Digging 6. Chewing 7. Fear of noises 8. Overprotective (family/property) 9. Escapes from yard	1. Aggression 2. Inappropriate elimination 3. Destructive behavior 4. Excitability/unruliness 5. Barking 6. Fears and phobias 7. Excessive submission 8. Compulsive and stereotypic behaviors	Aggression to pets or people Barking Destructive behavior Inappropriate elimination Excitability/unruliness (no order defined)	1. Hyperactivity 2. Housesoiling 3. Biting 4. Chewing 5. Fearful 6. Barking

[i] Campbell (1986)
[ii] Adapted from Landsberg (1991)
[iii] Patronek et al (1996a)
[iv] Miller et al (1996)

Figure 1.2 The most common behavior problems in dogs.

Most common problems seen by owners in cats housed indoors[i]	Most common problems seen at referral practices[ii]	Problems leading to increased risk for relinquishment[iii]	Problems leading to shelter surrender[iv]
1. Anxiety	1. Elimination	Elimination	1. Fearfulness
2. Scratching furniture	2. Aggression	Scratching	2. Scratching
3. Feeding problems	3. Compulsive disorder	Aggression	3. Elimination
4. Aggression	4. Separation anxiety		4. Objects to being
5. Inappropriate urination	5. Vocalization		held
6. Inappropriate defecation	6. Wool eating		
	7. Fear		
	8. Other		

[i] Heidenberger (1997)
[ii] Halip et al (1998)
[iii] Patronek et al (1996b)
[iv] Miller et al (1996)

Figure 1.3 The most common behavior problems in cats.

with the economics of the service, to clearly demonstrate that practicing good behavioral medicine is also fiscally sound.

The fact is that the addition of any 'profit center' to a veterinary practice depends on the service being able to deliver a 'profit.' While there are many factors that go into creating a profit, behavior counseling provides one of the best – encouraging the human–animal bond and the retention of the pet within the family unit. As has been previously described, a well-loved pet will typically remain with a family for the rest of its life. With any luck, you'll provide medical support to have that life extended to its fullest and most productive. Maintaining a pet within your veterinary practice, with regular care, for its entire life, is the most economically positive thing you can do for your bottom line.

Even if you never offer in-depth behavioral consultations, it is critical to hospital profits for you to counsel owners effectively about preventable problems. One of the easiest things to do is initiate pre-selection services, so you can advise clients and prospective clients before they ever acquire a pet. Too often, veterinarians wait until owners acquire a pet before they ever see the animal, and get a chance to give advice. This is often too late. Before the pet has been adopted is the best time to talk about suitable breeds, places to find a pet, cautions, temperament testing, and responsibilities of the parenting job. In some cases, the family may decide, based on your advice, that it is not the right time and circumstances to adopt a pet. You won't have lost a client – you will have gained a future client who will be a better owner when the time is right. Even if you decide not to charge for this service, providing this service will generate increasing revenues over time. This is the least expensive public relations and marketing opportunity that you will ever be offered. Once again, profit in a veterinary hospital is not dependent on a one-time sale of services; life-long quality care is always the best business decision.

Another venue for adding behavioral services involves encouraging proper socialization, habituation, and training. While this is covered in more detail within other chapters of the book, realize that these are critical factors in forging a life-long bond between owner and pet. Since veterinarians examine pets for other medical purposes (e.g., vaccination, neutering) during the critical socialization period and afterward, providing suitable instructions regarding socialization, habituation, and training is a natural extension of regular veterinary services. This is also an excellent opportunity to offer services such as puppy socialization classes, basic training, and even life skills training (brushing teeth, trimming nails, cleaning ears, basic grooming) that make pets more used to being handled, which in turn make pets better patients because they are used to being manipulated (e.g., to examine ears, check teeth, perform venipuncture, etc.). It is reasonable to assume that a pet that will easily allow a complete physical examination is more likely to receive a complete physical examination. Since veterinary revenues are dependent on being able to examine, diagnose, and treat, providing these behavioral services allows more patients to willingly benefit from your medical expertise. Best of all, from a profit standpoint, most of these services can be performed by well-trained paraprofessional staff, so they are extremely cost-effective for the hospital to provide.

Another important consideration is to detect behavioral problems early, when they can be most easily managed. Many surveys have documented that owners don't always share information about behavioral problems with their veterinarians. It is therefore important to regularly query owners specifically about behavior problems during any scheduled examination, food or accessory sale, prescription refills, or any other opportunity that avails itself. This is something to which all staff should be alerted. Since more animals will be euthanized for behavioral problems than from all medical conditions combined, do not underestimate the value of detecting behavioral problems early and addressing them immediately and completely.

Although it has been difficult to track, it is likely that point-of-purchase displays for collars, leads, halters, and various training devices can provide consistent revenue streams for a veterinary hospital, especially if doctors and staff regularly reinforce training and behavior issues. Markup on some of these items, especially the more expensive ones, tends to be less than other veterinary products because of competition from retail outlets.

Dealing with problems such as inappropriate elimination in single-cat households, coprophagia, or early cognitive dysfunction evaluation should be routine for the general practitioner, by first doing a complete medical workup to discern potential medical contributions to the problem, since determining organic causes is a logical first step. There are also safe medical therapeutic options for these types of disorders, making them very suitable for general veterinary practices.

While many behavioral problems can be successfully managed in general practice, the economics of providing advanced behavioral counseling are not nearly as enticing as the services already mentioned. Dealing with severe aggression, phobias, and compulsive behaviors cannot be managed within typical scheduled appointments and relies almost entirely on very direct veterinary involvement. This can be problematic for general practices, because few are set up to charge based on billable hours. If you would like to tackle some of these tough conditions, and feel you have the expertise to do so, be prepared to bill in multiples of your typical clinical examination. If you charge x for a routine examination (i.e., lasting 15–20 minutes), expect to charge 4–$6x$ for most initial behavioral sessions (e.g., inappropriate elimination, compulsive disorders, separation anxiety, etc.), and 6–$8x$ for aggression just to cover your time. Follow-up visits need to be billed similarly, but even behaviorists have a difficult time getting clients back in for recheck visits. While clients are often amenable to telephone re-evaluations, it is often difficult to charge appropriately for this service. If you decide to handle your cases as house calls, your in-house behavioral charges should be increased by at least 50%, or bill separately for travel time. In any case, handling advanced behavioral cases, fitting them into a standard veterinary schedule, and billing clients honestly for the visits and follow-up is a difficult task. Even though the charges may seem high (e.g., six to eight times a regular office visit for seeing an aggressive dog), it often takes up to two hours of initial consultation, there are liability concerns for safety of not only the owner and staff, but also those in your reception area, and you will likely deal with ongoing communications for which billing is difficult. Using current econometric evaluations of standard veterinary practices, advanced behavioral consultation is not one of the better profit centers to incorporate into a busy general practice. For most

CANINE BEHAVIOR CHECKLIST

Name: **Today's Date:**
Pet's Name: **Age:**   **Sex: M/F**   **Neutered: Y/N**
Scoring: 0 - none, 1 - exhibits problem but not a concern, 2 - mild, 3 - moderate, 4 - severe

	Score	If yes, when did problem begin? Briefly describe:
1. Destructive (e.g., digs, chews) ____		
2. Steals food items ____ Raids garbage ____		
3. Appetite: picky/poor ____ voracious ____		
4. Pica (eats non-food items) ____ Eats stool: Y/N own ____ other dog ____ cat ____		
5. Constantly follows family members ____ Overly demanding ____		
6. Anxious/destroys/salivates when left alone ____		
7. Fearful/shy (non-aggressive) – people/animals People: family ____ strangers ____ Dogs: family ____ unfamiliar ____ Other pets ____ other animals ____		
8. Fearful/timid (non-aggressive) – inanimate Objects/situations: ____ Describe: Phobias (e.g., thunder, noises) ____		
9. Threatens/aggressive: Y/N People: family ____ strangers ____ Dogs: family ____ unfamiliar ____ Other pets ____ other animals ____		
10. Housesoiling: stool ____ urine ____ Incontinence (lack of control) during: sleep ____ excitement ____ fear ____ Marking (vertical) ___		
11. Unruly/overly excitable/won't settle ____ Pulls/lunges on leash ____ Jumps up ____		
12. Difficult to train: poor with commands sit ____ down ____ stay ____ come ____ heel ____		
13. Pushy/disobedient/demands own way ____		
14. Goes on furniture/in rooms not allowed ____		
15. Excessive vocalization: day ____ night ____		
16. Nips/grabs people or clothing ____		
17. Won't drop/give objects on command ____ Possessive of food/toys ____		

18. Stereotypic/repetitive: licking _____ pacing _____ circling _____ chases lights _____ snaps at air _____ fixed staring _____ other _____		
19. Self-directed/self-injurious: licks self _____ chews self _____ sucks flank _____ chases tail _____		
20. Chases people _____ animals _____ Predation _____		
21. Mounts _____ Roams _____ Masturbation _____		
22. Sleep disorders _____ Wakes at night _____		
23. Other:		
Please indicate if you would like some help changing any of these behaviors (list numbers):		

Figure 1.4   Canine behavior checklist (form #2 – printable from the CD).

veterinarians in general practice, referring these cases to a trained veterinary behaviorist makes much more sense economically. The most profitable behavior services for the general veterinary practice involve preventive services, and managing cases that require a thorough medical workup and less intensive behavioral modification regimes.

Setting up a consultation service

It is easier to set up a consultation service if clients are aware of your interest in behavior. This will happen naturally as you make inquiries about behavioral situations during the course of routine veterinary visits. This serves to encourage clients to bring all behavioral concerns first to the veterinary practice and to identify problems early. In addition, behavioral changes and emerging problems can be a clinical sign of disease. Therefore, discussion of potential problems should not be limited to the initial visit with the client but should take place during each examination (Figs 1.4, 1.5).

Use routine visits to identify patients in your practice with behavioral problems. There are probably more than you think. If you feel confident counseling them further on specific problems, set up a separate appointment for the problem and allow sufficient time for a thorough consultation. It is a mistake to try to counsel owners during the time allotted for a routine medical or vaccination visit. Scheduling a separate appointment also shows your concern and interest in working with the problem. The client who agrees to attend a behavior counseling session is committed to (or at least interested in) correcting the problem at hand.

Also encourage your clients to set up pre-selection consultations with you before they acquire a new pet. This is an excellent time to offer suggestions before they actually have the animal in their home. The new acquisition should be seen within 48 hours of purchase and given a thorough physical examination; the owners should be educated about behavioral concerns to help prevent problems from occurring.

When offering behavioral consultations you should design a protocol for behavior consulting. Figure 1.6 lists factors to be considered, and details can be found in Chapter 3.

FELINE BEHAVIOR CHECKLIST

Name: **Today's Date:**
Pet's Name: **Age:**   **Sex: M/F**   **Neutered: Y/N**
Scoring: 0 - none, 1 - exhibits problem but not a concern, 2 - mild, 3 - moderate, 4 - severe

	Score	If yes, when did problem begin? Briefly describe:
1. Destructive: scratching ____ other ____		
2. Destructive: eats non-food items (pica) ____ Sucks: wool ____ owners ____ other ____ Excess licking ____		
3. Appetite: picky/poor ____ voracious ____		
4. Garbage raiding ____ food stealing ____		
5. Affection: decreased ____ irritable ____ increased ____ demanding ____ clingy ____ does not like to be alone ____		
6. Fearful/shy (non-aggressive) – people/animals People: family ____ unfamiliar ____ Cats: family ____ unfamiliar ____ Other animals: ____		
7. Fearful/shy (non-aggressive) – inanimate Objects/situations ____ Noises ____		
8. Sleep: decreased ____ excessive ____ Wakes at night ____		
9. Aggressive: hiss/growl/bite People: family ____ unfamiliar ____ Cats: family ____ unfamiliar ____ Other animals ____		
10. Compulsive/repetitive Staring ____ Chasing ____ Rippling skin (hyperesthesia) ____		
11. Skin: self-injurious ____ Overgrooming ____ hair loss ____ Chews/licks self ____ tail chasing ____		
12. Excessive vocalization ____		
13. Activity: decreased ____ Overexuberant/hyperactive ____		
14. Roaming ____ Masturbation ____		
15. Housesoiling: stool ____ urine ____ Spraying/marking (vertical surfaces) ____		

16. Goes on furniture/counters ____		
17. Steals food items ____		
18. Predation (hunts) ____		
19. Climbs: indoors (e.g., drapes) ____ trees ____ other ____		
20. Other		
Please indicate if you would like some help changing any of these behaviors (list numbers)		

Figure 1.5 Feline behavior checklist (form #6 – printable from the CD).

1. History: will a questionnaire be utilized and returned prior to the consultation?
2. Medical workup: is the medical assessment complete? For referred cases, has the medical history been obtained?
3. Expertise: clinic consult (with or without behaviorist support) or refer?
4. Scheduling: number and length of visits?
5. Fee structure: fee based on time or flat fee per consult or problem; fee for follow-up?
6. Format: housecall or in clinic?

Figure 1.6 Behavior consultation – factors to be considered in designing a protocol.

Staff utilization and training – the team approach

Veterinarians have some valuable allies for pet behavioral counseling. Properly trained veterinary technicians, nurses, assistants, and front-office staff can provide owners with a wealth of information and can interface with clients on routine matters. A team approach taken by the veterinary practice instills confidence in owners and increases the probability of owner compliance. When owners receive consistent and timely information over many different office visits, they are more likely to understand the concepts and not to suffer from information overload. Placing a checklist of behavior topics to discuss during vaccination visits in the file of each new puppy or kitten allows the staff to prioritize the message and to avoid duplication of effort (see Fig. 3.2, form #12 – printable from the CD). Providing the client with a reading list, utilizing handouts, pamphlets and videos, and demonstrating behavior products and techniques can all help improve the client's understanding and retention of important behavioral concepts.

The key to the team approach is proper education of staff (Fig. 1.7). Office personnel and technical staff should be trained through veterinary instruction and continuing education seminars, and a resource library should be provided. Many veterinary and technician nursing texts contain information on animal behavior,

TRAINING AREAS FOR OFFICE STAFF AND TECHNICIANS/NURSES

- Normal canine and feline behavior
- Principles of learning and behavior modification
- Stages of behavioral development
- Socialization
- Training techniques
- Handling and restraint
- Common training and behavior problems
- Recognizing abnormal behavior

Figure 1.7 Topics to be covered in training for the office team.

and most major veterinary conferences provide behavior lectures for both veterinarians and staff. Well-trained staff do a great service, but poorly trained or misinformed staff can be devastating to building client confidence and loyalty. Similarly, when veterinary staff are providing training services, it is imperative that they not only demonstrate competence but also adhere to humane dog training techniques. A Humane Dog Training Initiative has been launched through the auspices of the American Humane Association and the Delta Society, which stresses that professionals engaged in dog training adhere to the following guidelines:

- Understand the basics of canine behavior, and use this knowledge to anticipate and prevent problems.
- Ensure that dogs are contained or controlled so they are not a danger to themselves or others.
- Manage the training environment so that it is not dangerous to people or dogs.
- Recognize the importance of understanding the behavior of dogs based on ethological interpretations, not anthropomorphic ones.
- Utilize humane training methods that stress positive reinforcement and avoid, or at least minimize, the use of punishment.

Veterinarians will not become experts in behavioral counseling overnight, or even from reading a book or two. Only by putting behavioral concepts into practice will these become second nature (Fig. 1.8). This book addresses the theory of counseling in addition to providing concise and practical information for the busy veterinarian. As with all aspects of medicine, the concepts of behavior counseling are not static but are constantly evolving. Most major veterinary conferences now provide behavior seminars and you are advised to attend as many as you are able. It would be advantageous for at least one staff member to belong to the American Veterinary Society of Animal Behavior, which is a profes-

---

STAYING UP TO DATE ON BEHAVIOR COUNSELING METHODS AND INFORMATION

- Residency program in the veterinary behavior specialty (in the USA a conforming residency program involves at least two years of postgraduate studies under a behaviorist at a veterinary school)
- Attending continuing education seminars
- Review of the literature (veterinary medicine, psychology, ethology, animal behavior)
- Joining veterinary behavior associations (e.g., American Veterinary Society of Animal Behavior; Companion Animal Behaviour Therapy Study Group)
- Subscribe to behavior newsletters and periodicals
- Use computer bulletin boards with an on-line behavior consultant (e.g., Veterinary Information Network (VIN))
- Reading and resources

Figure. 1.8 How to stay up to date on behavioral information.

sional organization of veterinarians interested in applied animal behavior. Newsletters of the society can provide you with useful information as well as a forum for information exchange. The Companion Animal Behaviour Therapy Study Group and the European Society for Veterinary Ethology provide similar services for veterinarians in Great Britain and Europe respectively. Veterinarians in France, Australia, England and the rest of Europe have certification programs that are either approved or in development at the time of writing, and veterinary technicians in North America can now become active in behavior through the Society of Veterinary Behavior Technicians.

There is additional help available for veterinary practitioners with difficult behavior cases. Specialists in behavior will accept referral cases and, in most instances, offer advice to veterinarians by telephone. These behaviorists provide an important extension of the veterinarian's own behavior counseling services.

For a list of reading material that might be beneficial to veterinarians and pet owners, see Appendix B (printable from the CD).

REFERENCES

Ackerman L 2002 Business basics for veterinarians. ASJA Press, New York, 293 pp

Adams CL, Bonnett BN, Meek AH 2000 Predictors of owner response to companion animal death in 177 clients from 14 practices in Ontario. Journal of the American Veterinary Medical Association 217(9):1303–1309

Alexander SA, Shane SM 1994 Characteristics of animals adopted from an animal control center whose owners complied with a spaying/neutering program. Journal of the American Veterinary Medical Association 205(3):472

Business Communications Company 2001 The Pet Industry: Food, Accessories, Health Products and Services. www.bccreseach.com

Campbell WE 1986 The effects of social environment on canine behavior. Modern Veterinary Practice February:113–115

Cloud DF 1993 Working with breeders on solutions to pet overpopulation. Journal of the American Veterinary Medical Association 202(6):912

Gehrke BC 1997 Results of the AVMA survey of US pet-owning households on companion animal ownership. Journal of the American Veterinary Medical Association 211(2):169

Gorodetsky E 1997 Epidemiology of dog and cat euthanasia across Canadian prairie provinces. Canadian Veterinary Journal 38:649–652

Halip JW, Vaillancourt JP, Luescher UA 1998 A descriptive study of 189 cats engaging in inappropriate elimination behaviors. Feline Practice 28(4):18–21

Hawn R 1998 Examining pet overpopulation. AAHA Trends January:13

Heidenberger E 1997 Housing conditions and behavioural problems of indoor cats as assessed by their owners. Applied Animal Behavioral Science 52:345–364

Howe LM 1997 Short-term results and complications of prepubertal gonadectomy in cats and dogs. Journal of the American Veterinary Medical Association 211(1):57

Howe LM, Slater MR, Boothe HW et al 2000 Long-term outcome of gonadectomy performed at an early age in cats. Journal of the American Veterinary Medical Association 217(11):1661–1665

Howe LM, Slater MR, Boothe HW et al 2001 Long-term outcome of gonadectomy performed at an early age in dogs. Journal of the American Veterinary Medical Association 218(2):217–221

Hunthausen W 1991 It's time to offer behavior services. Veterinary Economics November:52–57

Hunthausen W 1996 Behavior problems: find a long-term solution instead of a quick fix. Veterinary Economics May:39–40

Landsberg GM 1991 The distribution of canine behavior cases at three behavior referral practices. Veterinary Medicine October:1011

Lord LK, Wittum TE, Neer CA et al 1998 Demographic and needs assessment survey of animal care and control agencies. Journal of the American Veterinary Medical Association 213(4):483

MacKay CA 1993 Veterinary practitioners' role in pet overpopulation. Journal of the American Veterinary Medical Association 202(6):918

Miller DD, Staats SR, Partlo C et al 1996 Factors associated with the decision to surrender a pet to an animal shelter. Journal of the American Veterinary Medical Association 209(4):738–742

Nassar R, Talboy J, Moulton C 1992 Animal Shelter Reporting Study 1990 American Humane Association, 5.

National Council on Pet Population Study and Policy 2001 www.petpopulation.org

Olson PN, Moulton C 1993 Pet (dog and cat) overpopulation in the United States. Journal of Reproduction and Fertility Suppl 47:433

Patrick GR, O'Rourke KM 1998 Dog and cat bites: epidemiologic analyses suggest different prevention strategies. Public Health Reports 113(3):252

Patronek GJ, Dodman NH 1999 Attitudes, procedures, and delivery of behavior services by veterinarians in small animal practice. Journal of the American Veterinary Medical Association 215(11):1606–1611

Patronek GJ, Glickman LT 1994 Development of a model for estimating the size and dynamics of the pet dog population. Anthrozoos 7(1):25

Patronek GJ, Lacroix CA 2001 Developing an ethic for the handling, restraint, and discipline of companion animals in veterinary practice. Journal of the American Veterinary Medical Association 218(4):514–517

Patronek GJ, Glickman LT, McCabe GP 1996a Risk factors for relinquishment of dogs to an animal shelter. Journal of the American Veterinary Medical Association 209(3):572

Patronek GJ, Glickman LT, Beck AM et al 1996b Risk factors for relinquishment of cats to an animal shelter. Journal of the American Veterinary Medical Association 209(3):582

Posage JM, Bartlett PC, Thomas DK 1998 Determining factors for successful adoption of dogs from an animal shelter. Journal of the American Veterinary Medical Association 213(4):478

Scarlett J 1999 Reasons for relinquishment of companion animals in United States animal shelters: selected health and personal issues. Journal of Applied Animal Welfare Science 2(1):41

Seksel K, Mazurski EJ, Taylor A 1999 Puppy socialisation programs: short and long term behavioural effects. Applied Animal Behavior Science 62:335–349

Strand PL 1993 The pet owner and breeder's perspective on overpopulation. Journal of the American Veterinary Medical Association 202(6):921

Sturla K 1993 Role of breeding regulation laws in solving the dog and cat overpopulation problem. Journal of the American Veterinary Medical Association 202(6):928

Theran P 1993 Early-age neutering of dogs and cats. Journal of the American Veterinary Medical Association 202(6):914

Thornton G 1992 The welfare of excess animals: status and needs. Journal of the American Veterinary Medical Association 200(5):660

Trut LN 1999 Early canid domestication: the farm-fox experiment. American Scientist 87(2):160–170

Wenstrup J, Dowidchuk A 1999 Pet overpopulation: data and measurement issues in shelters. Journal of Applied Animal Welfare Science 2(4):1

Zawistowski S, Morris J, Salman MD et al 1998 Population dynamics, overpopulation, and the welfare of companion animals: new insights on old and new data. Journal of Applied Animal Welfare Science 1(3):1

2

Puppy and kitten development

One of the principle risk factors for dog and cat relinquishment is the lack of knowledge of what can be expected in raising and training a puppy or kitten. Although an understanding of training techniques, health care and housing is essential, some knowledge of the normal behavior of cats and dogs is also needed to be able to determine what is to be expected, and what is abnormal or unhealthy.

PRENATAL DEVELOPMENT

The influence of the environment on behavior may actually come into play even before birth. In fact, based on rodent studies, it has been found that if a pregnant animal is subjected to stimuli that maintain a constant state of fear, the offspring are more reactive or emotional later in life. In addition, emotional females tend to give birth to more emotional offspring. Decreased learning of the offspring has also been associated with disturbances during the latter term of pregnancy in rats. High levels of stress during pregnancy might also lead to changes in reproductive behavior of the offspring when they become adults. This effect is attributed to the activation of the mother's adrenal cortex and secretion of androgens that affect developing fetuses. Male rats of mothers exposed to stress during the last third of gestation display low levels of male copulatory behavior and sometimes high rates of feminine sexual behavior, likely due to suppression of gonadal testosterone secretion during stress. It is not unlikely that excessive stress on the canine and feline mother may also have deleterious effects on her offspring and should be avoided, especially during the third trimester of the pregnancy. On the other hand, providing the mother with a friendly environment that affords positive social contact will likely facilitate desirable emotional development of her offspring.

Studies have also shown that there may be a relationship between fetal position and the behavior of the adult animal. In rats and mice, in utero exposure of females to androgens leads to increased urine marking and mounting, and decreased reproductive success on reaching adulthood, while males located between two females may be less aggressive on reaching adulthood. This effect may be due to the secretion of androgens on adjacent fetuses, or from the androgens transported in the blood flow from a male fetus caudal to the female in the same horn. A similar effect may be seen in dogs, since prenatal exposure of the fetus to testosterone has been shown to prime the central nervous system, so that male behaviors such as leg lifting begin to emerge with maturation, independent of testosterone levels at the time of onset of the behavior. It has also been reported that dominance-related aggression is more likely to be seen in females from predominately male litters, and that females exposed to testosterone in utero were more successful when competing for a bone with females from a litter that were not predominantly male.

CANINE DEVELOPMENT

There are five developmental stages that have been described in puppies: the neonatal stage (birth to 13 days); the transitional stage (13 to 19 days); the socialization period (19 days until approximately 12 weeks); the juvenile period (12 weeks to sexual maturity); and the adult stage (from sexual maturity). The beginning and end of each phase of development varies somewhat from individual to individual.

Neonatal stage

During the neonatal period, the puppy spends most of its time nursing or sleeping. Puppies have limited motor ability and, up until about five days, movement is on the belly by paddling and stroking with the limbs. By six to 10 days, the forelimbs are capable of supporting weight and by 11 to 15 days, the hind limbs can support weight and walking begins. The rooting reflex is present from birth and begins to wane after about 14 days. A slow and sustained pain response to toe pinch is present from birth, but withdrawal and escape from pain does not develop until early in the transition period. Eyes and ear canals are closed at birth and open by 10 to 14 days, at which time the palpebral reflex to touch and light and the pupillary responses are already developed. Being unable to hear or see, neonatal puppies are effectively shielded from most psychological effects of the environment. Defecation and urination are reflexes that are elicited by the mother's licking and cleaning of the perineal region. Temperature regulation is poor at birth and puppies huddle together. By four weeks of age, puppies tend to sleep in groups and at six weeks, they sleep alone.

An important consideration during development is the effect of handling and strong stimuli on the behavioral and physical development of the puppy. One study showed that puppies that have been exposed to short periods of handling from birth to five weeks of age were more confident, exploratory, and socially dominant than controls. Handled puppies had increased nervous system maturation, more rapid hair growth and weight gain, earlier opening of the eyes, and enhanced motor development. Thus, early handling may lead to improved learning ability and a more emotionally stable puppy. It has been suggested that mild stressors such as early handling affect the pituitary–adrenocortical system in a way that helps the puppy better cope with stress later in life.

Transitional period

Toward the end of the second week, the pup enters the transitional stage of its neurologic and behavioral development. During this period, the puppy goes from a condition of complete dependence upon its mother to one of relative independence. Adult behavior patterns begin to appear at this time. The transitional period begins with the opening of the eyes and the opening of the ears. The auditory evoked startle response usually begins by 18 days and the puppy may begin to localize sound. The brainstem auditory evoked response (BAER) also attains the characteristics of the adult at this time. The electroretinogram has the basic features of the adult pattern by 15 days and is fully developed by 28 days. Visual and auditory orientation develops around 25 days.

During the transitional period, the puppy begins to walk rather than crawl, both forward and backward. Puppies begin to exhibit voluntary control of elimination, but the mother still continues to clean the excretions. By the end of the transitional stage, the pup's pain perception is fully developed. Many of the patterns of adult social behavior and their accompanying emotions appear at the same time. Gently exposing the pups to all types of stimuli for short periods each day during this period is likely to enhance development. A simple type of exercise involves allowing the pups to crawl or walk on surfaces with differing textures and temperatures. Objects of varying shapes can be moved in front of them in order to promote visual acuity and motor skills. Providing a variety of noise stimuli at low decibels and varied frequencies may facilitate auditory development. Whistles, rattles, music, recordings of environmental noises, and the human voice can be used to provide a variety of auditory stimulation. Play mouthing by puppies begins to develop and by four weeks of age, nipping can be quite painful.

Socialization period

The onset and early stages of the socialization period are closely associated with the maturation and myelination of the spinal cord. All sensory systems are functional during this period and learning capacity becomes more developed. Although the puppy can support itself and becomes more mobile during the transitional period, normal sitting and standing develop by about 28 days. Teeth erupt and the pups begin taking solid food for the first time. A puppy's performance on classical and operant conditioning reaches adult levels at about four to five weeks, but vision and brainwave function do not reach adult levels until about eight weeks. By four weeks of age, puppies tend to sleep in groups and at six weeks, they sleep alone. Weaning begins around four to six weeks of age. At first, the puppy begins to show an interest in food, and the mother will begin to decrease nursing contact and may regurgitate food to her young. This is a good time to begin offering canned or moistened food to puppies. Most puppies are weaned and eating solid foods by about 60 days of age. By eight to nine weeks of age, puppies are attracted by the odors of urine and feces to specific areas for elimination and begin to avoid soiling their den (sleeping quarters).

This period is one of rapid development of social behavior patterns. At the beginning of this period, the puppy begins to respond to the sight or sound of persons or other animals at a distance. The behavior of puppies during the early socialization period is characterized by a willingness to approach novel objects and, in particular, moving stimuli. Investigative behavior becomes apparent and puppies begin exploring away from the nest area. Social following and early signs of pack behavior emerge. During this time, there is a marked increase in interaction with littermates, the mother and the environment. Distance decreasing and increasing social signaling begins to appear. Gradually, as the mother spends less time with the puppies, the interaction and relationship between littermates strengthens.

The socialization period is an important time period for puppy development. Whatever happens here sets a general pattern that will affect almost everything in later life because, by the end of this period, the puppy has formed patterns of response to the major influences in any sort of future existence. At the end of the transition period, the puppy has sufficiently developed that it can begin to interact with other individuals. During the socialization period, the puppy develops attachments to its own and to other species that it encounters socially. It is also a time that the puppy begins to become familiar with and make attachments with places (localization or site attachment) and adapts to many of the stimuli around it (habituation). Because the socialization period is the time when social relationships are established, it is essential that puppies have contact with all potential future social partners (people and animals). Neither reward nor punishment need be involved, although excessive stimuli, whether positive or negative, before seven weeks of age appear to increase attachments.

Besides being a time for development of social relationships, this also appears to be a period of extreme sensitivity to psychological stress. The sensitivity necessary to facilitate the formation of social relationships also seems to make the puppy vulnerable to psychological trauma. Fear postures begin to emerge at about eight weeks of age, and by 12 weeks sociability begins to decrease and the unsocialized puppy may become increasingly fearful of novel situations and people. Startle reactions to sound and sudden movement become much more pronounced. With time, the puppies learn to discriminate between stimuli associated with dangerous situations and those that are insignificant. Frequent, gentle handling is important in order to decrease the fear response shown to humans.

During the socialization period, social play and exploration become increasingly important. Play between puppies not only aids in physical development but also appears to be a form of exercise as well as an important step in the development of adult behaviors including communication, predation, and sexual relationships.

Since learning by observation allows for tasks to be learned from the bitch and other dogs in the pack, this is another important reason why part of the socialization period should be spent with other dogs. Although solitary play does occur, most play is social, with biting, barking, chasing, pouncing, and mounting (especially in male puppies) being the most frequent components.

Juvenile period/adulthood

The juvenile period extends from the end of the socialization period to sexual maturity. By this time, basic learning capacities appear to be fully developed. Object and environmental exploration increases during this period. On the other hand, it is also a time of increasing avoidance so few if any new social contacts are likely to develop. The speed of learning begins to slow by about four months, likely because previous learning begins to interfere with new learning. By four to six months, males begin to show greater attraction to females showing signs of estrus. The final period, adulthood, begins at puberty, which is around seven months or older in males and six months or older in females. Dogs are generally considered to be socially mature at about 18 months of age and fully mature by about two years.

FELINE DEVELOPMENT

Kittens go through the same developmental stages as puppies, although the periods may be shorter and less easily defined. The timetable for development can be variable between individuals based not only on genetic factors but also on maternal factors, environmental factors such as handling and housing, and sexual differences. The neonatal period is a time primarily of nursing and sleep, in which the kitten is fully dependent on its mother. The transitional period, where locomotion and sensory development emerge, begins in the second week, and the socialization period begins in the third week and extends to seven to nine weeks of age. The juvenile stage ends between about six and 12 months of age at sexual maturity, although social maturity is not reached until two and a half to four years of age.

Neonatal and transitional period

During the neonatal period, the kitten is predominantly guided by tactile, thermal, and olfactory stimuli. Although the kitten is born with its eyes closed and is unable to hear, tactile sensitivity and the vestibular righting reflex develop prenatally. Olfaction is present at birth and is fully mature by three weeks. Hearing is present by the fifth day and the kitten begins to orient to sounds by two weeks; adult-like orienting is present by a month. Although the eyes open at around seven to 10 days, visual orienting and following don't develop until the third week, and visual orienting and obstacle avoidance are not developed until four to five weeks of age. Full visual acuity may not be achieved until three to four months of age. Self-grooming in the form of oral grooming and paw grooming begin to emerge in the second to third week of life.

At birth, kittens move toward warmth but cannot regulate their body temperature until around three weeks of age; full adult temperature regulation may not be achieved until seven weeks. During the first two weeks, the kittens are fairly immobile, and walking doesn't begin until around three weeks of age. Body righting, although present at birth, is not well developed until one month.

Good maternal behavior is essential for healthy kitten development. Kittens that are separated from their mother and hand raised from two weeks of age are more fearful of kittens and people, more sensitive to novel stimuli, and slower to learn. Hand raised kittens may still develop social attachments to other kittens, but this occurs much more slowly. Kittens from undernourished mothers can have growth deficits in some brain regions (cerebrum, cerebellum, brain stem), as well as delays in the development of crawling, suckling, eye opening, walking, play, exploration, climbing, and predation. These kittens may also show decreased learning ability, antisocial behavior toward other cats, and increased fear and aggression. Many of these changes don't arise until much later in the cat's development. Maternal malnutrition, from a low protein diet, can also lead to abnormalities in behavior and motor development.

The effects of early handling on kittens

Early handling of kittens by humans is not only beneficial for improving social relationships between kittens and humans, but also leads to accelerated physical and central nervous system development. Kittens that are held and lightly stroked daily for the first few weeks of life open their eyes earlier, begin to explore earlier, and are less fearful of humans. Kittens that are handled for 5 minutes daily from birth to 45 days are less fearful than non-handled kittens. They approach strange toys and people more frequently and are slower to learn avoidance. In a study in which $5\frac{1}{2}$- to $9\frac{1}{2}$-week-old kittens were handled by 0, 1, and 5 people, the 5-person kittens exhibited the least fear of strangers. In another study, kittens that were handled between three and 14 weeks of age would accept holding for longer and would approach humans faster than kittens that had received no handling and those that were handled between seven and 14 weeks of age. These studies indicate that the most receptive time for socializing kittens to people is up to seven weeks of age, and that the more handling the friendlier the kitten is likely to be toward people.

Socialization period

By four weeks of age, hearing, vision, temperature regulation, and mobility are sufficient for the kitten to begin moving away from the nest and developing social relationships with people and other animals in its environment. At this age, learning can be accomplished solely by visual cues. Body righting ability is fully mature by about six weeks of age. Running begins in the fifth week and most adult locomotion is developed by seven weeks of age. Complex motor abilities may not be fully developed until 10 weeks or older.

During the first three weeks, the mother initiates nursing, and teeth begin to erupt around two weeks of age. At four weeks, the kittens begin to eat some solid foods and weaning begins. From this point onward, the kitten initiates most bouts of nursing. At four to five weeks of age in a free-living environment, the mother may begin to bring prey to the kitten. Kittens may start to kill mice as early as five weeks of age. Deciduous dentition is fully developed by five weeks of age. Kittens generally share their mother's food choices, and this is most marked by seven to eight weeks of age. Similarly, the choice of prey is usually similar to that of the mother. By five to six weeks of age, the kitten has full voluntary control of elimination, and digging and covering on loose soil may begin. By seven weeks of age, most kittens are weaned, although suckling may continue intermittently for several more weeks. Defensive reactions to large prey and fearful reactions to threatening stimuli may begin to be displayed by six weeks of age.

Within the socialization period, social attachments are formed most easily and rapidly. Social play begins at this time, before the interest in object play. Attachments can be formed at other times, but the process is much slower and involves extensive exposure. Socializing kittens to other species, including humans, may begin as early as two weeks of age and may only extend to seven weeks of age. Studies have shown that kittens reared with rats did not kill their cage mates or similar rats even as adults, while kittens raised with puppies did not show fear toward adult dogs. However, kittens raised in the absence of puppies prior to 12 weeks showed avoidance and defensive responses when exposed to them. Because of genetic differences between individuals, and other factors such as early handling, maternal effects, and the cat's environment and experiences, kittens and adult cats can show a great variability in their friendliness toward people and other cats, regardless of the amount of early socialization. Studies on cat personality types have identified at least two personality types: (a) sociable, confident and easy-going; (b) timid and nervous. Factors that might influence these personality types include paternal genetics, early socialization, maternal genetics, and social or observational effects of mother and littermates.

Play and predatory behavior

Playful social interactions with siblings and mother begin at around four weeks and are generally well developed by seven weeks of age. Social play includes wrestling, rolling, and biting of conspecifics and may be directed at the human hand (or other moving body part). Predatory type behaviors may become a part of social play in the third month and agonistic social behavior also begins to emerge. Play between older kittens may become more serious and intense over time. Play, exploration of inanimate objects, and locomotor play begins to escalate around seven to eight weeks of age and peaks at around 18 weeks of age, before it begins to decline. Social play, on the other hand, may continue at a fairly high level until 12 to 14 weeks of age, before it begins to decline. Object play may be social or solitary and may consist of pawing, stalking, and biting of objects. This type of play also simulates a variety of aspects of the predatory sequence. Owners should provide an opportunity for their kittens to engage in object play by offering a variety of prey-like toys for their cats to attack and catch. Kittens that are weaned at an earlier age show earlier development of object play.

Predatory behavior may be affected by social or observational learning, age of weaning, early socialization, maternal behavior, observation of other cats, genetics, and possibly by competition with littermates. A kitten's mother will gradually introduce it to prey so that maternal effects can be an important factor in prey preferences and hunting ability. At first, dead prey is brought to the kitten and this then progresses to live prey which the mother releases for it. If the kitten loses control or pauses too long the mother may intervene so that the kitten's skills are more finely tuned through observation and interaction. Lack of familiarity with a species, or socialization to that species, may inhibit predation of that species. Despite a lack of familiarity with prey, and even in the absence of maternal experience and learning, many cats still develop into competent hunters. Early weaned kittens develop predatory behavior earlier and show an earlier increase in object play while normally weaned kittens are less likely to become predators and have a later onset of object play. Hunger has been shown to increase the incidence of killing prey, while increasing prey size reduced the probability of killing. Similarly, studies of object play found that hunger increases the motivation to play and reduces fear of larger toys.

Juvenile period/adulthood

The juvenile phase continues until sexual maturity, at which time the cat may become increasingly independent. Age of sexual maturity depends in females on genetics, breed, and the environment. Sexual maturity is usually observed at five to nine months of age, although the first heat cycle may occur as early as four months in some cats. Although male kittens may be mature enough for spermatogenesis by about five months of age, mating and sexual maturity is usually not observed until around nine to 12 months of age.

BEHAVIORAL GENETICS

With work done on the human genome project, as well as the canine genome project, major advances are being made in the linkage of traits (both physical and behavioral) with gene mutations. While we are currently not in a position to identify tail chasing in Bull Terriers or rage syndrome in Springer Spaniels with a direct DNA test, the time may not be far off. While dogs (and humans) are clearly a lot more than their collective DNA, the field of behavioral genetics is coming into its own as gene mutations are being recognized that have a direct effect on behavior.

In human medicine, a great stride was made when fragile X syndrome, the first single-gene cause of mental retardation, was identified. Since then a wide variety of syndromes and genes have been identified that have cognitive and personality sequelae. This is not surprising since we suspect that approximately 30% of the estimated 30 000 genes in the human genome are expressed primarily in the brain, and of course it is the brain that governs everything humans do, think, or perceive. Should we suspect otherwise in animals?

Grounds to suspect a genetic basis for behavioral problems

We have already clearly demonstrated several inherited behavior traits in animals, including the sophisticated herding ability of the border collie, the signaling antics of the Nova Scotia duck-tolling retriever, the tracking ability of many hounds, and the fetching ability of many retrievers. In fact, most of the breeds created today have unique physical and behavioral traits, which have been accentuated with each passing generation. There is no reason to suspect that many other behavioral traits, good and bad, are not heritable to at least some extent. The domestication of dogs has probably gone on for the past 12 000 years or so, and there is little to indicate that the process will not continue. Research done in foxes suggests that using docile behavior as the only selection criteria, domestication can occur in 30 generations.

In dogs, there is interesting evidence to suggest that the species was domesticated intentionally, with selection to retain juvenile traits, a process known as pedomorphosis. Thus, both physical and behavioral traits of the young, such as skulls that are unusually broad for their length, whining, barking, and submissiveness, are retained in dogs throughout their lifespan, but are typically outgrown by wolves as they mature. Domestication of many species has led to interesting traits not seen in the wild, such as the appearance of dwarf and giant varieties, piebald coat color, curly tails, rolled tails, shortened tails, floppy ears, and changes in reproductive cycles. It is reasonable to predict that selection for tameness may alter regulatory mechanisms for neurochemistry, and the developmental pathways they govern. It is not unreasonable to further conclude that anomalies in these behaviors could have both heritable and environmental components.

When it comes to traits like aggression, we suspect that heritability probably plays some role in addition to environmental causes. Nature versus nurture needn't be a zero-sum game. For several years investigators have examined how two neurotransmitters, serotonin and vasopressin, interact to control aggression. In many species, aggressive behavior is inversely correlated with the level of serotonin in the brain. Rats become much more aggressive when they are given drugs that interfere with the serotonin receptors and more docile when given drugs that increase serotonin levels (such as fluoxetine – Prozac) or stimulate serotonin receptors. Vasopressin seems to have the opposite effect. In male hamsters, blocking the vasopressin receptors in the hypothalamus makes the hamsters less aggressive toward intruders; injecting vasopressin directly into the hypothalamus makes them more aggressive. In fact, serotonin may decrease aggressive behavior, in part, by inhibiting the activity of the vasopressin neurons. Potentially, an inefficient serotonin system may let vasopressin build up in the central nervous system, priming the body for aggressive behavior. The important point to be made here is that there is unlikely to be an 'aggression' gene that codes for surly canines. It is more likely that a gene exists that codes for some protein that codes for variable functionality of serotonin and which, in turn, alters other neurotransmitters, including vasopressin and many others.

The other likelihood is that genetics alone is probably not sufficient for clinical manifestations of disorders like aggression. We know of the critical socialization period for dogs (and cats), and that tractability is directly related to whether or not animals were properly socialized during that period. This could serve as 'one' of the many potential triggers for clinical forms of aggression. So, theoretically, a dog could have a genetic predisposition toward aggression, but it only becomes clinically manifested if the dog was improperly socialized during the critical period, or affected by some other trigger, such as diet, hormonal levels, or any number of other potential moderators of behavior.

Does this likely occur in dogs? Probably. Recent studies have shown that supplementing the diet of a dog with dominance aggression with tryptophan (Trpn) and changing to a low-protein diet with a high relative tryptophan to large neutral amino acids (LNAA) ratio may reduce aggression. The rationale here is that tryptophan is a precursor of serotonin and that supplementation with tryptophan (or relatively increasing the ratio of tryptophan to competing amino acids) will increase brain serotonin levels and reduce aggression. The presumption is thus that aggression is somehow associated with defective neurotransmitter metabolism, which is likely (at least partially) a heritable event that can be moderated, at least in part, by diet.

Genes causing behavioral problems

Hoping that genetics will explain all behavioral problems seen is simplistic, and does not reflect the way that genes actually work. Genes don't cause disorders – they code for proteins that interact with other proteins and the environment to cause variable effects. Even in single-gene defects such as von Willebrand disease in Doberman Pinschers, the resultant level of von Willebrand factor is a continuous trait that does not match well with our clinical impression of the disorder. Thus, while an individual animal with this monogenic disorder is either clear, affected or a carrier, there is a huge overlap in von Willebrand factor levels between carrier and affected individuals. It is this variability in expressivity that keenly complicates our understanding of even 'simple' genetic disorders and confounds our ability to truly appreciate 'complex' relationships between genes, proteins, and environmental impact. So, while we have successfully navigated the genomic revolution, a much more complicated fate awaits us as we start to investigate the new field of proteomics, an arena in which we must contend not with 30 000 genes written in a four-letter alphabet, but the mind boggling world of a million proteins written in combinations of 20 amino acids. The structure of these proteins is important, but it is the patterns in which they fold three-dimensionally, and their interaction with other proteins and the universe around them, that produces almost infinite variability in presentation. Thus, in human medicine, having the 'gene for schizophrenia' may indicate at least a 50% risk of developing the condition, but it is not a foregone conclusion that having the gene mutation makes schizophrenia inevitable.

Another likelihood, as we explore the genetics of behavioral conditions, is that different mutations in different genes may cause the same end result. For example, familial Alzheimer's disease has been associated with at least three mutations, for presenilins 1 and 2, and for amyloid precursor protein. For most behavioral problems seen in animals, we are not expecting to find a single genetic mutation responsible for a major behavioral problem, say aggression. Even if aggression was controlled by a single genetic mutation in one breed, we would not expect it to necessarily be the same in other breeds. For example, the gene that causes progressive retinal atrophy (PRA) in the Irish Setter is significantly different from the gene that causes PRA in the Siberian Husky, or the Cardigan Welsh Corgi for that matter. Accordingly, while there are DNA tests for PRA in each of these breeds (and in several others), the mutation seen in one breed is rarely shared with other than closely related breeds. Thus, while Siberian Huskies share the same gene mutation with Samoyeds and the DNA test can therefore be used in both breeds, this is fortuitous rather than commonplace. So, even if we ever developed a DNA test for aggression (or a compulsive disorder, etc.) in a particular breed, we should not presume that the behavior results from that same mutation in other breeds as well.

Unfortunately, for the majority of behavioral problems seen in animals (and humans), we are not expecting to find a single genetic mutation to explain the problem. For these types of 'continuous' traits that exist along a spectrum of behaviors, attempts have been made to map contributing genes with quantitative trait loci. The first report of successful mapping of a behavioral trait was in a study of emotionality in mice by Flint & Corley (1996), who found that the genetic variance was accounted for by just three quantitative trait loci. Since then, a pattern has been found: that most 'polygenic' traits are usually caused by a relative handful of genes rather than many genes. This bolsters our hopes that genetic tests will eventually be available for most 'complex' problems, including aggression and compulsive disorders (as well as hip dysplasia and many other heritable problems). It remains possible, for these and other complex disorders, that there may be a small number of genes that have fairly major effects and a larger number of genes that play a more minor role. If this is true, it should make the task of finding at least the first few quantitative trait loci that much easier.

Allelic association studies have a potentially great advantage in the investigation of quantitative trait loci (QTL), in that they are capable of detecting genes of small effect, as little as 1% of the variance. On the other hand, they are somewhat shortsighted in that the marker must be close to the trait locus or have some direct effect on the trait, and this requires the use of many closely spaced markers. That is, they need to involve markers in or around genes coding for proteins that are likely to influence the trait. This is necessarily hampered by low-resolution maps, but greatly improved maps based on hundreds of thousands of single nucleotide polymorphisms (SNPs), rather than a few hundred, together with high-throughput genotyping, should make identification of these QTLs more routine.

CONCLUSION

It is likely that many of the behavioral problems noted in this book have at least some heritable component. This is most likely when a particular breed exhibits an abnormality that is exclusive to or significantly more common in that breed, such as flank sucking in Dobermans, spinning in Bull Terriers, and wool sucking in Oriental breeds (see Fig. 10.1). Similarly within families and lines of dogs, it is not unusual to see traits ranging from fear (e.g., German Shorthair Pointers) to aggression (e.g., Springer Spaniels), even when the dogs have been raised under a variety of environmental conditions (e.g., different homes). However, it is unlikely that a given disorder will have the same genetic mutation in every breed. It is also likely that many disorders may have a genetic predisposition, but that environmental triggers are necessary for full manifestation of the trait. As gene maps become more sophisticated, it is likely that several behavioral disorders will be able to be diagnosed with DNA tests, on a breed-specific basis. Knowledge of the precise genetic anomaly also presents intriguing possibilities for new and more effective forms of treatment.

REFERENCES

Ackerman L 2000 The genetic connection. A guide to health problems in purebred dogs. AAHA Press, Denver, CO, 279 pp

Adams MD, Kelley JM, Gocayne JD et al 1991 Complementary DNA sequencing: expressed sequence tags and human genome project. Science 252:1651–1656

Anderson RK 1990 At what age can dogs learn? Veterinary Forum August: 32

Angameier E, James WT 1961 The influence of early sensory–social deprivation on the social operant in dogs. Journal of Genetic Psychology 99:153–158

Appleby D, Bradshaw JWS 2001 The relationship between canine aggression and avoidance behaviour and early experience. In: Overall K, Mills DS, Heath SE et al (eds) Proceedings of the third international congress on veterinary behavioural medicine. UFAW, Herts, UK, p 23–29

Ashmead DH, Clifton RK, Reese EP 1986 Development of auditory localization in dogs: single source and precedence effect sounds. Developmental Psychobiology 19:91–103

Bateson P 2000 Behavioural development in the cat. In: Turner D, Bateson P (eds) The domestic cat: the biology of its behavior, 2nd edn. Cambridge University Press, New York, p 9–22

Beaver BV 1992 Feline behavior. A guide for veterinarians. WB Saunders, Philadelphia

Beaver BV 1999 Canine behavior. A guide for veterinarians. WB Saunders, Philadelphia

Blackshaw JK 1988 Abnormal behavior in dogs. Australian Veterinary Journal 65(12):393–400

Butcher J 2001 Behavioural genomics – where next? The Lancet 357(9255):534–535

Collard RR 1967 Fear of strangers and play behavior in kittens varied with social experience. Child Development 38:877

Coppinger R, Coppinger L 1996 Biologic bases of behaviour of domestic dog breeds. In: Voith VL, Borchelt PL (eds) Readings in companion animal behaviour. Veterinary Learning Systems, Trenton, NJ, p 9–17

Dahloff LE, Hard E, Larsson K 1977 Influence of maternal stress on offspring sexual behaviour. Animal Behaviour 25:958–963

Estep DO 1996 The ontogeny of behaviour. In: Voith VL, Borchelt PL (eds) Readings in companion animal behaviour. Veterinary Learning Systems, Trenton, NJ, p 19–31

Feddersenpetersen D 1994a Comparative studies of behavioural development of wolves (Canis lupus) and domestic dogs (Canis familiaris). Domestication traits and selective breeding. Tierarztliche Umschau 49(9):527–531

Feddersenpetersen D 1994b Social behavior of wolves and dogs. Veterinary Quarterly 16(Suppl 1):S51–S52

Flint J, Corley R 1996 Do animal models have a place in the genetic analysis of quantitative human behavioral traits? Journal of Molecular Medicine 74:515–521

Fogle B 1990 The dog's mind. Viking Penguin, New York

Fox MW 1965 Canine behavior. Charles C Thomas, Springfield, IL

Fox MW 1968 Socialization, environmental factors, and abnormal behavioral development in animals. In: Fox MW (ed) Abnormal behavior in animals. WB Saunders, Philadelphia

Fox MW 1969 Behavioral effects of rearing dogs with cats during the 'critical period of socialization.' Behaviour 35:273

Fox MW 1971 Overview and critique of stages and periods in canine development. Developmental Psychobiology 4(1):37

Fox MW 1978 The dog: its domestication and behaviour. Garland STPM Press, New York

Fox MW, Stelzner D 1966 Behavioral effects of differential early experience in the dog. Animal Behavior 14:273–281

Freedman DG, King JA, Elliot O 1961 Critical period in the social development of dogs. Science 133:1016–1017

Herrenkohl LR 1979 Prenatal stress reduces fertility and fecundity in female offspring. Science 206:1097–1099

Horwitz DF 1993 Feline socialization: how environment and early learning influence behavior. Veterinary Medicine August:14–16

Houpt KA 1985 Companion animal behaviour: a review of dog and cat behaviour in the field, the laboratory and the clinic. Cornell Veterinarian 75:248–261

Houpt K 1998 Domestic animal behavior for veterinarians and animal scientists, 3rd edn. Iowa State University Press, Ames, IA

Joffe JM 1965 Genotype and prenatal and premating stress interact to affect adult behavior in rats. Science 150:1844–1845

Kerby G, Macdonald DW 1988 Cat society and the consequences of colony size. In: D Turner, P Bateson (eds) The domestic cat: the biology of its behavior. Cambridge University Press, Cambridge, UK

Kuo ZY 1930 The genesis of the cat's response to the rat. Journal of Computational Psychology 11:1

Levine S 1967 Maternal and environmental influences on the adrenocortical response to stress in weanling rats. Science 156:258

Markwell PJ, Thorne CJ 1987 Early behavioural development of dogs. Journal of Small Animal Practice 28:984–991

McGuffin P, Martin N 1999 Behaviour and genes. British Medical Journal 319(7201):37–42

Mech LD 1981 The wolf: the ecology and behavior of an endangered species. University of Minnesota Press, Minneapolis, MN

Mendl M, Harcourt R 2000 Individuality in the domestic cat. In: Turner D, Bateson P (eds) The domestic cat: the biology of its behavior, 2nd edn. Cambridge University Press, New York, p 47–64

Nott HM 1992 Behavioural development of the dog. In: Thorne C (ed) The Waltham book of dog and cat behaviour. Pergamon Press, New York, p 65–78

O'Farrell 1986 Manual of canine behaviour. British Small Animal Veterinary Association, Cheltenham, UK

Overall KL 1997 Clinical behavioral medicine for small animals. Mosby, St Louis

Randon E, Beach F 1985 Effects of testosterone on ontogeny of urinary behavior in male and female dogs. Hormones and Behavior 19:36–51

Robinson I 1992 Behavioural development of the cat. In: Thorne C (ed) The Waltham book of dog and cat behaviour. Pergamon Press, New York

Scott JP 1962 Critical periods in behavioral development. Science 138:949–958

Scott JP, Fuller JL 1965 Genetics and the social behavior of the dog. Chicago University Press, Chicago

Scott JP, Marston MV 1950 Critical periods affecting the development of normal and maladjustive social behavior in puppies. Journal of Genetic Psychology 77:25–60

Seitz PFD 1979 Infantile experience in adult behavior in animal subjects. II. Age of separation from the mother and adult behavior in the cat. Psychosomatic Medicine 21:353

Seksel K, Mazurski EJ, Taylor A 1999 Puppy socialisation programs: short and long term behavioural effects. Applied Animal Behavior Science 62:335–349

Serpell JA 1987 The influence of inheritance and environment on canine behavior: myth and fact. Journal of Small Animal Practice 28(11):949–956

Serpell J, Jagoe JA 1995 Early experience and the development of behavior. In: Serpell J (ed) The domestic dog: its evolution, behavior, and interaction with people. Cambridge University Press, Cambridge

Simonson M 1979 Effects of maternal malnourishment, development and behavior in successive generations in the rat and cat. In: Levitsky DA (ed) Malnutrition, environment and behavior. Cornell University Press, Ithaca, NY

Slabbert JM, Rasa OAE 1997 Observational learning of an acquired maternal behavior pattern by working dog pups: an alternative training method? Applied Animal Behavioral Science 53:309–316

Smith BA, Jansen GR 1977 Maternal undernutrition in the feline: behavioral sequelae. Nutrition Reports International 16:513

Stur I 1987 Genetic aspects of temperament and behavior in dogs. Journal of Small Animal Practice 28(11):957–964

Thompson WR, Melzack R 1956 Early environment. Scientific American 194:38–42

Thorne C 1992 The Waltham book of dog and cat behaviour. Pergamon Press, New York

Trut LN 1999 Early canid domestication: the farm-fox experiment. American Scientist 87(2):160–169

Turner DC 2000 The human–cat relationship. In: Turner D, Bateson P (eds) The domestic cat: the biology of its behavior, 2nd edn. Cambridge University Press, New York, p 193–206

Wahlsten D 1999 Single-gene influences on brain and behavior. Annual Review of Psychology 1999:599–621

Ward I 1968 Prenatal stress feminizes and demasculinizes the behavior of males. Science 15:82–84

Willis MB 1987 Breeding dogs for desirable traits. Journal of Small Animal Practice 28(11):965–983.

3

Prevention: the best medicine

WORKING WITH NEW PUPPIES AND KITTENS – THE TEAM APPROACH

Providing timely behavioral advice to new puppy and kitten owners can help prevent undesirable behaviors, as well as help correct existing problems before they become resistant to change. The first veterinary visit is the time to begin reinforcing important concepts and to make sure that the owner and the pet are on the right track. Some veterinarians may prefer to address only those problems or concerns that are raised by the pet owner. However, preventive advice should be offered to all new pet owners, so that they know what is needed and what to expect when raising a new pet. Since unrealistic owner expectations, insufficient counseling and reading material, lack of obedience training (dogs), allowing outdoors (cats), failure to neuter and housesoiling have been shown to increase the risk of owner relinquishment, then these are issues that need to be discussed with all owners. A list of topics that should be discussed can be found in Figure 3.1.

To make matters more expedient during those initial few veterinary visits, it is useful to have a 'new pet checklist', so that points can be addressed in an orderly manner and so important topics don't get missed. Advice to owners can be provided over the course of the puppy and kitten visits. As long as the information is properly prioritized, and given at an appropriate time in the pet's development, not all informa-

TOPICS FOR NEW PET OWNERS

- Socialization with people and animals of all types
- List of appropriate reading material and videos
- Providing a safe environment by pet proofing the home and yard
- Supervision, confinement, crate training
- Housetraining, litterbox training
- Basic handling techniques
- Exercise and play
- Chewing, scratching, and destructive behaviors
- Reward-based training
- Shaping behaviors and maintaining control
- Basic grooming needs, nail trimming
- Outdoor safety and pet ID (e.g., microchip)
- Health advice – vaccinations, nutrition, parasites, dental care, neutering
- Pet health insurance
- Training tools (e.g., head collars, leads, harnesses, toys)

Figure 3.1   These are topics that should be discussed with each new pet owner, and can be a major focus of staff training and involvement in preventive behavior counseling.

tion needs to be provided at once (Fig. 3.2). If the owner also schedules a pre-selection consultation and/or attends puppy or kitten classes (discussed below), then these are also additional opportunities to educate and counsel the new pet owner.

We wish to emphasize again that the veterinarian need not be the only person in the practice qualified to provide behavioral advice to family members with new pets. Properly trained staff can be very effective in this role, and also reinforce the practice's team approach to health care. Depending on the hospital set-up and the amount of training the staff have received, a great deal of behavioral education can and should be handled by trained office staff and technicians. However, it is the veterinarian's responsibility to ensure that the information the staff provides is correct and appropriate. In some hospitals, a practice member with a particular interest in behavior might be assigned to coordinate the preventive behavior counseling services as well as the protocol for treating behavioral problems that are presented to the practice.

Proper use of hospital staff will give the veterinarian more time to concentrate on important aspects of behavior and training within the time frame of a typical initial office visit. Veterinary staff can be trained to cover all of the topics in Figure 3.1. In addition, the use of a variety of personnel, as well as a variety of resources (e.g., handouts, videos, reading lists) may be a more practical way for the owner to be presented with information that will be retained and utilized. In addition to the handouts available throughout this text (also reprintable from the CD), two of the best resources for client handouts are those available from the American Animal Hospital Association (co-authored by Dr Hunthausen and Dr Landsberg) and a set of 62 client behavior handouts reprintable from a CD from Lifelearn co-authored by Dr Debra Horwitz and Dr Landsberg (www.lifelearn.com). This is also an important time for the veterinarian to provide a thorough physical examination to detect any medical conditions that might contribute to or exacerbate behavior problems.

Take the time during initial visits to address and correct problems early. Ask clients about problems at each visit, since they will not always volunteer the information. Many owners do not realize that members of your veterinary staff are important resources for behavioral advice, or that early intervention may prevent the development of more serious problems. You should also observe the pet for any undesirable behavior that it might exhibit (e.g., fear, aggression, unruliness) and advise on how these might best be handled. If the pet shows evidence that it may become dangerous to family members, it is incumbent upon the veterinarian to inform the owners fully and give them appropriate options. When behavioral advice is given, it is important to follow up by phone or in person at the next scheduled visit to ensure that sufficient improvement is being made.

When the clients leave the office, it is likely that they have been overwhelmed with medical and behavioral advice and might have trouble digesting and remembering it all. So, whenever possible, provide them with handout materials and pamphlets that can be taken home. Book and video suggestions may also be appreciated. Most pet food companies provide 'puppy packs'

CHECKLIST FOR NEW CLIENTS (To be completed and kept in file)

Owner: Pet's Name: Date of birth:

Species: Breed:

		Visit 1 Date: Age:	Visit 2 Date: Age:	Visit 3 Date: Age:	Visit 4 Date: Age:
Client Education					
1. Behavior	Socialization				
	Safety/pet proofing				
	Crate training				
	House/litter training				
	Reward training				
	Control/handling				
	Destructive chew/scratch				
	Play biting/nipping				
	Puppy/kitten classes				
	Neuter				
2. Health care	Vaccines				
	Deworm/fecals				
	Heartworm				
	Fleas				
	Grooming – ears/skin				
	Feeding/nutrition				
	Microchip/licensing				
	Dental				
3. General advice	After hours care				
	Clinic services				
	Insurance				
Handouts/samples	Puppy/kitten kit				
	Reading list				
	Rabies tag				
	Clinic brochure/handout				
Products	Food/treats				
	Heartworm treatment				
	Flea control				
	Training – head halter				
	Grooming				
	Behavior: chew/play				
	Dental				
	Microchip				
	Books/videos/pamphlets				
Send/follow up	Welcome letter/package				
	Magnet/business card				

Figure 3.2 New puppy or kitten checklist. Each should be initialed and dated by the staff member or DVM when discussed with the client (form #12 – printable from the CD).

or 'kitten kits' that contain free samples and literature, which can be supplemented with your own customized forms, including the ones found in this book, or on the aforementioned Lifelearn CD. Remember that the family often focuses on the new pet during the visit, and may not fully comprehend every message the veterinarian tries to relate.

PET SELECTION

One of the most valuable services a veterinarian can perform for clients is to assist them in picking the pet that best suits their home and lifestyle. This is an extremely useful but underutilized facet of veterinary practice. Insufficient effort and forethought about the selection of a pet, and about the preparation for its arrival, are major factors associated with later relinquishment and euthanasia. Some owners spend more time picking a houseplant than they do a pet that will live with them for over a decade.

A selection consultation is the best way to determine the needs of the prospective owner. There are several ways of determining whether the family is suited to pet ownership and, if so, which type of pet would be most compatible. There are numerous pamphlets (e.g., AVMA's A Veterinarian's Way of Selecting a Proper Pet), books and questionnaires (e.g., AVMA's Pet Selection Fact Sheet) to aid in the process. Most kennel associations, breed clubs, and humane societies have also produced useful handouts and/or have websites on the subject. Everyone has a stake in making sure the right pet ends up in the right household.

Some veterinarians feel uncomfortable discussing pet selection because they don't know much about the process, other than the medical consequences. Acquiring a pet is an emotional experience, and veterinarians would do well to put themselves in the place of clients when considering what recommendations to make. You may need to consider what kind of pet would be best for a young family that has never owned a dog before? How about a family without children whose home is lavishly and expensively decorated? Consider the widow on a pension who loves animals but can't afford to spend much on the purchase and upkeep of a pet (Fig. 3.3).

Because the pet selection consultation is so important, a questionnaire that provides all the necessary information for making an informed recommendation can be very helpful. Appendix C, Figure 1 (form #13 on the CD) is a client handout that can be utilized to collect information that will need to be considered for the pet selection consultation. It should be made clear to the client, however, that it is not the role of the consultant to choose a particular breed, age, or sex. Rather, the consultant should discuss the advantages as well as any concerns or warnings about each breed, and give suggestions on sex, age, and how to choose an individual dog or cat. With a variety of pets and hundreds of breeds to choose from, it can be very useful to have the owners first narrow the selection process down to the species and a few breeds that appeal to

- Type of pet (dog, cat, other)
- Breed (purebred vs mixed)
  - heritable medical problems
  - heritable behavioral tendencies
- Age (puppy or kitten vs adult)
- Physical characteristics
  - general appearance
  - size
  - haircoat
- Behavioral characteristics
  - temperament
  - activity requirements
  - sociability
  - protective behavior
  - tendency to bark
  - behavior with children
- Sex (male vs female; neutered vs intact)
- Source (breeder vs shelter vs retail shop)
- Parent assessment (behavior, physical appearance)
- Client considerations
  - expense (high maintenance vs low maintenance)
  - ages, limitations of family members (allergy, disabilities, etc.)
  - schedules and activities of family
  - family's experience with pets
  - environment – type of home, location, fencing

Figure 3.3 Factors for consideration in pet selection.

them before attending the consultation (see breed considerations below).

Be certain to utilize the time at the selection consultation to also provide the owners with the health, behavior, feeding, housing, and training information that they will need to get started on the right track.

Breed considerations

By selecting a mixed breed animal from a shelter, an abandoned animal can be saved from death, and the initial cost is very reasonable. One can even argue that there are genetic advantages to obtaining mixed breed animals. This is often referred to by geneticists as 'hybrid vigor.' However, the best way to predict the behavior, size, health, coat, and other attributes of an adult dog or cat is to obtain a purebred animal of known parentage. Because there is such wide genetic variation in size, shape, behavior, and health amongst dog breeds, the selection process for purebred dogs is not always a simple task.

With several hundred recognized purebreds and many more rare breeds, it is certainly not possible to help the owners work through all possible breeds. Therefore, before attending a selection consultation, the client should be encouraged to narrow the selection process down to a few breeds that they are most interested in. This can be accomplished by providing suggested reading and websites (see Appendix C, Fig. 1, form #13 on the CD), as well as having the client attend some dog or cat shows to see a variety of breeds and meet some breeders or handlers. The owners might also be encouraged to contact groomers, trainers, and kennel clubs to get their input. Another option is to visit one of the computerized selection services on the Internet. At this point, with a few breeds under consideration, the owner should be encouraged to attend a consultation in person at your clinic.

Two of the most important aspects of pet selection include determining the family's reason for owning a pet as well as any family limitations for owning certain types of pets. This may not only dictate the type of pet to be obtained but also eliminate certain breeds from consideration. For example, a family that is interested in obtaining a pet primarily for companionship may be interested in agility training or flyball, or might be a sedentary couple incapable of providing intensive exercise or training. Similarly, potential pet owners may want to consider breeds for a particular type of work (herding, hunting, household protection), for a particular size range, or because a family member has allergies.

If an owner then has a query about a breed with which you have less familiarity, be prepared to do the research before you make your recommendations. If you take the time to document pros and cons for each breed as you experience or read about them, eventually you will have an impressive array of facts for the would-be owner. In addition, you should collect a good library of books and journals, and a list of websites since the owners will need information on:

- Breed standards (physical requirements)
- Breed function (i.e., the selection pressures on this breed when it was developed)
- Any potential genetic and health problems
- Generally accepted breed behavioral characteristics
- Documented breed behavior problems

Although there are a number of books that provide breed behavioral profiles, there can be a great deal of variability between different lines, across different geographical areas, and amongst individuals within the same litter. Veterinarians should have some idea of the characteristics that are most predictable (e.g., watchdog ability in Rottweilers, vocalization in Siamese cats, low activity level of Basset Hounds), and which traits are more affected by environment and training such as destructiveness and housesoiling. Veterinarians should also be cognizant of potential problems such as tendencies toward aggression, high activity level, fear, sensitivity to pain and noise, and specific conditions such as flank sucking in

Doberman Pinschers, wool sucking in Siamese cats, and spinning in Bull Terriers.

Pet age

Puppies and kittens are most receptive to socialization, adapting to new environments and habituating to a variety of new stimuli. Conversely, they require a committed family to provide the appropriate time and energy to properly socialize and train the puppy or kitten at this highly impressionable age. Adult dogs and cats may already be insufficiently socialized or improperly trained so that problems may be difficult or impossible to correct. Adult pets may have difficulty adapting to an environment or social group that is dissimilar from their previous household. On the other hand, adult pets may be able to handle longer owner departures, may present fewer problems with overexuberant play, nipping and chewing, and may already have some basic training. This is an age where testing (see below) may be a relatively accurate way to determine whether the pet is likely to adapt to a new home.

Pet gender

Male dogs and cats are slightly larger in stature than females. Male dogs are also somewhat more assertive and more active. Females may be easier to train and to housetrain. Castration or spaying of dogs and cats reduces sexually dimorphic behaviors. However, surgery won't always eliminate the behaviors. For example, about 10% of spayed female cats and 5% of castrated males will mark territory with urine. After castration, male dogs may show decreases in behaviors such as mounting, roaming, urine marking, and aggression toward other male dogs. Castration of male cats reduces urine odor and decreases sexually dimorphic behaviors such as fighting, spraying, and roaming, but has no effect on hunting. Spaying of queens and bitches reduces estrous behavior and associated urine spraying.

Source

The best source of a purebred pet is a reputable breeder, although rescue groups and shelters may also be good sources. In general, retail outlets should be avoided. If puppies and kittens are obtained directly from the breeder, the buyer can better assess and ensure that they have been properly cared for and have had sufficient human contact. The breeder also may have the parents available so that their health and behavior can be assessed. In particular, studies of cats have clearly demonstrated that the paternal (father's) genes are more likely to influence boldness, the cat's resistance to handling or restraint, and perhaps even friendliness. Therefore, whenever there is a chance to observe and handle the father this is likely to be most valuable. Reputable breeders should be happy to provide references (veterinarians, previous buyers) and should be proud to show you their kennel and other dogs.

The buyer should pay close attention to the health and behavior of both parents since the temperament, size, coat, and personality of a puppy or kitten will often resemble those of its parents when grown. Purebred dogs and cats that are obtained from pet stores, breeding farms, puppy mills, and animal shelters usually have unknown medical and genetic histories. They are highly stressed by weaning, transport, handling, and housing, and have high levels of exposure to other animals at a time when their resistance is low or suspect. The risk of respiratory and intestinal diseases is highest in these animals. Saving the life of a pet from a breed rescue organization or shelter could be seen as a gallant gesture and should be considered, but the owner must be counseled about the potential risks. Sometimes the background (i.e., previous household and previous health) is known, but often the pet's health and behavior are unknown commodities and may have been a factor in relinquishment. Families wishing to obtain a cat for rodent control should select a kitten from parents that are known hunters; those who want a social animal should choose a kitten from highly social parents.

To find a pet, the first step is to use personal references. Many owners have decided on a particular breed because of a pet that they have met through a relative, friend, or acquaintance. If the pet is healthy and has a desirable personality, it might be possible to contact the breeder to see if brothers or sisters from more recent litters might be available. Veterinarians might also consider collecting listings of breeders who have proven to produce problem-free pets. In addition, the kennel clubs of most countries (e.g., American Kennel Club, Canadian Kennel Club, Cat Fancier's Association, The Kennel Club, Fédération Cynologique Internationale – FCI, United Kennel Club) publish directories of breed and rescue associations either in print or on the web. Annual directories, such as Dogs in USA Annual, Cats in US Annual, Dogs in Canada Annual, are available in many countries. Monthly magazines and weekly newspapers aimed at the pet-owning community contain useful information. There may be a local Breeder Referral Service, such as that run by various corporations and pet organizations.

Temperament testing

Temperament testing is another useful function that can be performed during the selection process. The value of this type of evaluation is in determining the current temperament and social nature of the animal, not in predicting adult behavior patterns. Testing young puppies and kittens that are still developing behaviorally and physically is unlikely to predict behavioral changes or problems that will arise through behavioral development, as well as those that will be affected primarily by training and environmental stressors. Some of the factors to consider in the selection of young puppies are listed in Figure 3.4. Although testing of puppies prior to three months of age may have little predictive value, as puppies proceed through the different stages of development, assessments become increasingly more accurate. In fact, testing of adult dogs and cats may be a relatively accurate way to assess the pet's personality and potential for behavior problems, and has proven to be

---

Factors to consider in puppy assessment tests:
a) Primary socialization period continues to 12 weeks or older
b) Fear begins to emerge at 8 to 12 weeks and may begin to become predictive at 3 months or older (but is increasingly predictive with age)
c) Dominance hierarchies do not begin to emerge until 15 weeks or older
d) Sexual maturity is not attained until 6 to 12 months of age
e) Social maturity may not be reached until 18 to 24 months of age
f) In police dog testing, retrieval could be predicted at 8 weeks of age but testing for aggression was not significant at 9 months

Figure 3.4

valuable for improving placement success in adult animals in shelters.

There are some traits that are identifiable in young animals, but more research is needed before specific recommendations can be made. A specific form of temperament testing used to screen potential guide dogs at six to eight weeks of age has increased the success of guide dog selection from 30% before tests were initiated, to almost 60% after temperament testing. Therefore a common sense approach to testing may be useful in identifying undesirable traits that may have already begun to emerge, such as shyness, overactivity, or uncontrollable biting and growling. These may be warning flags for potential future problems.

Keeping in mind that the testing is likely to be more accurate with increasing age, dogs should first be observed and evaluated for overall healthiness, sociability, fearfulness, and activity level. Tests might include social attraction to people, how the dog gets along with any other dogs or animals that might be present, possessiveness (taking away food or a chew toy), response to handling and restraint (e.g., lifting, handling the muzzle, stroking over the head, brushing, nail trimming), reactivity to sound, touch or sudden movement (e.g., opening an umbrella), and energy level (Fig. 3.5).

A number of shelters have been able to improve rehoming success and reduce further relinquishment using assessment testing of

What is being assessed?	Tests
Health	• Observation for lethargy, respiratory signs (eye or nasal discharge or cough), gastrointestinal upset (e.g., vomit, diarrhea), skin disease (e.g., hair loss, scabs, irritation, scratching), overall weight and appearance • Although some problems may be evident in puppies, many genetic problems may not begin to emerge until adulthood
Sociability	• Test approach, handling and stroking by a stranger • Walk away and observe response • Greater validity with increasing age
Excitability	• Take the animal to a quiet area and observe • Attempt to calm down in sit or stay position – assess pet's response • May note extremes with puppies but greater validity with increasing age
Fear or aggression	• Observe facial expressions and body postures during approach by strangers • Identify fearful responses, overly submissive responses (retreat, avoidance, ears back, cowering, lateral recumbency, and submissive urination) • Identify any threats or attempts to bite (other than play biting) and discontinue testing immediately • Watch for unusual startle responses to loud or sudden noises or visual stimuli (e.g., umbrella, hand movement, running) • Response to handling – stroking, lifting, gentle restraint, brushing, handling feet or muzzle • Observe response to other pets • Test response to a doll • Observing excessive fear or aggression is a serious concern regardless of age, but may not yet be evident in assessing puppies
Possessiveness	• Give food or toy and observe response to approach/removal • Consider using an artificial hand for assessment if any potential for aggression

Figure 3.5   Some tests that can be used to assess behavioral traits.

adult pets and matching these pets to an appropriate home. In one standardized, validated test developed in the Netherlands (MAG-test), a set of 16 subtests are utilized to assess a dog's potential for aggression. The tests are done outdoors with eight carried out in the presence of the owner and eight in the owner's absence. The dog is approached and petted in a friendly manner by a stranger using an artificial hand, in an unfriendly manner, confronted with a doll, an unfamiliar dog of a different breed but the same gender, and with both visual and acoustic stimuli. The dog is surrounded by three people, once at a normal pace and once at a running pace. If no biting occurred, the test proved to be 82% accurate when compared to the known history of the dog.

It may prove to be more accurate to assess the temperament of cats, since their primary socialization period ends at a much earlier age. At least

two common personality types have been identified: (1) sociable, confident and easy-going; (2) timid, nervous and unfriendly. A third personality type – active and aggressive – has also been suggested. Fearful, timid, or aggressive cats should be avoided. As with dogs, testing is likely to be more accurate with increasing age. Cats can be observed and evaluated for overall health, sociability, fearfulness, and activity level. Tests might then include social attraction to strange people, social relationships with other animals, response to handling and restraint (e.g., stroking, lifting, grooming, nail trimming), energy level, and reactivity to novel stimulus such as moving wand toys, novel odors, or sounds. In general, a healthy, affectionate cat will make the best pet whereas shy, withdrawn, fearful, or aggressive cats should be avoided. If the cat tolerates handling, lifting, and petting with minimal resistance, it is likely to be a good family pet. As many as

15% of cats may not be able to be socialized to people successfully.

SOCIALIZATION AND HABITUATION

Socialization has been discussed in Chapter 2 but is mentioned again here since it is one of the most important concepts for the veterinarian to relay to the family with a new pet. Socialization is the process in which pets develop a relationship with animals of their own species and others. The most critical period for socialization in puppies is between three and 12 weeks of age, while the most receptive period for kittens is from two to seven weeks of age. During these periods, dogs and cats make attachments to individuals of their own species, other species, and new environments most rapidly. Pets that develop social relationships during these periods are often capable of maintaining these relationships for life. If they have not been properly socialized with people and other pets by the end of this period, they are likely to be fearful, defensive, and potentially aggressive when exposed to them at a later age. Although these are sensitive stages for primary socialization, continued socialization is also necessary for these social relationships to be maintained.

For proper social development, the breeder should begin providing handling experience and environmental enrichment shortly after birth. Puppies and kittens that lack sufficient auditory, tactile, and visual stimuli may be slower learners, less social, and more fearful than properly stimulated littermates. Adequately stimulated puppies and kittens have superior coordination, higher sociability toward people, better problem-solving scores, and are less fearful in novel situations. Breeders who isolate puppies or kittens and deprive them of sufficient early handling may produce pets that are overly fearful and lack desirable social behavior.

Another critical factor in the early development of dogs and cats is the role of the mother. Bitches and queens with good maternal behavior produce offspring with better digestion, better resistance to disease, and better weight gain,

which develop and mature faster than puppies born to bitches with poor maternal instincts. Dogs and cats that have been deprived of maternal and peer interactions form poor social bonds later in life. For example, if a puppy or kitten is removed from the litter at birth and hand-reared, it may be unable to mate or care for its own litter later in life. Dominant and submissive signaling and controlled aggression may also not develop normally if there is insufficient early social interaction with conspecifics, and there are often reports of solely hand-reared pets being overly rambunctious and less inhibited in their social interactions with family members.

Puppies or kittens removed from the litter at four weeks of age or younger may not be able to relate appropriately to members of their own species at a later age. Therefore, it is generally recommended that puppies remain with their mother and littermates until approximately seven weeks of age, so they can develop communication skills, develop social skills, and have an opportunity to play and interact with other dogs. It is equally important for kittens to develop and maintain proper social relationships with other cats. However, since the critical socialization period for cats begins to wane by as early as seven weeks of age, social contact with people and other species must begin before this time. In order to accomplish good intraspecific socialization skills, continued socialization with members of the species should continue throughout the socialization period, even after the pet moves into the new home. Having more than one dog or cat in the home, visiting with the pets of friends and relatives (provided the pets are healthy, sociable, and up to date on vaccinations), along with puppy or kitten classes are often the best ways to maintain good social skills with conspecifics (Fig. 3.6).

By seven weeks of age, puppies are least inhibited and therefore best able to adapt to new experiences. This is also just prior to the start of the primary fear period. Although continued socialization with other dogs is important, the focus of socialization should now be shifted toward as many new people and situa-

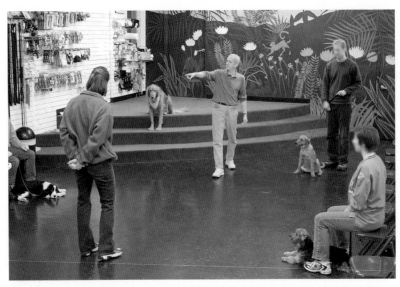

Figure 3.6 Puppy classes are an excellent way to encourage proper socialization. Dennis Bastian teaches puppy classes at the Westwood Animal Hospital.

tions as possible. Dogs that have had no social contact with people by 14 weeks of age are unlikely ever to make adequate family pets and tend to behave more like their wild counterparts.

Every attempt should be made to introduce the puppy to people, animals, and environments that it might be likely to encounter in adulthood (Fig. 3.7). When reviewing the examples, be certain to have the family concentrate on stimuli that differ from those in the daily household (Fig. 3.8). An excellent way for owners to socialize their puppies to new people is to use the concept of 'socialization biscuits' (Appendix C, Fig. 2, printable handout #3 on the CD). The owner should take the puppy into novel situations armed with a box of small biscuit treats. The puppy should be encouraged to approach everyone it meets along the way (e.g., children, joggers, cyclists, postal delivery people). When the puppy responds appropriately (e.g., responds to the 'sit' command given by the stranger without showing any apprehension), the owner gives the stranger a biscuit treat to give to the puppy. A treat, some play, and a few friendly pats are usually all that is required to socialize puppies. The same can be done with the staff in the veterinary clinic and visitors com-

ing to the home (Fig. 3.9). The owner should also be told that properly socializing a puppy does not mean that it won't protect their home and family at a later date. Not only is this a time when social relationships need to be established, but this is also a time when the puppy is most adaptable to new stimuli (habituation) and to making attachments with places (localization or site attachment). On the other hand, unsocialized the puppy becomes increasingly fearful starting at about eight weeks of age while sociability begins to wane at 12 weeks of age, so that excessively fearful situations and stimuli must be avoided. Socialization before 14 weeks of age is critical, but continued socialization after that time is also very important.

Overall the factors for optimum socialization and prevention of fear and avoidance in adulthood include (a) a domestic maternal environment, (b) socialization throughout the socialization period, and (c) continued socialization through the juvenile period. Puppies with a non-domestic maternal environment (kennel, barn, garage) and insufficient socialization are at increased risk for developing avoidance behavior (unfamiliar people, dogs, noises, and places) and fear aggression.

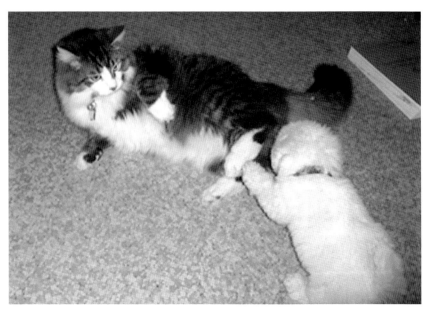

Figure 3.7 Buffy the Bichon meets Switch. Early socialization during the first few months of life will help ensure that pets will get along with members of other species when they are adult.

Animate stimuli – should be exposed to sights, sounds, smell, and contact with the following:
People of differing ages (children/babies, teenagers, adults, males/females, elderly persons)
Men with beards
People with differing complexions, color
People with uniforms, backpacks, hats, headgear, or glasses
People with physical disabilities (wheelchairs, walkers, canes, altered mobility)
People and associated activity/noise (e.g., playing sports, skateboards, roller blades, bicycles)
Veterinarians/veterinary clinics
Other animals of own and other species (cats, dogs, birds, rabbits, etc.)

Inanimate stimuli – should be exposed to sights, sounds, smell, and contact with the following:
The new household
Unfamiliar locations – veterinary clinic, visit to family members or neighbors
Cars, trucks
Roadway/pavement (sidewalk)
Park
Lifts (elevators)
Crate/kennel
Vacuum cleaners, trains, cars, etc.
A variety of tastes to avoid unhealthy or excessive preferences
Stimuli that are novel/unique to the new environment (e.g., planes, trains, hot air balloons)

Figure 3.8 Stimuli for socialization and habituation of puppies and kittens.

1. Choose breeding animals that exhibit desirable social behavior
2. Provide social interaction with conspecifics
3. Provide regular and positive early human handling
4. Provide opportunities for socialization to humans and other species prior to the end of the primary socialization period
   – optimum age for canine pet adoption may be 7 to 8 weeks (less inhibited, pre-fear period)
   – optimum age for feline pet adoption is prior to end of primary socialization at 7 to 9 weeks
5. Habituate to as many stimuli and environments as practical during the early months of life
6. Consider any and all people, animals, stimuli, and locations (see Fig. 3.8) that the pet may be exposed to at a later age but are not presently in the household and try to seek out exposure. Be particularly diligent about exposure to children, the elderly, or people who have other physical or behavioral differences from the family
7. Avoid excessively fearful situations and exposures – keep all meetings and greetings positive and use toys or treats to ensure a positive association
8. Continue exposure to conspecifics into adulthood to maintain healthy social relationships
9. Consider puppy and kitten classes for early training and a variety of socialization opportunities in a controlled environment

Figure 3.9   Steps for optimum social development of puppies and kittens.

Cats that have had no social contact with people by seven to nine weeks of age may never be able to develop a healthy social relationship with humans. Therefore, for a kitten to develop a healthy social relationship with people, other animals, and new environments, the kitten should either be removed from the litter and taken into its new home by seven weeks of age, or the potential owner must ensure that the kitten has had adequate exposure and handling by people before it is obtained. Again, concentrate on socialization and habituation to all aspects of the new household, as well as those people and pets that differ from the present household and family. Wherever possible provide treats when meeting or greeting new people or pets, so that a positive association can be made (Fig. 3.10). A client handout on

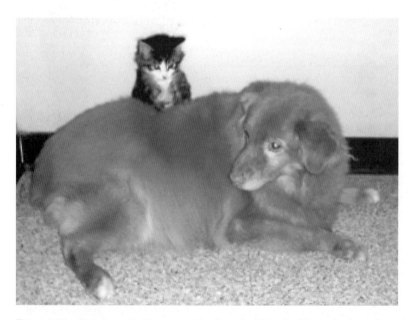

Figure 3.10   Switch meets Grace: socialization of a kitten to other animals such as dogs helps to reduce the possibility of fear of dogs as the cat grows and matures. Using treats can help to ensure a positive association.

kitten socialization can be a useful tool (Appendix C, Fig. 3, printable handout #18 on the CD). Also have the owners try and maintain their kitten's good social skills with other cats, by having more than one cat in the home, visiting friends with healthy, vaccinated, sociable cats, or by attending kitten kindergarten (discussed below).

PUPPY CLASSES AND KITTY KINDERGARTEN

One way to achieve socialization to a variety of people and other pets is to take puppies to puppy classes and kittens to kitty kindergarten (see Fig. 3.6). If your clinic has sufficient room and a staff member who has sufficient knowledge to 'run' these classes, they can be held on site. The goals of these classes are to provide continued socialization to a variety of people and pets, and to educate owners in the training of pets and prevention of behavior problems. These classes help emphasize your clinic's interest and expertise in

providing behavioral advice, and expand the clinic services you offer. The classes should have between four and eight puppies or kittens per instructor. During the sessions, puppies and kittens should have some structured play (Fig. 3.11) and social interaction with people and other pets as well as some demonstration and guidance on reward-based training techniques. Any emerging problems should be identified and appropriate management and solutions discussed. Studies to date have not shown a clear correlation between puppy classes and improved socialization, but puppies in these classes are better trained and have had early and effective behavior problem intervention compared with puppies that did not attend puppy classes. In addition, puppies attending well-designed puppy classes had higher rates of retention as adults. An outline of what might be covered in these classes is listed in Figures 3.12 and 3.13.

Veterinary hospitals that do not have sufficient space to run these classes might consider having a one- to two-hour puppy or kitten socialization

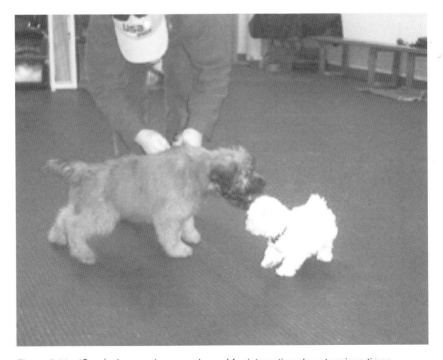

Figure 3.11 'Go play' – puppies are released for interactive play at various times throughout the puppy class at 'The Puppy People,' Thornhill, Ontario.

PUPPY CLASS TRAINING OUTLINE
(adapted from Wayne Hunthausen DVM and Dennis Bastian, Westwood Animal Hospital, Westwood, KS)

LESSON 1
  1. **Introduction**
     A. Have fun
     B. Don't take good behaviors for granted
     C. Set the puppy up to succeed
     D. Schedule and think ahead and try to prevent mistakes before they happen
     E. Reward/correction principles
     F. Consistency
  2. **Play Period** – puppies only
  3. **Housetraining** – see handout on housetraining
  4. **Confinement Training** – see handout on confinement training
  5. **Food Lure–Reward Training** – see handout on basic training
  6. **Sit and Lie Down on Command** – practice in class
  7. **Socialization Discussion** – see handout on socialization
  8. **Socialization Period** (puppies and people)

LESSON 2
  1. **Play Period** – puppies only
  2. **Review**
  3. **Chewing** – see handout on destructive behavior
  4. **Fetch Command**
  5. **Settle** – see settle handout
  6. **Gentle Leader Head Collar** – for additional physical control of large, unruly, distracted, or hard to train puppies, see handout on head halter application for details
  7. **No-Pull Harness** – a body harness that stops tugging and pulling on the leash
  8. **Socialization Period** (puppies and people)

LESSON 3
  1. **Play Period** – puppies only
  2. **Review**
  3. **Bite Inhibition** – see handout on mouthing
  4. **Teaching Off** – see handout on mouthing
  5. **Basic Handling Exercises (level 1)** – see handout on handling
  6. **Unruly Behavior – Jumping Up** – see handout on unruly behavior
  7. **Socialization Period** (puppies and people)

LESSON 4
  1. **Play Period** – puppies only
  2. **Review**
  3. **Come When Called** – see handout on basic training
  4. **Come–Sit Exercise**
  5. **Round Robin Exercise** – recall exercise between two or more people
  6. **Teach the Puppy to Go to Someone on Command and Play 'Hide and Seek'**
  7. **Leadership** – see handout on leadership
  8. **Heel On Lead** – see handout on basic training
  9. **Socialization Period** (puppies and people)

LESSON 5
  1. **Play Period** – puppies only
  2. **Review**
  3. **Feeding exercises** – see handout on handling
  4. **Stay on Command** – see handout on basic training

LESSON 5 (*continued*)
   5. **Handling Exercises (level 2)** – see handout on handling
   6. **Pass the Puppy** – puppies passed from family to family for gentle handling
   7. **Teach to Turn a Circle and Shake for Graduation**
   8. **Socialization Period** (puppies and people)

LESSON 6
   1. **Play Period** – puppies only
   2. **Review**
   3. **Unruly Behavior**
      Getting on the furniture – see handout on unruly behavior
      Barking – see handout on barking
      Digging – see handout on destructive behavior
   4. **Tricks**
      A. Shake hands
      B. Jump through a hoop
      C. Poison trick
      D. Crawl
      E. Play dead and roll over
   5. **Canine Communication**
      A. Facial expressions
      B. Body postures
   6. **Neutering, Behavior and Health**
   7. **Furthering your Dog's Education and Fun: Obedience Training, Agility, and Flyball**
   8. **Conclusion**
      A. To get reliability at home, integrate training into every activity that the puppy enjoys
      B. Training must go on for the rest of the dog's life
      C. Training must be done in all rooms, environments, and situations
      D. Socialize, socialize, socialize
      E. Handle, handle, handle
      F. Don't get discouraged. Hang in there. Whatever investment you make in training your puppy will pay off ten times more in good adult behavior
   9. **Graduation**
  10. **Socialization Period** (puppies and people)

Reference: *Sirius Puppy Training* – video by Ian Dunbar. Very helpful if you plan to start your own puppy classes. Includes control of play biting, bite inhibition, handling exercises, establishing leadership and socialization. It also contains some tips on housetraining, chewing problems, and obedience training for puppies. James and Kenneth Publishers, 2140 Shattuck Ave. #2406, Berkeley, CA 94704; (510) 658-8588.

Figure 3.12   Puppy training outline (form #14 – printable from the CD).

party in the reception area every couple of months (see Fig. 3.14). During this get together, families can bring their new pets, meet the staff, take a tour of the hospital, get additional information on nutrition, grooming and dental care, and have some social and play time with other people and pets. A few refreshments for owners and pets and some free samples might also be a good way to encourage attendance. If your clinic then recommends a trainer in the neighborhood for continued socialization and training classes, you could have the trainer attend the open house to give a brief demonstration, supervise some puppy or kitten socialization games, and sign up pets for the next set of classes.

One major concern of some veterinarians and pet owners is the risk of disease to puppies and kittens that have not yet finished their vaccination series. However, in order for socialization classes to be optimally effective, they should

KITTEN KINDERGARTEN CLASS OUTLINE

As with young puppies, early socialization, training, and owner education are important in preventing behavior problems and decreasing the chances of future relinquishment. Although less popular than puppy classes, a set of kitten socialization classes over two to four weeks can be a valuable socialization and training tool for kittens and their owners as well as a public relations tool for the practice.

Kittens should be under 13 weeks of age, and free from external parasites and any evidence of potentially infectious diseases, and have at least one set of vaccinations before entry into the program. The kitten class outline below can be combined into two sessions or expanded over four classes.

CLASS ONE

This class could take place with or without the kittens. It is primarily intended to explain kitten care, discuss normal cat behavior, and help the owners design an environment that meets all of the kitten's needs while preventing the development of behavior problems. Handouts and a reading list should be distributed so that owners can review the information at home.

1. The cat – normal outdoor behavior – adapting the cat to be an indoor family pet
2. Socialization
3. Developing an indoor environment to meet all of the cat's needs
   a) Litterbox training/elimination
   b) Sleeping/bedding
   c) Object play/exploration
   d) Social play
   e) Scratching and other destructive behaviors
4. Setting the pet up to succeed
   a) Avoiding problems through prevention
   b) Kitten-proofing/confinement
   c) Interrupting undesirable behavior and booby traps
5. Play, training, and control products
6. Discuss medical basics – parasites, vaccinations, feeding
7. Carrying, traveling, and restraint – discuss before next session

CLASS TWO (can be combined with class one)

1. Discussion: Q&A
2. Discuss normal play and when/how to intervene/interrupt
3. Kitten session: play and socialization
4. Discuss individual differences observed during play and socialization session
5. Discussion and demo: rewards, reinforcer assessment, and reward-based training
6. Kitten session: holding, handling, and getting attention for rewards
7. Second socialization and play period

CLASS THREE

1. Discussion: Q&A
2. Kitten session: play and socialization
3. Discussion and demo: reward-based training – lure–reward training and demo
4. Kitten session: reward-based training – sit, give me five, give me ten, come
5. Discussion and demo: nail trimming, grooming, pilling, dental care
6. Kitten session: nail trimming, grooming, pilling, and dental care
7. Discussion of neutering, and adult health care
8. Second play and socialization session
9. Graduation

Figure 3.13   Kitten kindergarten class outline (form #11 – printable from the CD).

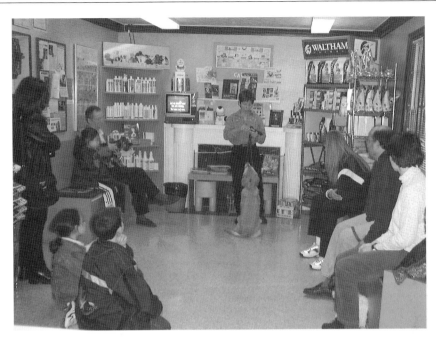

Figure 3.14 A puppy party can combine an open house with an entertaining and informative session about puppy socialization, play, and training. The trainer demonstrates the power of positive reinforcement at a puppy party at the Doncaster Animal Clinic.

begin well within the primary socialization period (i.e., before 12 weeks of age). Therefore the risk of disease must be weighed against the potential benefits of early socialization and training. If puppies and kittens have been examined and found to be in good health and free of parasites, have been vaccinated at least 14 days earlier, and continue to receive their vaccinations in a timely manner, then bringing them into an indoor training environment with other pets their own age should be a minimum risk compared with the benefits that might be achieved. In fact, this type of well-screened and supervised environment might be less risky than a walk along the street, or a trip to other areas frequented by pets. Risk can be further reduced by ensuring that the pet has been in the new home for a reasonable length of time (e.g., beyond the incubation period for common infectious diseases) before beginning classes. Training could begin later in areas where infectious diseases with high morbidity or mortality are endemic or epidemic, and earlier in areas where they are uncommon.

EXERCISE, PLAY, AND STIMULATION

Dogs should be given sufficient exercise to dissipate energy and prevent or greatly reduce behavior problems. This is especially true of breeds bred for endurance or work (e.g., Siberian Huskies, Labrador Retrievers, German Shepherd Dogs). A 15-minute exercise period once or twice daily may be suitable for many dogs, but working dogs may need much more. Obedience training, long walks, jogging, and games of chase or tug of war appeal to most dogs. Although there has been some controversy about whether games that involve pulling, tugging, and rough play might be problematic, studies have shown that these types of play do not lead to the development of other behavior problems, except perhaps in dogs that cannot be controlled because they become too excitable, use their mouths inappropriately to grab and bite arms, legs, hands, or clothing, and those that cannot be sufficiently calmed down at the end of the play session. Selection of an appropriate type and amount of play should be based on the breed (and the work for which it was bred), the owners, the household, and the dog's age and activity level. For example, pulling carts might be more appropriate for dogs bred for this purpose, while retrieving breeds might be more suited to games of fetch and flying disk. Highly energetic breeds, from terriers to the herding breeds, that do not have the opportunity to perform the work for which they were bred could have their energy channeled into flyball or agility training. Less active dogs, such as Basset Hounds, may be satisfied with a brief walk and some owner contact. In general, a dog has had enough exercise if it settles down and rests following its outing and remains settled and relaxed between play and exercise sessions. Whereas some owners jog, run, or take long walks to satisfy their dog's needs, more sedentary owners can accomplish the same goals by throwing a ball, toy, or flying disc for the pet to retrieve. It should be borne in mind that unrestricted exercise may not be healthy for all dogs. For example, it has been hypothesized that rapidly growing large-breed dogs should not be strenuously exercised for fear of exacerbating developmental orthopedic problems such as hip dysplasia.

Play and exercise sessions should be part of the daily routine. Insufficient play and stimulation can be an underlying cause for many behavior problems (Fig. 3.15), while play with owners has been shown to build confidence and obedience. Caution should be taken however that the owners are the ones to initiate play sessions (rather than the dog), to avoid excessively overdemanding, excitable, and attention-seeking behavior. Toys and play sessions are a highly desirable reward, and therefore play might also be used as reinforcement if it is provided for housetraining, obedience training, or for counterconditioning and never for demanding or overly excitable behavior. Dogs should also be given the opportunity to play with other dogs to help develop and maintain good intraspecific social skills. Play with owners does not entirely substitute for play with other dogs, while play with other dogs does not suppress the dog's motivation to play with humans.

It is also not sufficient to allow your dog to sit around all week and then take it for a long run on the weekend. Owners should make plans to spend time with their dogs and then honor the commitment – both will benefit. Exercise periods are not only healthy for owner and pet, but are wonderful interactive sessions that help in the bonding process and can also prevent unwanted attention-getting behaviors. When owners provide a routine program of interactive, owner-initiated daily exercise to their dog's schedule, this provides a more predictable daily routine, and a dog that may be calmer and more relaxed between outings. Well-exercised dogs may be easier to train and may exhibit less anxiety-induced and attention-getting behavior problems.

If a kitten's needs for play, exercise, and social contact are provided, undesirable behavioral consequences such as excessive nocturnal activity, destructive exploration, scratching, overly exuberant activity sessions, play aggression, and annoying attention-getting behaviors are less likely to develop (Fig. 3.15). The kitten should be provided with an appropriate scratching post and toys for self-play. A play center with perches, ledges, dangling toys, and a variety of surfaces for scratching can be either purchased or constructed. Some cats enjoy investigating and playing in empty cardboard boxes or paper bags.

Since predation is a highly innate behavior in most cats, some play sessions should be

---

Behaviors that might arise from insufficient outlets for play and exercise

- Destructive chewing, digging, and scratching
- Investigative behavior, garbage raiding
- Hyperactivity, excitability, nocturnal activity
- Unruliness, knocking over furniture, jumping up
- Excessive predatory and social play
- Play biting, rough play
- Attention-getting behaviors, such as barking and whining

Figure 3.15 Some examples of behaviors that might be reduced or prevented by adequate play and exercise.

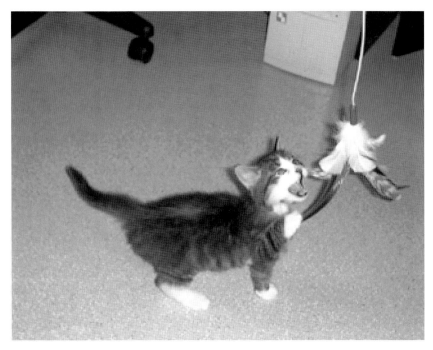

Figure 3.16 A cat toy serves as an outlet for play and a substitute for mousing.

designed to provide active chase-and-pounce targets. Battery-operated rolling toys, small plastic balls, walnuts, or ping-pong balls will work for some cats. Cat toys that dangle from a door handle or scratching post, and those mounted on springs, can also provide good outlets for predatory play. Interactive play, however, can be the best outlet for most cats' needs. Interactive cat toys include long wands, ropes, or sticks with toys attached to the end that resemble prey (Fig. 3.16). When these needs for play, attention, and exercise are satisfied during the day and evenings, most cats will sleep through the night. Allowing cats access to the outdoors is generally not essential, provided the owner presents the cat with sufficient outlets for its investigative, predatory, and playful instincts.

Some cautions are needed when counseling owners about toys and playing with their pets. Be certain that the toys are not so small or fragile that they can be chewed and swallowed. Be particularly vigilant to keep string and thread away from cats and that all toys are large enough and sturdy enough that they cannot be broken or ingested. Since some dogs have such a strong desire and ability to chew, be certain that all chew and play toys are either safe for chewing and ingestion or large and indestructible enough that they cannot be swallowed. A number of such toys are available from commercial companies. Many dog chew toys are made of durable rubber and may have grooves or holes where chew products, food, or treats can be stuffed (Figs 3.17, 3.18). Some toys are designed to be manipulated by rolling or chewing to 'deliver' the food that has been placed inside, while others are made of compressed edible products which may also prove useful for dental care. Articles of clothing, hands and feet, or household items (such as old towels or blankets) should not be used for play, since some pets will generalize their chewing to possessions that the owner does not want damaged. Other family possessions that might appeal to the puppy must be kept out of reach (Fig. 3.19). Never allow a pet to initiate play sessions by barking, grasping, pouncing, or performing other forms of 'demanding' behavior, as this

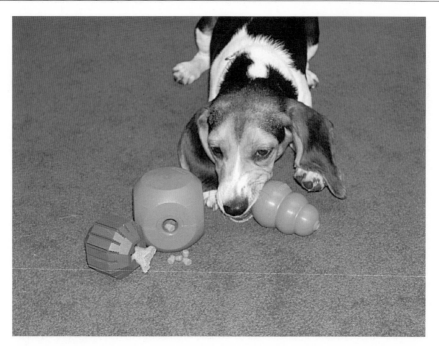

Figure 3.17   Many chew toys have been designed so that food can be used to stimulate interest by coating the toy or by stuffing food or treats within the grooves or openings.

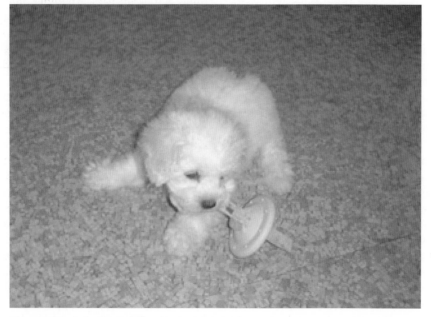

Figure 3.18   A Goodie Ship® toy is made of durable rubber and can be stuffed with dental chew strips or rawhide to keep the interest.

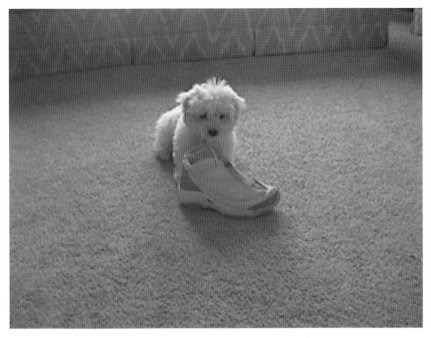

Figure 3.19 Keep the puppy away from the owner's possessions, such as shoes, and do not give old shoes or clothing as toys.

may encourage attention-getting behavior and more intense mouthing and biting.

SOCIAL RELATIONSHIPS – DOGS

Dogs are pack animals and as such readily establish social relationships with other members with which they live. Although dogs are capable of vocalization, most of their social communication is accomplished by means of facial expressions, body postures, and occasionally by using body contact. This type of communication is innate, shared by virtually all members of the species, and is very important in establishing and maintaining the social hierarchy. Within the living group, there is a dominant leader dog (alpha) holding the top position and subordinates holding lower ranking positions in a fairly linear hierarchy. The ability of one dog to become dominant over the others depends on inherited traits, sex, size, hormonal status, and the relative dominance of other pack members. The dominant position affords the alpha individual such benefits as better access to food, mates, and resting areas. Assertive young dogs will challenge the leader of the pack and, if they are dominant enough, may eventually usurp the role. The same may happen in the home environment with other family pets. Longevity in the household provides a certain degree of authority, but will not deter an assertive newcomer from challenging.

When we adopt dogs into a human family, they must learn to interpret the body postures, actions, words and wishes of their owners. Understanding canine behavior, canine communication and basic learning principles are therefore important concepts for dog owners if they are to be able to successfully shape and train desirable behavior. A lack of understanding of what the owners are trying to communicate, inconsistencies in how the owners respond, inconsistencies in training, and the use of punishment can lead to conflict, increasing anxiety and uncertainty in the puppy. Rewards should be used to teach the puppy the desired response to commands, to accept and enjoy handling, to give up resources such as food or toys on demand, and to defer to the owners. The family should control the initiation of all that might be positive including food, play, and attention, and never defer to the dog's demands. Catch phrases such as learn to earn, nothing in life is free, who's training who, deference training, and leadership help owners to be better aware of when rewards should and should not be given (Fig. 3.20, client handout #19 – printable from the CD).

The concept that a dog fits into the human family in a way that is analogous to a dog within a pack is a somewhat oversimplified and outmoded concept. Dogs can only communicate and interact within the framework for which they have been genetically programmed. Therefore, the human response to the dog's actions, vocalization and body postures teaches the dog what can be expected in future encounters. This can be a particular problem with chil-

---

LEADERSHIP

Leadership and control

Positive and consistent training, both in action and in attitude, are needed to gain control of your puppy. In the dog pack, a dog will assume a position in the hierarchy based on its genetics and the results of its ongoing social interactions with other pack members. Although the human household may not be entirely representative of a dog pack, any dominant displays, postures, or attitudes toward the owners (e.g., nipping, excessive mouthing, mounting, jumping up) must be discouraged, while obedience or deference to the owners should be encouraged. At the very least, if these behaviors have been reinforced or are allowed to continue unabated, they become increasingly difficult to resolve and may even progress to more intensive displays of overexuberance, disobedience, dominance, and aggression.

A. Be fair
   1. Be consistent with rewards and corrections. Set rules that everyone observes. This is the only way that the puppy can learn what is acceptable and what is not acceptable.
   2. Don't take good behaviors for granted.
   3. Be generous with praise; give much more praise than scolding.
   4. **Never** hit the puppy or use any type of physical punishment.
B. Make the puppy aware of your importance in its life
   1. Feed it on schedule at specific times.
   2. Make the puppy say please by responding to a command before it gets anything it wants or needs (dinner, treats, toys, picked up, walks, petting, play). It may help to keep in mind one of these two catch phrases: 'Learn to earn' or 'Nothing in life is free.'
   3. Once it learns to stay, ask it to stay for a second or two before following you around the home, in and out of rooms, and in and out of the home.
C. Do not allow the puppy to take control
   1. Do not allow it to constantly solicit attention.
   2. Do not defer or give in to the puppy's demands, unless the behavior is desirable (e.g., barking at the door to eliminate outdoors).
   3. Teach the puppy to stop play biting on command.
   4. Curb excessive barking.
D. Show your leadership in actions
   1. Train your puppy to learn commands and then insist that he or she is immediately responsive. If the puppy ignores you or refuses to obey, gently but immediately show the puppy what is expected.
   2. Be certain that you are the one to initiate all that is positive. This means that the puppy should not get affection, attention, or treats on demand, but rather when they are initiated by you or when you are using them to reward a desired behavior. Deferring to the owner should be encouraged.

Figure 3.20 Establishing leadership and control (client handout #19 – printable from the CD).

dren, who might be less able to read the dog's body language and signals and may be less consistent in their responses. In fact, if the puppy learns that its actions (e.g., nipping or biting), postures or vocalization are successful at getting attention, play or rewards, then problems may develop if the cute, playful puppy grows into a stubborn, defiant adult.

Dogs with assertive personalities, those that are unruly or excitable, those that have a high resource-holding potential (i.e., possessive) and those that are difficult to motivate might be most likely to develop into hard-to-control adults. When aggression does emerge it may be a result of learning, anxiety, conflict and resource-holding potential. Where the dog sleeps and when the dog eats are unlikely to have any impact on the development of dominance hierarchies with family members. Dominance aggression might be a consideration in those cases where the owner has deferred to the dog by allowing it to gain resources and privileges on demand, but then challenges this position by expecting the dog to defer or give up privileges in other situations (see sociopathy in Ch. 21).

SOCIAL RELATIONSHIPS – CATS

As individual hunters feeding on small prey, cats are capable of living a rather solitary existence, particularly when food and resources are scarce. Being solitary, however, does not preclude social behavior. Over the past few years, our knowledge of cat social structure has slowly evolved away from the widespread belief that cats are exclusively a very asocial species. Recently, there have been numerous studies that demonstrate wide diversity in sociability and social structure in groups of cats. In free-living feline groups, the fundamental social unit is typically a group of females and successive generations of descendants. Relationships between neutered males are more similar to those among females than among uncastrated males. Adult males and some females are more solitary and, as such, do not form social groups. There is a great deal of individual variability based on genetic factors, early social interactions

during the sensitive period (two to seven weeks of age), sexual status, and food availability. Encounters between solitary cats are rare, while group-living cats display frequent social interactions. Even cats that spend most of their time alone may occasionally be seen in the company of other cats, particularly a mother cat and her offspring.

Social relationships between cats and humans also show widespread diversity. Cats differ greatly in personality and temperament. Genetic variability and the amount and quality of exposure to humans during the critical socialization period are important factors determining how social a cat will be with humans. Some cats are independent, with little desire for contact with humans or other cats. Others maintain social relationships with people or other family pets throughout life. Approximately 15% of cats seem resistant to socialization with humans. Most cats adapt well to sharing a home or apartment with people, other cats, and other pets. On the other hand, it is not unusual for some cats to have difficulty adjusting to changes in the household, particularly the introduction of a new cat.

The concept of dominance or status in the cat's relationship with people is not analogous to dogs in that a similar dominance hierarchy does not exist within most cat groups. However, when cats are housed in a group in a relatively restricted environment, such as indoors within a home, there may often be one or more cats that the other cats defer to or avoid. This may be a function of personality, learning, or both. These cats may control resources or may chase other cats in the home, while the more 'subordinate' cats may avoid confrontation and retreat for the most part, but may maintain their position or even challenge the more dominant cat over some resources or when they are first to enter an area. Similarly, active and confident cats may also gain control if the owner's responses are ambivalent or inconsistent. For example, if these cats are successful when they solicit petting, affection, attention, food, or play, then they learn that they can control the acquisition of these resources. Furthermore, inconsistency in the owner's responses can lead to anxiety. This can lead to problems within the human–cat social relationship. Some cats that exhibit play biting, chasing, and petting-induced aggression toward owners may only exhibit this behavior to those owners who have been overly compliant in their responses to the cat's demands. Whether this is truly a form of status-induced aggression or whether these behavior problems are an effect of personality and learning is open to discussion. Therefore, as with dogs, family member initiation of play and affection, some simple handling exercises (see below) and training exercises (see food lure training below), and consistency in response to the cat's demands will help to maintain a healthy cat–owner social relationship.

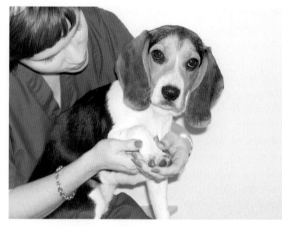

Figure 3.21 Owners need to gradually accustom puppies to accept all forms of gentle handling, especially those that might become a source of anxiety or resistance (paw handling).

HANDLING AND RESTRAINT

It is essential that puppies and kittens learn to accept and enjoy all forms of handling from every family member as well as other humans with which they will come into contact. The family should be advised to expose the pet frequently to all types of handling in the context of gentle play and social attention (Figs 3.21, 3.22). Handling exercises should include gentle handling of the face, ears, feet, collar, skin, and haircoat (Fig. 3.23). Provided there are no signs of anxiety or resistance, the owner should gradually proceed to tooth brushing, grooming, lifting, nail trimming, and handling the muzzle and nape of the neck. The young pet should also be taught to tolerate all approaches and handling by family members while it is eating or playing with a toy. A pet that is not accustomed to being handled may resist or become fearful or aggressive when handled by a groomer, veterinarian, trainer, or child.

Any handling that leads to fear, resistance, threats, or aggression must immediately be identified and terminated. Training should then be undertaken to condition positive responses to these forms of handling. Whatever interaction causes resistance or anxiety should be performed in a manner that is so mild and muted that no anxiety is elicited, while the handler provides something highly desirable, such as a toy, food, or calm talk. The length and intensity of the sessions should gradually increase.

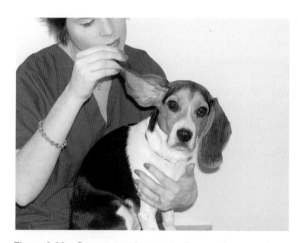

Figure 3.22 Owners need to gradually accustom puppies to all forms of gentle handling, especially those parts of the body that might become a source of anxiety or resistance (ear handling).

HANDLING AND FEEDING EXERCISES

The first goal (Level 1) of handling exercises is to teach the puppy to tolerate and enjoy all types of handling from family members and friends. The second goal (Level 2) is to teach the pet to tolerate more intensive, firm, or unfamiliar forms of handling that might be necessary for restraint, grooming (including nail trimming, ear cleaning, and combing), teeth brushing, veterinary care, or that might arise in greeting or play with new people or children. If the puppy can be trained to associate these forms of handling with rewards and play, it may not become problematic when they are experienced later. The goal is to 'proof' the puppy to prevent it from getting upset if it is handled roughly or caught by surprise.

Similarly, feeding exercises are intended to help the pet accept and enjoy approach and handling during feeding.

PRECAUTIONS
1. Avoid any type of handling during these exercises that causes the pet to become agitated or anxious.
2. If you observe threats or aggression during any of these exercises, seek guidance from a trainer or behaviorist before proceeding.
3. Reaching out for the puppy should always be positive. Hand contact must always be considered a friendly (non-aversive) gesture. Never hit the pup or roughly grab its muzzle or neck.

HANDLING EXERCISES

A. Level 1: Teaching tolerance
The goal of handling exercises is to accustom the puppy to accept and enjoy all types of handling from friends and family members.
1. Begin by only working with the puppy when it is calm.
2. Inspect its ears, mouth, paws, belly, and haircoat.
3. Initially interact for only one second and end with praise or food (the pup's dinner time is a good time to do this).
4. Anticipate the puppy's mood and reaction and always stop before the puppy stops you.
5. Frequently repeat the exercises, gradually lengthening the interaction time.
6. Always praise the puppy whenever it doesn't resist handling.
7. Progress slowly enough to avoid eliciting resistance, aggression, or anxious behaviors. Don't ever force the puppy to endure handling, especially if it seems uncomfortable or stressed.

B. Level 2: Proofing puppies for more intensive handling
1. Act jolly; offer food or a toy.
2. Gently touch, pet, stroke, or massage various areas of the body and collar while giving the pet food or a toy.
3. Gradually increase the intensity of touching, pushing, patting, and grasping different areas of the body (e.g., face, feet, muzzle, ears) as the puppy gets more used to it.
4. Always praise the puppy and intermittently give favored treats whenever it doesn't resist handling.
5. Start with short sessions, anticipate the puppy's attention span and stop before the puppy gets tired of the exercise.
6. Consider your dog and lifestyle and adapt and progress with your handling exercises (gentle, positive, reward association) to what the puppy might one day be expected to encounter (e.g., brushing the teeth, lifting and carrying, bathing, grooming, cleaning ears, wiping feet, nail trimming, etc.).

FEEDING EXERCISES
Food bowl handling is intended to teach the puppy to feel comfortable and even learn to enjoy the presence of people while it is eating or near its food bowl.
A. Don't put the food bowl down and ignore the puppy while it eats. Sit down, visit with the pup, talk to it, and spend some quality social time.

(continued)

Figure 3.23 Handling and feeding exercises for puppies (client handout #12 – printable from the CD).

FEEDING EXERCISES (*continued*)
B. Food bowl handling (teach that the hand is coming to give, not to take away).
   1. Walk by the puppy while it is eating and drop a piece of canned food, meat, or cheese-flavored treat into the food bowl. Ask visitors to do the same.
   2. Occasionally reach down toward the bowl and put a food treat in it.
   3. Place the bowl in your lap or on the floor in front of you. Feed the puppy. Handle the food, gently pet the puppy. Act jolly.
   4. Take the bowl away. Put a highly desirable food treat in the bowl and give it back.
   5. Gently touch and handle the puppy while putting a food treat in the bowl.

Figure 3.23 (*continued*)

PREVENTION OF PROBLEMS – DOG PROOFING, CAT PROOFING, AND CONFINEMENT

The simplest form of prevention of undesirable behaviors involves separating the pet from the site of the problem, or confining it so that the undesirable behavior cannot be performed. A common misconception is that confinement is cruel or unfair. On the contrary, leaving a pet unsupervised to investigate, destroy, and perhaps get injured is far more inhumane. For kittens, caging may be useful but most kittens can be housed in a 'safe room' with toys, a scratching post, and litterbox, provided there are no objects that can be damaged by climbing or chewing. Child locks, secured cupboards, and motion-activated alarms are useful in designing a cat-proof room.

Crate training is certainly not a necessity for all families and all pets. Owners who seldom leave their pets alone, and those that house their pets outdoors when they cannot be supervised, may require little or no indoor confinement. However, when owners must leave a new pet unsupervised, it is essential that it be confined to an area where it will not injure itself, cause household damage, or eliminate in unacceptable locations. Some homes can be successfully dog proofed by closing off doors to areas where the pet is not allowed, by placing child gates across areas that are out of bounds, or by using one or more of the indoor avoidance devices (see environmental punishment in Ch. 5).

Although dog proofing a room might be successful for some dogs, a cage, run, or pen is usually the safest and most secure form of canine confinement. Crate training is an excellent way to curb many behavior problems, including housesoiling, destructiveness, digging, escape behavior, and garbage raiding. As long as a crate is big enough for the pet to stand up and turn around in comfortably, the dog gets sufficient exercise and attention, and it is not left in the crate longer than it can control elimination, it can be a safe, secure, and humane place to confine a pet when it is unsupervised. The goal of crate training is to teach the pet to use its crate for napping, relaxing, and security as it might a bed or favored easy chair. In turn, the owners must attempt to schedule confinement only at times when the pet has had sufficient interactive play, training, and exercise, has used its elimination area, and is now ready to relax, nap, or chew on some favorite toys.

When a crate is used as a daily confinement area, its use should be limited to sleeping during the night and for periods not exceeding four to five hours during each day. Use of a crate is excessive if the pet is confined all night as well as eight to 10 hours each day when the family is away from home. Also, the crate should not be regarded as a prison cell where a dog is sent if it misbehaves. At each feeding time during the day, the owner should encourage the pet to go into the crate by repeatedly tossing pieces of dry food for the pet to chase into the crate (Fig. 3.24). If the owner says 'Go to your crate' each time the pet runs into the crate, it will eventually be conditioned to run into the crate on command. Toys should also be placed in the crate periodically throughout the day, and occasionally a biscuit should be left in the crate so the pet is tempted to go into the crate on its own. This provides plenty of positive associations with the crate. It is ideal to start with short confinement periods and gradually lengthen them. The owner should ignore vocalizations and should not allow the pet out if it is barking, whining, or scratching. If it needs to be released to eliminate, but continues to vocalize, the owner can try providing a distracting noise (whistle, hand clap, thump the wall) in an attempt to get the pet to orient toward the sound and be quiet for 10 seconds or more before it is released. However, the crate is simply a tool. It does not replace sound behavioral modification techniques, but is a helpful adjunct. Introducing the pet to a confinement pen can be done with the same approach used for crate training. As the pet becomes consistent about using a proper elimination area and can be trusted not to explore or damage the home, the confinement door can be left open during short departures and gradually the time left out of the confinement can be increased (see Fig. 3.25 – handout #5 printable from CD).

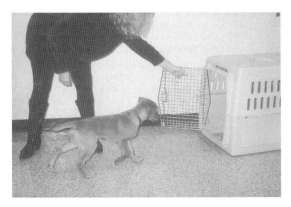

Figure 3.24 A puppy can be taught to go to its crate on command by tossing dry food and saying 'Go to your crate!'

For details on housetraining puppies and litterbox training kittens see Chapters 17 and 18.

SETTING THE PET UP FOR SUCCESS

Owners must be taught that it is far more productive and effective to train and guide the puppy or kitten into acceptable responses (e.g., what to chew, where to scratch and eliminate, etc.) rather than trying to punish the pet for every behavior that might be undesirable. A few simple rules will greatly increase the chances of success while minimizing the need for punishment.

1. *Reward-based training:* using positive reinforcement (food lure–reward training) to teach the pet to understand and immediately obey a few basic commands is the first step in gaining control through verbal communication.
2. *Supervision:* young and new pets should constantly be within eyesight of a family member. Using basic training commands and, if needed, a leash left attached to a neck collar, head halter, or body harness, the pet can be encouraged to engage in appropriate and desirable behaviors, while interrupted and redirected if exhibiting undesirable behavior.
3. *Understanding the pet's needs:* overall success is only likely to be achieved if all of the pet's innate needs are considered and met. For example, chewing and scratching are normal behaviors for young dogs and cats. The pet must be provided with acceptable outlets for these behaviors, and taught what forms of chewing, climbing, scratching, exploration, and play are acceptable. Pets should also be provided with access to acceptable elimination areas as needed. Other needs the family must provide for include mental stimulation, physical exercise, and social interaction.
4. *Prevention and confinement:* prevent access to areas and objects that might be targets of undesirable behavior when the owner is not

GUIDE TO CRATE/CONFINEMENT TRAINING

Confinement training is intended to provide a comfortable bed, den, or play area for the dog, while restricting access to areas where it might housesoil, do harm to itself, or cause damage. Crate training should be considered akin to placing a young child in a playpen or crib for playtime or sleeping. Other alternatives for confinement include housing the dog in a pen, run, or dog-proofed room, where it might have more freedom to stretch out, chew, or play with its toys. If you don't provide a safe confinement area at times that you cannot supervise, your dog will wander the home unsupervised and will likely engage in destructive chewing, roam through restricted areas, eliminate in undesirable locations, and get into potentially dangerous situations.

The location and techniques used for training should be designed to keep the experience positive. For example, the dog should be encouraged to sleep, nap, or play with its chew toys in its confinement area. On the other hand, if the dog is confined at a time when it is in need of play, attention, or elimination, then escape attempts and anxiety are to be expected. If a dog's attempts at escape are ever successful, then future, more ambitious attempts to escape are likely to occur. Therefore a secure, inescapable form of confinement should be utilized.

Benefits of a crate/confinement trained dog
1. Security – a specific area that serves as a den or resting area for the dog.
2. Safety for the pet.
3. Prevents damage (chewing, investigation, elimination, etc.).
4. Aids in the training of proper chewing and elimination by preventing failure and encouraging success.
5. Traveling: accustoms the dog to confinement for traveling and boarding.
6. Improved relationship with your pet: fewer problems and therefore less discipline for the pet and less frustration/anxiety for you.

Crate training
1. A metal, collapsible crate with a tray floor or a plastic traveling crate works well, provided it is large enough for the dog to stand and turn around. Some dogs adapt quicker to a small room, run, or doggy playpen.
2. Because dogs are social animals, an ideal location for the crate is a room that the family frequents such as a kitchen, den, or bedroom, rather than an isolated laundry or furnace room. If you have observed your dog choosing a particular corner or room to take a nap, or you wish your dog to sleep in a particular location at night, then this might be the best location for the crate.
3. For the crate to remain a positive retreat, it should not be used for punishment. If social isolation (time-out) is used, consider placing the dog in a laundry room or bathroom.
4. A radio or television may help to calm the dog and may help to mask environmental noises that can trigger barking.

Puppies
1. Introduce the puppy to the crate as early in the day as possible. Place a few treats, toys, or food in the crate so that the puppy is motivated to enter voluntarily. Command training (e.g., 'Go to your kennel') can also be useful.
2. The first confinement session should be after a period of play, exercise, and elimination (i.e., when the puppy is ready to take a nap). Place the puppy in its crate with a toy and a treat and close the door. Alternatively, if the puppy lies down to take a nap, move the puppy to the crate for the duration of the nap.
3. Leave the room but remain close enough to hear the puppy. Some degree of distress vocalization is to be expected the first few times the puppy is separated from its family members. Never reward the pet by letting it out when it cries or whines. Ignore it until the crying stops. Release the puppy when it wakes or if you need to awaken your puppy for feeding, play, or elimination (e.g., prior to your departure).
4. If crying does not subside on its own, a mild interruption may be useful. Any interruption that causes fear or anxiety must be avoided since it is not mentally healthy for the pet and could aggravate the vocalization or cause elimination in the crate. During the interruption, you should remain out of sight, so that the puppy does not learn to associate the interruption with your presence. A sharp noise, such as that provided by a shaker can containing a few coins, can be used to interrupt barking. A squirt from a water gun may also be effective. Another way to discourage barking is to use a commercial bark-activated device that produces an alarm or distracting spray when the puppy vocalizes.

Figure 3.25 Crate training (client handout #5 – printable from the CD).

Puppies (*continued*)

5. Repeat the confinement training procedures a few more times before bedtime.
6. Prior to bedtime, the puppy should be exercised and secured in its crate for the night. Again do not go to the pet if it is crying. If the puppy cries in the middle of the night, it should be ignored or a brief interruption can be utilized (as above). Then release the puppy when it is quiet and time to get up. Puppies under four months of age may not be able to keep their crate clean for the entire night, so an early morning walk may be necessary for the first few weeks. Sometimes the best way to reduce distress vocalization is to locate the crate in the bedroom.
7. Never leave the puppy in its crate for longer than it can control itself or it may be forced to eliminate in the crate. If the pup must be left for longer than it can control elimination, a larger confinement area with paper for elimination, a puppy litterbox, or access to an elimination area outdoors by dog door will be necessary.
8. Until a puppy has been housetrained (no accidents for at least four consecutive weeks) and no longer destroys household objects in your absence, it should not be allowed out of its confinement area except under direct supervision. While the puppy is out of its confinement area, constant supervision is required so that undesirable behaviors can be interrupted and desirable behaviors can be rewarded.

The adult dog

1. The most important principles for effective crate training include locating the crate (or confinement area) in a location where the dog feels comfortable about sleeping or napping and gradually introducing the dog to confinement in as positive a manner as possible.
2. Set up the crate in the dog's feeding area or sleeping area with the door open for a few days. Place food, treats, and toys in the crate so that the dog enters the crate on its own. Once the dog is entering the crate freely, it is time to close the door.
3. Follow steps 1 to 4 in puppy training above to accustom the dog to confinement. Repeat these procedures for a few days, gradually increasing the amount of time the dog must remain quietly in the crate before it is released.
4. Finally, the dog should be left in its crate during bedtime or during departures. Try short departures first, and gradually make them longer.
5. Some dogs may adapt quicker to crate training by having the dog sleep in the crate at night.
6. If you are away from home four or more days per week, the pet should not be left in the crate for more than about four hours during the day each day when you are gone.

Crate training problems

If your dog is particularly anxious or eliminates in its crate, then it may be an indication that some part of the crate training technique needs to be revisited.

1. It may be possible that the dog is being left in its crate longer than it can control elimination. Confine the dog for a shorter time and be certain that it has eliminated prior to confinement.
2. If the crate is overly large some dogs may sleep in one end and eliminate in the other. Consider a smaller crate or a divider.
3. If your dog is anxious or attempts to escape when left in its crate, then he or she may not have been accustomed to its crate in a gradual and positive enough manner. Review the steps above to ensure that the crate is in a comfortable bedding location, that each crate introduction is positive, and that the crate is not used for punishment.
4. If the dog has previously escaped from its crate, this serves to encourage further escape attempts. Change to a more secure confinement area or ensure that the crate is inescapable. It may then be necessary to supervise the dog in its crate for a period of time to help reduce anxiety and deter further escape attempts.

Figure 3.25   (*continued*)

available to supervise. This can range from confinement options such as crate training, a dog run or a pet-proofed room, or closing off or booby trapping areas where problems might occur. Confinement should only be implemented after there has been ample opportunity for attention, play, exercise, and elimination. The family should provide the pet with toys for chewing and play within its confinement area. Pets that must eliminate during the time that the owners are away will also need to be provided with access to an elimination area.

THE ROLE OF REWARDS AND PUNISHMENT

The effective use of rewards and punishment is discussed in detail throughout this book as they apply to learning principles and in the correction of undesirable behavior. Rewards should be used to reinforce desirable responses and to turn potentially anxious situations and events into ones that are positive. Just because something is appealing does not mean that it will be a form of positive reinforcement, unless it is consistently associated with the behavior and properly timed. For rewards to be successful as reinforcers, they should be highly appealing, given immediately when the desired response is exhibited (contiguous), and only when the response is exhibited (contingent).

To ensure that certain objects or food are successful for reinforcing the pet, the owner should first consider what rewards would be most appealing and then withhold or deprive these rewards except for training. It is essential that owners be taught to identify all rewards and only to give them immediately following desirable responses. If rewards are given at any other time they may lose their motivational value and may inadvertently reinforce undesirable behavior. For example, a dog might be given attention for growling or barking in an attempt to calm it down. Dogs that solicit play and affection by whining, mouthing, chasing, or jumping up often get the very attention they are seeking, and this ensures that the behavior will be performed in the future. In addition, owners that use physical forms of punishment in an attempt to stop attention-seeking behaviors might either serve to reinforce these behaviors, or make the dog increasingly fearful, anxious, and conflicted about whether or not to approach during greeting depending on how the 'punishment' is applied. See Figure 3.26 for our handout on reward training. For more details and defini-

tions on rewards, punishment, and behavior modification, see Chapter 5.

Reward selection and timing

Anything that the pet finds appealing can be a reward. In both dogs and cats, the value of any particular item as a reward will vary from pet to pet, based on individual differences, previous experience, and degree of deprivation. The dog that enjoys attention, playing ball, going for a walk, having its head or belly rubbed, or the food that you are eating will effectively get a reward when these are given. Cats can also be trained using the same reinforcement principles, but it may be more difficult to find rewards that are sufficiently motivating. Novel and favored food treats may be effective for some cats (fresh cooked chicken, liver, tuna, shrimp, dried fish), as might catnip treats and favored toys. Some cats are also motivated by affection or play. Deprivation may be especially important to sufficiently increase motivation. For example, food should be given at meal times rather than free choice, and play and affection periods can be withheld until training times. Some of these reinforcers may also have limited duration of appeal in cats, so that short affection and play sessions may be all that can be utilized.

Reinforcer assessment is the process during which we determine which rewards might best motivate our pets (and we save these exclusively for the retraining program). Although the pet's favored food might be sufficiently appealing, other special food items (cheese, popcorn, meat for dogs, chicken, fish paste, fish pieces for cats) might be more motivating and therefore better for reward training. Similarly, favored toys, walks, and affection can be used as rewards, but only if the owner is willing to save these mainly for training. As the family progresses through new commands and more difficult training, the favored rewards or a jackpot of rewards are given to immediately mark the desired response. It is essential that these rewards be deprived except for training, since we want to maintain the high motivating value of these rewards.

REWARD-BASED TRAINING

The key to the effective use of rewards involves giving the reward immediately when the desired response is exhibited (contiguous) but only when the response is exhibited (contingent). For positive reinforcement to be effective, the reward must be given immediately following the desired response so that it increases the chance that the response will be repeated.

Reward selection and timing
1. Anything that your pet enjoys can be a reward. This can include treats, food, a toy, attention, play, affection, going for a walk, or even a rub of its head or belly. Since there is a great deal of individual variation you must first choose the rewards that most appeal to your pet.
2. Whenever you give the pet something it enjoys, you are positively reinforcing whatever behavior the pet is performing at that time, whether desirable or undesirable. Therefore, never give a reward unless it immediately follows a behavior you wish to encourage. If you do so, the very problems that you need to correct (e.g., fearful responses, grasping and biting, barking, etc.) may inadvertently be rewarded by your responses.
3. Learn to earn: rewards should be used only as positive reinforcement for desirable responses. Rewards must be withheld at all other times. In fact, before getting anything of value you should use a training command to ensure that the dog is behaving appropriately.
4. Depriving the dog of rewards at all times except for training increases their motivational value. In principle, depriving a pet of a reward increases the pet's 'hunger' for the reward, while rewards that are given too often may lose appeal. For example, food rewards are most effective when the pet is most hungry, around meal time. Therefore, if your pet is fed free choice, it might be better to switch to a feeding schedule. Training can be held just prior to meal times in order to increase the appeal of the food rewards.
5. Reinforcer assessment: assess the motivating value of rewards and place them in order from most desirable to least desirable. Use your dog's most favored rewards or multiple rewards (reward jackpot) to shape and reward newer, more difficult, or more exact training responses and use lesser rewards for intermittently reviewing and rewarding previously learned responses or less exact responses.
6. Timing: dogs learn fastest if the rewards are given every time, immediately as the dog displays the desirable behavior. Later, a switch to a variable intermittent reward schedule will help to ensure that the pet continues to perform indefinitely.
7. Secondary reinforcers: a clicker can be paired to a food reward by consistently sounding it just prior to giving the food until it becomes a conditioned stimulus for food. The value of a clicker is that it can then be used as a reward to immediately mark correct responses in a convenient and precise manner, with the food being given shortly afterwards. While they can become effective enough to reinforce responses without the need for food, intermittently giving the food treat following these secondary reinforcers will help continue to maintain their value. In addition to clickers, favored food rewards can be paired with praise, stroking, or petting.
8. Extinction: if you stop reinforcing a previously reinforced behavior, it will eventually stop being performed. This is often the best way to stop undesirable behaviors that have been reinforced by attention, praise, affection, or food (e.g., jumping up, barking). However, behavior problems that have been rewarded intermittently will take much longer to become extinct.

Command–response–reward training
There are a number of training methods that might be considered and your veterinarian or trainer can help to determine which might be most suited to you and your dog. In simple terms you need to give a command and reward the desired response immediately and every time until the pet consistently responds. Begin the training in an environment with few distractions when the pet is calm. Start with simple commands, and gradually progress to more difficult commands in more difficult environments. Use mildly appealing treats at first, and save the highly favored rewards for later when the pet is giving more improved responses in difficult situations. This will encourage the dog to progress and improve.

If your dog doesn't obey immediately, it may be that the command is not understood or that the pet is distracted. If the pet does not immediately respond to the command, there are two alternatives: either to give no reward and try to progress a little more slowly or to consider a physical control device such as a leash and head halter to physically guide the dog into the correct response. Punishment should not be used for training. Punishment for

(*continued*)

Figure 3.26   Using rewards effectively (client handout #22 – printable from the CD).

Command–response–reward training (*continued*)

incorrect responses may lead to fear and anxiety, and while it may stop the inappropriate response, it in no way encourages the pet to display the desired response.

Training with rewards: command–response–reinforce

If a command is paired with a response and there is immediate reinforcement, the pet should learn the desired response for each command. Once a response can consistently be achieved on command, shaping can be used to progress to more difficult responses in a variety of environments.

1. Food lure training
   a) The movement of food is used to lure the pet into performing the desired behavior. Holding and wiggling the food in front of the dog should lure the dog into a come, while moving the food upward and back should lure the dog into a sit, while down and forward should lure the dog into a down.
   b) A cue word (command) is spoken as the pet is performing the movement.
   c) The food is given **immediately** upon completion.
   d) As training progresses, the lure is made less obvious by being presented in a closed hand, and praise and stroking are intermittently substituted for the food reward.
2. Observe and reward
   Observe the pet for desired behaviors and reward immediately. If a behavior can be anticipated, a command can be given just prior to the behavior and then an immediate reward can be given once the behavior is completed. Some dogs can learn to eliminate on command with this technique.
3. Physical prompt and fade
   Give a command as you use a prompt such as a head halter or hand prompt (e.g., guiding the pet into a sit position) to get the desired response, and then reinforce. Over time, the prompt can be faded (i.e., gradually removed).
4. Negative reinforcement
   Apply a prompt or correction that the subject dislikes until the desired response is achieved, and then immediately remove it to indicate that the correct response has been achieved.
5. Shaping
   Determine the desired response and reward behaviors that approximate the response. Once successful, only behaviors that are slightly closer to the desired goal are rewarded, while less accurate responses are no longer rewarded.

Punishment

1. **No physical punishment should be used. Never** hit the pet, throw it on its back, shake it by the scruff, push the lips against the teeth forcefully, or use any other type of physical correction.
2. If you observe the pet doing something that is undesirable, interrupt the behavior in a manner that is sharp, startling, and strong enough to immediately stop the undesirable behavior without causing the puppy to be overly anxious.
3. If you cannot generate enough volume with a loud '**no**' to stop the pet, then a shake can, air horn, alarm, citronella spray, or water bottle may be used immediately as the word '**no**' is given. Care should be taken when scolding cats. Many cats will begin avoiding family members if yelled at loudly or frequently. It is preferable to use a neutral stimulus (e.g., water gun) without saying anything or even looking at the cat when attempting to interrupt misbehavior.
4. After interrupting the undesirable behavior, you should guide your pet into the proper behavior and reward it, if possible.
5. A leash and head halter can be used to guide the dog into position if it does not immediately obey, and a release of pressure and positive reinforcement given for success.
6. If the undesirable behavior occurs when you cannot interrupt and guide your pet into the proper behavior, an unpleasant consequence associated with the behavior may deter recurrence. Aversive noises and devices (e.g., Snappy Trainer™, spray avoidance devices, motion detectors) and aversive odors and tastes may be effective deterrents depending on the pet and the problem.

Figure 3.26 (*continued*)

Reward control – learn to earn

Each time we give our pets a reward we must ensure that it has been earned. This program, referred to by William Campbell as 'Learn to earn,' is not only a means of improving our training and control, but also reminds us that training, shaping, and progression are accomplished through positive means.

Each time we give attention, food, play, treats, or anything else the dog 'wants' we need to ask ourselves what the pet has just done to earn the reward. As mentioned, if the pet has initiated the sequence that achieves the reward then we may be rewarding inappropriate behavior, and giving away a potential reward (reducing its motivating and rewarding ability). Therefore, keeping in mind phrases such as 'Nothing in life is free' (Victoria Voith) or 'No free lunch' helps to remind us that not only do we need to withhold these rewards when the dog is asking for them, but we need to save them for our training programs when they are earned.

Pushy pets

When the pushy pet approaches for attention, play, food, or affection, it is usually best to completely ignore it. This includes refraining from any verbal or physical contact interactions with the dog. Any response on the part of the owner may otherwise serve to reinforce the behavior and allows the pet to control how and when the reward is obtained. If the pet persists to a point where the owner can no longer ignore the behavior, then it might be possible to walk out of the room, and even close the door until the pet ceases the behavior. Another more immediate option is to give a command (down, quiet time, go to your mat) to get an appropriate response; i.e., the pet must obey a command (nothing in life is free) or learn a new task (learn to earn) before any reward is given (see Figs 3.20, 3.26). After the pet has settled for a sufficiently long period of time (this should gradually be increased), the owner can go to the dog to give a reward. Another option is to keep a leash and head halter attached to the

pup while it is being supervised, so that the behavior can immediately be stopped and success can be achieved (Fig. 3.27).

Clicker training and secondary reinforcers

Sometimes it is not possible to immediately reward an appropriate behavior at the most appropriate time, so we resort to secondary reinforcers, signals that tell the dog that he did the right thing and will receive a reward later. For example, clicker training pairs the neutral sound of a clicker with a very favored primary reward, such as a food treat, so that the clicker soon becomes a consistent predictor of food. It can be referred to as a conditioned stimulus as soon as the clicker leads to salivation, excitement, and food anticipation, even before the food is presented (Fig. 3.28).

The clicker can be used as a potent and immediate reinforcer of desirable behavior. During training there may often be a delay between the pet's response and the presentation of the primary reinforcer (affection or food). The advantage of a secondary reinforcer like a clicker is that it can be given immediately to mark the correct response. The food treat or affection could then be briefly delayed, but the pet would still be in anticipation of its 'reward' and would likely still understand what it has been rewarded for. In this context the clicker might be referred to as a bridging stimulus. In practice, other devices such as horns, whistles, or the use of a phrase such as 'good dog' or 'good kitty' can also become secondary reinforcers if they are immediately and regularly preceded by primary reinforcers such as stroking, food, treats, or affection.

Punishment

Punishment is intended to reduce the chance that a particular behavior will be repeated. Animals quickly learn to avoid unpleasant or aversive situations in nature. Similarly, we can teach our pets to avoid certain areas and behaviors with the proper use and application of

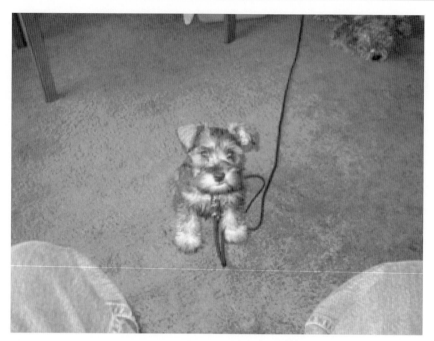

Figure 3.27 A long lead and head halter are left attached for immediate control.

punishment. Under no circumstances should the owner ever strike the pet with a hand or anything in a hand. Owners must understand that if they strike their pet, the consequences can be disastrous. Since the human hand should only be associated with affection, play, or rewards, physical punishment (hitting) is never indicated. Physical punishment can lead to handshyness, fear biting, avoidance of humans, aggression, and submissive urination. Remote punishment techniques and booby traps that are of appropriate intensity for the pet's temperament are the preferred forms of punishment, since they cause no fear of the owner and they teach the pet to avoid an area or behavior whether the owner is present or not. In addition, for punishment to be successful it must be sufficiently aversive to deter the pet immediately, and must be applied immediately and consistently until the behavior ceases to be performed. Punishment (such as an abrupt, loud noise) is sufficiently aversive if the undesirable behavior stops immediately, the pet shows a slight startle response without any sign of fear, and will readily come to the owner without any hesitation. Anything the owner does to

stop a behavior that results in any sign of fear is inappropriate (for further details see Ch. 5).

BASIC TRAINING

There are limits to what should be expected in the training of puppies and kittens. Some animals have natural aptitudes while others are more limited. Learn to work with what you've got. Don't expect a bloodhound to walk perfectly on a leash immediately, because it has been bred to track a scent. The excitable pet will probably train better after it has had the opportunity to play and vent some of that energy. Also be aware that certain medical conditions and a variety of drugs can interfere with the learning process.

All dogs should learn basic obedience command responses such as 'come', 'sit', 'stay,' and 'down'. The dog that learns to roll over or play dead may be fun at parties, but the basic skills could mean the difference between life and death. Dogs that will not stay or come when called may end up in front of a car on the road. There are numerous books and videos

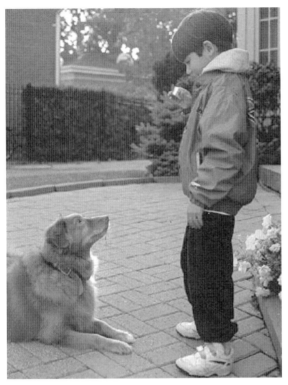

Figure 3.28 Clicker training is effective for dogs of all ages. This 14-year-old Nova Scotia Duck Tolling Retriever 'Grace' has minimal hearing and sight but is still immediately responsive to the clicker.

of learning and conditioning. In simple terms we need to give a command, ensure success, and reward the desired response immediately and every time. The trainer needs to proceed slowly with simple commands in quiet environments and gradually progress to more difficult commands in more difficult environments. By rewarding each response, and saving more favored rewards for each new step along the way, the pet will continue to progress and improve. Clicker training, target training, and lure–reward training are highly effective, but if additional physical control is needed, a leash and head halter can be used to prompt the dog to respond and ensure immediate success. Regardless of the method used, once the command is given, the goal is to get the desired response and reward the response, while unsuccessful responses earn no rewards. Punishment can be a dangerous tool for training. If it is too harsh, inconsistent, or poorly timed, it may lead to fear and anxiety, and while it may stop the inappropriate response, it in no way encourages the pet to display the desired response.

Food lure training

Dogs can be taught to come, sit, and lie down using food lure–reward training. This can even be done during a routine veterinary examination. Standing about 60 cm away from the puppy, a piece of food is held between the thumb and forefinger and extended. As the puppy approaches, its name is called, followed by the command 'come!' (Fig. 3.29). When the puppy reaches the food, it is slowly moved above its head. Avoid moving the food too high over the pet's head or it will jump up instead of sit. As the puppy lifts its head up toward the food, it moves naturally into a sitting position (Fig. 3.30). As it begins to sit, the command 'sit!' is given. Holding the food reward on the ground entices the pet into the 'down' position (Fig. 3.31). Even this basic start helps the owner establish leadership and gain control, and serves as a tool for socializing. It also decreases jumping up and handshyness because the puppy associates greeting with sitting and an outstretched hand with a food

dealing with training, but formal obedience classes are still the best way to learn. This puts family members under the supervision of a trainer, where they are less likely to make fundamental errors. It also affords an opportunity for socialization with new people and other dogs, an important part of behavioral development. Take the time to visit training classes personally so that you don't inadvertently refer a family to a trainer who is not reputable.

Command–response–reward training

There are a number of training methods that might be considered, based on the needs of the pet and the owner and the expertise of the trainer. Training techniques should be based on the use of positive reinforcement and the principles

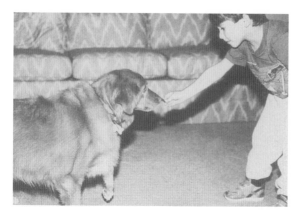

Figure 3.29 Food lure training is an excellent way to teach a 'come' command. The owner stands about 60 cm from the dog, extends the hand with a food morsel, and says 'come!'

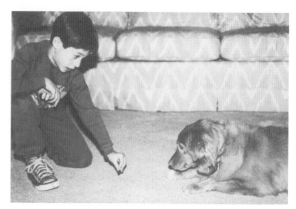

Figure 3.31 Food lures can also be used to entice a dog into the 'down' position.

reward. Making the dog come and sit before it gets anything also helps define a leadership role for the owner. Some basic training procedures using food lure techniques are reviewed in Appendix C, Figure 4 (client handout #2 – printable from the CD).

Rewards can also be used to train cats to perform a variety of tasks and respond to a number of commands. Cats are no more difficult to train than any other animal, but kittens may be easier to train because they may be more highly motivated by play, toys, and novel food treats. All one needs to do is associate a reward with a particular action, and the cat is likely to want to repeat or continue that action. For example, if the cat approaches its scratching post, uses its cat litter, comes to the owner, or sits up on its hind legs, a desirable reward should be provided and the cat will want to perform the behavior time and time again. On the other hand, if the owner calls the cat over to be punished for inappropriately scratching or chewing, it is less likely that the cat will respond to further 'come' commands.

Lure–reward techniques work effectively for most cats. Hold out a piece of food or cat toy, and say 'come.' Repeat this exercise a few times and the cat will learn to associate a reward with the 'come' command. Hold out a piece of food or toy above the cat's scratching post, and use a different command (e.g., 'scratch') and the cat should soon learn to go to its scratching post on command. Similarly, the cat can be taught to sit up and beg, go to its bedroom, or even go to particular people in the home by using the lure–reward technique.

Ensuring the correct response

Over time, as the training improves, the dog should learn to respond quickly to the given

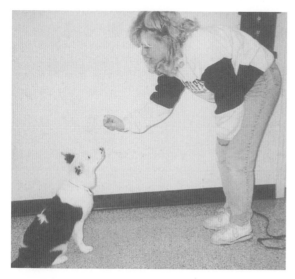

Figure 3.30 A puppy will quickly sit when a piece of food is moved over the top of its head.

command and then can earn the reward. However, a dog may not obey for a variety of reasons. At first, it may not clearly 'understand' the command. Then, even when the command is understood, the reward may not be sufficiently motivating for the dog to entice it to respond. Often owners think that these dogs are disobeying a command, when in fact they may not yet have entirely learned the word, or they are not interested in the reward at this time. These pets must be immediately encouraged to respond so that they clearly understand what is expected of them, and so that they do not learn that ignoring the command is acceptable. Unfortunately, many owners then threaten or punish the dog for not obeying, which in fact may make them more fearful rather than more obedient the next time the command is given. Therefore, in order to ensure that the owners consistently give an immediate and correct response, they could have a leash and head halter attached to the dog, or have a strong enough lure to ensure that the dog is sufficiently motivated to obey.

SELECTING AN APPROPRIATE TRAINING COLLAR: TO CHOKE OR NOT TO CHOKE

The goal of training is to teach the pet to respond to a variety of commands. To be successful, the owner must first be able to get the pet to exhibit the desired response when the command is given. To achieve this, the owner can use a lure such as food or a toy (lure–reward training) or a closed hand target (target training) to encourage or lead the dog to the correct response. Alternatively, a training device such as a head halter and leash can be used to prompt the appropriate response from the dog. The dog should then be immediately rewarded upon performance of the desired response. Although primary reinforcers such as food or a favored toy are generally used first, secondary reinforcers (e.g., clicker, praise) should replace these over time. Clicker training pairs a clicker with food so that the clicker soon becomes a consistent predictor of food. It can then be used to imme-

diately mark and reward desired responses. In time, the training can then gradually progress to more complex or more accurate responses (shaping).

Unfortunately, many training techniques still rely heavily on punishment, which is intended to discourage or 'reduce' undesirable behavior rather than train and encourage desirable behavior. This is not a very efficient approach to training, because punishment does not teach the dog what it is 'supposed' to do. Punishment can also cause fear, anxiety, aggression, and discomfort, or even actual harm to the pet. Some dogs may even respond by attacking the person who is administering the punishment. Therefore, the use of punishment alone is generally not an acceptable method of training, and may in fact be counterproductive.

What is perhaps confusing is that many dogs appear to have been successfully trained with punishment. In fact, many of these dogs have actually been trained with negative reinforcement, where the pain or discomfort is released as soon as the desired behavior is exhibited. This is a difficult concept to teach, and requires 'impeccable' timing. In addition, dogs that have been trained with punishment may be fearful of misbehaving in the trainer's presence. Some of these dogs are then labeled as 'one-person dogs,' because the dog is only responsive to a trainer who can successfully administer the punishment. On the other hand, dogs trained with rewards and shaping should respond to the commands of any family member as long as the commands are consistent and positive.

Neck control vs body control

Ideally, it is the goal of training to have a pet that is entirely responsive to commands, without the need for any form of physical restraint. However, dog owners may not be able to immediately achieve sufficient control and training for the pet to consistently come, stay, or heel on command, especially when it is distracted or highly motivated to perform an alternative response (e.g., chase, greet, play, fight, defend, run away). Therefore, some form of physical restraint is necessary to protect these pets from possible injury to themselves or others, and to ensure that they learn the appropriate response to each command (at least until they are better trained or are in an environment where there is no risk). In fact, a control device is often mandatory in many urban municipalities.

There are a wide variety of leash, halter, and harness systems that can be used for walking and training. Traditionally, a leash attached to a collar around the dog's neck is the most common form of physical control used in most countries. However, concern is growing about the safety and logic of controlling our pets with devices that encircle (and tighten around) the neck and trachea. Therefore, it is becoming increasingly more common for head halters and body harnesses to be used for routine control (Fig. 3.32).

Choke, pinch, and prong devices

Choke, pinch, and prong collars have been designed to control and train in a manner that makes it increasingly uncomfortable if the dog does not obey. The more forceful the owner's pull, the more discomfort for the pet. Choke collar training may be useful as a means of applying negative reinforcement. This can be accomplished by issuing a command, pulling on the choke collar to get the desired response, and then immediately releasing as soon as the dog complies (obeys). In other words, release from discomfort indicates to the dog that the desired response is now being exhibited. Unfortunately, since many owners are unskilled, untrained, or unsuccessful in the use of negative reinforcement, they may escalate to pinch and prong collars to correct or punish undesirable behavior. In the short run, these corrections may cause sufficient discomfort for the behavior to cease. However, with repeated exposure and training, the dog's fear and anxiety may actually increase each time it is exposed to the stimulus because previous exposures have been uncomfortable or aversive. Conversely, some dogs may become so accustomed (desensitized) to the effects of the choke or pinch device that it

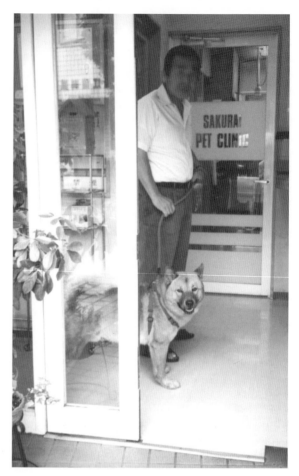

Figure 3.32 At this Japanese veterinary practice, dogs are most commonly controlled by body harnesses rather than devices that encircle the neck.

becomes ineffective. Although many trainers still train with devices that are intended to pull, jerk, choke, or punish, the most effective and humane means of training is through motivation, positive reinforcement, and shaping.

Remote collars

Some devices utilize shock or other forms of discomfort to stop the undesirable response. Ideally, the shock should then be terminated as soon as the desired response is achieved (negative reinforcement). While this may be a successful form of training in experienced hands, these products not only cause undue discomfort to the pet, but are often unsuccessful as a training aid. Their use may also result in undesirable responses (e.g., fear, escape, aggression) and may lead to a conditioned fear or anxiety if the shock is paired with a particular stimulus. A remote citronella collar may be more successful at interrupting the undesirable response without causing excessive fear or anxiety, so that the desirable behavior can then be reinforced. In fact, the collar also has a remote-activated tone that can be used as a conditioned reinforcer (see clicker training). Another new product is a remote collar that gives a mild vibration, which has been designed for training deaf dogs, but could be used as a conditioned reinforcer for training any dog.

Body harnesses and head halters

Body harnesses or head halters are two alternatives to neck collars. Some body harnesses merely serve as restraint devices (Fig. 3.32), while others such as the K9 Pull Control™, Lupi™, and No Pull Halter™ have been specially designed to apply pressure in such a way as to prevent the pet from lunging forward. However, these devices do little to aid in controlling an unruly dog that throws itself about, or getting a dog to focus toward the owner as the head halters do.

There are a number of devices that utilize head control. Since the Gentle Leader™ head halter (previously known as the Promise System™) has both a neck and nose strap adjustment, it can be used either to control the dog when the owner is holding the leash, or with a 2- to 3-m-long leash or 'drag' line left attached (while supervising the dog) for immediate 'remote' control. The Halti™ is a head halter which is an effective leash control device but cannot be fitted so as to be left attached to the dog. The Snoot Loop™ is a head halter with side adjustments to allow for a snugger muzzle fit, thereby reducing the chances that the pet can remove it. This makes it a good choice for brachycephalic breeds. Other products such as the NewTrix™ head halter are designed to stop pulling but are less effective at controlling the muzzle and getting the dog to focus on the owner.

One of the most effective means of gaining control, and ensuring that the pet responds quickly to each command, is to use a leash and head halter such as the Gentle Leader™ for training. With the Gentle Leader™, the owner gains control naturally through pressure exerted behind the neck and around the muzzle. The head halter acts as a tool to help achieve the desired response without punishment, and to communicate the owner's intentions. The proponents of head halters point to the fact that horses can be successfully and humanely controlled with head devices since 'where the nose goes the body follows.' With a head halter the owner can gain eye contact and reorient the dog to perform the desirable response (sort of a power steering option for dogs). With the head halter properly fitted and the leash slack, the dog is not restricted from panting, eating, drinking, chewing, barking, jumping up, biting, lunging forward, or stealing from the table or the garbage. On the other hand, since the halter encircles the head and muzzle, a pull on the leash can immediately curtail pulling, barking, chewing, stealing, stool eating, and even some forms of aggression. The head halter and leash can also be used to prompt the dog to respond to a command (e.g., 'quiet' for barking, or 'off' for puppy nipping, or 'watch' to get the dog to focus on the owner and calm down) (see Figs 3.33–3.36). A release indicates to the dog that it is performing the desired behavior. With a 10-ft leash attached, the head halter also provides the owner with a mechanism for interrupting and deterring undesirable behavior immediately (e.g., garbage raiding, jumping up, housesoiling). A longer rope can be used for outdoor training. The key to success with a head halter, as with any training device, is a good understanding of its fitting and use, as discussed in Figure 3.37 (client handout #13 – printable from the CD).

Dogs wearing head halters might paw at their noses more, which can be disconcerting for some

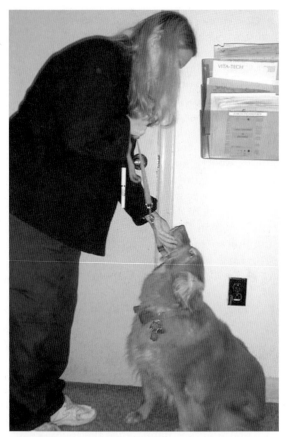

Figure 3.33 The Gentle Leader™ head halter can be used with a hand for support to get the dog into a sit position focused on the owner (as in the sit, quiet, or watch commands).

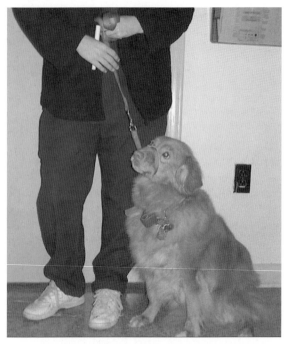

Figure 3.35 In this sequence the Gentle Leader™ is used to prompt the dog into a calm, sitting position without the hand support while facing forward.

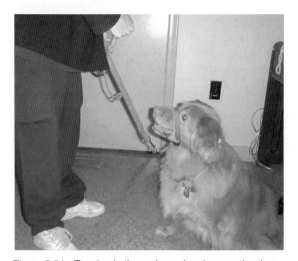

Figure 3.34 Tension is then released as long as the dog remains focused and in the sit position.

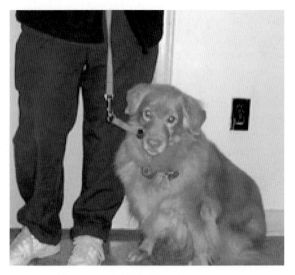

Figure 3.36 Tension is released as long as the dog stays in the controlled sit position.

HOW TO USE THE HEAD HALTER FOR TRAINING AND CONTROL OF UNDESIRABLE BEHAVIOR

Pets tend to oppose or pull against pressure. Dogs that walk or lunge ahead of their owners are therefore more likely to pull even harder if the owner pulls back on the leash. There are three basic ways of pulling on the head halter to achieve most goals. If the dog is walking at your side or slightly behind you with a minimum of slack on the leash, all you have to do is pull forward to get the dog to back up (heel, follow). A pull upward will close the mouth (barking, nipping) while continuing to pull up and forward will back the dog into a sit. With the leash attached to the head halter, you can immediately turn the head to achieve eye contact. A continuous pull rather than a tug or jerk should be used until the desired behavior is achieved. Immediately releasing tension as soon as the pet complies indicates to the dog that it is now responding acceptably. With the second hand, the dog's head can be cradled into position by gently cupping the hand under the jaw.

Training should begin in calm environments with minimal distractions. The dog is given the command and if it responds appropriately, a reward is given. A lure reward or closed hand target can be used to help guide the pet into the correct response. Rewards for training might include something the pet values (food, walk, or play toy) along with praise and stroking. After a few successful responses, the special treat can be phased out and given intermittently, but the praise and stroking should continue. Clicker training would be another option. If the command is given and the desired response cannot be achieved, an immediate pull on the head halter can be used to guide the pet into the desired position and ensure success. The tension is then released and the dog rewarded.

There are five key elements to successful head halter training.

1. Ensure proper fit
Be certain to review the manual or video or have a demonstration on fitting. If the strap around the neck is not high and snug enough and the nose strap adjusted properly, the head halter may either be too tight around the nose or so loose that the dog may pull it over the nose. To ensure that the pet adapts quickly to the head halter, it can be helpful to offer food treats as the dog slips its nose through the nose loop and as the collar is fitted. The dog can then be taken for a walk or played with to keep it distracted while getting used to the head device.

2. Be prepared for immediate action
If the dog does not instantaneously respond to a command, then the owner must immediately ensure success. This means that the head halter should be on, there should be minimal (perhaps 1 to 2 inches) of slack on the leash, and it should be pulled instantaneously to get the desired response. A pull up and forward can get eye contact (for target training, control, and calming), close the mouth, and get the dog to back up, follow, or heel. Continuing to place tension on the leash should get the dog to sit. Using the second hand to guide or support the head can help the dog to respond faster and calm quicker.

3. Motivate
Although the halter gives the owner the physical control to get the desired response, an encouraging voice, holding up a target (e.g., closed hand with food inside), appealing eye contact, and rewards are critical for motivating the pet to respond. Of course the rewards (stroking, clicker, food, toy) are not given until the dog responds appropriately.

4. Release tension as soon as the desired behavior is exhibited
The owner gives the command and pulls quickly to achieve the desired response (sit, heel, quiet) if the pet does not immediately obey. Just as quickly, the owner begins to release as soon as the pet obeys.

5. Repeat or reward
As the owner releases (a very small amount of slack is given), the dog will either respond appropriately (at which point the reward can be given) or will resume the undesirable response (e.g., tries to stand, lunge ahead, bark).

(continued)

Figure 3.37   How to use the Gentle Leader™ head halter for training and control of undesirable behavior (client handout #13 – printable from the CD).

5. Repeat or reward (*continued*)

If the latter is the case, the owner should immediately take up the slack and pull to achieve the desired response. The pet is then again released and the sequence repeated as often as necessary until the desired behavior can be maintained without pulling. While it may take numerous repetitions of the pull and release to get the desired response, the total time to achieve success might range from a few seconds to a few minutes. Remember that by releasing only a small amount of slack, it will require only a slight pull to regain control. A hand can be used to help support and guide the pet into position. It is important to understand that the pulling is a prompt to get the desired behavior while a release indicates that the desired behavior has been achieved. The reward (food, clicker, toy, praise, stroking) is intended to mark and acknowledge the correct response so that future success is ultimately driven by rewards.

Once these steps are accomplished, the owner can proceed to more complex tasks or more difficult environments. For example, the dog can be taught to sit and stay for gradually longer periods of time before the reward is given. The owner can gradually move farther from the dog (still maintaining only an inch or two of slack) to train the dog to stay and not to follow or lunge forward. The dog can be trained to quiet down at the front door. Once the dog will walk by the owner's side, the heel or follow command can be given at times when the dog might lunge forward on a walk or jump up at visitors at the door or bark.

Figure 3.37 (*continued*)

owners, but there was no difference in measurements for physiological stress while wearing either type of collar. In recent studies dogs wearing neck collars were more unruly and disobedient and pull on the leash more than those wearing head halters. In addition, puppies that attended puppy classes and used head halters were less likely to be relinquished by their owners.

REFERENCES CONTAINING INFORMATION ON PET SELECTION

Ackerman L 2001 The contented canine: pet parenting for dog owners. ASJA Press, New York

Adams GJ, Clark WT 1989 The prevalence of behavioural problems in domestic dogs: a survey of 105 dog owners. Australian Veterinary Practitioner 19:135–137

Bartlett M 1987 Follow-up: puppy aptitude testing. Pure-bred Dogs/American Kennel Club Gazette May:36–42

Beaudet R, Daillaire A 1993 Social dominance evaluation: observations on Campbell's test. Bulletin on Veterinary Ethology 1:23–29

Beaudet R, Chalifoux A, Daillaire A 1992 Mise au point d'un test d'valuation du temperament applicable... la selection de chiens de compagnie. Proceedings of 6th international conference, animals and us, Montreal

Beaudet R, Chalifoux A, Dallaire A 1994 Predictive value of activity level and behavioural evaluation on future dominance in puppies. Applied Animal Behavior Science 40(3&4):273–284

Benjamin CL 1990 The chosen puppy: how to select and raise a great puppy from an animal shelter. Howell Book House, New York

Blackshaw JK 1988 Abnormal behavior in dogs. Australian Veterinary Journal 65(12):393–400

Campbell W 1992 Behavior problems in dogs, 2nd edn. American Veterinary Publications, Goleta, CA

Cargill J 1994 Temperament tests as puppy selection tools. Dog World April:40–49

Carricato AM 1992 Veterinary notes for dog breeders. Howell Book House, New York

Dietrich C 1984 Temperament evaluation of puppies: use in guide dog selection. In: The pet connection: its influence on our health and quality of life. Center to Study Human–Animal Relationships and Environment, Minneapolis, MN

Fisher GT, Volhard W 1979 Puppy personality profile. Pure-bred Dogs/American Kennel Club Gazette March:31–42

Goddard ME, Belharz RG 1984 The relationship of fearfulness, sex, age, and experience on exploration and activity in dogs. Applied Animal Behavior Science 12:267

Goddard ME, Beilharz RG 1986 Early prediction of adult behavior in potential guide dogs. Applied Animal Behavior Science 15:247

Goodloe LP 1996 Issues in description and measurement of temperament in companion dogs. In: Voith VL, Borchelt PL (eds) Readings in companion animal behavior. Veterinary Learning Systems, Trenton, NJ, p 32–39

Ledger RA 1997 The development of a validated test to assess the temperament of dogs in a rescue shelter. In:

Proceedings of the first annual conference on veterinary behavioural medicine. Universities Federation for Animal Welfare, Potters Bar, UK, p 87–91

Netto WJ, Planta DJU 1997 Behavioural testing for aggression in the domestic dog. Applied Animal Behavior Science 52:243

Overall K 1994 Temperament testing and training – do they prevent behavioral problems. Canine Practice 19(4):19–21

Penny N, Reid PJ 2001 Predicting canine behavior through early assessment. In: Overall K, Mills DS, Heath SE et al (eds) Proceedings of the third international congress on veterinary behavioural medicine. UFAW, Herts, UK, p 92–95

Planta DJU 2001 Testing dogs for aggressive biting behavior. The MAG test (sociable acceptable behavior test) as an alternative for the aggression test. In: Overall K, Mills DS, Heath SE et al (eds) Proceedings of the third international congress on veterinary behavioural medicine. UFAW, Herts, UK, p 142–147

Scott JP, Fuller JL 1965 Dog behavior: the genetic basis. University of Chicago Press, Chicago

Slabbert JM, Odendaal JSJ 1999 Early prediction of adult police dog efficiency – a longitudinal study. Applied Animal Behavior Science 64:269–288

Van der Borg JAM, Netto WJ, Planta DJU 1992 Behavioral testing of dogs in animal shelters to predict problem behavior. Applied Animal Behavior Science 32:237

Weiss E, Greenberg G 1997 Service dog selection tests: effectiveness for dogs from animal shelters. Applied Animal Behavior Science 53:297–308

Wilsson E, Sundgren PE 1996 The use of a behaviour test for the selection of dogs for service and breeding, I: Method of testing and evaluating test results in the adult dog, demands on different kinds of service dogs, sex and breed differences. Applied Animal Behavior Science 53:279–295

Wilsson E, Sundgren PE 1997 Behaviour test for eight-week old puppies – heritabilities of tested behaviour traits and its correspondence to later behaviour. Applied Animal Behavior Science 58:151–162

Young MS 1988 Puppy selection and evaluation. In: Dogs: companions or nuisances. Public seminars, Werribee Veterinary Clinical Center, Princess Highway 22:8–15

REFERENCES ON BREEDS AND BREED SELECTION

Ackerman L 2001 The contented canine: pet parenting for dog owners. ASJA Press

Ackerman L, Landsberg G, Hunthausen W (eds) 1996a Cat behavior and training: veterinary advice for owners. TFH Publications, Neptune, NJ

Ackerman L, Landsberg G, Hunthausen W (eds) 1996b Dog behavior and training: veterinary advice for owners. TFH Publications, Neptune, NJ

Alderton D 1992 The eyewitness handbook of cats. Dorling Kindersley, New York

American Kennel Club 1989 Complete dog book. Howell House, New York

American Veterinary Medical Association – A veterinarian's way of selecting a proper pet (pamphlet)

Baer N, Duno S 1995 Choosing a dog: your guide to picking the perfect breed. Berkly Publishing, New York

Beaver BV 1993 Profiles of dogs presented for aggression. Journal of the American Animal Hospital Association 29:564–569

Beaver BV 1994 Owner complaints about canine behavior. Journal of the American Veterinary Medical Association 204(12):1953–1955

Borchelt PL 1983 Aggressive behavior of dogs kept as companion animals: classification and influence of sex, reproductive status, and breed. Applied Animal Ethology 10:35–43

Canadian Kennel Club 1988 Book of dogs. Stoddart, Toronto

Clark RD 1992 Medical, genetic, and behavioral aspects of purebred cats. Veterinary Forum Publications, St Simons Island, GA

Clark RD, Stainer JR 1994 Medical and genetic aspects of purebred dogs. Veterinary Forum Publishing, St Simons Island, GA

De Prisco A, Johnson JB 1990 The mini-atlas of dog breeds. TFH Publications, Neptune, NJ

Gebhardt RH (consultant editor) 1979 A standard guide to cat breeds. McGraw-Hill, New York

Hart BL, Hart LA 1984 Selecting the best companion animal: breed and gender specific behavioral profiles. In: The pet connection – its influence on our health and quality of life. Center to Study Human–Animal Relationships and Environments, Minneapolis, MN

Hart BL, Hart LA 1985 Selecting pet dogs on the basis of cluster analysis of breed behavior profiles and gender. Journal of the American Veterinary Medical Association 186(11):1181–1185

Hart BL, Hart LA 1988 The perfect puppy. WH Freeman, New York

Hart BL, Miller MF 1985 Behavioral profiles of dog breeds. Journal of the American Veterinary Medical Association 186(11):1175–1180

Howe J 1980 Choosing the right dog. Harper & Row, New York

Houpt KA 1985 Companion animal behaviour: a review of dog and cat behaviour in the field, the laboratory and the clinic. Cornell Veterinarian 75:248–261

Landsberg GM 1991 The distribution of canine behavior cases at 3 referral practices. Veterinary Medicine 86:1081–1089

Lowell M 1990 Your purebred puppy – a buyer's guide. Henry Holt, New York

Palmer J 1987a A practical guide to selecting a small dog. Tetra Press, London

Palmer J 1987b A practical guide to selecting a large dog. Tetra Press, London

Project Breed: Breed Rescue Efforts & Education 1989 Network for Ani-males & Females, Germantown, MD

Siegal M (ed) 1983 Simon and Schuster's guide to cats. Simon and Schuster, New York

Siegal M, Margolis M 1991 Good dog, bad dog. Henry Holt, New York

Tortora D 1983 The right dog for you. Simon and Schuster, New York

Wilkinson T 1985 Delinquent dogs. Quartet Books, London

Wright JC, Nesselrote MS 1987 Classification of behavior problems in dogs: distribution of age, breed, sex, and reproductive status. Applied Animal Behavior Science 19:169–178

REFERENCES AND SUPPLEMENTAL READING

(See also book list in Appendix B)

Anderson RK 1990 At what age can dogs learn? Veterinary Forum August: 32

Angameier E, James WT 1961 The influence of early sensory–social deprivation on the social operant in dogs. Journal of Genetic Psychology 99:153–158

Appleby D, Bradshaw JWS 2001 The relationship between canine aggression and avoidance behaviour and early experience. In: Overall K, Mills DS, Heath SE et al (eds) Proceedings of the third international congress on veterinary behavioural medicine. UFAW, Herts, UK, p 23–29

Ashmead DH, Clifton RK, Reese EP 1986 Development of auditory localization in dogs: single source and precedence effect sounds. Developmental Psychobiology 19:91–103

Askew HR 1994 How scientific is pet behavior therapy? Praktische Tierarzt 75(6):539

Ban B 1994 From growl to whimper: the spectrum of canine behavior modification. Journal of the American Veterinary Medical Association 204(1):7–12

Bateson P 2000 Behavioural development in the cat. In: Turner D, Bateson P (eds) The domestic cat: the biology of its behavior, 2nd edn. Cambridge University Press, New York, p 9–22

Collard RR 1967 Fear of strangers and play behavior in kittens varied with social experience. Child Development 38:877

Coppinger R, Coppinger L 1996 Biologic bases of behaviour of domestic dog breeds. In: Voith VL, Borchelt PL (eds) Readings in companion animal behaviour. Veterinary Learning Systems, Trenton, NJ, p 9–17.

Dahloff LE, Hard E, Larsson K 1977 Influence of maternal stress on offspring sexual behaviour. Animal Behavior 25:958–963

Duxbury M 2002 Puppy socialization class attendance and other factors related to post-weaning handling: the association with retention of dogs in their homes. In: Proceedings of the AVSAB scientific sessions, Nashville, TN, p 4

Estep DQ 1996 The ontogeny of behavior. In: Voith VL, Borchelt PL (eds) Readings in companion animal behaviour. Veterinary Learning Systems, Trenton, NJ, p 19–31

Feddersenpetersen D 1994a Comparative studies of behavioral development of wolves (*Canis lupus*) and domestic dogs (*Canis familiaris*). Domestication traits and selective breeding. Tierarztliche Umschau 49(9):527–531

Feddersenpetersen D 1994b Social behavior of wolves and dogs. Veterinary Quarterly 16(Suppl 1):S51–S52

Fox MW 1968 Socialization, environmental factors, and abnormal behavioral development in animals. In: Fox MW (ed) Abnormal behavior in animals. WB Saunders, Philadelphia

Fox MW 1969 Behavioral effects of rearing dogs with cats during the 'critical period of socialization.' Behaviour 35:273

Fox MW 1971 Overview and critique of stages and periods in canine development. Developmental Psychobiology 4(1):37

Fox MW, Stelzner D 1966 Behavioral effects of differential early experience in the dog. Animal Behavior 14:273–281

Hall SL, Bradshaw JWS 1998 The influence of hunger on object play by adult domestic cats. Applied Animal Behavior Science 58:143–150

Herrenkohl LR 1979 Prenatal stress reduces fertility and fecundity in female offspring. Science 206:1097–1099

Horwitz DF 1993 Feline socialization: how environment and early learning influence behavior. Veterinary Medicine August:14–16

Horwitz D, Mills D, Heath S 2002 BSAVA manual of canine and feline behavioural medicine. British Small Animal Veterinary Association, Gloucester, UK, 288 pp

Hunthausen W 1990 Giving new puppy owners practical tips to curb unruly behavior can save lives. DVM Magazine July:29

Joffe JM 1965 Genotype and prenatal and premating stress interact to affect adult behavior in rats. Science 150:1844–1845

Kerby G, Macdonald DW 1988 Cat society and the consequences of colony size. In: Turner D, Bateson P (eds) The domestic cat: the biology of its behavior. Cambridge University Press, Cambridge

Kuo ZY 1930 The genesis of the cat's response to the rat. Journal of Computational Psychology 11:1

Landsberg GM 1993 Confinement training. Veterinary Practice Staff 5(3):19–22

Levine S 1967 Maternal and environmental influences on the adrenocortical response to stress in weanling rats. Science 156:258

Markwell PJ, Thorne CJ 1987 Early behavioural development of dogs. Journal of Small Animal Practice 28:984–991

Mech LD 1981 The wolf: the ecology and behavior of an endangered species. University of Minnesota Press, Minneapolis, MN

Mendl M, Harcourt R 2000 Individuality in the domestic cat. In: Turner D, Bateson P (eds) The domestic cat: the biology of its behavior, 2nd edn. Cambridge University Press, New York, p 47–64

Milani MM 2000 Crate training as a feline stress reliever. Feline Practice 28(3):8–9

Miller DD, Staats SR, Partlo C et al 1996 Factors associated with the decision to surrender a pet to an animal shelter. Journal of the American Veterinary Medical Association 209(4):738–742

Nott HM 1992 Behavioural development of the dog. In: Thorne C (ed) The Waltham book of dog and cat behaviour. Pergamon Press, New York, p 65–78

Ogburn P, Crouse S, Martin F et al 1998 Comparison of behavioral and physiological responses of dogs wearing two different types of collars. Applied Animal Behavior Science 61:133–142

Randon E, Beach F 1985 Effects of testosterone on ontogeny of urinary behavior in male and female dogs. Hormones and Behavior 19:36–51

Robinson I 1992 Behavioural development of the cat. In Thorne C (ed) The Waltham book of dog and cat behaviour. Pergamon Press, New York

Rooney NJ, Bradshaw JWS 2002 An experimental study of the effects of play upon the dog–human relationship. Applied Animal Behavior Science 75:161–176

Rooney NJ, Bradshaw JWS, Robinson IH 2000 A comparison of dog–dog and dog–human play behaviour. Applied Animal Behavior Science 66:235–248

Scarlett JM, Saidla JE, Pollock RVH 1994 Source of acquisition as a risk factor for disease and death in pups. Journal of the American Veterinary Medical Association 204(12):1906–1913

Scott JP 1962 Critical periods in behavioral development. Science 138:949–958

Scott JP, Marston MV 1950 Critical periods affecting the development of normal and maladjustive social behavior in puppies. Journal of Genetic Psychology 77:25–60

Seitz PFD 1979 Infantile experience in adult behavior in animal subjects. II. Age of separation from the mother and adult behavior in the cat. Psychosomatic Medicine 21:353

Seksel K, Mazurski EJ, Taylor A 1999 Puppy socialisation programs: short and long term behavioural effects. Applied Animal Behavior Science 62:335–349

Serpell JA 1987 The influence of inheritance and environment on canine behavior: myth and fact. Journal of Small Animal Practice 28(11):949–956

Serpell J, Jagoe JA 1995 Early experience and the development of behavior. In: Serpell J (ed) The domestic dog: its evolution, behavior, and interaction with people. Cambridge University Press, Cambridge

Simonson M 1979 Effects of maternal malnourishment, development and behavior in successive generations in the rat and cat. In: Levitsky DA (ed) Malnutrition, environment and behavior. Cornell University Press, Ithaca, NY

Slabbert JM, Rasa OAE 1997 Observational learning of an acquired maternal behavior pattern by working dog pups: an alternative training method? Applied Animal Behavior Science 53:309–316

Smith BA, Jansen GR 1977 Maternal undernutrition in the feline: behavioral sequelae. Nutrition Reports International 16:513

Stur I 1987 Genetic aspects of temperament and behavior in dogs. Journal of Small Animal Practice 28(11):957–964

Thompson WR, Melzack R 1956 Early environment. Scientific American 194:38–42

Ward I 1968 Prenatal stress feminizes and demasculinizes the behavior of males. Science 15:82–84

Willis MB 1987 Breeding dogs for desirable traits. Journal of Small Animal Practice 28(11):965–983

4

Behavior counseling and behavioral diagnostics

CAUSES OF BEHAVIOR PROBLEMS

A knowledge of medicine, health, and pathology provides an important dimension for the veterinary behavior consultant in working up companion animal behavior problems that is not afforded to all consultants. Prior to performing the actual behavioral consultation, it is critical that a thorough physical examination be done and that underlying medical conditions are ruled out or treated. For example, using behavioral modification for a cat with inappropriate urination is counterproductive if the underlying cause is lower urinary tract disease. The various categories of medical conditions that might lead to behavioral signs are listed in Figure 4.1.

In general, the presenting signs may arise as a result of a disease process, primary behavior problems, or some combination of these factors. Medical causes become an increasingly important consideration with age, since the senior pet can be afflicted with a wide array of medical problems, including endocrinopathies, arthritis, alterations in the immune response, sensory decline, neoplasia, and age-related organ dysfunction including brain aging, each of which could have an impact on the pet's behavior. Medical conditions in senior pets and their potential effect on behavior are discussed in detail in Chapter 12. The presence of a medical problem does not necessarily mean that it is the cause of the behavioral signs. For example, a cat with a positive feline leukemia virus (FeLV) test

Type of medical condition	Example
Congenital/inherited	
• physiological	Narcolepsy; epilepsy
• structural/malformation/aplasia	Hydrocephalus; Wobbler syndrome
• hypoplasia/dysplasia	Cerebellar hypoplasia
• metabolic/genetic	Lethal acrodermatitis
Infectious	
• bacterial	Listeria
• viral	Rabies; canine distemper; Feline Immunodeficiency Virus (FIV); Feline Leukemia Virus (FeLV)
• fungal	Cryptococcus
• parasitic	Cuterebra; heartworm
• protozoal	Toxoplasma
Metabolic	
• hepatic encephalopathy	Congenital; acquired
• hypoglycemia	Insulinoma; malnutrition
• storage diseases	Fucosidosis; alpha-mannosidosis
• copper toxicosis	As seen in Bedlington Terriers
• multi-system neuronal degeneration	As seen in Cocker Spaniels
Toxic	
• drugs	Ibuprofen; levamisole; hallucinogens
• insecticides	DEET; fenvalerate
• toxins	Lead; mercury
Nutritional	
• deficiencies	Thiamin
• other	Adverse food reactions
	High-protein diet (??)
Neoplasia	Glioma; meningioma
	Metastatic disease
Immune/inflammatory	
• inflammatory	Steroid-responsive meningitides
• immune-mediated	Granulomatous meningoencephalitis
Hormonal	Hypo/hyperthyroidism; hyperestrogenism; hyperadrenocorticism
Degenerative	Aging
	Cognitive dysfunction
Traumatic	Head injury – glial scar
Vascular	Infarct; hemorrhage
Neural	Psychomotor epilepsy
	Receptor/neurotransmitter abnormalities (??)
Idiopathic	Rage syndromes (??)

Figure 4.1 Some medical causes of abnormal or unacceptable behavior (or changes in a pet's behavior).

might be aggressive or spraying for reasons independent of its positive viral state. Genetic, medical, and environmental effects could also contribute to a state of behavioral pathology, where neurotransmitter dynamics have been altered.

Assuming there is no obvious medical cause, most behavioral problems are a result of the owner's inability to manage and control an otherwise normal behavior, so that treatment will require a combination of owner education, behavioral management techniques, alterations to the environment, and perhaps surgery (e.g., castration) or concurrent allopathic or naturopathic therapy. However, to make an accurate diagnosis, practitioners must not focus solely on the presenting complaint, since this may represent only one sign (albeit the most serious for the owners) of a larger physical or behavioral problem. Therefore it is critical to look at the patient as a whole in making the behavioral diagnosis.

PREPARATION BEFORE THE SESSION

Since behavior counseling requires a knowledge and understanding of a wide variety of problems, it is seldom practical to perform a behavioral consultation without some advance preparation. Gathering information can be very tedious work. It is therefore advisable to request that the family fill out a history questionnaire so you can use this information to research the problem thoroughly before the counseling session. Using a history questionnaire will facilitate collection of data, keep information together so it can be readily referenced during follow-ups, and help the consultant avoid overlooking important questions. It is advantageous to have the questionnaire filled out and returned at least 48 hours prior to the consultation time, so that you have adequate time to review it beforehand. The 48-hour return policy also helps with the appointment schedule. When your receptionist notes that a form has not been returned in a timely manner (forgetful owner or cancellation without notification), a call can be made as a reminder, and if there is a cancellation the appointment time can be freed.

The behavior data sheet questions should explore a wide variety of pertinent information. You can design your own forms using the outline in Figure 4.2 as a guideline, or you can use the forms that accompany this book (Appendix C, Figs 5 and 6, which are printable from the CD as forms #3 and #7, respectively). If you do design your own forms, be certain to investigate all aspects of the pet's health and behavior, since the primary complaint may be only one sign of a more complex health or behavioral problem.

It is advisable to counsel and inform clients about simple behavioral concerns during their regular veterinary visits. However, for more involved problems it is best to schedule a separate appointment. This will allow the practitioner to spend an adequate amount of time discussing the problems rather than hurriedly trying to collect information and give treatment recommendations during a medical visit. Tackling more difficult problems, such as aggression or complex phobias, is best reserved for behavioral specialists or those veterinarians who have already acquired significant experience in behavior counseling. If you feel uncomfortable with your ability to handle some cases, consider referring them, or set up your own telephone consultation with a behavior referral center. Veterinarians should not attempt to counsel cases beyond their abilities. Incomplete, insufficient, or inaccurate advice could lead to worsening of the problem, potential liability, and loss of the client's confidence.

SCHEDULING THE BEHAVIOR CONSULTATION

A behavior consultation requires the time and commitment of both veterinarian and client. Rarely is it possible to offer any meaningful behavioral advice for a difficult problem during a 15–20-minute routine office visit. Behavior consultations need to be scheduled accordingly, allowing one to two hours for the initial interview. Whenever possible, have all members of the family present.

Fees may be structured in different ways: a set fee might be charged for the visit, no matter how long it takes; an hourly fee might be charged, or an hourly fee with a maximum amount (ceiling) imposed. The average hourly income should approximate at least the amount that would be received if the veterinarian were seeing medical patients during that time. So, if the veterinary practitioner typically schedules four to six office appointments per hour and a behavioral consultation is believed to require two hours, the

Family information	• Home, apartment
	• Rural, urban
	• Family size, ages, schedules
	• Physical/mental disabilities
	• Experience with pets
	• Other pets in the home
Pet information	• Signalment
	• Age at adoption
	• Source of pet, when obtained, previous owner information if known
	• Personality, temperament
	• Medical history (medications administered, any recent or pertinent laboratory tests)
	• Medical/behavioral information of parents, siblings, or littermates
	• Diet – including type of food and frequency, treats fed, who feeds, behavior around food
Training	• Methods used
	• Types of training tools used
	• Confinement training
	• Reward use and pet's response (reinforcer assessment)
	• Punishment use and pet's response (punisher assessment)
	• Training results
	• Use of behavior modification devices (and pet's response)
	• Use of control devices (e.g., head halter) and pet's response
Pet's environment, lifestyle, and daily schedule	• Pet's housing, where it stays during the day, night, and when the family is gone
	• Elimination areas, feeding areas, scratching or play areas
	• Play and exercise routines
	• Favorite toys
	• When and how long it is left alone
	• Time indoors and outdoors
	• Family members that care for the pet
Reactions to people and animals	• Family members
	• Unfamiliar people
	• Other pets in the household
	• Unfamiliar animals
	• How does pet react to other animals and non-family members on-property and off-property
	• Social postures, vocalizations, interactions, approach behaviors, fear, aggression
Response to handling	• Bathing, nail trimming, grooming, petting, etc.
Primary problem	• '5 W's'
	1. What happens?
	2. Where does it happen?
	3. When does is occur?
	4. Who is present (people, animals)?
	5. Why does the family think the behavior occurs?
	• Initial circumstances. Can the owner identify any events that might have caused the problem?
	• Environmental changes preceding appearance of problems
	• Duration
	• Frequency
	• Stimuli that trigger the behavior
	• Change in appearance
	• Treatment attempted and pet's response
Additional problems	• Are there any behavior problems that are separate from the principal problem

Figure 4.2 Basic information for a behavior data sheet.

income from that visit must at least approximate the eight to 12 office visits that could have been scheduled during the same time period or the veterinarian will be losing revenue by seeing behavioral cases. Additional fees should be charged for travel time when the consultation is a house call. Ultimately, the fees that are charged will depend on the demographics of the area and the perceived value of a behavior consultation for a pet.

There are also considerations as to where the behavior consultation should take place. Since the history with respect to the environment can be an important component for some problems, a house call can be a practical way to assess first hand where the pet lives, how it is housed, and the role that the environment might play in the management of the problem. However, a house call may be impractical for some practitioners and may not have a significant impact on the diagnosis, prognosis, or treatment plans. The advantages and disadvantages of each are discussed in Figure 4.3.

Behavior consultations are very much like any other medical consultation; there are rarely any quick fixes that you can offer to mend a long-standing problem. A significant amount of time is required to diagnose the problem, determine the prognosis, formulate a safe and effective treatment plan, and present the treatment plan. The family then needs to decide if such a plan is safe, practical for their home, family and lifestyle, and within their budgets and capabilities. It is critical that the owner understands all the options and alternatives at this time. Some families may decide the complexities, danger, or expenses entailed in the correction process are greater than they can manage, and elect to rehome or euthanize (or abandon the animal!). When all of these factors are considered, the prognosis may be poor to guarded, but this can-

not usually be determined until all factors related to the pet's health, the problem itself, the level of risk or danger, the environment, the family, and the owner's commitment to proceed have been assessed. If the case involves aggressive behavior, you may want to consider a liability release form before making treatment recommendations (Appendix C, Fig. 12 – printable as form #1 from the CD).

THE BEHAVIORAL AND MEDICAL HISTORY

An accurate diagnosis of the cause of any behavioral sign can only be made by assessing the behavioral history, the medical history, and the results of any laboratory tests that might be indicated by the history and physical examination. The examination should assess all organ systems, but in particular the nervous system, since any alterations in mentation or gait, and any cranial nerve deficits, might be indicative of a primary neurologic condition.

Behavioral history

Taking the behavioral history is the heart of companion animal behavior therapy. It usually takes between 30 and 90 minutes to complete, depending on the complexity of the situation. Complicated cases can require hours of informa-

Location	Advantages	Disadvantages
Clinic visit	• Ability to see the pet and family members • Distractions can be minimized • Can utilize clinic resources (staff, videos, books, handouts)	• Don't see environmental components • Pet's behavior may be dramatically altered in the clinic • History and questionnaire will need to be far more comprehensive
House call	• Can see the environment and problem at first hand • Increased investigator awareness of varying home environments	• Presence of the veterinarian may alter the behavior • Time-consuming and expensive • May be interruptions and distractions • Staff and resources not available
Telephone consultation	• Increased accessibility	• Cannot observe or examine animal • Cannot learn as much about owner • Must rely much more on the history • No opportunity to demonstrate techniques, products, literature

Figure 4.3 The advantages and disadvantages of different locations for behavioral consultations.

tion collecting. The consultant needs to have good information-collecting skills in order to pull together the necessary information. You should have as many family members, caretakers, or acquaintances of the pet as possible present during the consultation. This is important for two reasons: it helps ensure that you gather the most information, and it is advantageous to have everyone involved with the pet to hear the same instructions at the same time. You will find it helpful to have a behavior data sheet or history form completed by the family and returned to you prior to the actual consultation. This allows you to have some idea of what to expect. This can be especially important when dealing with very aggressive pets.

It is important to keep in mind that the goal of history taking is to obtain sufficient information to make a diagnosis, prognosis, and treatment plan. To do this, the consultant must get an accurate description of all pertinent aspects concerning the pet, the family, the environment, and the behavior problem. The process of obtaining information should be structured enough to avoid missing critical facts, but flexible enough to allow the interviewer and family to pursue novel lines of thought that might reveal unforeseen information. The family should be guided through various areas of importance without actually being led into certain answers.

Oftentimes, the family comes into the consultation a bit apprehensive, not knowing what to expect. It is important to show understanding and compassion. You'll have a better chance to gather a complete history if you are warm and take an understanding interest in the family's problems, rather than coolly and clinically collecting facts. Do your best to include the whole family in the discussion, so that all dimensions of the problem can be explored. You will also get a better idea of everyone's emotional investment in the pet as well as their commitment to solving the problem.

The demeanor of the consultant can be extremely important in determining the quality and amount of information obtained. The interviewer should strive to be friendly and open. Appropriate smiles, eye contact, and gestures of understanding are usually helpful in gaining trust. Leaning in with relaxed arms and hands sends signals that encourage communication, while leaning back with arms and legs crossed suggests you are less open to listening and may be more critical. In some cases, the interviewer can help the family relax by showing an appropriate sense of humor.

Many pet owners feel vulnerable discussing personal details about the family and the pet. Some may feel a sense of failure that they are unable to correct the pet's problems without professional help. So, it is very important to remain non-judgmental. An indiscreet comment, facial expression, or body gesture can quickly inhibit communication and close your access to important facts. For example, owners frequently use particular correction methods that are not only inappropriate, but may actually have contributed to the problem. Inconsiderate comments about their behavior may make them uncomfortable, so that they are less likely to be forthcoming with other pieces of important information. You will get better cooperation if you convey to the owner that 'There are better methods to get the job done,' rather than telling them 'What you did was wrong.' As you might imagine, good consultants should have as much knowledge about human body language and communication as they do about animal body language and communication.

One of the problems encountered during history collection is that clients often provide information that is overly subjective or anthropomorphic. When the owners say that the pet was mad, jealous, upset, or unhappy, the consultant must ask exactly what was observed that brought them to that conclusion. As you progress through the interview, terms may need to be defined for the client. You can't take for granted that you and the family are talking about the same thing when it comes to behavioral terms. For example, aggression might mean a snarl or growl to some owners, while others only consider the dog aggressive if it exhibits a full-blown attack. In other cases, you might find that family members refer to any type of urination outside of the litterbox as 'spraying.'

Information that needs to be collected:

I. The family and environment
II. The pet
III. The problem itself

For sample canine and feline history forms, see Appendix C, Figures 5 and 6 (printable from the CD as forms #3 and #7, respectively).

I. The family and environment

Information needs to be collected about the family and the environment in which they live. You'll want to know if they live in a house or an apartment, as well as if the area is rural or urban. Find out about the yard, how big it is and what kind of fencing is present. Ask about the type of animal and human foot traffic that passes nearby. For urine marking, feline redirected aggression, or territorial aggression problems, you should ask if stray animals frequently visit the yard.

Aspects about the family, such as size, ages, and schedules, can be important. For example, a large, busy family may not be providing enough supervision, exercise, or attention to a young dog that is destructive. The age, as well as mental and physical capabilities of family members can influence the treatment plan, as well as the risk of danger in aggression cases. Find out if family members are experienced or naïve about raising dogs and cats. Knowing the primary caretaker(s) for the pet can help you make the decision about who will be assigned training responsibilities. Determine the family's daily schedule and whether the problem consistently occurs at a specific time in relationship to this routine. Changes in the home environment or in the owner's schedule can contribute to the development of some behavior problems and should be discussed, exploring in particular how the changes affected the pet. Find out about what other pets are in the family and how they interact. If the problem only occurs when no family members are present, the pets may need to be separated to determine for sure which one is the perpetrator. You may also want to explore whether previous family pets have been euthanized or abandoned due to behavior problems, and if the problems were similar to the present ones.

II. The pet

You need to know the signalment of the pet, including the sexual status (male vs female; intact vs neutered). Some behavior problems are more likely to be seen at certain ages. For example, a three-month-old pet that is biting is more likely to be playing, while a three-year-old pet that bites probably has a much more serious problem. Even the name of the pet can be an important piece of information. If the Young family tells you their miniature Schnauzer is named 'Harold Young,' you gain some insight into the family's relationship with the pet. Another way of getting similar information is by asking the family to describe the pet's personality. Basic information about why, when, and where the pet was adopted, as well as how old it was when adopted may also be important. If possible, find out if any related pets had similar problems.

Ask the family to describe how the pet spends an average day. Find out where it is kept when they are home, away, or sleeping, as well as where the pet spends time when friends visit. If it is confined away from guests, you need to find out why this is done. In most cases, the pet is separated from visitors because of some problem with the pet's behavior. Enquire about how much exercise the pet gets. Does it have favorite toys? Does it play with them? When and what does it eat? Housesoiling may begin for a variety of reasons following a dietary change. You'll want to enquire about the social nature of the pet, including how it gets along with other pets, and whether it is relaxed, nervous, or aggressive when it meets unfamiliar people. You will also want to find out about the type and success of training, the tools used for training, and to what commands the pet will respond.

Behavior issues with an underlying medical etiology are unlikely to be resolved unless the medical problem is successfully diagnosed and treated. The medical history can be very important in some cases that involve aggression, housesoiling, and cognitive function. The owners of pets that are aggressive when reached for or touched should be queried about any painful medical or surgical problems. If the pet housesoils, you need to know if there is anything abnormal about the act of elimination or the appearance of the pet's stool and urine. You'll also want to find out if the pet is on any medication, since some medications can cause polyuria/polydypsia and subsequent housesoiling. Some medications, such as corticosteroids, may cause behavior and personality changes.

III. The problem itself

When asking about the behavior problem, remember the 'Five W's.' What occurs? Where does it occur? When does it occur? Who is present when it occurs? Why do you think the pet does it? Ask the family for a complete description of the problems including when they first appeared and how long they have existed. Ask for details of the initial circumstances during which the problem was first noted. They should give a detailed account of what the pet does, including body postures and facial expressions. You will want to know when, where, and during what time period they are most likely to occur, and who is present. An attempt should be made to identify all stimuli that precede or trigger the behaviors. When working up an aggression case, you will want the family to make a list of everything that makes the pet act either aggressive or anxious. You will also want complete descriptions of facial expressions and body postures preceding, during, and following aggressive incidents. Including all family members in the discussion will help you put together a more complete picture of the problem.

Explore the sequential development of the problem to get a handle on what is going on and how things have progressed. Begin with the most recent incident, which should be freshest in the family members' memories, and then ask them to sequentially go back in time, describing the details of each instance of problem behavior. Alternatively, they can be asked to begin with the first incident and progress to the present. Find out if there were any changes in the pet's environment or in its interaction with family members just prior to the appearance of the problems, and what was the pet's general response to these changes. Ask about the frequency of the problem behaviors and whether there has been a change in frequency. If there has been some change, find out why. When a problem occurs sporadically without any apparent stimulus, it may be helpful for the owner to keep a diary that lists the date, day, time, appearance of the problem, as well as anything of interest associated with the occurrence of the problem.

The family should describe all methods that have been used in an attempt to correct the problem behaviors, and what results were seen. If they mention that an approach you are considering has not worked, be sure to get details about exactly what the family did in case the technique simply was not applied correctly. Asking questions about punishment should be done carefully. If you ask, 'Have you ever hit the pet to correct the problem?' an owner might be reluctant to admit this and respond, 'No.' It may be better to matter-of-factly ask, 'Has spanking the pet helped?' Finally, be sure to explore any behavior problems the pet might have beyond those for which it was presented. For example, it would be important to know that a pet displaying fear-related aggression is also housesoiling. This could be helpful information to pursue because the family might be frustrated with the housesoiling, using harsh punishment and, therefore, contributing to the fear-related aggressive behavior.

Medical history

The medical history should focus on those signs that might be indicative of a pathologic process or a chronic state of anxiety, such as tachycardia, tachypnea, salivation, gastrointestinal disturbances, skin diseases, self-injurious behavior, and stress or excitement-induced elimination. Increased drinking and urination, a change in appetite (increased or decreased), obesity, marked weight loss, alterations in grooming, diminished responsiveness to stimuli, and changes in sleep pattern could all be indicative of more generalized behavioral or medical disorders. Behavioral changes such as aggressiveness, altered sexual, maternal, or exploratory behaviors, decreased learning ability, decreased performance or a decline in cognitive function, a loss of self-control (inhibition), and unpredictable or excessive responses to stimuli should be considered in combination to accurately diagnose the underlying problem.

MEDICAL AND PHYSICAL HEALTH AND ITS EFFECTS ON BEHAVIOR

For each behavior problem, it is important to consider all medical and physical conditions or anomalies that might play a role in the development or manifestation of the problem (Fig. 4.1). For example, aggression can be due to primary diseases of the central nervous system, primary diseases of other organ systems, painful conditions (otitis, arthritis, anal sacculitis), or sensory dysfunction (loss of vision or hearing).

Any condition that might affect the central nervous system and its function, whether directly or indirectly, might affect behavior. Brain tumors are commonly associated with alterations in behavior and mentation, but are usually accompanied by neurologic signs such as circling, seizures, head tilt, ataxia, and cranial nerve deficits. Inflammatory, infectious, toxic, and metabolic diseases can affect behavior as can any disease process that impedes blood flow to the central nervous system. Alterations in hormones related to productive tumors, destructive diseases, and aging may also have a significant impact on behavior. Disease processes that affect urine or stool output might contribute to the development or perpetuation of a housesoiling problem, while diseases that caused polyphagia and those that affect nutrient absorption may induce picas or coprophagia. Sensory deficits, painful conditions, and neuromuscular problems could also lead to behavior changes.

There is controversy and uncertainty about the role that some medical conditions might play in behavior. Often results are inconsistent between research centers, and diagnostic tools and techniques that might be available in human medicine are either impractical or too costly to utilize in pets. The relationship between seizures and behavioral signs is also unclear. Partial seizures are a form of epileptic disorder due to a focal acquired lesion. These might be produced in people by glial scars, congenital abnormalities, neonatal hypoxia, infarction, vascular abnormalities, degenerative diseases, or neoplasia, and may be static or progressive. Generally, seizure episodes are recurrent, intermittent, repetitive, and abnormal, and generally have a normal interictal period. Depending on the cause, most seizure foci would improve when therapeutic levels of anticonvulsant medications (such as phenobarbital or potassium bromide) are achieved. In experimental studies, stimulation of the hippocampus in cats led to episodes of glancing, or staring, while stimulation of the hippocampus and amygdala led to episodes of fear, including autonomic signs such as piloerection, salivation, and pupillary dilatation. Psychomotor seizures have been induced by bilateral necrosis of the hippocampus or pyriform lobe in the dog, with signs of barking, growling, and piloerection with the dog unable to be interrupted. A complex partial seizure has been implicated as a possible diagnosis for the following:

- Sudden onset of fear and panic
- Fly biting
- Staring
- Jaw snapping
- Spinning–tail chasing
- Head bobbing
- Feline hyperesthesia
- Self-injurious behaviors
- Unprovoked aggression
- Sudden appearance of apparent pain (e.g., tucked abdomen).

For a more detailed look at some examples of how medical problems might have an impact on behavior, see Figure 4.1 and Figure 12.12 on medical causes of senior behavior problems. Based on the history and results of the physical examination, the necessary diagnostic tests to rule out possible medical causes for the presenting signs will then need to be ordered. Although a minimum database for diagnostics (and prior to any drug dispensing) might include a complete blood count, biochemical profile, urinalysis, and some baseline endocrine screening (e.g., total/free T_4, urine cortisol–creatinine for dogs), more extensive testing may be indicated based on the initial assessment and the results of any previous laboratory testing.

Another area that is not yet clear is the effect of the endocrine system on the development and treatment of behavior problems. Thyroid hormones are likely to have an effect on behavior, but their role is still unclear. Hyperthyroidism in cats may lead to increased irritability and increased appetite, and hypothyroidism in dogs may cause lethargy and weight gain. However, there are also reports in the behavior literature of decreased thyroid levels in dogs leading to aggression, extreme shyness, and other aberrant behaviors that improve with thyroid supplementation. It is not surprising that thyroid supplementation may affect behavior; what is questionable is whether (i) adequate diagnostic testing was done to confirm these diagnoses, (ii) the lowered thyroid levels 'caused' the behavioral signs, or (iii) the lowered thyroid levels were caused by some other underlying disease or even by the behavioral problem itself. Activation of the hypothalamic–pituitary–adrenal axis that occurs in stress will lead to increased glucocorticoid output which in itself can have medical and behavioral effects and inhibit learning. Cortisol can then lower the baseline levels of circulating thyroid hormones, perhaps by inhibiting secretion of thyroid releasing factor. Sex hormones also have an important effect on behavior, yet dogs and cats that are spayed or neutered may still show apparent sexual dimorphism. This may be the effect of learning, so that a dog that is neutered may continue to mount and fight with other male dogs. On the other hand, some forms of sexually dimorphic behavior, such as leg lifting, may arise at sexual maturity, even if the dog has been previously neutered, indicating an effect of either learning and environmental influences or androgenation of the brain prior to neutering. In addition, there are conditions in which sex hormone abnormalities are the result of adrenal disorders (e.g., alopecia X, 21-hydroxylase deficiency, adrenal sex-hormone dermatosis), so sex hormone-related problems can actually occur, even in the neutered animal.

Does the disease cause the behavior signs or does the behavioral disorder cause disease?

There appears to be such a close relationship between stress and disease, it is often difficult to determine which comes first. For example, the relationship between inflammation and stress seems to be accepted in human medicine, with problems such as urticaria (hives) sometimes being attributed to stress when no other underlying allergic component can be identified. Cats with psychogenic alopecia and hyperesthesia may have an underlying medical cause, but when no such cause can be identified, a presumptive behavioral diagnosis (displacement behavior, compulsive disorder) is made. Cats with psychogenic alopecia that improve with injections of repository corticosteroids are presumed to have allergies. However, a link has been found in humans between stress and an increase in epidermal permeability. Therefore, if percutaneous absorption of allergens leads to pruritus in the atopic patient, stress might actually predispose the patient to exacerbation of the allergic predisposition. In addition, the T-cell response in cats with allergic dermatitis is similar to that found in humans and rodents that are exacerbated by stress. It has also been suggested that some behavior problems such as acral lick dermatitis in dogs, tail attacking, and feline hyperesthesia may be sensory neuropathies that might improve with anticonvulsants such as gabapentin or tricyclic antidepressants such as amitriptyline. However, stress and immune responses are known flare factors for sensory neuropathies in humans. Therefore, is the condition due to a sensory neuropathy or does the sensory neuropathy arise due to stress? In cats with feline lower urinary tract disease, 65% of non-obstructed and 30% of obstructed cats have no identifiable cause. Because of the similarity in presentation to interstitial cystitis in women, including the fact that glycosaminoglycan reduction and an increase in mast cells are common to both, a diagnosis of feline interstitial cystitis has been suggested. Complicating matters even more are the anecdotal reports of FLUTD responding to hypoallergenic diets. In interstitial cystitis, stress has been identified as a flare factor in women, which may be precipitated by increased sympathetic activity during acute stress. This theory has also been suggested for cats with idiopathic cystitis and studies have found some correlation between stress and the onset of FLUTD. In short, it seems that not only can medical problems be a cause of behavioral signs, but stress and anxiety can induce medical problems as well.

Medical contributing factors: surpassing the threshold

The threshold theory, as it applies to dermatology, is that each animal will tolerate a certain number of pruritic stimuli without itching. However, when stimulation exceeds a certain threshold, or when multiple stimuli (e.g., allergens) act together, clinical pruritus may be exhibited. Similarly, it may take multiple stimuli to 'push' the pet beyond a threshold to where a behavior problem is exhibited. Medical conditions might also lower the threshold or level of tolerance. This is especially important in aging pets, where organ decline, sensory decline, painful conditions, age-related nervous system pathology, and an increasing number of medical problems can all affect behavior. For example, a pet that is fearful of children, but has never before displayed aggression, may begin to threaten or bite as it becomes more uncomfortable (as with dental disease) or less mobile (as with arthritis). Similarly, the hyperthyroid cat might be more irritable and hence more likely to spray when exposed to the sights,

sounds, or odors of new cats on the property, or more likely to be aggressive when handled by a stranger.

Response to therapy

For some medical and behavioral problems, a therapeutic trial may be the most expedient or accurate way to reach a diagnosis. For the cat with self-induced alopecia, a novel protein or hypoallergenic diet food trial, a trial with a parasiticide, and allergy testing would be a valuable diagnostic approach. The pet that is anorexic due to dental disease, the dog that begins to housesoil due to cystitis, or the dog that is aggressive due to arthritis should improve when these underlying medical problems are treated. However, this is not always the case, since the consequences of the pet's reactions might lead to newly learned or conditioned behavioral responses. For example, even if the aggression arose out of pain, the pet may continue to bite because (i) it has learned that the children will retreat if aggression is displayed and (ii) there may be continued fear of being handled because the pet might still be protective of any patting around the head. Similarly, if the pet begins to housesoil due to cystitis when the owners are out, the pet will have learned that there is an indoor site where it can successfully relieve itself when the owners are out (with no untoward consequence). In addition, the odor and texture may continue to attract the pet back to the site.

Primary behavior problems

Assuming there are no primary medical problems, the North American approach to behavioral problems has generally been to diagnose and treat most behavioral complaints as normal behaviors that are undesirable to the owners in the context that they are being displayed. As pets grow and develop, the innate and species-specific behaviors begin to emerge and are affected by experience (positive, negative, or absent). The behavior problems that arise as puppies and kittens grow and develop into adulthood may be normal behaviors that the owners cannot control or accept because of inappropriate expectations, their lifestyle, or the pet's environment, may arise as a result of learning (consequences) or conditioning (associations), or may be due to stress, conflict, or frustration-evoking situations. For the most part these problems require pet owner education as to what is normal canine and feline behavior and how these problems can best be managed using behavior modification and learning principles and modifications to the pet's environment or daily routine. Although drugs may be useful in some problems, they may not be used initially if there is no underlying pathology. Behavior problems that arise in adult pets not due to medical problems are generally related to changes in the pet's environment that lead to anxiety, conflict, frustration, or new consequences. Schedule changes, a new member of the household (e.g., baby, spouse), a new pet, or moving can have a dramatic impact on a pet's behavior. Some examples of these normal but unacceptable behaviors might include protecting toys and food, protective aggression toward visitors to the household, digging, chewing, and intraspecific aggression. Although a far less frequent diagnosis in the North American model, abnormal behaviors must also be considered. Abnormal behaviors are those that are considered dysfunctional. They may be associated with extreme anxiety, may be out of context or inappropriate with respect to the stimuli, or may be excessive, uninhibited, or impulsive. These types of problems might be due to inherited factors, the effects of endogenous factors (endocrine, metabolic, inflammatory, immunological, and aging changes) and exogenous factors (such as the effects of deprivation or repeated or chronic exposure to situations of stress, anxiety, or conflict). Compulsive disorders, excessive fear, panic and phobias, aggression arising from dyscontrol or lack of inhibition (rage?), and learning deficits associated with hyperactivity might all fall into the category of abnormal behaviors. In these cases an alteration in neurotransmitters may be present and drug therapy may be a necessary part of the therapeutic program.

THE BEHAVIORAL CONSULTATION

The protocol for each behavior case or behavior problem is to make a diagnosis, determine all factors that may have caused the problem or may be further perpetuating (maintaining) the problem, discuss the prognosis with the owners, develop an appropriate treatment plan for the pet and the home, and follow up each case to modify the program (and prognosis) as needed and determine the ultimate outcome.

Figure 4.4 shows the sequence of events from the initial consultation to the treatment plan.

Diagnosis

The diagnosis is based on the patient history, observation of the pet, and physical examination. It is made by matching this information with criteria for a specific behavior problem. Diagnostic tests may need to be conducted to rule out organic causes for the problem. Although medical abnormalities are less likely causes of most primary behavior problems, it is always important to assess all patients thoroughly for medical problems before rendering a behavioral diagnosis, or recommending therapeutic intervention. During a behavior consultation there is also the opportunity to observe and interact with the pet for an extended period of time. Observations of the pet from previous visits as well as from any video provided can also give important diagnostic information. A temperament evaluation form such as the one in Appendix C, Figure 7 (form #15, printable from the CD) can be used to help collect data during consultations.

Occasionally, the consultant may have to rely on sketchy information from an emotionally involved owner who may view the pet a bit too anthropomorphically and who may not have been present when much of the undesirable behavior occurred. This can make a firm diagnosis difficult in some cases and impossible in others.

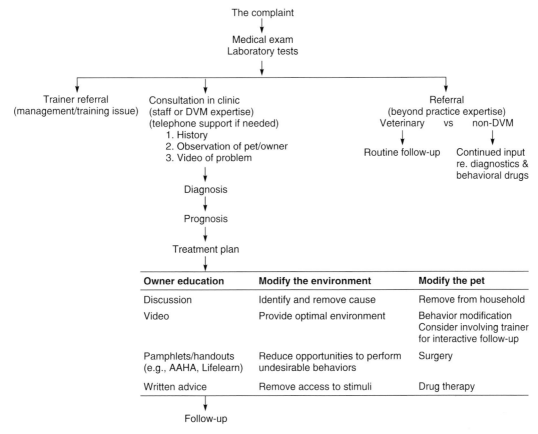

Figure 4.4   Handling a behavior consultation.

Prognosis

After historical information has been collected and a diagnosis has been made, the consultant must give some thought to the prognosis. Predicting the outcome of behavioral therapy and estimating time costs is an essential part of the consultation and provides important information for the family. The prognosis may determine whether the pet will be treated or removed permanently from the home. Factors that contribute to the ultimate prognosis include the pet itself, the owners, and the environment in which the pet lives, the type and extent of the problem, the consultant's diagnostic and communication skills, and whether a practical correction program can be implemented safely and practically for the problem at hand (Fig. 4.5).

Most cases have difficult as well as simple aspects to address. The opportunities for successful, safe treatment become less when the difficult areas outweigh the straightforward areas. The temperament and signalment of the pet must be appraised. If the pet's temperament varies significantly from the norm, such that intense degrees of fear or aggression are exhibited, the chances for a successful outcome are lessened. Problems that develop because of early social deprivation may also be extremely difficult to overcome. If the behavior is significantly influenced by sexual hormones and the pet is not (and will not) be neutered, you can expect that the prospect for a good prognosis will be diminished. Behaviors that are especially typical for the species or breed may be more difficult to eradicate since the frequent appearance of beha-

Good prognosis	More guarded or grave prognosis
• The problem can readily and accurately be diagnosed	• The problem or the cause of the problem is poorly understood
• All stimuli can be identified, controlled, or removed	• Inability to identify, control, or remove initiating stimuli
• Mild problem of short duration	• Severe or advanced problem of long duration
	• High level of intensity or severity
	• High or unpredictable frequency
• Low motivation for the behavior	• Very strong motivation to perform behavior
• Low level of arousal, easy to get the pet's attention and interrupt	• High level of arousal, difficult to interrupt
• Conditioned behavior problem	• Strongly innate factors, type of behavior is common for the species or breed
• Simple, single problem	• Complex, multiple problems
• Historically, a good prognosis for the diagnosed problem	• The type of problem responds poorly to conventional therapy
	• Appropriate correction techniques have been attempted, but were unsuccessful
• Degree of danger is low	• Marked danger
	• History of uninhibited behavior and severe damage
• Commitment and ability of family members is high, family communicates well	• Inability or unwillingness of owners to treat
	• Complex family situation, poor family communication
	• Weak bond with pet
	• Desire of family to remove pet from household
• Good understanding and ability to follow necessary correction techniques	• Owners unable to generalize prevention or treatment techniques to similar situations
	• Owners cannot comprehend nature of problem or principles of treatment

Figure 4.5 Prognostic considerations.

vior in a related group of individuals suggests a possible genetic component.

The type of problem itself may dictate how easy or difficult it will be to resolve. Normal behaviors and learned behaviors are more easily treated than abnormal (e.g., compulsive disorders, psychomotor epilepsy) or innate behaviors (e.g., predation). The prognosis might be somewhat improved when a drug is available that historically has been helpful for treatment. The complexity of the situation is another factor, since a pet with a single behavior problem has a better chance of being successfully treated than one with multiple problems. Problems that have existed for a relatively short time without worsening merit a better prognosis than those with a long duration that have been progressively getting worse. Problems involving fear or aggression that consistently involve very high levels of arousal have a guarded prognosis. The frequency of occurrence can affect a case in different ways. Behaviors that occur very frequently often develop into habits that are difficult to

obliterate. However, problems that have been occurring at a low frequency can also be problematic. For example, some destructive problems occur so infrequently that uncovering the exact cause(s) for the behavior can prove to be very difficult and the prognosis remains guarded to poor.

The environment in which family members live, as well as their ability to control or modify that environment, can be important. Treating territorial aggression will be difficult if the pet is chained in the yard next to a busy sidewalk all day. The prognosis for safe resolution of dominance-related aggression is better if there are no children or irresponsible adults in the home. The prognosis for resolving a urine-spraying problem is better if neighborhood cats can be prevented from entering the yard. The inability to control severe, frequent, and unpredictable storms makes treatment of thunderstorm phobias more of a challenge.

Many aspects about the family have an important impact on the prognosis. Success is more likely if the family has a strong commitment to the pet and a good record in following through with instructions (e.g., obedience training, medical treatments, and so on). For many types of problems, the more control the family has or can establish over the pet, the better the prognosis. If the family has unrealistic goals or if there is poor cooperation, the chances for satisfactory resolution are reduced. The family must have the aptitude to understand the conditions influencing the existence of the problem and the basic principles of the treatment program. The physical size and assertiveness of family members may be important for some cases. For example, a small, passive person is more likely to have problems with a pet that has a dominance-related problem, while a large, assertive family member with little patience will likely compromise the treatment of a fearful cat, or a dog that urinates submissively. Chances for injury are higher when the family is composed of individuals who are unable to understand or unwilling to comply with safety recommendations (e.g., young children, physically challenged, individuals with learning disorders, elderly, teenagers). The therapist must consider all characteristics of the family in order to make recommendations that are the most practical for the home situation.

And finally, the attributes of the therapist also play a role in contributing to the prognosis. The therapist's level of skill, familiarity with the type of problem, ability to communicate, and compatibility with the pet and its family can all influence the outcome of the treatment program.

For some households it is not practical to improve the pet's problem to the satisfaction of all parties concerned. In these cases, the owners and consultant will need to determine whether the pet can be left in the home, or whether the best option is to remove the pet from the household. In some cases, it might be possible to find a more suitable home for the pet, but when there is a risk of injury, when the pet is 'suffering,' or when an appropriate alternative home cannot be found, euthanasia may need to be considered.

Treatment of behavior problems

The treatment of behavioral problems utilizes a variety of approaches either to modify the pet's behavior or modify the environment to better suit the needs of the owners and the pet. The following treatment techniques are discussed in detail elsewhere in the book:

- Education of the family – what the problem is, why it has developed, what might be achieved (prognosis), the limitations on what might be accomplished, and the treatment options (Ch. 5)
- Modification of the environment (Ch. 5)
- Behavior modification (Ch. 5)
- Behavior management aids/products (Ch. 5)
- Surgery (Ch. 5)
- Drug therapy (Ch. 6)
- Alternative therapy (Ch. 7)
- Dietary considerations (Ch. 8)
- Pain management (Ch. 9)

Follow-up

Another important opportunity for educating and interacting with the family occurs during the follow-up. It is essential that the consultant continues to monitor each case to be sure that the family is correctly following treatment recommendations, and that the case is progressing as expected. This also provides an opportunity to gather more information about the situation in general. This is particularly important when there are multiple treatment options and the initial diagnosis was tentative. When drugs have been discussed or dispensed, regular follow-up is essential. For some cases, additional diagnostic tests and owner information will be required following the initial consultation, so that a formal follow-up telephone call or session may need to be scheduled. For most cases, initial follow-up contacts at two, four, and 12 weeks will provide good assessment of progress. The actual frequency will depend on the type of problem, the family, and the pet (see Appendix C, Fig. 8 – form #9, printable from the CD).

BEHAVIORAL MEDICINE: A FRENCH APPROACH

The French approach to behavioral medicine, as ascribed to by Dr Patrick Pageat, differs from the North American approach in that there have been many different forms of behavioral pathology proposed that may be linked to alterations in neurotransmitter systems. These behaviors are considered pathologic when they lose their plasticity and their adaptive function and are no longer capable of returning to equilibrium or homeostasis at the end of the action. In his book (Pathologie du comportement du chien, now in its second edition), Dr Pageat, a French behaviorist, classifies behavioral disorders by paying close attention to both the behavioral and somatic signs, and the age at which they arise. Behaviors should not be considered separately but rather categorized together with other presenting signs into syndromes. The pet may fall into one of a number of pathological states, including pathological emotional states, phobias, and pathological anxiety, pathological states concerning mood, acute and chronic depression, mood instabilities, and the state of instrumentalization. Drugs are then selected to treat the neurotransmitter system that might cause these groupings of signs and are utilized along with behavioral therapy. Throughout this text, with the aid of Dr Pageat, we have attempted to describe some of his diagnostic and treatment protocols. Pheromone therapy is discussed in Chapter 7, French considerations for stereotypic behavior are discussed in Chapter 10, and Dr Pageat's approach to geriatric behavior is integrated into Chapter 12. Dr Pageat reviews additional details of his French approach to diagnosis and treatment of dogs in Chapter 21.

FURTHER READING

Breazile JE 1987 Physiologic basis and consequences of distress in animals. Journal of the American Veterinary Medical Association 191(10):1212–1215

Buffington CAT, Chew DJ, Kendall MS et al 1997 Clinical evaluation of cats with non-obstructive urinary tract disease. Journal of the American Veterinary Medical Association 210:46–50

Cameron ME, Casey RA, Bradshaw JWS et al 2001 A study of the environmental and behavioral factors involved in the triggering of idiopathic cystitis in the domestic cat. In: Scientific proceedings of the BSAVA congress, Birmingham, UK

Casey RA 2001 Pathological consequences of environmentally induced stress in the domestic cat. In: Overall K, Mills DE, Heath SE et al (eds) Proceedings of the third international congress on veterinary behavioural medicine. Universities Federation for Animal Welfare, Herts, UK, p 30–36

Chapman B 1993 Geriatric behaviour. In: Animal behaviour. The TG Hungerford refresher course for veterinarians. Postgraduate Committee in Veterinary Science, University of Sydney, Sydney, p 133–143

Chapman BL, Voith VL 1990 Behavioural problems in old dogs: 26 cases (1984–1987). Journal of the American Veterinary Medical Association 196(6):944–946

Chrisman CL 1989 Neurological disorders producing abnormal behavior. In: Proceedings of the 56th annual AAHA meeting, Denver, CO

Chrisman CL 1994 Seizures and behavioral abnormalities in dogs and cats with neurological dysfunction. Veterinary Quarterly 16(Suppl 1):S28–S29

Dannerman PJ, Chodrow RE 1982 History taking and interviewing techniques. Veterinary Clinics of North America, Small Animal Practices 12(4):587–592

Dehasse J 1994 Pathological anticipatory defense behavior in dogs. Veterinary Quarterly 16(Suppl 1):S49

Hart BL 1985 Animal behavior and the fever response: theoretical considerations. Journal of the American Veterinary Medical Association 187(10):998–1001

Hart BL, Barrett RE 1973 Effects of castration on fighting, roaming, and urine spraying in adult male cats. Journal of the American Veterinary Medical Association 163:290–292

Heath S 1994 Commonly encountered feline behavior problems. Veterinary Quarterly 16(Suppl 1):S51

Hewson CJ, Luescher UA 1996 Compulsive disorders in dogs. In: Voith VL, Barchelt PL (eds) Readings in companion animal behavior. Veterinary Learning Systems, Trenton, NJ, p 153–158

Hopkins SG, Schubert T, Hart BL 1976 Castration of adult male dogs: effects on roaming, aggression, urine marking, and mounting. Journal of the American Veterinary Medical Association 168:1108–1110

Hornhfeldt CS 1994 Nepeta cataria (catnip) 'poisoning' in cats. Veterinary Practice Staff 6(5):1–7

Hunthausen W 1994a Collecting the history of a pet with a behavior problem. Veterinary Medicine 89(10):954–959

Hunthausen W 1994b Identifying and treating behavior problems in geriatric dogs. Veterinary Medicine 89(9):688–700

Jaggy A, Oliver JE, Ferguson DC et al 1994 Neurological manifestations of hypothyroidism – a retrospective study of 29 dogs. Journal of Veterinary Internal Medicine 8(5):328–336

Kalkstein TS, Kruger JM, Osborne CA 1999 Feline idiopathic lower urinary tract disease – Part 2. Potential causes. Compendium on Continuing Education for the Practicing Veterinarian 21:15–26

Knol BW 1994 Social problem behavior in dogs – etiology and pathogenesis. Veterinary Quarterly 16(Suppl 1):S50

Kohlke HU, Kohlke K 1994 Animal behavior therapy – characteristics and specific problems from the psychological point of view. Kleintierpraxis 39(3): 175–180

Krawiec DR 1988 Urinary incontinence in dogs and cats. Modern Veterinary Practice 69(1):17–23

Lieberman DA 1993 Learning, behavior and cognition, 2nd edn. Brooks/Cole, Pacific Grove, CA, p 134–143, 227–233, 315–357

Luescher UA 1993 Hyperkinesis in dogs: six case reports. Canadian Veterinary Journal 34:368–370

Mook DG 1987 Motivation. The organization of action. WW Norton, New York, p 226–239

Nielson J, Eckstein RA, Hart BL 1997 Effects of castration on problem behaviors in male dogs with reference to age and duration of behavior. Journal of the American Veterinary Medical Association 211(2):180

Nolan K 1994 Flea collars may cause erratic behavior. Irish Veterinary Journal 47(5):230

Overall KL 1994 Stereotypic and ritualistic behaviors. In: Proceedings of the North American Veterinary Conference, p 55–57

Owren T, Matre PJ 1994 Somatic problems as a risk factor for behavior problems in dogs. Veterinary Quarterly 16(Suppl 1):S50

Polsky RH 1993 Does thyroid dysfunction cause behavioral problems? Canine Practice 18(4):8–11

Polsky RH 1994 The steps in solving behavior problems. Veterinary Medicine 89(6):504–507

Rapaport JL 1989 The boy who couldn't stop washing. EP Dutton, New York

Reisner I 1991 The pathophysiologic basis of behavior problems. Veterinary Clinics of North America, Small Animal Practice 21:207–224

Reisner IR, Erb HN, Houpt KA 1994 Risk factors for behavior-related euthanasia among dominant-aggressive dogs: 110 cases (1989–1992). Journal of the American Veterinary Medical Association 205(6):855–863

Roosje PJ, van Kooten PJS, Thepen T et al 1998 Increased numbers of CD4+ and CD8+ T cells in lesional skin of cats with allergic dermatitis. Veterinary Pathology 35:268–273

Salmeri KR, Bloomberg MS, Scruggs SL et al 1991 Gonadectomy in immature dogs: effects on skeletal, physical, and behavioral development. Journal of the American Veterinary Medical Association 198(7):1193

Seksel K 1993 Feline elimination problems. In: Animal behaviour. Proceedings of the TJ Hungerford refresher course for veterinarians. Postgraduate Committee in Veterinary Science, University of Sydney, Sydney, p 147–153

Steigerwald ES, Sarter M, March P et al 1999 Effects of feline immunodeficiency virus on cognition and behavioral function in cats. Journal of Acquired Immune Deficiency Syndrome and Human Retrovirology 20:411–419

Towell TL, Shell LG 1996 Endocrinopathies that affect the central nervous system of cats and dogs. In: Voith VL, Berchelt PL (eds) Readings in companion animal behavior. Veterinary Learning Systems, Trenton, NJ, p 116–121

Voith VL 1996 Interview forms. In: Voith VL, Berchelt PL (eds) Readings in companion animal behavior. Veterinary Learning Systems, Trenton, NJ

Voith VL, Borchelt PL 1985 History taking and interviewing. Compendium of Continuing Education for the Practicing Veterinarian 7(5):433

Voith VL, Borchelt PL 1996 (update by Debra F Horwitz) History-taking and interviewing. In: Voith VL, Berchelt PL (eds) Readings in companion animal behavior. Veterinary Learning Systems, Trenton, NJ

5

Treatment: behavior modification techniques

INTRODUCTION

In the next five chapters we will discuss techniques for treating behavior problems including behavior counseling (client advice on behavior and environmental management) in this chapter, drug therapy in Chapter 6, complementary and alternative therapy in Chapter 7, diet-related behavior problems and their management in Chapter 8, and pain assessment and treatment including the use of adjunctive drugs for behavior therapy in Chapter 9.

EDUCATION OF THE FAMILY

The ultimate success of treating the problem is directly related to the degree of owner comprehension and compliance. Since family members themselves will carry out the behavioral modification in most cases, they must understand their roles and the techniques they will be required to perform.

The family must understand normal needs and behavior for cats and dogs. Providing pets with appropriate outlets for play, exercise, elimination, chewing, and digging may be all that is required to solve some problems. It is often necessary to provide some explanation of how animals communicate and learn. The principals behind the use of some behavior modification tools will also likely need to be discussed.

When clients are educated, they realize more clearly which problems are most likely to be completely eliminated, which are likely to only be decreased, and which are unlikely to be changed. Once the family is well informed about the situation and treatment options, the decision may be made to live with the problem rather than institute the necessary steps for corrections, while others may decide that rehoming or euthanasia are safer, more appropriate choices for their circumstances (Fig. 5.1).

MODIFICATION OF THE ENVIRONMENT

Environmental modification involves manipulating various aspects of the pet's environment in order to diminish the performance or intensity of the behavior. A number of variables can be controlled, including confinement areas, exposure to eliciting stimuli, access to people, access to other animals, access to targets of the behavior, and modification of targets (Fig. 5.2).

MODIFICATION OF THE PET'S BEHAVIOR
Change the behavior or the response with surgery

Castration of male dogs and cats not only helps stem the pet population but also has valuable behavioral and medical benefits. Castration can decrease unacceptable sexual behavior, aggressiveness, urine marking, and prevent breeding. With respect to behavior, it should be clearly understood that the only behaviors affected by castration would be those that are influenced by male hormones. Thus, castration affects sexually dimorphic behaviors, those seen predominantly in males (Fig. 5.3). There are medical benefits of castration as well. Since castration can help curtail roaming, castrated dogs and cats are less likely to be endangered by viral, bacterial, parasitic, or environmental dangers. In dogs, castration is useful in the prevention or treatment of prostatic disease, testicular cancer, and in the reduction of perianal tumors.

Other surgical procedures that have been used for certain behavior problems include olfactory tractotomy for refractory spraying cases, dental disarming, declawing, and devocalization. Many of these procedures are only considered as a last-resort alternative to euthanasia, and in some countries may be unacceptable or illegal. Surgery or medical therapy might also be necessary when an underlying medical condition (e.g., hyperthyroidism, anal sacculitis, chronic otitis) is causing or contributing to the behavioral signs.

Modify the pet with behavioral modification techniques

Behavioral modification is the principle means of correcting or controlling undesirable beha-

Problem	Owner education required
Dominance aggression	• Pack structure, social communication, dominant and subordinate signaling, the dog in the family pack
Canine housesoiling	• How dogs learn, crate training, relationship between eating and eliminating, supervision and confinement
Feline housesoiling	• Normal elimination behavior, substrate preferences, odor elimination
Feline spraying	• The role of neutering, social behavior and communication of cats, influence of cat density, pheromones
Unruly dog	• Normal greeting behavior, obedience training, halter devices, principles of conditioning
Canine destructive behavior	• Importance of play and exercise, pros and cons of adding a playmate, discussion of appropriate chew toys, the concept of guilt, principals of applying an appropriate correction, the role of anxiety
Feline play aggression	• Normal feline play behavior, feline predatory behavior, feline social behavior, how to properly play with a cat, adding a second cat

Figure 5.1   Examples of problems and information for owners.

Change	Example
Identify and remove the cause	• For urine marking, reduce the number of cats in the home or close drapes to reduce exposure to outdoor trigger stimuli • For inappropriate elimination, stop using unacceptable litter substrate • Ignore the pet when exhibiting excessive attention-soliciting behaviors
Reduce the opportunity to misbehave	• Provide a safe confinement area • Keep within eyesight with a leash • Place objects out of reach to stop destructive chewing • Build a privacy fence to reduce territorial barking
Provide an environment conducive to the pet's needs	• Install a dog or cat door to manage housesoiling by providing continuous access to the outdoors • Provide stimulating and interactive toys to decrease destructive behavior • For feline housesoiling, move the litterbox to a quiet area or decrease noisy activity in the room with the box • Provide an acceptable scratching post for cats that scratch unacceptable surfaces • More exercise and social contact for the young, unruly dog
Change the behavioral function of an area	• Place food, toys, or bedding in areas where the owner does not want the pet to eliminate
Make the area or object aversive	• Motion-activated alarms to keep the pet off furniture and counters • Aversive tasting sprays to stop chewing

Figure 5.2   Ways to manipulate the environment.

vior. Therefore it is critical for the consultants to understand the basic principles of learning and motivation if they intend to perform behavioral counseling in practice. It is also recommended that books on training and behavior be consulted for more basic instruction on these techniques. Learning and behavior modification techniques are discussed later in this chapter.

The use of behavior products to modify behavior

There are a wide variety of products that can be useful in the prevention and management

of undesirable behavior in pets. These are described throughout the text and a list of some of the product manufacturers can be found in Appendix B. For a client handout (also printable from the CD) reviewing the use of these products see Figure 5.4.

Modify the pet's behavior with psychoactive drugs, pheromones, and alternative remedies

Although medication is being used more and more frequently to treat companion animal behavior problems, there are very few drugs

Behavior	Effects of castration
Undesirable sexual behavior	• Can reduce attraction to females, roaming, mounting, and masturbation • Roaming in cats can be reduced in over 90% of cases and 70–80% of dogs have a reduction in roaming but only about 40% are completely resolved • Mounting in dogs is reduced in 70–80% of cases but resolved in only 25%
Marking	• Marking with urine is a common territorial behavior in dogs and cats • Castration reduces marking in about 70–80% of dogs but only about 40% are completely resolved. Marking by spraying urine is reduced in 90% of cats
Aggression	• Intermale aggression can be reduced in about 60% of dogs and 90% of cats • Aggression toward family dogs and family members may be reduced in about 30% of dogs • Aggression toward unfamiliar dogs and intruders may be reduced in 10–20% of dogs

Figure 5.3   Behavioral benefits of castration.

PRODUCTS FOR MANAGING AND CORRECTING UNDESIRABLE BEHAVIOR

Note that products are mentioned by name because of author familiarity, and not because they are necessarily superior to other products.

There are a wide variety of products that can be useful in correcting or managing undesirable behavior in pets. Devices that are activated by the owner can be used to disrupt a behavior so that the desirable response can be achieved or may serve to punish the undesirable behavior so that the pet is less likely to repeat the act in the future. However, devices that are activated by the owner may only allow the owner to manage the problem behavior when the owner is present, since the pet will learn that there are no unpleasant consequences for the behavior when the owner is absent. In fact, if the behavior is enjoyable (e.g., garbage raiding, sleeping on a couch) or provides relief from discomfort (e.g., housesoiling, chewing) then the pet will be highly likely to repeat the behavior in the owner's absence. Therefore remote forms of punishment or environmental punishment ('booby traps') may be more effective.

DISRUPTIVE STIMULI (EXTERNAL INHIBITION)
The goal of the disruptive stimulus is to inhibit the undesirable response and achieve a desirable response, which can then be reinforced (negatively and/or positively). If the disruption is preceded by a command, and then the desirable response is achieved, these devices can be a useful training aid. If the device, on the other hand, causes fear, anxiety, or discomfort, it might meet the definition of a punisher since it should decrease the likelihood that the pet will repeat the behavior (at least when the owner is present).

Remote punishment
Remote punishment can be used to deter undesirable behavior without causing fear of, or association with, the owner. Punishment can be administered remotely with any of the direct intervention devices or with any device activated by a remote switch. Garbage raiding and jumping onto counters are problems that might be corrected with a properly and consistently applied remote device. As soon as the inappropriate action begins it can be stopped, disrupted, or deterred with one of these products. Using negative reinforcement principles, the owners should also be taught to withdraw the punishment/discomfort as soon as the undesirable action ceases. Desirable responses can then be rewarded.

Environmental punishment and avoidance
Environmental punishment or booby traps can be used to deter undesirable behavior or entry into restricted areas even in the owner's absence. The effect is for the pet to learn that the area or the behavior itself is associated with unpleasant consequences. This type of punishment resembles the learning that occurs when pets are exposed to unpleasant or fearful aspects of their environment such as cars, predators, porcupines, toxic plants, barbed wire, sprinklers, etc.

Shock and discomfort
Most pets quickly learn to avoid situations or locations that lead to fear or discomfort. Similarly, some training devices use varying levels of discomfort or shock, such as electronic avoidance devices (e.g., Invisible Fencing®, Scat Mat®), and bark-activated shock collars. These devices are considered inhumane and are therefore illegal in certain countries, but are still widely available in North America. In principle, pet owners should be able to find successful alternative training methods and products to correct or manage most behavior problems. However, when all other practical solutions have been exhausted, these products offer another alternative that may quickly and effectively resolve the problem, but could also be unsuccessful or lead to excessive fear and discomfort. Therefore when the problem is sufficiently severe (i.e., euthanasia or rehoming may otherwise be considered), the pet's safety is at risk, and there is a product that will successfully resolve the problem with a minimum of discomfort, the potential benefits will need to be weighed against the risks and potential harm to the pet.

Figure 5.4 Useful products to manage undesirable behavior (handout #21 – printable from the CD).

Disruption and punishment devices

Owner-activated devices

a) Direct devices include commercial devices such as audible trainers (Barker Breaker™, Sonic Pet Trainer™), ultrasonic trainers (Pet-Agree™, Easy Trainer™, Ultrasonic Pet Trainer™), or a citronella spray (Direct Stop™). Other devices that might be homemade or modified from other applications include a can full of pennies (shake can), pocket rape alarms, air horns, a water rifle, or a can of compressed air.

b) Remote devices: commercially available products include remote-controlled citronella (Master Plus™, Spray Commander™) and shock collars and a remote-control vibrating collar (PetPager™, for training deaf dogs). Homemade products include long-range water rifles and remote-controlled switches that can be used to activate an alarm, hair dryer, water sprayer, or tape recording. By placing these devices in the area where the pet might misbehave (e.g., plant, garbage) and activating them with a remote switch, the pet should quickly learn to avoid the area.

Pet-activated devices

1. Outdoor devices. Electronic containment systems can be used to keep dogs within selected boundaries, or away from selected areas. A transmitter wire is buried along the boundary, and a radio transmitter sends a signal that is received by the collar. As the pet approaches, there is first a warning tone, and then activation of the collar (e.g., citronella spray or shock) if the pet does not retreat out of range. Motion-activated alarms (Critter Gitter™), ultrasonic deterrents (The ScareCrow™ – a motion detector sprinkler), and pet repellents might also help to keep the owner's pet out of selected areas on the property (e.g., gardens) or stray animals off the property.

2. Indoor devices. Commercial devices designed to keep pets away from areas (or confined to specific areas) include indoor electronic containment systems that use citronella (Spray Barrier™) or shock collars that are activated by a transmission dish. The Scraminal™ is a motion detector alarm, and there are mats that set off an alarm (SofaSaver™, Scratcher Blaster™) or give mild static-type shocks (e.g., Scat Mat™, Pet Mat™) that can deter entry into areas or onto furniture and windowsills. The Snappy Trainer™ has a plastic flap that fits over the end of a mousetrap, which serves as a safer approach to using mousetraps as booby traps. A spray device that is activated by the approach of a pet (Ssscat™) is a useful product for keeping dogs and cats away from selected areas (e.g., garbage, counters). Commercial chew deterrents (e.g., Ropel™) and pet repellents are also available. Motion detectors designed for home security use may also be effective. Homemade or modified deterrents might include less appealing substrates (e.g., aluminum foil, plastic, or rubber mats), uncomfortable substrates (e.g., upside down vinyl carpet runners, double-sided tape), or bitter or 'hot' tasting sprays (menthol, oil of eucalyptus, cayenne pepper mixed with water). With a little innovation and forethought owners can set up a stack of empty cans, a bucket of water perched to fall when disturbed, or balloons set to pop on contact when the pet enters the area.

3. A number of dog and cat doors have been designed to be activated only by the pet wearing the activation collar or 'key'. These products allow only one selected pet to access areas that require entry through the pet door.

4. Bark deterrents: for a bark-activated device to be effective, it must immediately interrupt the barking, must be sensitive enough to detect each undesirable vocalization (whine, bark), and specific enough that it is not activated by extraneous stimuli. The Super Barker Breaker™ and K-9 Bark Stopper™ are audible bark-activated alarms that are designed to be placed on a counter or table in an area where a dog might bark (front hall, cage, etc.). Bark-activated collars emit an audible or ultrasonic noise or a spray of citronella with each bark. The audible and ultrasonic devices are seldom sensitive, specific, or noxious enough to be effective. The most effective antibark collars have proven to be the Gentle Spray™ or Aboistop™ collar, which emits a spray of citronella with each bark. A bark-activated scentless spray is also now available, which may be equally effective for some, but not all dogs.

Figure 5.4 (*continued*)

labeled for this application (see Ch. 6 for details). Synthetic pheromones have been developed for the treatment of urine spraying in cats, marking, scratching, reducing feline aggression, as well as reducing anxiety in dogs and cats (see Ch. 7 for details).

Remove the pet from the household

Removing the pet from the home may be an unfortunate but important option, especially if there is significant danger posed to family members or if the owners are completely resistant to appropriate behavioral modification techniques. Although removal of the pet may seem like a failure, it is desirable if it prevents the animal from hurting members of the household or being inhumanely treated by the owners with inappropriate correction strategies. New owners must, however, be aware of the situation and be in a position to manage the pet.

BEHAVIORAL MODIFICATION TECHNIQUES AND TERMS

Although environmental modification, drugs, pheromones, alternative therapy, dietary management, behavior modification products, and surgery may all be useful in the treatment of a behavior problem, the pet's behavior generally needs to be modified through proper application of learning principles and training techniques. The behavior modification techniques discussed below are utilized throughout the text in various treatments of individual behavior problems.

Aversion therapy

Aversion therapy is a procedure for eliminating undesirable behavior by pairing the unwanted behavior with a sufficiently unpleasant stimulus. For example, by pairing an aversive stimulus such as bitter taste, a foul odor, or irritating noise with the behavior (e.g., rock eating, destructive chewing, compulsive licking), the behavior may be eliminated. In humans, associating shock or a nauseant such as apomorphine with smoking, or a bitter compound

with nail biting, may successfully stop the undesirable habit. To be successful, the degree of noxiousness or discomfort must outweigh the motivation to perform the behavior. Taste aversion (see below) is a specific form of aversion therapy.

Avoidance and escape

In avoidance conditioning the animal learns to avoid the aversive stimulus, while in escape conditioning the correct response terminates an aversive stimulus. To be effective, the stimulus must be of sufficient intensity to produce the desired response. Timing is the critical element. If the aversive stimulus is applied as soon as the behavior begins, the pet can learn that escape terminates the stimulus. On the other hand, if the aversive stimulus is immediately preceded by a brief neutral stimulus (e.g., a buzzer), the animal may learn to avoid the neutral stimulus. When a warning stimulus is followed by the aversive event (e.g., shock) and the shock is not presented if the pet withdraws, this is known as signaled avoidance. Avoidance learning depends on both classical conditioning of fear (warning stimulus plus aversive stimulus) and negative reinforcement (since the stimulus is terminated by the avoidance response).

Motion detector alarms and noxious tastes and odors can be used to teach animals to avoid particular objects or areas. A dog that jumps off a couch to avoid a shock mat is escaping from the aversive stimulus itself. However, if an unpleasant event (noxious taste, shock, alarm) is paired with a warning stimulus (tag odor, visual cue, audible cue), the pet can learn to avoid objects that are paired with the warning stimulus without having to experience the unpleasant event. For example, by pairing a neutral tone with the shock of electronic fencing or by placing a white pillowcase in any area where a shock mat or motion detector is employed, the pet can learn to avoid an area by just responding to the warning stimulus. Similarly, by applying a tag odor such as vinegar to a more aversive event (cap device that pops, stack of cans that tumbles down, water trap, upside down mouse trap), the pet can quickly be taught to avoid the tag odor itself. It is interesting to note that although early in avoidance training the warning sound or odor may indeed provoke fear, fear diminishes as the avoidance response is learned. Ultimately, the pet learns to avoid the stimulus without fear, and the avoidance behavior is maintained in the absence of the unpleasant stimulus.

Avoidance conditioning is most likely to be successful when the desired response to the fear-evoking stimulus is compatible with the animal's expected defensive or survival reaction (fight, flight, or freeze). The response of a dog or cat is likely to differ from the reaction of a pigeon or a hedgehog. These instinctive responses, which are often referred to as species-specific defensive reactions (SSDRs), are related to the species, the stimulus, and the environment. Behaviors that are compatible with the animal's innate defensive reactions are learned most quickly. In practice, most of our applications for avoidance involve training the pet to avoid or retreat from an object (couch, garbage can) or an area of the home (windowsill, dining room). However, in some situations, freezing or attacking the fear-eliciting stimulus may be a more likely response for some pets.

Classical conditioning

This type of learning begins with an unconditioned stimulus (US) that elicits a reflex behavior called an unconditioned response (UR). A neutral stimulus (NS) that has no influence on the reflex is repeatedly paired (just prior to the US) until it becomes a conditioned stimulus (CS) that is able to elicit the response by itself. The response to a CS is referred to as a conditioned response (CR).

This type of conditioning is also known as Pavlovian conditioning, after the scientist who conditioned dogs to salivate when they heard a bell. Salivation is a reflex response (UR) to the stimulus of food (US). The researcher conditioned the dogs by repeatedly ringing the bell (NS) as the dogs were about to be fed. In time, they began to salivate whenever they heard the

bell even when no food was present. At that point, the sound of the bell became a conditioned stimulus (CS) which triggered salivation (CR). The experiment is duplicated daily in many households, whenever a pet hears the sound of a can opener or the food cupboard being opened. Similarly, the dog may become excited or anxious each time the doorbell rings (depending on what association has been made) or may become anxious when taken in the car, or on arriving in the parking lot of a veterinary clinic (if there have been previous unpleasant experiences). Dogs with separation anxiety will soon identify cues that are predictive of being separated from the owner (e.g., getting car keys, picking up a purse or laptop), and these become conditioned stimuli for anxiety. An inhibitory conditioned stimulus is a stimulus that is predictive of the absence of the unconditioned stimulus. Using a clinical example, if a neutral stimulus such as a music CD, tag odor, or piece of owner clothing is associated with reward training and relaxation exercises, then this formerly neutral stimulus becomes both pleasant and predictive of the owner being at home (an absence of owner departures). Therefore, counterconditioning anxiety-evoking stimuli as well as developing a set of inhibitory stimuli can both be valuable retraining tools in separation anxiety.

An example of the use of classical conditioning is the technique of clicker training. By repeatedly giving food to a dog immediately following a specific cue such as a clicker or tone, the cue will eventually become a conditioned stimulus. Similarly by pairing an aversive stimulus with a neutral cue, the cue will become a CS for fear and anxiety. This can be of practical and humane importance, since the use of more noxious stimuli such as shock can be greatly reduced by pairing an audible or visual cue with the shock so that the pet soon learns to avoid the cue (signaled avoidance).

Conditioned punisher

By pairing a neutral stimulus (such as a 'no' command, tone) with an unpleasant or aversive stimulus then the neutral stimulus becomes a conditioned stimulus that can be used for punishment. Similarly if a neutral stimulus ('no,' tone) immediately and consistently precedes punishment then it becomes predictive of the punishment (conditioned punisher) and can be used as a bridging stimulus for punishment. For example, just prior to activating the spray on the remote citronella collar, the owner can command no or stop in a harsh voice. If the command consistently precedes the spray the command itself takes on the deterrent effect of the spray. In fact, the pet may learn that by stopping the behavior on command it can avoid being sprayed (escape).

A novel odor or taste can also be used as a conditioned punisher, by pairing it with an aversive event such as spraying the odor across the dog's nose or squirting some into the dog's mouth, as long as the product is safe and not too aversive. Alternatively the odor or taste might be paired with something more aversive (a spray from a can of citronella, an air spray, an audible alarm, or a booby trap of cans set to topple). Once the more neutral stimulus has been paired on multiple occasions (or even a single occasion in the case of one-event learning discussed below), the taste or odor alone should be sufficient to lead to avoidance.

Conditioned reinforcer (bridging stimulus)

By repeatedly pairing a neutral cue such as a clicker or whistle prior to the presentation of a favored food treat, the neutral stimulus becomes a conditioned stimulus which leads to the same reflexive response as the unconditioned stimulus. This conditioned stimulus can then be used to immediately reinforce a desirable behavior, as long as it continues to be paired with the unconditioned stimulus. Similarly, if a neutral stimulus (duck call, the phrase 'good dog,' whistle) immediately precedes a primary reinforcer, it becomes predictive of the treat (conditioned reinforcer) and can be used as a substitute for the primary reinforcer. At this point the phrase, clicker (or tone,

duck call, etc.) can be used to immediately reinforce (or mark) the desirable response until the primary reinforcer can be given. Since the conditioned reinforcer bridges the time and serves to reinforce the response until the primary reinforcement can be given, it can be referred to as a bridging stimulus.

Controlled exposure

When flooding (see below) is utilized in behavioral therapy, exposure to the full stimulus may be so traumatic to the pet that effective control may be impractical and habituation therefore does not occur. A more practical technique is to reduce the stimulus so that fear is minimized to a point where the pet can be controlled safely and effectively. Once habituation to the stimulus occurs, the pet can then be exposed to progressively more intense stimuli at subsequent training sessions. Controlled exposure techniques differ from systematic desensitization in that the pet is exposed to low or controlled levels of the fear-evoking stimuli rather than levels of stimuli that approach but are below the threshold that would evoke fear (see systematic desensitization below). Inhibitors such as distraction devices (shake can, ultrasonic alarm), control devices (such as head halters or cages), and counterconditioning techniques may all be useful in combination with exposure techniques to ensure that the pet habituates to the stimulus before it is withdrawn or increased.

Counterconditioning

This technique involves conditioning an animal to alter its emotional response to a stimulus (i.e., a response that is independent of voluntary control). When a behavior problem is associated with an aversive or negative emotional component, the goal is to pair the stimulus or event with a strong opposite emotional response (i.e., highly positive). Counterconditioning is often used to modify the behavior of fearful pets. The goal is to take the conditioned stimulus that incites the response and pair it with an unconditioned stimulus that evokes the desirable and opposite (positive) response.

Similarly, aversive counterconditioning can be used when the pet is attracted to an item or location that is potentially dangerous or considered 'out of bounds.' In this form of counterconditioning, a noxious (aversive) stimulus is paired with the response, whether learned, conditioned, or unconditioned (mounting, marking, sleeping on couch, chewing on shoes), to bring about avoidance. However, when the stimulus is food, it is unlikely that repeated pairing of any aversive stimulus other than a nauseant (see taste aversion below) can deter the behavior.

Countercommanding

This term might be used to describe the situation where a pet is taught to respond to a particular command that is incompatible with the undesirable behavior. For example, sitting for a food reward is a behavior that would be incompatible with jumping up at the door. Since the use of commands is not a necessary prerequisite of changing the undesirable response to one that is acceptable or desirable, we will utilize the terms 'response substitution' and 'differential reinforcement' to describe this retraining technique.

Differential reinforcement

Differential reinforcement is one of the most practical means of reducing and eliminating undesirable behavior. The goal is to reinforce a competing alternative behavior (differential reinforcement of an alternative behavior) while ignoring (not reinforcing) the undesirable behavior. In practice the dog or cat would be rewarded for exhibiting any behavior other than the undesirable behavior. For example, the cat that is aggressive during petting would be reinforced after a predetermined period of time for any behavior other than biting. The owners must first determine the length of time that the cat will tolerate petting before it might

bite so that the reinforcement can be administered successfully. Over time the length of petting should be gradually increased, while reinforcing the cat for any behavior other than biting.

One of the most practical techniques for correcting, altering, or eliminating undesirable behavior is to train the pet to exhibit a response that is acceptable, and both motivationally and physically incompatible with the unwanted behavior. This technique, which is also known as response substitution (training the pet to display an acceptable response instead of the undesirable response), is accomplished through differential reinforcement of an incompatible (DRI) response. If a dog or cat has been trained to immediately respond to a few simple commands, it might then be possible to train a dog to sit, settle, dance, or even fetch during greeting rather than jump up (countercommanding). The desirable (incompatible) response is then reinforced with the most potent form of reinforcement available, which in the case of greeting might be affection. Equally important is that the undesirable response is no longer reinforced (contingency management). Using favored rewards and training sessions that are designed to ensure success (planned greetings) can more quickly help the pet to learn the desirable response. In addition, physical control devices such as a leash and head halter, or disruption devices such as a citronella spray collar, can help ensure that the desirable behavior is exhibited, before any reinforcement is given.

Although extrinsic rewards such as food or a favored toy might be withheld until the desired response is exhibited, intrinsic rewards such as social interactions and play might be more difficult to control so that the most practical strategy would be to redirect the behavior to a more desirable target. For example, a puppy might be given a favored toy to carry and chew, rather than nipping on the owner's hands, or a cat might be encouraged to chase and pounce on a favored chase toy rather than the owner's feet or hands.

Discriminative stimulus (command cue)

Generally, pets are trained to respond appropriately to a specific stimulus through the use of reinforcement. When the dog responds to a specific command or cue with a consistent and predictable response, the cue or command is a discriminative stimulus. When owners respond predictably and consistently and the outcome is desirable for the dog (e.g., when the leash is picked up, a walk is coming), the dog may learn that the leash is a discriminative stimulus for going for a walk. Yet, when commands are used for training, the owner may be inconsistent in providing rewards or in the use of these commands, so that they do not become clear discriminative stimuli (commands). For example, the owner that calls the dog to come to administer a punishment will have difficulty in achieving a positive outcome and response to the come command. Yet most pets will quickly learn and retain commands associated with tricks (e.g., play dead, roll over) because these commands are always used in the same positive context, and associated with rewards until they are consistently displayed.

Disruption and diversion

A device that is sufficiently startling or novel to interrupt either a conditioned or a learned response might be considered a disruptive device (also see external inhibition below). Dog whistles, noise devices, ultrasonic trainers, a shake can, compressed air, and citronella spray products might be effective for disrupting the undesirable response so that the appropriate response can be trained. However, if the device is sufficiently aversive to reduce the probability that the behavior will be repeated, then it is actually serving as a punishment device. Similarly, a favored squeaky toy might be used to divert or distract the dog so that the appropriate response can be achieved.

Drug desensitization

When the stimulus cannot be effectively controlled or muted, drugs may be effective for reducing the pet's anxiety, fear, or aggressiveness, so that a desensitization program can be implemented (see Ch. 6 for details). As the desired response and emotional state is achieved, the drug is gradually reduced at subsequent training sessions. In effect the stimulus intensity is reduced by the effect of the drugs and the intensity is gradually increased as the drug dosage is reduced.

External inhibition

This occurs when a novel stimulus is presented immediately following the conditioned stimulus so that it subdues the conditioned response. For example, if the goal is to change the anxiety-evoking response of a doorbell to one that is calm or positive, a high-pitched whistle or shake can may be sounded as soon as the bell rings, but before the barking begins. The barking response will be inhibited as the pet orients to the noise.

Similarly, external inhibition or a disruptive stimulus can be used to interrupt a response to a stimulus so that an acceptable response can be achieved and reinforced. For example, a disruptive device such as a bark-activated citronella spray collar might immediately disrupt the barking that might occur as a stranger arrives on the property. If the dog is then taught to come to a family member and play ball or have its tummy rubbed, this new response, along with a positive association with visitors, might be achieved. Similarly, a dog that exhibits coprophagia immediately following each bowel movement might be immediately disrupted with a noise device or citronella spray, which would provide a window of opportunity in which the dog could be taught an alternative acceptable response such as coming to the owner's side and sitting for a food reward (i.e., DRI, response substitution).

Extinction

The withholding of reinforcers leads to the elimination of a behavior. For example, an owner may inadvertently reward a nuisance behavior (e.g., whining or begging at the table) by giving the pet a piece of food. If the reward for the soliciting behavior is taken away (food is no longer given), the behavior will cease. The use of extinction may not be sufficient on its own to correct many behavior problems, but it is an important part of the approach. Behaviors that have been rewarded intermittently are much more resistant to extinction. Once extinct, it takes very little encouragement for the behavior to resurface. In some cases, spontaneous recovery can occur after a rest period between extinction trials. Therefore for more permanent resolution, differential reinforcement should be used to replace the response being extinguished with an incompatible response.

Extinction burst

When reinforcement is first removed, the animal's behavior may initially intensify as the pet tries even harder to achieve the reward. Owners must be aware that this increase in behavior, known as an extinction burst, must also be ignored, or the new and more intense behavior will be reinforced.

Flooding (response prevention)

Flooding involves the continuous exposure of the subject to a stimulus at a level that evokes a response, until the response to the stimulus ceases. Pets that have learned an avoidance response to a fear-evoking stimulus can be retrained to overcome conditioned fears by exposing them to the stimulus so that they cannot escape. To be effective, the animal must be continuously exposed to the stimulus until the fear subsides and the stimulus itself must no longer be associated with fear. If the pet is unable to perform the avoidance response, and the previously fear-eliciting stimulus is no longer threatening, the fear response will undergo extinction. If the stimulus is removed before signs of fear abate or if the owner provides patting or attention (in the belief that it might help calm the pet), fearful behavior may be reinforced rather than diminished. Similarly, if the pet retreats before the fear abates, the threat will have been removed by the escape behavior (negative reinforcement). Flooding can potentiate problems if used improperly and is most practical for the treatment of mild fears, since full exposure of a pet to a very strong fear-eliciting stimulus may severely traumatize it. Controlled flooding (controlled exposure) techniques, where the pet is exposed to mild, and then to progressively more intense stimuli, may be more useful for overcoming intense fears.

Habituation

Habituation is the process by which animals learn to adapt to novel sounds and experiences, provided they suffer no consequences from such exposure. During habituation, the subject is repeatedly exposed to the stimulus without the presence of negative or positive reinforcers until the response ceases. The animal that is initially anxious during car rides usually settles down after it takes several car rides and realizes nothing aversive is going to happen. During the primary socialization process, it is important to expose young dogs and cats to as many different environments and experiences as possible (e.g., cars, veterinary clinics, stairs), so that they do not become fearful of these situations. When using disruptive and punishment devices, they must be sufficiently startling or aversive, as well as contiguous with and contingent on the behavior. Improper or excessive use may lead to habituation of the punishment or disruptive device.

Latent learning

This type of learning occurs without the presence of purposeful reinforcement and is usually not readily obvious. Latent learning will facilitate the relatively rapid acquirement of accurate performance of a behavior at a later time when reinforcement is introduced. Rats that are allowed to investigate a maze, but receive no reinforcement, are quicker to learn to run the maze for a food reward than are rats that have had no previous experience with the maze. A dog that is being taught to find an object on command will learn more quickly in an environment that it has previously had the opportunity to explore than in an unfamiliar environment.

Learning

Dogs learn through the consequences of their acts. They are motivated to repeat and increase those behaviors that have positive outcomes and minimize or avoid those behaviors that have aversive or unpleasant outcomes.

Motivation

Motivation is an animal's drive or desire to perform a behavior. The pet's level of motivation is a key consideration in training and in trying to reduce behaviors through behavioral modification. Motivation is dependent on the degree of deprivation, as well as the attractiveness of the reward. Deprivation of food, for example, leads to the increased drive to attain food. One might even say that deprivation of a needed resource leads to arousal, and that the pet is then motivated to perform behaviors to achieve de-arousal or homeostasis.

When selecting rewards for training (and counterconditioning), the strongest possible motivator (see reinforcer assessment) should be used to overcome the pet's desire to perform an alternative behavior, and to ensure that the pet performs the desired behavior.

Another practical aspect of behavioral therapy is that the pet's motivation to perform an undesirable behavior can be reduced to a level where the pet is less likely to perform the undesirable response. Desensitization and controlled exposure techniques involve the manipulation of stimuli so that the pet's motivation to perform the undesirable behavior (barking, aggression) or response (fear) is reduced. Then, through the

use of differential reinforcement, the pet can be motivated to perform an alternative competing behavior or through counterconditioning can develop an alternative acceptable emotional state.

When the pet is highly motivated to perform an undesirable behavior (Fig. 5.5), stringent control mechanisms and a deterrent of high intensity will likely be required. However, for behaviors that have low levels of motivation (or when the motivation can be reduced by modifying the stimulus or reducing the pet's desire for the stimulus), less intense deterrents and a lower level of control might suffice.

Observational learning

Observational learning refers to learning that occurs passively by watching others. Studies have been carried out in many species, including great apes, dolphins, rodents, birds, and puppies. However, there is some question as to whether dogs can learn by observation, although there are aspects of social facilitation or group-facilitated behavior that might occur with eating, hunting, chasing, greeting, or barking. In addition, dogs and cats are likely to respond to the same cues as other pets in the household (e.g., jumping into a car, escaping from a confinement area). Allelomimetic behavior, especially in the young dog, may also be confused with observa-

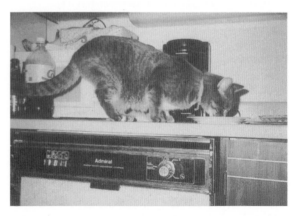

Figure 5.5 Food left on worktops is a powerful motivator for cats to climb onto those surfaces.

tional learning. In allelomimetic behavior, however, the animal learns because of its social inclination to follow the lead or join in the activities of its conspecifics and other members of the social group (hence the importance of early socialization to humans).

One-event (trial) learning

If a situation is particularly startling or noxious the pet may learn with a single association to become fearful of the stimulus in the future. This is only likely to occur on initial exposure to the stimulus, since any previous experience with the stimulus, which might have been neutral or positive, will have already molded the pet's response. One-event learning can be an effective way to teach the pet to avoid particularly dangerous or undesirable activities from the outset by pairing a neutral stimulus with a strongly aversive stimulus. For example, the use of a highly noxious taste may deter chewing of electrical cords, while a spray of citronella when the pet sits on a couch may teach the pet to permanently avoid the couch.

Operant conditioning (instrumental conditioning)

This is the type of learning that occurs when the results of a behavior influence the probability of that behavior recurring. Giving praise or food for the desired response to an obedience command is a common use of operant conditioning. Although training programs are designed to provide the pet with reinforcers for appropriate behavior (and punishment for inappropriate behavior), a great deal of operant learning occurs independent of owner interactions. Pets that knock over a bin/trash barrel and obtain food or even relieve themselves in an inappropriate location in the owner's absence will increase the likelihood of these behaviors recurring, since they are rewarding to the pet at the time. However, when eliminating on the carpet or raiding the rubbish can result in an immediate severe scolding, the probability of the pet

eliminating in front of the owner in the future diminishes.

Overlearning

This involves the continued reinforcement of a behavior that has already been learned. The consequence of overlearning is an increased resistance to extinction and longer retention of learning once all reinforcement stops. Also, responses are more dependable and consistent in the presence of stressful or distracting stimuli.

Prevention – setting the pet up to succeed

Preventive techniques are some of the most valuable tools in behavior therapy for pets with behavior problems. By preventing access to problem areas or targets for misbehavior, the desirable effects of these acts (whether intrinsic or extrinsic) can be avoided so that the problem is not further reinforced. For example, once the pet eliminates in an inappropriate area, or begins to chew on the owner's possessions, the problem is much more likely to reoccur. Preventive techniques can also help to direct pets to utilize appropriate and desirable outlets for their acts. Prevention may also be the most practical way to prevent injury and avoid damage to the owner's possessions.

Problems might be prevented in a number of ways. By keeping the pet occupied with appropriate and acceptable activities (chew toys, play toys), inappropriate forms of chewing and play can be prevented. Confinement to a safe area such as a crate or pen can also be effective, if appropriate confinement training methods are utilized (see Ch. 3 and handout #5 on the CD for details). For some pets it may be more practical to deny access to problem areas rather than to use overly restrictive confinement techniques. While closing a few doors or placing a few child gates might be effective, electronic avoidance devices can be used to keep pets away from potentially problematic areas (see environmental punishment techniques below). A number of dog and cat doors have been designed to be activated only by the pet wearing the activation collar.

Punishment

Punishment involves the application of an aversive stimulus during or immediately (within one to three seconds) following a behavior to decrease the likelihood that the behavior will be repeated. To be effective and at the same time humane, the stimulus must be intense enough to reduce the pet's desire to repeat the behavior, without causing physical harm or undue discomfort. Timing and consistency are critical (Fig. 5.6). If punishment is not immediately successful at stopping the behavior, it should not be used at all. Application of a stimulus that decreases the chance of the behavior being repeated is actually referred to as positive punishment. Removal of a stimulus or event that is positive can also be used to lower the probability that a behavior will be repeated, and this is known as negative punishment. For example, if a dog expects a piece of food for an action and

that food is withheld because the dog's behavior is inappropriate or not sufficiently accurate, the behavior will be less likely to be repeated.

Punishment can be a useful tool in behavioral modification but its inappropriate use can exacerbate the situation and cause other behavior problems. It is important that the form of punishment be tailored to each pet. If the punishment is too weak, it can lead to habituation as well as not remedying the problem. In fact, it may even serve to reinforce the problem by providing a form of attention. If it is too harsh, punishment can cause additional behavioral problems. Physical punishment should always be avoided since it can lead to fear of the owner, handshyness, and fear biting, and could be potentially harmful to the pet.

By initially pairing a minimal aversive stimulus (e.g., a harsh 'no') with a more aversive stimulus (e.g., shake can or air horn), it may be possible to use the command alone for future punishment (conditioned punisher). Commonly used forms of punishment include direct owner-initiated techniques (e.g., noise, verbal), remote

Type of failure	Reason for failure
The pet does not associate the punishment with the act The pet learns to avoid an area instead of learning to avoid the performance of a behavior The behavior problem continues but targets may change, e.g., chews different items, raids other garbage cans	• Punishment is applied too late or inconsistently • The pet is punished in some locations where undesirable behavior occurs but not in others • When the pet is highly motivated to perform a behavior or the outcome of the behavior is desirable (extrinsic or intrinsically reinforced), the pet will continue to perform the behavior or similar ones until it is taught an acceptable substitute behavior
Punishment reduces a desirable response	• The pet that is punished by the owner as it eliminates indoors becomes fearful of eliminating in front of the owner in any location (including outdoors)
Punishment is unable to overcome fear or excessive submission	• Punishment leads to an increase in submissive behavior • Punishment may cause fear and avoidance of the owner or defensive aggression toward the owner • Punishment may worsen the fear response to a fear-eliciting stimulus
The behavior continues in the owner's absence	• The owner punishes an action when supervising but the behavior continues without consequence in the owner's absence
Punishment leads to an increase in behavior	• Punishment that does not immediately stop or suppress the behavior may be insufficiently aversive and may even serve to reinforce the response

Figure 5.6 Punishment failures.

owner-initiated techniques (e.g., sprays of water), and environmental techniques (leading to avoidance and escape) such as bitter tastes or smells or motion-activated deterrents.

Punisher assessment

Punisher assessment involves predicting which form of punishment will be most practical, appropriate, and successful for an individual pet. The ultimate success or failure of punishment techniques depends on the individual pet's sensitivity to the punishment, the motivation to perform the particular behavior, as well as the behavior for which it is being punished. One might anticipate that the more aversive the stimulus the more effective the punishment, but this is not necessarily true. For example, many dogs continue to hunt porcupines and skunks even after they have experienced the ill effects of such a meeting.

Punishment techniques

(i) **Direct interactive punishment**. Direct interactive punishment should only be considered when the pet performs an undesirable act in the presence of the owner. An immediate, startling reprimand or loud noise is often effective and all that is necessary for young or sensitive pets. On the other hand, if punishment causes excessive fear, submission, or any threats or aggression it should be discontinued immediately. A quicker and more effective control can often be achieved by leaving a long leash attached to the pet for applying a gentle correction. This not only allows the owner to interrupt or deter the undesirable behavior, but also to direct the pet into a more acceptable behavior. There is no indication for the use of physical techniques (especially hitting) for punishment. This can lead to handshyness, fear of the owner, and defensive aggression. In addition, the pet may not be able to associate the punishment with the act, except in those cases where the behavior is directed toward the owner, such as jumping up, mounting, or play biting, and the owner responds during the act. When the owner

is not present to supervise, problematic behaviors must be prevented by controlling the pet's environment or by using alternative forms of punishment (e.g., booby traps).

The use of a deterrent device rather than the human voice may be a more practical and effective means of punishment, since it may be more aversive or startling than verbal reprimands, is less likely to lead to habituation, and is less likely to cause fear of the owner. Most devices emit noises that the pet finds unsettling. Some are audible to people, but many of the new products are in the audible range of pets alone. An aversive device is most practical when it is used during the undesirable behavior, and is withdrawn as soon as the problem behavior ceases. Using a verbal command (such as 'no!' or 'quit!') at the same time as the primary punishment often results in the command alone being sufficient punishment in the future (conditioned punishment).

Examples of direct punishment devices include commercial devices such as audible trainers (Barker Breaker™, Sonic Pet Trainer™), ultrasonic trainers (Pet-Agree™, Easy Trainer™, Ultrasonic Pet Trainer™), and citronella sprays (Direct Stop™). Other devices that might be homemade or modified from other applications include a can containing pennies (shake can), pocket rape alarms, air horns, a water rifle, or a can of compressed air.

(ii) **Remote interactive punishment**. Remote interactive punishment involves the application of an aversive stimulus to the pet by a person the pet cannot see. Peeking around corners, using mirrors, video cameras, or following the situation with an intercom, child monitor, or pet monitor (an electronic device that emits a signal when disturbed) will be necessary to ensure that the pet is immediately caught as the inappropriate behavior begins. If punishment can then be meted out while the owner remains out of sight, the pet should associate the punishment with its behavior rather than with the owner (Fig. 5.7).

Owners can rig up noisemakers, buckets of water, hoses, and sprinklers that they can control and activate from out of sight as the undesirable behavior begins. There are also a number

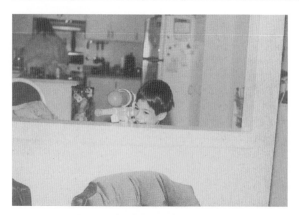

Figure 5.7 Remote punishment is where the owner is not associated with the punishing behavior (e.g., use of a water rifle). It is important that the person administering the punishment remains out of sight.

of gadgets that can be activated by remote control to provide aversive stimuli. For example, remote-control switches can be plugged into an electrical outlet and connected to a variety of devices including vacuum cleaners, water piks (spray small quantities of water), strobe lights, sirens, alarm clocks, and hair dryers. As soon as the behavior stops, so should the punishment. Remote-control shock and citronella spray collars work on the same principle. The remote citronella collar has two levels of spray, as well as a neutral tone (that can be paired with a

favored reward so that it can be used as a conditioned reinforcer or bridging stimulus. If a command such as 'stop' precedes each spray, it may soon become a quicker and more effective way of stopping undesirable behavior (conditioned punishment). However, when the longer, more intense spray is used to interrupt undesirable behavior (without a warning command), it may be an effective form of remote punishment for some behavior problems (e.g., garbage raiding, climbing onto furniture, etc.) (Fig. 5.8). Using a long lead attached to a halter device is another effective way to interrupt or punish undesirable behavior 'remotely.'

The primary advantage of remote punishment is that the person is not directly associated with the act of punishment. This means that the pet may learn to cease the behavior, even when the owner is not present. In addition, the risk of the pet becoming fearful of that person is eliminated. This is especially important with cats. Cats are much less likely to tolerate interactive punishment, such as a stern scolding, than are dogs. A cat that is directly punished repeatedly by the owner may quickly learn to avoid the person providing the punishment and the relationship deteriorates.

(iii) **Time out**. The goal of time out is for the pet to learn that misbehavior leads to temporary

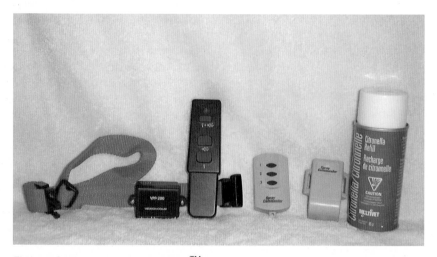

Figure 5.8 Remote trainers: PetPager™ remote-activated vibration collar (left) and Spray Commander™ remote citronella spray collar (right).

isolation and removal of rewards. When the pet first starts to misbehave (e.g., barking), it is given a command (e.g., quiet) and given the opportunity to respond appropriately. If it does, it should be rewarded and praised immediately. If unsuccessful (e.g., the barking continues), the pet is relocated to a confinement area for a period of about three minutes. It is only released when it is quiet. To be effective, the isolation room should not be the feeding, sleeping, or play area of the pet. A laundry room, basement, or bathroom is a good choice. Since the pet may not make the association that the confinement is a consequence for the behavior, time out may merely serve to separate the pet away from the site and stimuli for the problem until it settles down.

(iv) **Environmental punishment**. Environmental punishment does not rely on the owner monitoring the situation. The environment is rigged so that an unpleasant consequence occurs when the pet misbehaves. Booby traps, or home security and child safety alarms can be set to go off when they are triggered by the pet. This can be as simple as taping balloons to a couch (Fig. 5.9), setting a mousetrap upside down in a plant, or stacking a set of empty tin cans or cups where a cat might scratch. New technology has provided us with other intriguing devices that are triggered when the pet misbehaves or enters an area where the misbehavior occurs.

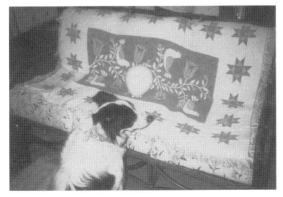

Figure 5.9 A balloon can be rigged to pop when the dog attempts to get on to the couch. Photo courtesy of Dennis Bastian.

Commercial devices designed to keep pets away from areas in the home (or confined to specific areas) include indoor electronic containment systems (citronella or shock) which use transmitter dishes to activate the collar (or the home can be wired as with the outdoor confinement systems) (see Fig. 5.9). Motion or touch-activated devices include free-standing motion-activated alarms (Scraminal™), mats that set off an alarm (SofaSaver™ and Scratcher Blaster™), and mats that give a mild 'static' type shock when touched (Scat Mat™ and Pet Mat™). Motion detectors designed for home security use may also be effective. The Snappy Trainer™ has a plastic flap (resembling a flyswatter) that fits over the end of a mousetrap which serves as a safer approach to using mousetraps as booby traps (Figs 5.10, 5.11). A spray device (Ssscat™) activated by the approach of a pet has just recently been introduced which can keep cats and occasionally dogs from selected areas. Commercial chew deterrents (e.g., Ropel™, ChewGuard™) and pet repellents are also available. Also see Figure 5.4 on behavior products (client handout #21, printable from the CD) and the list of behavior product manufacturers in Appendix B (and on the CD) for further details.

Homemade or modified deterrents might include less appealing substrates (e.g., aluminum foil, plastic, or rubber mats), uncomfortable substrates (e.g., upside down vinyl carpet runners, double-sided tape), or bitter or 'hot' tasting sprays (menthol, oil of eucalyptus, underarm deodorant, cayenne pepper mixed with water). With a little innovation and forethought owners can set up a stack of empty cans, a bucket of water perched to fall when disturbed, or balloons set to pop on contact when the pet enters the area.

For outdoor use, electronic containment systems can be used to keep dogs within selected boundaries, or away from selected areas. A transmitter wire is buried along the boundary, and a radio transmitter sends a signal that is received by the collar. As the pet approaches, there is first a warning tone, and then activation of the collar (e.g., citronella spray or shock) if the pet does not retreat out of range. Motion-

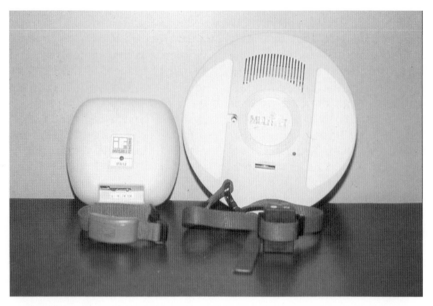

Figure 5.10   Environmental punishment: indoor avoidance units – transmitter dish and shock collar (left); Spray Barrier™ transmitter dish and citronella spray collar (right).

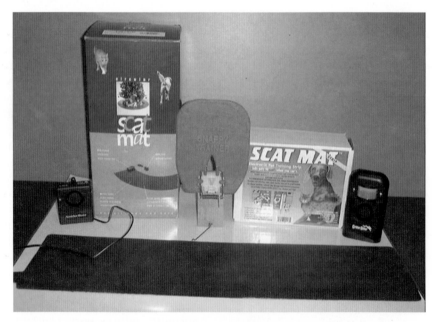

Figure 5.11   Environmental punishment: a variety of commercial devices have been developed to keep pets away from selected area. Front – Scratcher Blaster™ mat produces an audible alarm when contact is made. Rear (from left to right) – 1. Alarm unit that attaches to Scratcher Blaster™. 2. Scat Mat™ produces a mild electronic shock when contact is made. This is the semicircle shape for placing around plants or trees. 3. Snappy Trainer™ is a mousetrap with plastic covering to protect against injury. 4. Scat Mat™ also comes in windowsill and sofa sizes. 5. Scraminal™ (motion detector alarm).

activated alarms (Critter Gitter™), The ScareCrow™ (a motion-activated water sprinkler), and pet repellents might also help to keep the owner's pet out of selected areas on the property or stray animals off the property.

There are several different bark-activated devices that are designed to control and inhibit barking. For any bark-activated device to be effective, it must be sensitive enough to detect each undesirable vocalization, specific enough that it is not activated by extraneous stimuli, and must immediately interrupt the barking. The Super Barker Breaker™ and K-9 Bark Stopper™ are audible bark-activated alarms that are designed to be placed on a windowsill or table in an area where a dog might bark (front hall, doorway, cage, etc.). Bark-activated collars emit an audible sound, an ultrasonic sound, a spray of citronella, or deliver a shock with each bark. The audible and ultrasonic devices are seldom sensitive, specific, or noxious enough to be effective. The most effective and humane antibark collars have proven to be the Gentle Spray™ (formerly ABS™) or Aboistop™ collars, which emit a spray of citronella with each bark. A bark-activated scentless spray is also now available which may be equally effective for some, but not all, dogs.

Shock and discomfort

Most pets quickly learn to avoid naturally occurring situations or stimuli that cause fear or discomfort. Similarly, some training devices use varying levels of discomfort or shock for conditioning, such as bark-activated shock collars and remote-activated shock collars. To be an effective punishment, a device must be noxious enough to immediately deter the behavior and reduce the chance of it being repeated. Devices that inflict pain or shock are considered inhumane and are therefore illegal in certain countries, but are still widely available in North America. In practice, most problems can be effectively prevented or corrected without the need for shock. However, when all other practical solutions have been exhausted, when the pet's safety is at risk, or when the problem is sufficiently severe that the pet may have to be removed from the home,

these products provide another option that might be effective. Ideally, products that have a warning signal might be preferred since they can lead to signaled avoidance where the pet avoids the signal without the need for further shock. Although shock devices might be a quick and effective deterrent, they can cause excessive fear and anxiety, and for some pets and some problems (especially those that are highly motivated) shock may not even be effective.

Reinforcement

Positive reinforcement

Positive reinforcement involves the application of a stimulus immediately following a response that increases the likelihood of the response being repeated. Anything that the dog or cat finds desirable can be a primary reinforcer. Whether a particular reinforcer will be effective depends on the history of previous reinforcement, as well as the motivational state of the dog in relation to the reward. While food is a primary reinforcer for most pets, its efficacy will vary with the pet's interest in the food. The motivational value of any reward is likely to be increased by deprivation (e.g., using food as a reward when a meal is due) and by use of special treats or toys for which the pet has shown a strong desire (reinforcer assessment). Petting and attention, playing with family members or other pets, a favored toy, going for a walk, a car ride, or a chew toy can all be used for reinforcement but will have varying appeal depending on the pet's temperament and personality, previous experience, and degree of deprivation. For example, the pet's sociability, fearfulness, familiarity, and attachment to a person will determine whether affection and attention from that person will be reinforcing.

An event or stimulus that is not initially a primary reinforcer can become a reinforcer if it is paired with other events or stimuli that are already reinforcing. For example, praise ('good dog'), or events (going for a walk) can become conditioned reinforcers if they are paired with primary reinforcers such as a favored food treat or social play.

For rewards to be effective they must be contingent on the behavior (given only when the desired response is performed). If the reinforcement is also provided non-contingently, the behavior will be unlikely (or much slower) to change. For example, if a dog or cat gets affection or treats with no regard for the behavior that they follow, they may lose their effectiveness or ability to act as reinforcers. In order to use these desirable resources and activities as reinforcers they must be saved and timed properly for effective learning and training.

Of even greater concern is that these reinforcers may follow undesirable behavior such as jumping up, barking, whining, begging, play biting, or care soliciting. Since these acts have a desirable outcome (attention, affection, treats, play), they are inadvertently being reinforced. Owners who then try to discourage these actions by ignoring the acts most (but not all) of the time provide a variable and intermittent reinforcement schedule, making the undesirable behavior far more resistant to extinction (see reinforcement schedule below). Similarly, the owner who tries to comfort the fearful or aggressive pet by patting, saying 'calm down,' or having a heart-to-heart talk with the pet may actually be rewarding the fearful or aggressive response. Owners must also be cautioned that mild punishment (stop, get down, light hitting) is unlikely to dissuade the pet, and may inadvertently be rewarding the problem with attention. For example, the owner who attempts to dissuade play biting or scratching with a light swat will usually be unsuccessful and the interactive contact may actually encourage further play. If the physical reprimand is then increased in intensity, the pet could either learn to enjoy rougher and rougher handling, or may desist but become fearful and handshy of the owners.

Rather than use punishment techniques to decrease the performance of those behaviors that the owner considers undesirable, it is much more practical and humane to closely supervise the pet and provide it with desirable outlets for chewing, play, feeding, elimination, etc., and reward the desired response. In this way, little if any punishment or discipline should ever be required.

Since the pet's actions are successful at achieving their goal, they are constantly being reinforced. For more information, refer to Figure 3.26 (printable handout #22 on the CD).

Negative reinforcement

Negative reinforcement is a form of reinforcement that increases the probability of a behavior being repeated by escaping from an aversive stimulus. In practical terms, the pet learns to cease a behavior or avoid a situation that it finds unpleasant. For example, when a dog has had its tail pulled by young children, it might learn to retreat to its crate for a rest. When outside during a storm, a dog will learn that by seeking shelter under the porch the unpleasant stimulus will be removed (escape behavior). When the aversive stimulus has been associated with specific cues, the pet may learn an avoidance response so that in time the cues themselves may initiate the avoidance response (avoidance conditioning). Although not recommended, squeezing a dog's or cat's lips until the mouth opens or using a remote-controlled shock collar and terminating the shock at the instant the dog displays the appropriate behavior are examples of negative reinforcement that have been used in training applications.

Because punishment and negative reinforcement involve aversive stimuli, they are often confused. With punishment, the application of the stimulus during or immediately following the behavior leads to a decreased likelihood that the pet will repeat a behavior. In negative reinforcement the withdrawal of the stimulus increases the chance of a behavior recurring. Thus, punishment involves the aversive stimulus being applied during or immediately following the behavior, while negative reinforcement consists of the aversive stimulus preceding the behavior and being withdrawn when the behavior occurs.

Timing and schedules of reinforcement

Reinforcement that occurs immediately after the response promotes the most effective and fastest learning. Therefore when a new response is being developed, immediate reinforcement is essential. During initial training, the desired behavior should be reinforced regularly (continuous schedule of reinforcement). Once the response is performed consistently, delayed reinforcement is acceptable. However, if any other response occurs in the intervening period between the desired response and the reward, it will be the intervening response that is rewarded. For example, if the pet eliminates in an appropriate location outdoors and the owner gives a reward as soon as the pet comes back indoors, coming indoors is reinforced, not eliminating.

Reinforcement delivered after every response is referred to as continuous reinforcement while reinforcement delivered after only some of the responses is referred to as intermittent reinforcement. During initial training, a behavior will be learned most quickly with continuous reinforcement while intermittent and variable reinforcement promotes a response that is stronger and more resistant to extinction.

Intermittent reinforcement can be scheduled as either fixed or variable. Either the ratio can be fixed (a response is reinforced after a fixed number of repetitions) or the interval can be fixed (the first response after a fixed interval of time is rewarded). Similarly, the ratio can be variable (a response is rewarded after a variable number of repetitions) or the interval can be variable (the first response after a variable length of time is rewarded). Performance and responding are higher with variable ratios and intervals

compared with fixed ratios and intervals, and the learned behaviors are more resistant to extinction. Unfortunately, many undesirable behaviors (e.g., begging, jumping up, vocalization) are rewarded variably and intermittently so that they are highly resistant to extinction.

Reinforcer assessment

The more valuable the reward, the faster the learning. Since an individual pet's response to any specific reinforcer may vary, it is essential that pet owners determine which rewards (play, toys, food, or affection) are most likely to motivate their pets. The effectiveness of the reinforcer can be enhanced by withholding it at all times other than during training. Reinforcers should be used sparingly during training, so that shaping can be used for more difficult and complex learned behaviors (Fig. 5.12).

Shaping (successive approximation)

Shaping refers to the process whereby pets can be trained to perform increasingly complex tasks by building on their existing knowledge. This is accomplished by gradually withdrawing rewards for general behaviors and progressively rewarding only the behaviors that more closely approximate the desired behavior. For example, shaping can be used to encourage a dog to bark when someone is at the front door. The initial process involves simply rewarding the dog for barking. Then, rewards are only given when the barking occurs near the front door, and nowhere else. Finally, the barking is only rewarded when someone is actually at the front door.

	Reinforcement **Increases probability of behavior recurring**	**Punishment** **Decreases probability of behavior recurring**
Positive	Behavior increased due to positive consequence of behavior	Behavior decreased due to unpleasant consequence of behavior
Negative	Behavior increased due to removal, termination, or avoidance of an unpleasant consequence	Behavior decreased due to removal or termination of a reinforcing (positive) consequence

Figure 5.12 Punishment and reinforcement.

Systematic desensitization

Systematic desensitization refers to exposing pets repeatedly to stimuli that cause fear, anxiety, or aggression in sufficiently small doses so as not to cause the response. The stimuli are then gradually increased at increments that do not lead to a recurrence of the response. The stimuli are repeated so many times with no effect that they become inconsequential.

Systematic desensitization is often used in conjunction with counterconditioning to facilitate training. For example, a pet may be fearful of thunder but not fearful when a tape recording of thunder is played at low volumes. If the pet listens to the recording and shows no signs of anxiety, it is paired with a highly positive motivator such as a food treat. By gradually increasing the volume over a period of time, the pet can be desensitized systematically to the fear-evoking stimulus and counterconditioned to be in a happy, food-anticipatory state when it hears the sound of thunder. The key is to expose the pet to a level of the stimulus that is below its threshold for anxiety, and then very gradually increase the intensity until it mimics real-life circumstances.

Taste aversion

Taste aversion is a specific form of aversive conditioning, in which the animal develops an aversion to a particular odor or taste that is associated with illness, following a single taste–illness pairing. Taste aversion is likely to be an innate defense mechanism, so that the animal learns to avoid potentially toxic substances. Taste aversion differs from other forms of aversion therapy or avoidance conditioning in that it generally takes a single event, and the illness may take place a considerable time following the ingestion of the substance. In avoidance conditioning, immediate timing of the aversive stimulus with the unconditioned stimulus, and numerous repetitions, may be required before the aversion is conditioned.

APPLICATION OF BEHAVIORAL MODIFICATION TECHNIQUES

Training a dog to settle or relax on command is an important aspect of most canine retraining programs. There are a number of ways that this can be achieved, but the key element is that the dog will not only sit, stay, or go to a selected location but will be relaxed and calm in that area. This command could then be used if the dog tends to be out of control or overly excited during homecomings, when visitors arrive, or even prior to departures for the dog with separation anxiety. A command that achieves a relaxed state is also an important component of desensitization and counterconditioning programs. Training the dog to steady (not pull at the end of a leash), look or focus (with attention paid to the owner for successively longer periods of time), to lie down in a relaxed position, or to go to a selected relaxation location can be achieved by lure–reward techniques and shaping, head halter control, or physical relaxation training such as SOFT exercises (Fig. 5.13 – handout #23 on the CD).

Systematic desensitization and counterconditioning are used in combination to change the pet's response to a stimulus from one that evokes fear, anxiety, or aggression to one that is positive. All stimuli that incite the undesirable response must be identified and a means of control must be established. For example, a distance gradient (i.e., exposure at sufficient distance to minimize the response), a volume gradient (e.g., a recording of the stimulus that can be reduced to a low enough volume), or a similarity gradient (using a video of the stimulus or a family member rather than a stranger) can be used to begin exposure. In addition, the person training and handling the pet and the environment in which the pet is trained can be altered to reduce the response. Favored rewards should also be placed along a gradient, with the favored rewards paired with the presentation of the muted stimulus. The mild stimuli are paired with presentation of the favored reinforcers and as the pet makes positive associations with the stimulus, the intensity is gradually increased until counterconditioning

TRAINING A DOG TO SETTLE OR RELAX

An important training exercise is to teach a dog to settle down or relax on command. The goal is to train the dog to achieve a state of physical and mental relaxation on command. For calming and settling a dog as a training command (e.g., STEADY, LOOK, FOCUS), the goal is to teach the dog to focus on the owner. Another form of settle (SOFT, GO TO YOUR MAT) is intended to calm the dog that is overly anxious, aroused, excitable, or fearful in the home.

Once the dog has learned to settle, the command can be used to help achieve a calm response during the correction or management of a wide variety of behavior problems. It can be used to get the dog to focus when it might be overly excited or anxious in greeting family members, strangers, or other animals. It can also be used with dogs that become anxious as the owners prepare to depart or become overly excited when company arrives or when preparing for a walk.

Training a dog to settle and focus should begin in an environment where your dog is calm and there are minimal or no distractions. The sequence for training is to give a 'settle' command (or other suitable word), get the desired response (using one of the techniques described below), and then give clear and immediate reinforcement. Food, affection, or a favored toy can all serve as rewards if they are consistently given immediately following the behavior. Later, they can be given on an intermittent schedule and slowly phased out.

Calming exercises for any location

1. Puppy training – teaching 'steady'
   - While you are standing still, give the puppy three to four feet of the leash. If the leash remains loose, occasionally give the puppy a food or social reward and say 'steady.'
   - When the puppy starts to walk away, the 'steady' command is given as a warning. As the puppy gets to the end of the leash and starts to tug and pull against the leash, a final warning of 'steady' is given, immediately followed by a slight tug on the leash by the owner to get the puppy's attention and stop it. Then, slack is returned to the leash.
   - Upon compliance (loose leash) immediately give a food or social reward.
   - After several repetitions, the puppy learns that it is rewarded for keeping the leash loose.
   - Practice a couple of times a day in the home with few distractions. As the puppy gets better, gradually add distractions and start working outside.
   - This can also be used to stop tugging and pulling on the leash while walking.

2. Teaching 'look' or 'focus'
   - Show your dog a favored toy or treat and then hide it behind your back. Have your back against the wall or be in a corner so the dog can't get behind you. An alternative method is to hide the treat in your closed hand in front of your chest in a line between your dog's eyes and your eyes.
   - Say 'look' or 'focus' and as soon as your dog stops its attempt to get the treat and makes eye contact, use your reward word or clicker and give the treat. Repeat to improve consistency and immediacy.
   - Gradually increase the amount of time you require eye contact to last and then start adding distractions in the background like people playing or a fridge door opening, etc. Your dog ONLY gets rewarded after maintaining (i.e., not breaking) eye contact with you. Once the dog is consistent in giving the correct response even when there are distractions, go to other places (outside) and add mild distractions, such as another dog nearby or children playing. After each successful session gradually increase the distractions and work in busier environments.
   - The goal is for your dog to maintain eye contact for several minutes, regardless of the amount of distraction and background activity.

(continued)

Figure 5.13   Training a dog to settle or relax (handout #23 – printable from the CD).

Calming exercises for any location (*continued*)

3. Teaching settle in a down position
   - Another method is to use food lure training to train the dog to lie down in a relaxed position, on its belly with both hind legs on the same side.
   - Gradually progress to longer down stays in a variety of environments and then gradually increase the background noise and distractions.

4. Head halter training
   - The head halter can be used concurrently with lure–reward training, or by itself, to teach the pet to assume a relaxed position.
   - The head halter is used immediately following the command to get the dog to focus and pull (or prompt) it into the settle position (steady, focus, down).
   - As soon as the pet relaxes, the tension on the leash is relaxed and a favored reward is given.
   - See our head halter training handout for further details.

Indoor exercises

Although any of the above exercises can also be used for indoor training, there are additional techniques that might help the dog to calm down quickly and effectively when indoors. These techniques can be used to help reduce anxiety associated with owner departures or fearful stimuli such as thunder, as well as calm dogs that are unruly and excitable or overly aroused when visitors come to the home.

1. Teaching a settle location
   - Training the dog to settle indoors can sometimes be more easily accomplished by using a settle down area. The dog can be taught to 'go to a mat' or 'go to a kennel' where it learns to stay calmly for progressively longer periods of time for affection and food rewards.
   - Food lure training, with or without the aid of a head halter, can be used to achieve the initial response. The dog is taught to stay calmly for progressively longer periods of time before the reward and affection are given.
   - At first the owner may need to take the dog to the area to ensure success, but as the training progresses the dog should learn to go to the area on command to receive its rewards.
   - If the dog is also taught to sleep in this area and favored toys are kept in the area, it may soon learn to go to this area to relax on its own.

2. Physical exercises – SOFT exercise
Techniques that use physical contact can help to increase the enjoyment and decrease any fear associated with handling and restraint. While the physical contact and attention may provide sufficient reinforcement for some dogs, food treats can also be used to mark and reward the desirable response.

IMPORTANT: Physical exercises are intended to be used <u>only</u> with friendly, non-aggressive dogs. If you think your dog might become aggressive, <u>do not begin</u> without first discussing this with your behavior consultant. If your dog growls or attempts to bite, becomes fearful, or struggles excessively during these exercises, immediately discontinue them and seek the advice of a behaviorist or trainer.

The SOFT exercise (based on techniques of Dr David Tuber, 1986)

- The SOFT exercise is designed to achieve a calm or settled response on command.
- The SOFT exercise uses gentle physical manipulation to get the dog in a position on its side with its back against the owner's knees and its head resting on the floor.
- The most practical method to achieve this is to kneel on the floor with the dog standing sideways to you. Say 'SOFT' as you reach over the dog's back and grip the front and back legs closest to you, near the paws. The limbs are then gently raised which pulls the dog back onto your lap, preventing it from falling.
- With the ramp provided by the knees, the dog is then gently eased to the floor and is maintained in this position using gentle pressure from both forearms and a soothing voice.

(continued)

Figure 5.13 (*continued*)

Indoor exercises (*continued*)

- The legs should continue to be held so that they cannot make contact with the floor until the dog is settled and relaxed.
- Some resistance can be expected and this will need to be overcome with a firm but gentle approach.
- Once the dog begins to relax and its resistance decreases, pressure should be gradually released but reapplied if the dog begins to struggle or rise. The goal is for the dog to learn that relaxation leads to pressure release.
- Once there is no further resistance, the pressure can be entirely removed and replaced by gentle stroking along the neck, shoulder, and back.
- Massage and stroking should continue for at least a minute after the dog has stopped resistance.
- Finally, the hands should be removed with the dog remaining in place before the exercise ends. During subsequent practice session, the length of massage should gradually be increased.
- Each time you begin the exercise, the 'SOFT' command should be given.
- By practicing this exercise multiple times a day, the dog should initially learn to assume the relaxed posture with a minimum of restraint and ultimately learn to assume the SOFT position on command.

Training aids

Training devices that interrupt undesirable behavior (e.g., unruly, excitable, aroused) without causing excessive fear or anxiety can be useful for providing a window of opportunity to get the pet's attention so that it can be successfully trained. Citronella spray collars (whether bark-activated or remote), a surprising noise (e.g., a squeaker, ultrasonic device, or duck call), or a leash and head halter can be very helpful for interrupting the undesirable response.

Figure 5.13   (*continued*)

has been successful with the full stimulus. In practice, it may be difficult to implement all aspects of counterconditioning because it may not be possible for owners to identify and control all stimuli and to prevent exposure to the stimuli until counterconditioning is complete.

Controlled exposure techniques are intended to expose the pet to a muted or reduced intensity of the stimulus where an acceptable response can still be achieved (response substitution). For systematic desensitization, exposure should begin at a level below that which would lead to fear or anxiety. However, with controlled exposure the pet is exposed to levels of the stimuli that lead to some degree of fear and anxiety. The session must continue until the acceptable response is achieved, either by allowing the pet to habituate or through reward-based training commands. A control device such as a leash and head halter for dogs, a leash and harness for cats, or an open crate might be most practical to prevent injury and ensure a successful outcome. Distraction devices such as a squeaky toy, shake can, or citronella spray may also be useful to get the pet's attention. A favoured treat (consider clicker training) should then be given to mark the acceptable response and ensure a positive association with the stimulus (counterconditioning). As with desensitization, it will be necessary to identify and control each stimulus so that they can be exposed at gradually increasing intensity. The owner must remain positive and calm as owner anxiety and punishment will further aggravate the problem. The stimulus itself should not be threatening and neither the pet nor the stimulus should be removed until a successful outcome is achieved and reinforced. At subsequent sessions, the pet should be exposed to gradually higher levels of intensity as long as a positive outcome can be achieved. With good control of the pet and stimulus, and proper contingency management that includes making favored reinforcers contingent on exhibiting an acceptable response in the presence of the stimulus (and ensuring no reinforcement for undesirable responses), success can usually be achieved. See Figures 11.3, 11.8, 11.9 (handouts #8, #9, #10, respectively, printable from the CD) for details.

FURTHER READING

Adler L, Adler H 1977 Ontogeny of observational learning in the dog (*Canis familiaris*). Developmental Psychobiology 10:267–272

Askew HR 1993 Use of punishment in animal behavioral therapy. Praktische Tierarzt 74(10):905–909

Beaver BV 1981 Modifying a cat's behavior. Veterinary Medicine Small Animal Clinic 76:1281–1283

Beaver BV 1994 The veterinarian's encyclopedia of animal behavior. Iowa State University Press, Ames, IA

Borchelt PL, Voith VL 1985 Punishment. Compendium of Continuing Education for the Practicing Veterinarian 7:780–788

Borchelt PL, Voith VL 1996 Punishment. In: Voith VL, Borchelt PL (eds) Readings in companion animal behavior. Veterinary Learning Systems, Trenton, NJ, p 72–80

Crowell-Davis SL 1990 Negative reinforcement is not punishment – help clients know the difference. Veterinary Forum March:18

Gustavson CR 1996 Taste aversion conditioning vs. conditioning using aversive peripheral stimuli. In: Voith VL, Borchelt PL (eds) Readings in companion animal behavior. Veterinary Learning Systems, Trenton, NJ, p 56–67

Hart BL 1985 The behavior of domestic animals. WH Freeman, New York

Hart BL 1991 Effects of neutering and spaying on the behavior of dogs and cats: questions and answers about practical concerns. Journal of the American Veterinary Medical Association 198(7):1204

Hart BL, Eckstein RA 1997 The role of gonadal hormones in the occurrence of objectionable behaviours in dogs and cats. Applied Animal Behavioral Science 52:351

Hart B, Hart L 1985 Canine and feline behavioral therapy. Lea & Febiger, Philadelphia, PA

Hengst A 1994 Animal behavior therapy. Praktische Tierarzt 75(12):1138

Houpt K 1991 Domestic animal behavior. Iowa State University Press, Ames, IA

Keller FS, Schoenfeld W 1968 Principles of psychology. Appleton-Century-Crofts, New York

Kirkpatrick M, Rosenthal GG 1994 Animal behavior – symmetry without fear. Nature 372(6502):134–135

Landsberg G 1994 Products for preventing or controlling undesirable behavior. Veterinary Medicine 89(10):970

Lindsay SR 2000 Handbook of applied dog behavior and training – volume one. Iowa State University Press, Ames, IA, p 410

Lindsay SR 2001 Handbook of applied dog behavior and training – volume two. Iowa State University Press, Ames, IA, p 410

Marder A, Reid P 1996 Treating canine behavior problems: behavior modification, obedience and agility training. In: Voith VL, Borchelt PL (eds), Readings in companion animal behavior. Veterinary Learning Systems, Trenton, NJ, p 62–71

Mills DS 1997 Using learning theory in animal behavior therapy. Veterinary Clinics of North America, Small Animal Practice 27:617–636

Nobbe DE, Niebuhr BR, Levinson M et al 1978 Use of time-out as punishment for aggressive behaviour. Canine Practice 5:12–18

Overall KL 1993 Treating canine aggression. Canine Practice 18(6):24–28

Overall KL 1994 Management-related problems in feline behavior. Feline Practice 22(1):13–15

Owren T 1987 Training dogs based on behavioural methods. Journal of Small Animal Practice 28(11):1009–1029

Reid P, Marder A 1996 Learning. In: Voith VL, Borchelt PL (eds) Readings in companion animal behavior. Veterinary Learning Systems, Trenton, NJ, p 62–71

Spreat S, Spreat SR 1982 Learning principles. Veterinary Clinics of North America 12:593–606

Thorndike EL 1911 Animal intelligence: experimental studies. Macmillan, New York

Thorpe WH 1963 Learning and instinct in animals. Harvard University Press, Cambridge, MA

Voith VL 1979a Learning principles and behavioral problems. Modern Veterinary Practice 60:553–555

Voith V 1979b Multiple approaches to treating behaviour problems. Modern Veterinary Practice 60:651–654

6

Pharmacological intervention in behavioral therapy

INTRODUCTION

The timely and appropriate use of drugs may allow the pet owner an opportunity to resolve the pet's behavior problem successfully, or modify its behavior sufficiently to allow the pet to remain in the home. Failure to identify and suggest potentially helpful pharmacological agents may mean the difference between a safe and healthy pet–owner relationship, and the pet's demise. Drug selection requires an accurate diagnosis of the behavior problem and a comprehensive knowledge of which drug(s) would be the safest and most effective for resolving the problem at hand (Fig. 6.1).

Drug prescription must proceed in agreement with local regulations and licensing requirements. In the UK, for example, the drug of first choice should be one that is licensed for the species being treated, provided there is a suitable choice available. The second choice of drug to consider should be one that has been licensed in another animal species. The third choice should be one that has been licensed for use in man, and the final choice, when the other three choices are not possible, would be a drug that is available (perhaps on trial or through another country) but is as yet an unlicensed drug.

Although some of the old favorites (relatively speaking), such as acepromazine and the progestins, are still in frequent use, newer drugs that are non-addictive, relatively free of poten-

PRETREATMENT CONSIDERATIONS

1. Complete medical workup
2. Accurate behavioral diagnosis
3. Age and health of pet
   - Concurrent medical problems
   - Concurrent medications
4. Potential side effects and adverse effects
5. Owner compliance
   - Cost
   - Dosing frequency
   - Mode of administration – owner's ability to comply
6. Expected time to efficacy/improvement
7. Monitoring requirements – when, what tests, how often
8. Need for concurrent behavioral and environmental management

Figure 6.1

tial organ toxicity, and cause minimal sedation are now available. Many of these so-called 'smart drugs,' exert their effects on the specific behaviors that may need to be altered with little or no alteration of other behaviors. Side effects are less common since most selectively target specific neurotransmitter systems. In fact, in cases of behavioral pathology where there may be alterations in neurotransmitter levels or function, these drugs may help to re-establish normal neurotransmission. Most of these medications have been used widely in humans but have not been approved for use in animals. While disposition and metabolism for some of these drugs have been determined for dogs and cats, this is not always the case. **Therefore direct extrapolation to animal use of human psychotropic drugs may not be accurate as drug metabolism (including metabolites, half-life, route of excretion) as well as neurotransmitter effects and receptor effects may vary between species.** In fact, for some drugs the active metabolites in humans may not be produced in the same amount and routes of excretion may vary. Drug dosage information is provided in Appendix D.

There are four situations where drug therapy might be indicated.

(1) Psychotropic drugs are most commonly used as an adjunct to behavior therapy. Factors to consider include whether there may be a drug that could help to more quickly resolve the problem, potential adverse effects of the medica-

tion, the owner's commitment to the behavioral program, and the humane considerations for the pet (i.e., whether the pet's interests might be better served with medication). The treatment of separation anxiety, fears and phobias, and aggression are examples of where a drug may help to facilitate the initiation and implementation of behavior therapy. For example, studies in the use of clomipramine for separation anxiety showed that there was greater improvement and faster improvement in the group with drugs and behavior modification compared with the group with behavior modification alone (i.e., placebo group). Choosing an appropriate drug may provide an opportunity to resolve the problem in a quicker or safer manner. However, without concurrent behavioral modification, the problem may not improve significantly and is likely to recur when the drug is removed.

(2) Drug desensitization is a technique that can be applied when the stimulus cannot be effectively controlled or reduced, or when there are multiple stimuli that lead to fear or aggression. The drug should be given at sufficient dosage so that the pet is relaxed and calm when exposed to the stimulus. By pairing exposure to the stimulus with favored treats, the association can be made even more positive (counterconditioning). Even if the drug alone does not completely calm the pet, it may still be possible to reduce its arousal enough to get the pet to respond to a training command such as focus, sit/stay, or settle, and this response can then be reinforced (response substitution). Drug-aided desensitization should be combined with other behavioral modification techniques such as systematic desensitization, controlled flooding, counterconditioning, and differential reinforcement so that behavioral techniques, rather than the drug itself, are the principle methods of altering behavior. As soon as the successful response (and mood) can be consistently achieved in the presence of the stimulus, the drug can be gradually reduced at subsequent training sessions.

(3) A third indication for drug use is when a behavior problem is unlikely to be corrected by behavioral modification techniques alone. This

might be the case for urine marking, and compulsive disorders such as acral lick dermatitis (granuloma) or tail chasing. Not only might these behavioral problems require drugs to help control the condition, but it may never be possible to withdraw the drugs without recurrence of the condition.

(4) A final indication for drug use is when underlying pathology, whether medical or behavioral, is present. Medical problems that might lead to behavior problems could include endocrinopathies (hyperthyroidism, hypothyroidism, and hyperadrenocorticism), epilepsy, hepatic encephalopathy, interstitial cystitis, cognitive dysfunction syndrome, chronic painful conditions, or neuropathic pain. Similarly, behavioral pathology (i.e., where behavioral changes may be due to altered neurotransmitter function) may only improve with appropriate drug therapy. Compulsive disorders, attention deficit hyperactivity disorders, and some of the European classifications of behavior disorders (such as hypersensitivity–hyperactivity and dissociative disorders) may require medication to effectively treat the problems.

Since most drugs used in canine and feline behavior therapy are not licensed for use in pets, they should be used cautiously. In the United States, the owner should sign a release where appropriate, advising that the drug is considered investigational and that its use is 'extra-label' with respect to the manufacturer's recommendations (see Appendix C, Fig. 9 – printable form #5 on the CD). Owners should monitor their pets for a reduction in severity, frequency, or intensity of the targeted behaviors. Adverse or unexpected effects should be reported immediately. Veterinary literature should be regularly reviewed for reports of adverse effects or changes in dosage recommendations. Although potential adverse reactions in humans cannot necessarily be extrapolated to animals, it is also advisable to consult the human literature and manufacturers' data, to determine areas of potential concern. Ideally, blood and urine tests should be performed before any behavioral drug is dispensed to rule out underlying medical problems and establish

a baseline against which future tests can be measured. Testing should be repeated at regular intervals (at least once a year) based on the pet's age and health and the potential side effects of the medication being used.

When there is more than one potentially effective treatment regimen, the safest course of action should be followed. Accurate doses have not yet been established for many of the drugs used in pet behavioral therapy so that, in some cases, wide dosage ranges can be found in the veterinary literature. For most cases, dispensing a drug that is licensed for use in that species would provide the best opportunity for safety and accurate dosing. When treatment fails or untoward side effects are identified, it should first be determined whether a dosage adjustment is practical and whether a longer duration of therapy might be indicated. Alternative regimens, which might be potentially more harmful to the pet, must be weighed against all other options.

NEUROTRANSMITTERS

In order to make an intelligent decision when choosing a psychoactive drug for behavioral therapy, it is important to have an understanding of central nervous system (CNS) neurotransmitter activity. The classic view of neurotransmission suggested that the presynaptic neuron transmitted a single substance that had an activating or inhibiting effect on the postsynaptic receptors. However, there may actually be many neurotransmitters released. Neurotransmitters are responsible for the transmission of impulses from one neuron to another or to a non-neuronal cell. Neurotransmission can be increased or decreased to accommodate any physiological situation. Alterations in the levels of neurotransmitters can be responsible for neurological and behavioral disorders and these alterations can sometimes be modified by the administration of certain drugs. While drugs can be used to manage disease conditions they can also result in aberrations of neurotransmitters causing adverse effects.

Following stimulation of the presynaptic neuron, the nerve impulse travels along the axon to the nerve ending, where neurotransmitters are released from the terminal endings (synaptic boutons). The neurotransmitter diffuses across the synaptic cleft to the postsynaptic membrane (which is on the dendrite or cell body of the postsynaptic neuron, where it binds to specific receptors – Fig. 6.2). If enough neurotransmitter diffuses across to the receptors an action potential can be generated by the postsynaptic neuron. The neurotransmitter is then broken down by enzymes in the synaptic space or attaches to re-uptake receptor sites on the presynaptic neuron where it re-enters the neuron from which it was released. Re-uptake blockage therefore prolongs the effect of the neurotransmitter and this is the basis for the action of many of our psychoactive drugs.

Receptors are cell membrane proteins that react with specific neurotransmitters. Primary messenger transmission occurs when the neurotransmitter–receptor complex results in a change in membrane potential. Secondary messenger transmission is a delayed indirect intracellular process in which cell membrane proteins relay 'messages' from the neurotransmitter–receptor complex to the neuroplasm of the cell. Secondary messenger systems can activate a variety of intracellular mechanisms that alter the transcription of receptor proteins.

Neurotransmitters are considered to be excitatory if they increase the firing of the postsynaptic neuron, and inhibitory if they decrease its firing. In addition, receptors that are stimulated continuously by neurotransmitters or drugs (agonists) can become hyposensitive or 'down-regulated,' whereas receptors that are not stimulated by their neurotransmitters or are blocked by drugs (antagonists) can become hypersensitive or 'up-regulated.' The result is a decrease or increase in the physiological response of the effector cell.

Psychotropic drugs act at varying sites, presynaptically, postsynaptically, and within the synapse. The production and release of neurotransmitter may be enhanced; drugs may block the effects of the neurotransmitter at the postsynaptic receptor; drugs may affect receptors on the presynaptic neuron; drugs may stimulate the postsynaptic receptor; and drugs may block the re-uptake of neurotransmitter into the presynaptic neuron. Drugs may also act by inhibiting the breakdown of neurotransmitters within the presynaptic neuron or within the synapse. The neurotransmitters that are altered by behavioral medications are primarily serotonin, norepinephrine, dopamine, acetylcholine, gamma-amino butyric acid (GABA), and excitatory amino acids such as glutamate.

The cholinergic system

Acetylcholine

Acetylcholine is synthesized from the union of acetylcoenzyme-A (acetyl-coA) and choline in the axonal boutons and is stored in the synaptic vesicles. Acetylcholine action is rapidly terminated by the enzyme acetylcholinesterase and

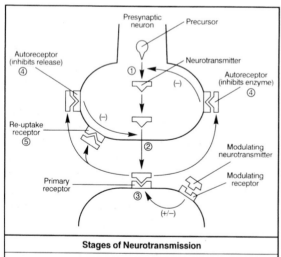

Stages of Neurotransmission

1. Synthesis of neurotransmitter in the prejunctional neuron
2. Release of neurotransmitter in response to an action potential
3. Interaction of neurotransmitter with the receptor
4. Auto-regulation
5. Re-uptake

Figure 6.2   The stages of neurotransmission and receptor sites.

most of the choline necessary for the production of acetycholine is obtained through re-uptake from the synaptic cleft. It is the only major neurotransmitter not derived directly from an amino acid. In vertebrates, acetylcholine is the neurotransmitter at all neuromuscular junctions and is involved in preganglionic to postganglionic neurotransmission for both the sympathetic and parasympathetic nervous systems (nicotonic synapses). Nicotonic receptors are excitatory. There are both N-m nicotinic receptors, which are located at the neuromuscular junction leading to muscle contraction, and N-n receptors, which are found in the brain, adrenal medulla, and autonomic ganglia. Acetylcholine is also the postganglionic neurotransmitter of the parasympathetic nervous system (muscarinic synapses). Muscarinic stimulation leads to a decrease in heart rate and cardiac output and arteriole vasodilation, and an active digestive system. Five subtypes of muscarinic receptors have been identified, each acting on a different secondary messenger system. Acetylcholine is present in subcortical structures above the brainstem, especially in the area of the lower part of the basal ganglia named the nucleus basalis of Meynert. A defect in central cholinergic transmission may lead to learning and memory deficits and has been found in human patients with Alzheimer's disease.

Atropine blocks muscarinic synapses and therefore the effect of the parasympathetic system at the target organs, while curare blocks nicotonic synapses, thereby paralyzing skeletal muscles. Acetylcholinesterase inhibitors, such as some organophosphate compounds, potentiate the effects of cholinergic activity, while atropine acts as an antidote by blocking cholinergic receptors in the brain. The side effects of many of the psychotropic medications are to block muscarinic acetylcholine receptors.

Monoamines

This neurotransmitter group is divided into catecholamines, indoleamines, and histamine. The catecholamines noradrenaline (norepinephrine), adrenaline (epinephrine), and dopamine are all synthesized from the amino acids tyrosine and phenylalanine, and share a common chemical structure. The indoleamines serotonin (5-hydroxytryptamine) and melatonin are synthesized from tryptophan.

Catecholamines are the neurotransmitters associated with the arousal of the autonomic nervous system. Catecholamine depletion in the brain results in mood changes and locomotor deficits. During stressful or fearful moments, the catecholamines dopamine and noradrenaline are released, resulting in CNS stimulation and anxiety. Chronic stress might lead to exhaustion and depletion of noradrenaline and dopamine and resultant depression. Almost all classes of psychotropic drugs interact in one way or another with the monoamine system. There are numerous catecholamine receptors including five dopaminergic receptors and four noradrenergic receptors. Many of the receptors affect the postsynaptic neurons by stimulating adenylate cyclase to convert adenosine triphosphate (ATP) to cyclic adenosine monophosphate (cyclic AMP), an important secondary messenger.

Dopamine

Dopamine is a neurotransmitter that is synthesized from tyrosine by dopaminergic neurons. Tyrosine is converted to levodopa and then dopamine and stored in prejunctional vesicles. After release, dopamine interacts with dopaminergic receptors. This is followed by re-uptake by the prejunctional neuron. Levels are held constant by changes in tyrosine hydroxylase activity and not by levels of tyrosine. Therefore drugs that reduce the activity of the enzyme will lead to a reduction in catecholamine production. Dopamine is inactivated by the enzymes monoamine oxidase (MAO), primarily MAO B and by catechol-O-methyltransferase (COMT) into dihydroxyphenyl acetic acid and homovanillic acid (HVA). HVA is used as a marker of dopamine turnover in humans. Dopamine neurons in the midbrain extend into the limbic system and cortex. Excessive dopamine may be associated with stereotypies and schizophrenia, while altered dopamine transmission may lead to behavioral changes such as decreased alertness, cognitive decline, anxiety, depression, extrapyramidal signs, Huntington's chorea in humans, Parkinsonian-like tremors, and may be a contributory factor in certain forms of pituitary-dependent hyperadrenocorticism. The selective MAO B inhibitor, selegiline, may therefore be useful in the treatment of some of these conditions. In fact, the neurotoxin MPTP, which depletes the brain of dopamine, will cause irreversible Parkinsonian signs in humans and alterations in circadian rhythms and increased cortisol output in dogs.

Noradrenaline (norepinephrine)

Noradrenaline is the primary catecholamine neurotransmitter in the central nervous system. It is synthesized from tyrosine in noradrenergic neurons. The locus ceruleus, which is located in the gray matter of the pons, is the principal noradrenergic nucleus. Noradrenergic neurons in the locus ceruleus send their processes into the thalamus, cerebral cortex, cerebellum, and spinal cord. Noradrenaline is also the neurotransmitter of the sympathetic postganglionic neurons. In monkeys, stimulation of the locus ceruleus leads to the fear response while the drug clonidine or lesions of the locus ceruleus nucleus decrease fear. Similarly in cats, stimulation of the hypothalamus or exposure to a dog or an aggressive cat leads to defense reactions that are associated with increased firing of the locus ceruleus noradrenergic neurons. Suppression of firing can be achieved through clonidine administration. Following synthesis, dopamine is taken up into storage vessels where it is converted to noradrenaline. Noradrenaline is stored in prejunctional vesicles and, when released, interacts with noradrenergic receptors. The effects of noradrenaline are primarily terminated by re-uptake at the prejunctional neuron, similar to dopamine. Noradrenaline is also broken down by monoamine oxidase A (MAO A) and by catechol-O-methyltransferase (COMT). Noradrenaline decreases in depression and increases in mania. Drugs that inhibit noradre-naline uptake (e.g., tricyclic antidepressants) and drugs that inhibit MAO increase noradrenaline availability and have been used to treat depression in humans.

Adrenaline (epinephrine)

In response to noradrenaline release, adrenaline is secreted from the adrenal gland and together they cause sympathetic effects, e.g., pupillary dilation, piloerection, tachycardia. There are both alpha- and beta-adrenergic receptors. Activation of alpha-receptors leads to vasoconstriction, increased cardiac contractile forces, iris dilation, intestinal relaxation, pilomotor contraction, contraction of the intestinal and bladder sphincters, and inhibition of the parasympathetic nervous system. Stimulation of beta-one (b1) receptors leads to an increase in cardiac output while b2 receptor stimulation causes vasodilation, intestinal relaxation, uterine relaxation, and dilation of coronary vessels as well as bronchodilation. Drugs that block beta-receptors, such as propranolol, may therefore block some of the physiological signs associated with fear. Nicergoline is a competitive antagonist to alpha-adrenoreceptors that has recently been marketed for the treatment of a variety of behavior problems by increasing cerebral blood flow.

Serotonin

Serotonin (5-hydroxytryptamine) is synthesized from tryptophan by serotonergic neurons and is found mainly in cells in the midline raphe. Its molecular structure is very similar to the psychedelic agent lysergic acid diethylamide (LSD). There are 14 different classes of serotonin receptors. Serotonin plays a major role in the sleep–wake cycle, mood and emotion, and in other functions mediated by the limbic system. 5HT1A receptors affect mood and behavior while 5HT1D receptors affect cerebral blood flow. Urinary 5HIAA (5-hydroxyindoleacetic acid) excretion in the urine may be indicative of serotonin turnover.

Serotonin levels are controlled by cellular uptake of tryptophan and the action of tryptophan hydroxylase, which is involved in the rate-limiting step in serotonin synthesis. Inactivation is by re-uptake or by breakdown by MAO. An increase in serotonin may be associated with an activation of the pituitary adrenal axis. A decrease in serotonin may lead to depression, increased anxiety, aggression, and decreased food intake. In humans, altered serotonergic system function is associated with hyperaggressive states, schizophrenia, affective illness, major depressive illness, and suicidal behavior. Increasing or normalizing serotonin levels may be useful in the treatment of depression in people, compulsive and stereotypic disorders, and some forms of aggression and anxiety. Specific serotonin re-uptake inhibitors and tricyclic antidepressants increase serotonin availability by decreasing re-uptake, and MAO inhibitors increase serotonin by decreasing serotonin breakdown. Serotonin agonists have been shown in rat studies to reduce offensive aggression, without blocking defensive aggression. Impulsivity (disinhibition, unpredictability, prolonged arousal) may be correlated with the presence of low serotonin metabolites (5HIAA). This is also true in human studies of impulsive violent offenders. Serotonin re-uptake inhibitors may decrease these forms of aggression while cyproheptadine (serotonin agonist) may increase aggression. In studies of non-human primates increased serotonin was correlated with higher social rank but inversely correlated with aggression. In fact, in dogs aggression seems to be more common in middle-ranking individuals. In rodent studies, fluoxetine inhibited offensive aggression in resident–intruder studies and mice lacking the 5HT1B receptor were more aggressive while mice lacking 5HT1 receptors were more anxious. Serotonin may act to inhibit aggression, at least in part, by antagonizing the aggression-promoting effects of vasopressin. It has also been suggested that there is a relationship between dopamine and serotonin levels in that higher levels of 5HT may inhibit dopamine

release. In fact, one factor in schizophrenia in humans may be decreased inhibition of the release of dopamine by 5HT in the mesencephalon and frontal cortex and that treatment should help to normalize the relationship between 5HT and dopamine.

Histamine

Histamine is found in low quantities in the brain. Its precursor is histidine. Histamine receptors are found primarily in the hypothalamus. Histamine receptors initiate secondary messenger systems. Histamine may help to regulate body rhythms, thermoregulation, and neuroendocrine functions.

Amino acids

Amino acids are the most prevalent of the CNS neurotransmitters. They are involved in rapid point-to-point communication. Glycine, glutamate, and aspartate are three of the most important of the 20 amino acids that function as neurotransmitters. Glycine is an inhibitory neurotransmitter of the hindbrain and spinal cord. Glutamate and aspartate are excitatory neurotransmitters, which may be produced in abnormal levels in schizophrenic, impulsive, and aggressive disorders.

GABA – Gamma amino butyric acid

GABA causes mostly inhibitory effects and is the most widespread neurotransmitter in the brain. It is synthesized from glutamic acid. After it interacts with its receptor, there is active re-uptake by the prejunctional neuron. GABA is metabolized by GABA transferase (GABA T). Seizure activity and Parkinson's disease may be associated with GABA decreases or disorders, so that GABA agonists such as benzodiazepines can be useful in the treatment of these conditions. GABA agonists may also be helpful in the treatment of anxiety disorders.

Neuropeptides

Endorphins and neurokinins (substance P and NK1)

This group is composed of molecules that are short-chained amino acids. They mainly function as modulators of other neurotransmitters, evoking facilitation or inhibition of neurotransmitter activity at the postneuron receptor site. Central nervous system endorphin release has been implicated in some compulsive disorders involving stereotypic behavior, although the role is still not too well understood. Substance P is a neuropeptide that is found in the spinal cord and central nervous system, which is a modulator of nociception involved in signaling the intensity of noxious stimuli. Along with neurokinin 1 (NK1), substance P is likely involved in the body's response to stress, anxiety, invasion of territory, and noxious or aversive stimuli. Substance P is present in the limbic system, including the hypothalamus and amygdala, and may play a role in emotional behavior. NK1 is present in the hypothalamus, pituitary, and amygdala, which play a role in affective behavior and response to stress. In fact, mice lacking an NK1 receptor were less aggressive toward intruders. The development of substance P antagonists might provide new alternatives for the treatment of anxiety and emotional responses.

Other neurotransmitters

There are numerous other mediators of neurotransmitter release (e.g., encephalins, nitric acid), but further discussion is beyond the scope of this text.

HORMONES

Endogenous compounds such as hormones or other substances that are naturally produced by the body have gained increased interest for the treatment of human psychiatric disorders. The idea is that if we administer substances that the body already has we can rebalance underlying deficits. Recent studies have shown that estrogen supplementation, growth hormone, and even secretin, which is used in the treatment of autism, may have beneficial effects in depressed patients. Although some may consider that using substances already found in the body is somehow safer, hormone excess can also lead to serious medical problems.

VASOPRESSIN

Vasopressin, in addition to its effects as an anti-diuretic hormone, affects a variety of functions including cardiovascular regulation, antipyresis, learning, memory, and arousal. In hamster and rat studies, injections of vasopressin in multiple CNS sites led to offensive aggression, while vasopressin receptor antagonists inhibit aggression. It has been hypothesized that, at least in the hamster, serotonin inhibits fighting by antagonizing the aggression-promoting action of vasopressin. A similar reciprocal relationship between vasopressin and serotonin may also exist in humans, so that in some personality disorders associated with aggression there may be elevated vasopressin, which may be inhibited by serotonin.

RECEPTOR PHARMACOLOGY

It has been suggested that since many of the psychotropic drugs (such as antidepressants) act to increase the availability of neurotransmitters, such as norepinephrine, serotonin, or dopamine, the abnormal or undesirable behavior might be caused by an alteration in these neurotransmitters (Fig. 6.3). While this might sometimes be the case, it seems to be an oversimplification. It is likely that the drugs we give do not affect the amount of neurotransmitter available as much as they affect the receptors. Therefore, when we suggest that there is a net increase in the amount of a neurotransmitter such as serotonin due to re-uptake blockade, it is perhaps more accurate to say that they affect the serotonin transporters in the cell membranes. In fact each SSRI may have a slightly different application because they may bind differently to serotonin transporters. In addition, there is some

Condition	Proposed neurotransmitter involvement
Alzheimer's disease – memory and learning deficits	Decline in cholinergic transmission
Anxiety – experienced in anticipation of an unpleasant or stressful experience. May be a component of panic, phobic, or obsessive–compulsive disorders. May be seen in a variety of syndromes or disorders	May be associated with reduced action of GABA. Benzodiazepines increase GABA binding and the inhibitory action reduces anxiety
Depression – feelings of worthlessness, despair, or self harm – may be accompanied by somatic disorders	Associated with reduced norepinephrine and serotonin levels, combined with increased number of beta-adrenergic and serotonergic receptors. Antidepressants may work by increasing neurotransmitter levels, inhibiting monoamine oxidase, or inhibiting the re-uptake system
Mania – euphoria, hyperactivity, flight of ideas, and pressured speech	Associated with increased noradrenaline, decreased serotonin, and a decreased number of adrenergic receptors. Lithium increases noradrenaline uptake
Parkinson's disease	Associated with loss of specific brain cells, loss of dopaminergic function, depleted GABA, and an overactive cholinergic system. l-DOPA increases dopamine levels, bromocriptine stimulates dopamine receptors, and anticholinergic drugs counteract the overactivity of the cholinergic system
Schizophrenia – social withdrawal and disturbances in thought, motor behavior, and interpersonal function	Possibly associated with overactivity of the dopaminergic system. May also be associated with serotonin abnormalities. Antipsychotic drugs block dopamine receptors and reduce dopaminergic overactivity

Figure 6.3   Human conditions with defects in neurotransmission.

question as to whether the oral administration of these drugs and hormones actually reaches the target tissues and, even if they do, whether they are effectively utilized. Therefore, while we might speculate on the mode of action of a particular drug, hormone, or supplement, this may one day prove to be inaccurate.

Some drugs have more general effects on the behavior of an individual (e.g., phenothiazines, anticonvulsants, antihistamines), while others are more selective in their results (e.g., selective serotonin re-uptake inhibitors). Use of drugs in the latter category can be advantageous in that desirable behaviors, like play and social interaction, are less likely to be sacrificed for the benefit of altering a single undesirable behavior, such as fear or aggression.

A drug is able to act in a selective manner when the drug's chemical configuration allows for a unique fit with a distinct neurotransmitter receptor macromolecule on the surface of the effector cell. A number of distinct neurotrans-

mitter receptor sites exist on the surfaces of pre- and postsynaptic cells. Activation of these sites can result in a wide variety of cellular responses. Any of these receptor sites provides a potential location for drug interaction.

The primary receptor sites on the postsynaptic cell interact with the neurotransmitter from the presynaptic neuron, resulting in major biological changes within the postsynaptic cell. Activation of these sites may influence a variety of physiological activities including ion movement across the cell membrane, changes in cell membrane potential, and activation of intracellular enzymes. Drugs that have molecular conformations similar to that of the primary neurotransmitter can attach to the receptor sites and either mimic neurotransmitter activity or block normal neurotransmitter activity, depending on the specific character of the molecule.

After detaching from postsynaptic receptor sites, the neurotransmitter molecules are either enzymatically degraded or diffuse to re-uptake receptor sites on the presynaptic neuron, where they attach and are transferred into the cell. In addition to decreasing the neurotransmitter's interneural concentration by physically removing molecules from the interneural space, re-uptake indirectly results in a decrease in interneural concentration by increasing the intracellular storage pool. This occurs because an intracellular feedback system inhibits neurotransmitter synthesis as the concentration of neurotransmitter increases within the neuron. Thus, the re-uptake receptor site provides an excellent target for drug action by effectively increasing the amount of neurotransmitter available to interact with the postsynaptic cell.

The influence of the primary neurotransmitter on the effector cell may be modulated by secondary neurotransmitters, such as polypeptides, as they interact at separate modulator receptor sites on the postsynaptic cell membrane. Attachment of modulatory neurotransmitters at these sites can result in the inhibition or facilitation of the effect of a primary neurotransmitter on the postsynaptic cell. Drugs with a correct fit can also work at these sites to regulate neurotransmitter effect.

Other locations on the presynaptic neuron where drugs can modulate neurotransmitter activity are the autoreceptor sites. Activation of these sites following attachment of neurotransmitter molecules diffusing through the intercellular space provides negative feedback probably by having an inhibitory influence on neurotransmitter synthesis and release. Inhibition of neurotransmitter synthesis occurs due to decreased activation of the synthesizing enzyme from its inactive to active form or by directly downgrading the enzyme's activity. Autoreceptor activation can also have an inhibitory effect by directly decreasing the amount of neurotransmitter that is released from the presynaptic cell. This is an effective feedback system that results in less synthesis and release as extracellular neurotransmitter concentration increases. Pharmacological blockage or desensitization at these sites results in less inhibition and increased synthesis and release of neurotransmitter molecules. It is interesting to note that

when a strong serotonergic re-uptake blocker, such as fluoxetine, is given, the initial increase in serotonin results in activation of inhibitory autoreceptors which actually decreases the release of neurotransmitter from the presynaptic cell. With time, the overstimulated autoreceptors become hyposensitized and inhibition of serotonin synthesis and release wanes so that the net effect is an increase in serotonin transmission. This is the likely reason for the delayed effect of fluoxetine and other re-uptake blockers.

Another way that a drug might increase the interneural concentration of a transmitter is by having an inhibitory effect on enzymes involved in the catabolism of that neurotransmitter. An example of a drug that works in this way is an MAO inhibitor which inhibits the enzyme that metabolizes monoamine transmitters (Fig. 6.4).

NEUROLEPTICS/ANTIPSYCHOTICS

Neuroleptics are drugs that block dopamine receptors in the brain. Classical neuroleptics include the phenothiazines, haloperidol, and thioridazine. Neuroleptics are most commonly used in veterinary medicine as tranquilizers. They decrease motor function at the level of the basal ganglia in the brain, elevate prolactin levels, and may reduce aggression through their action as dopamine antagonists. Many are effective antiemetics. Phenothiazine tranquilizers, such as acepromazine, chlorpromazine, or promazine, have been used for a variety of fearful, anxious, and phobic behaviors, but their effect is through a non-specific depression of the central nervous system. Since they decrease motor function, cause a reduced awareness of external stimuli, and are effective antiemetics, they have also proven to be useful for motion sickness and distress during traveling, some forms of aggression, and when a decrease in exploratory or investigative behaviors is desired. These drugs are most useful when sedation is required, but this is an undesirable effect when behavior modification is needed. Tranquilized pets should be cautiously assessed as phenothiazines have a variable effect on aggression, and some patients may be more reactive to noises and may

Neurotransmitter	Drugs that increase effects	Drugs that decrease effects
Acetylcholine	Carbachol, neostigmine, physostigmine, cholinesterase inhibitors, arecoline (muscarinic), black widow spider venom	Atropine, botulinum toxin, curare (blocks N-m nicotinic synapses), trimethaphan (blocks nicotinic N-n receptors)
Dopamine	l-DOPA, amphetamine, apomorphine, bromocriptine, selegiline, MAO inhibitors	Neuroleptics (e.g., thioridazine, acepromazine, risperidone), lithium
GABA	Benzodiazepines, sodium valproate	Tetanus toxin, picrotoxin, flumazenil
Noradrenaline	Alpha-adrenergics (ephedrine, phenylpropanolamine), amphetamine, MAO inhibitors	Metyrosine, reserpine, lithium, beta-blockers (pindolol, propranolol), clonidine, risperidone
Serotonin	Tryptophan, selective serotonin re-uptake inhibitors, sumatriptin, MAO inhibitors, eltoprazine, buspirone	Cyproheptadine, methysergide, nicergoline, risperidone

Figure 6.4 Drugs that affect neurotransmitters.

easily startle. Classical antipsychotics may also be useful in calming anxious pets, and might be considered for pets with productive signs such as destruction, escape and agitation such as in thunderstorm phobias and separation anxiety. However, as mentioned above, they are not useful as adjuncts for behavior modification therapy.

Low levels of neuroleptics such as chlorpromazine or thioridazine may be effective at reducing anxiety associated with specific situations and, in people, are less likely to generate drug dependency. However, benzodiazepines are preferable to neuroleptics for treatment of anxiety because they more specifically target anxiety and do not have the potential for extrapyramidal signs, as do neuroleptics.

Potential side effects of phenothiazines include hypotension (due to alpha-adrenergic blockade), decreased seizure threshold, bradycardia, ataxia, and extrapyramidal signs such as muscle tremors, muscle spasms, muscle discomfort, and motor restlessness. Caution should be taken in patients with liver disease because of slow hepatic clearance.

Higher-potency neuroleptics, such as perphenazine, fluphenazine, and haloperidol are less sedating, less hypotensive, and less anticholinergic, but have a higher potential for extrapyramidal signs. They are potent and specific antagonists of amphetamine and apomorphine and bind with high affinity to D2 receptors.

They are used for psychotic and aggressive states in people and may be a consideration for some forms of aggression and stereotypies in pets, although their doses and effects have not been entirely established.

Metoclopramide and promethazine are antidopaminergic emetics that also have the potential for side effects, as other neuroleptics. Pimozide blocks D2 receptors. It is mildly sedating, mildly anticholinergic, and should be used cautiously due to the potential for extrapyramidal signs. It should not be used in patients with cardiovascular disease or respiratory diseases. Pipamerone is not available in North America but has been used for behavior therapy in pets in Europe (see Ch. 21), in combination with clomipramine for the treatment of separation anxiety and primary dissocialization and in combination with other drugs for the treatment of some sociopathies. It is a weak dopamine antagonist, which may improve disturbed sleep, social withdrawal, and symptoms of chronic schizophrenia with little chance of extrapyramidal effects. Amisulpride is also only available in Europe and selectively binds D2 and D3 receptors as well as presynaptic dopamine receptors. This presynaptic dopamine blockade may account for the clinical efficacy of amisulpride against the negative symptoms of schizophrenia at low doses. Another atypical neuroleptic available in Europe is sulpiride, which may also be effective against the negative symptoms of schizophrenia with a low incidence of adverse effects.

The atypical antipsychotics clozapine, olanzipine, and risperidone may have less potential for extrapyramidal signs since they have a lower affinity for the D2 receptor. Higher levels of D2 blockade can lead to elevated prolactin levels and extrapyramidal signs. These drugs act as both dopamine and serotonin antagonists.

Risperidone does block the D2 receptor, which may help to control the positive symptoms of schizophrenia, and the 5HT2 receptor, which may help to liberate dopamine in the cortex for the treatment of negative symptoms. It is an effective antiemetic, which lasts a full day in humans with a single oral dose. It has minimal anticholinergic, sedative, and antihistaminic effects. Clozapine is also a dopamine and serotonin antagonist. It weakly blocks D2 receptors and has the least potential of the antipsychotics for extrapyramidal effects. It is sedating and anticholinergic. Clozapine may be superior to risperidone and haloperidol in human schizophrenia patients with hostility and aggression. Because of the significant risk of agranulocytosis with clozapine in people, human patients must have a white cell and differential count prior to therapy and should be monitored weekly throughout the course of therapy. It also has the potential for gastrointestinal effects and seizures. It should be used with caution in patients with underlying cardiovascular disease. Olanzipine, a newer antipsychotic, may have less potential for agranulocytosis. It has a high affinity for 5HT2, serotonin, dopamine (D1, D2, D4), adrenergic (alpha 1), and histamine (H1) receptors. The elimination half-life in dogs is about nine hours and most excretion is through the feces. These drugs may have anti-aggressive effects in human schizophrenic patients and may therefore be a consideration for some forms of aggression, self-injurious, and hallucinatory type behaviors in dogs. Anticholinergic effects and confusion are potential side effects.

In humans, antipsychotics are used to treat schizophrenia, which can be associated with positive symptoms (hallucinations, delusions, thought disturbances) or negative symptoms (decreased motivation, decreased drive, lack of energy, decreased attentiveness, inability to experience pleasure, speech and memory problems). Drugs that treat positive symptoms primarily act to reduce dopamine activity in the limbic system. For negative symptoms, drugs that antagonize 5HT2 may help to normalize dopamine levels in the cortex. Thioridazine has been suggested for use in aberrant motor behavior including aggressiveness, flybiting, and acral lick dermatitis in dogs. French behaviorists utilize neuroleptics for a number of behavior problems (see Ch. 21). A dissociative syndrome characterized by decreased receptivity to the environment and hallucinatory type signs, similar to human schizophrenia, has been described that is treated with risperidone. Risperidone has also been used in Europe to treat recently developed sociopathies toward people. Neuroleptics have been utilized in stage 3 deprivation syndrome (deprivation depression associated with sleep disturbances and self-injurious behaviors), in separation anxiety when there are motor disturbances (pimpanerone in combination with clomipramine), in some cases of primary dissocialization, in social phobias (thioridazine or fluphenazine), and in stage 2 sociopathies toward humans (in combination with cyproterone and carbamazepine).

Combining antipsychotics with other medications: phenothiazines may be combined with anxiolytics such as benzodiazepines, but their cumulative effects are additive so that profound sedation may result. Since both tricyclic antidepressants and phenothiazines are anticholinergic, there may be an intensification of both sedative and anticholinergic effects if these drugs are used together. Since antidepressants can take several weeks to achieve the desired effect, benzodiazepines may be used concurrently in the initial stages of therapy. However, for dogs that do not respond to the benzodiazepine or become more agitated, using a phenothiazine in combination with the TCA may be helpful.

BENZODIAZEPINES

Benzodiazepines can be considered for the treatment of any condition that may have a fear or anxiety component, including fear aggression and some forms of feline inappropriate elimination. They potentiate the effects of GABA, an inhibitory neurotransmitter. Like phenothiazines, benzodiazepines lack behavioral specificity. In general they cause decreased anxiety, hyperphagia, muscle relaxation, decreased locomotor activity, and varying degrees of sedation. Benzodiazepines act as mild sedatives at low doses, as anti-anxiety agents at moderate doses, and as hypnotics at high doses. They may also act as anticonvulsants. Studies of animal models of anxiety have shown that the inhibition related to fear and anxiety can lead to a decrease in eating, drinking, and exploratory behaviors, and an increase in avoidance or aggression, while treatment with benzodiazepines leads to disinhibition resulting in increased exploration, resumption of appetite, and a decrease in avoidance and aggression. However, in some instances this disinhibition could lead to an increase in aggression.

Benzodiazepines might be used on an as-needed basis for the treatment of situational anxiety such as with thunderstorms, fireworks, car rides, visits to veterinary clinics, or the anxiety associated with departures in dogs with separation anxiety. In humans, low-potency longer-acting benzodiazepines such as clonazepam or chlordiazepoxide are more commonly used for generalized anxiety since they are less likely to produce a rebound effect between doses as might occur with the high-potency shorter-acting benzodiazepines such as alprazolam. While all of the benzodiazepines act as anxiolytic medications, muscle relaxants, and to varying degrees hypnotics (sleep-inducing agents), clonazepam, alprazolam, or perhaps diazepam might be more useful in panic attacks, either alone or in conjunction with antidepressants such as sertraline. Alpraxolam, clonazepam,

and lorazepam might be useful as adjunctive therapy in the treatment of compulsive disorders, clonazepam and chlordiazepoxide for generalized anxiety disorders, and alprazolam for agoraphobia.

Wherever possible, the benzodiazepine should be administered about an hour prior to the 'event' and repeated where necessary before the drug 'wears off.' Because it can take several weeks for drugs such as antidepressants to achieve their therapeutic effects, benzodiazepines might be used during the initial stages of antidepressant therapy to more immediately control the clinical signs. In addition, benzodiazepines can be used in conjunction with antidepressant therapy when situations of more intense anxiety arise while the pet is on antidepressant therapy. Benzodiazepines have amnesic effects so they may be useful for the short-term treatment of fearful or phobic situations but may have a detrimental effect on the success of training and behavior modification programs.

Although most benzodiazepines have similar therapeutic effects, onset of action, duration of effect, intensity of effects, and metabolism differ, so that a particular benzodiazepine might be more suited to a particular application. Benzodiazepines are absorbed unchanged from the gastrointestinal tract with the exception of clorazepate, which is converted to its intermediate metabolite nordiazepam (desmethyldiazepam) in the gastrointestinal tract prior to its absorption. Most benzodiazepines, such as diazepam, are metabolized by the liver and some have active intermediate metabolites that may be more active than the parent compounds. The metabolites are then conjugated by the liver and excreted in the urine. Nordiazepam, which in turn is converted to the active metabolite oxazepam, is an active metabolite of chordiazepoxide, diazepam, and clorazepate. Alprazolam and triazolam have short-lived metabolites with minimal activity. On the other hand, oxazepam and lorazepam have no intermediate metabolites and therefore may be safer for the obese, elderly, or those with liver disease and have less chance of residual or cumulative effects. Flurazepam, which is primarily used in people for sleep induction, has three active metabolites, is sedating, and may have a longer duration of effect. Triazolam is also used for sleep induction but has a rapid oral absorption and a shorter duration of action. Alprazolam, diazepam, and the active metabolite of clorazepate have rapid oral absorption and therefore faster initiation of effect, while oxazepam has slower oral absorption and slower onset of action. Lipid solubility also affects the rate at which the drug becomes active, with diazepam, clorazepate, and triazolam having higher lipid solubility, and chlordiazepoxide, lorazepam, oxazepam, alprazolam, and clonazepam lower solubility and slower onset of action but perhaps a more sustained effect. In humans, oxazepam and lorazepam are considered short-acting benzodiazepines, alprazolam is intermediate acting, and diazepam, chlordiazepoxide, and clorazepate are longer lasting. Clonazepam is also a long-acting benzodiazepine that has no active intermediate metabolite and is indicated for the control of seizures in humans. It may lead to less sedation than some other benzodiazepines. In general, clorazepate, clonazepam, and perhaps oxazepam, might be preferable when a longer duration of action is required.

In the past, **diazepam** has been the benzodiazepine of choice for anxiety in cats, but due to rare cases of fatal hepatopathy attributed to the drug, it is now used less frequently and with much more caution. Anorexia can be a sign that the cat is having a hepatic reaction and should be cause for immediate cessation of the drug. In cats, diazepam has been used successfully for spraying, anxiety-motivated inappropriate elimination, anxieties, and fears (including fear aggression). It has also been used successfully to stimulate appetite, to control seizures, and to treat feline hyperesthesia. As with any anxiolytics it might lead to disinhibition and an increase in aggression. Diazepam may also decrease predation through its inhibitory effect on acetylcholine. Because of the relatively short half-life in dogs (two and a half hours compared with five hours in cats), as well as the short half-life of its active metabolite nordiazepam (three hours in dogs compared

with 21 hours in cats), it has limited value for long-term use or ongoing maintenance. Since diazepam has such a short half-life in dogs (two and a half hours), it may be a useful adjunct to desensitization programs for fears and fear aggression, and may be useful for departure anxiety and noise phobias of short duration.

Alprazolam is a benzodiazepine that has indications in humans for fear and anxiety and is one of the more useful benzodiazepines for the treatment of panic situations and agoraphobia. Because of its short duration of action and high potency, it is most useful for acute fears. In pets, it has been used successfully for some forms of fear or anxiety-related aggression, but may lead to disinhibition and increased aggression. It may also be useful for pets that wake up anxious at night, and in refractory cases of feline inappropriate elimination. At low doses, it may successfully reduce fear and aggression with less effect on motor function than diazepam.

High-potency longer-acting benzodiazepines such as **clonazepam** (see anticonvulsants below) are also less sedating than diazepam. In addition to its use as an anticonvulsant, clonazepam may be useful in the treatment of panic and obsessive–compulsive disorders in people, because of its longer duration of action and less frequent dosing. **Oxazepam** is an effective appetite stimulant for cats and provides a longer duration of action than diazepam. In people oxazepam is a favored benzodiazepine in the elderly and in patients with impaired hepatic function. **Lorazepam** provides more sustained release in people but has a slower onset of action. In dogs it has been reported to maintain therapeutic blood levels for 90 minutes at a dose of 0.2 mg/kg. It has been used for the control of acute agitation and aggression in people and may be effective for an overly fearful victim cat in cases of intercat aggression.

Clorazepate might be used in pets for either its anxiolytics effects or as an adjunct to anticonvulsant therapy. It may have a longer duration of effect than other benzodiazepines, with a peak duration of effect of up to six hours. In pharmacokinetic studies, a sustained release form has been shown to have no longer duration of effect in dogs. **Chlordiazepoxide** has also been used for urine spraying in cats. Chlordiazepoxide combined with clinidium may be effective for stress-induced colitis.

In addition to sedation and hyperphagia, benzodiazepines may cause a paradoxical increase in aggression or excitement (which generally resolves within a few days). Long-term use may lead to dependence. Therefore, all benzodiazepines, particularly those of high potency, should be withdrawn slowly (e.g., 10–25% per week). This is especially true in patients administered benzodiazepines for the control of seizures, as status epilepticus may be precipitated if the drug is not tapered slowly. Behavior problems may recur when the drug is withdrawn. In one study, 91% of cases of inappropriate urination in cats recurred when the diazepam was discontinued. As mentioned, since fear may be a factor inhibiting aggression, pets on benzodiazepines may become more aggressive. Since some benzodiazepines have been associated with hepatic failure, liver function should be assessed prior to therapy and pets should be monitored closely throughout the course of therapy. Rare cases of fulminant hepatic failure, within three to five days of onset of diazepam therapy, have recently been reported in cats. Baseline screening with close attention to ALT and reassessment three to five days after onset of therapy is recommended.

Benzodiazepines are commonly used to complement behavioral modification techniques such as desensitization, controlled flooding, and conditioning techniques. In general, short-acting high-potency benzodiazepines such as alprazolam are preferred for acute fear situations such as those associated with a visit to the veterinarian, car travel, or a temporary visitor to the home, while longer-acting benzodiazepines such as clorazepate or chlordiazepoxide might be used for ongoing treatment of anxiety. Although there is now a reluctance to use benzodiazepines in cats due to the potential for liver toxicity, they may be the most effective drugs at reducing anxiety and may be most practical to induce appetite for counterconditioning programs. Perhaps the choice of oxazepam or lorazepam may reduce this potential for toxicity.

Although drugs such as tricyclic antidepressants may be more appropriate for chronic anxiety situations, such as separation anxiety, shorter-acting drugs that do not require several weeks to reach a therapeutic state, such as benzodiazepines, may be better suited to anxieties of shorter duration such as a boarding situation, thunderstorms, fireworks, or for a few days after a move or other changes in the household.

For immediate control of panic or phobic states, injectible lorazepam or the intrarectal administration of diazepam may help to gain a more calm, controlled state.

Benzodiazepines have been combined with tricyclic antidepressants or fluoxetine in people for panic attacks, obsessive–compulsive disorders, and as an adjunct to antipsychotic therapy with phenothiazines or lithium. Benzodiazepines such as alprazolam or clonazepam have been used in combination with propranolol in people for treating social phobias (e.g., stage fright), and in panic disorders that have not responded to other forms of drug therapy. Combination therapy of benzodiazepines plus tricyclic antidepressants, propranolol, or phenothiazines has also been used occasionally in veterinary medicine (e.g., separation anxiety, thunderstorm phobias).

HYPNOTICS AND SLEEP DISORDERS

Another group of benzodiazepines, the hypnotics, exert their effects on sleep. The goal of use of these medications is to help re-establish a proper sleep schedule over the short term. In general benzodiazepines decrease REM sleep. Disruption of stage 4 sleep by benzodiazepines may suppress the release of growth hormone. In people, the primary use for hypnotic benzodiazepines such as flurazepam and triazolam is for the treatment of insomnia. Flurazepam has rapid absorption, a long half-life, and may sedate during the next day (in people). At low doses it may not affect REM sleep in humans. Triazolam has slower absorption and a very short half-life. When used for pets that wake during the night, flurazepam may be preferable if pets wake too early on triazolam or alprazolam. Triazolam has also been reported to be effective in some cases of aggression in cats. Benzodiazepine marketed for anxiety can also be used for sleep induction. Clorazepate, diazepam, clordiazepoxide, and clonazepam resemble flurazepam but may have a faster onset of action and shorter duration. Clonazepam may also be a useful sleep agent, because it decreases REM sleep while stage 4 sleep is increased on the night of medication but decreased the night following medication (in humans). It might be most useful when cognitive decline or other forms of neurological disease are associated with decreased sleep. Oxazepam may help to sustain sleep but is not an effective sleep inducer. Sedating antihistamines such as diphenylhydramine and cyproheptadine may also induce sleep. Similarly, amitriptyline, doxepin, and trazodone may be effective. Trazodone may increase sleep time, decrease night-time waking, but unlike tricyclic antidepressants may not increase stage 4 sleep. Neuroleptics such as thioradazine and acepromazine may cause sedation and help pets to sleep. Tryptophan, although now off the market as a human supplement, may also be effective for inducing sleep, and melatonin has been useful in people with jet lag to re-establish normal sleep–wake schedules (see Ch. 7 for more on alternative therapy). Other sleep disorders include enuresis and night terrors. These may be improved with tricyclic antidepressant therapy (amitriptyline, nortriptyline, or imipramine), or perhaps with benzodiazepines. Natural therapies such as valerian, kava, and melatonin may also be useful (see Ch. 7 on alternative therapy).

Zolpidem (USA) and zopiclone (Canada) are non-benzodiazepine hypnotics. Although they may also be useful for sleep induction, dose and duration for dogs and cats has not been established. It appears that for zolpidem, low doses such as 0.2 mg/kg may be effective but, as with benzodiazepines, paradoxical excitation including hyperactivity and tachycardia may be seen, especially at higher doses (0.6 mg/kg). These drugs may have less residual effects than some of the hypnotic benzodiazepines. In addition to its hypnotic effect, zopiclone may

have muscle relaxant, anxioloytic, and anti-aggressive activity and at higher doses may lead to sedation.

ANTICONVULSANTS

The most commonly used anticonvulsant in veterinary medicine is phenobarbital, although KBr (potassium bromide) is quickly gaining increased favor as a first choice therapeutic by veterinary neurologists. Anticonvulsants have few applications for clinical veterinary behavior, unless an epileptic component to the behavior problem (psychomotor epilepsy) is suspected. Spinning in Bull Terriers, hyperesthesia syndrome in cats, and sporadic behavior changes with no obvious stimuli (e.g., so-called 'rage' syndromes) may be responsive to anticonvulsants. Phenobarbital may also be useful for mild cases of overactivity and excessive vocalization. It may be useful in combination with other drugs such as clomipramine or propranolol for conditions such as separation anxiety and some forms of aggression. Reported side effects of phenobarbital and propranolol combinations include increased thirst and night wetting in spayed bitches. Phenobarbital may reduce the effects of beta-blockers while antihistamines and phenothiazines may potentiate the sedative effects of phenobarbital. During initiation of therapy, ataxia and sedation may be noticed, which generally resolve with continued treatment. Lipemia and hepatotoxicity may develop with long-term use.

Clonazepam, clorazepate, and carbamazepine are three other anticonvulsants that may have behavioral applications in veterinary medicine. Clonazepam and clorazepate may be useful where the chronic use of a benzodiazepine is needed for the treatment of generalized anxiety states in dogs and cats, and may be useful in the control of behavioral signs that are associated with partial complex seizures. Clonazepam may be used for the first three to four weeks of antidepressant therapy for severe anxiety, phobic and panic disorders, until the full effect of the antidepressant can be achieved. Clonazepam has a slower onset of action and may be safer for pets with compromised hepatic function since it has no active intermediate metabolite. Peak concentrations are achieved in one to three hours. The elimination half-life is approximately one to two hours at low doses, but with higher doses and long-term therapy, therapeutic serum concentrations for seizure control (as established for humans) seem to be maintained with a dose of approximately 0.5 mg/kg bid to tid. It may be effective in the treatment of panic disorders. Clorazepate has a more rapid onset of action and has not been associated with the anticonvulsant tolerance that may be seen with clonazepam. These drugs can be used in combination with phenobarbital or KBr for seizure control, but doses of both clonazepam and clorazepate may need to be increased if treating concurrently with phenobarbital, which increases their elimination through microsomal enzyme induction. Due to the possibility of physical dependence, withdrawal should be gradual. Signs of abrupt withdrawal might include 'wet dog shakes,' increased temperature, listlessness, and seizures.

Anticonvulsants such as gabapentin and carbamazepine might also be useful in the treatment of neuropathic and chronic pain disorders and in mood disorders (discussed in Ch. 9). **Gabapentin** is structurally similar to GABA, but unlike GABA it has been formulated to cross the blood–brain barrier. However, gabapentin does not appear to have any effect on GABA receptors and may actually affect the glutamate system. In addition to its anticonvulsant effect, gabapentin might be useful in behavior therapy for the treatment of generalized anxiety disorders, mood disorders, panic disorder, and as adjunctive therapy in compulsive disorders. It may also be effective in some cases of neuropathic or chronic pain that have not been responsive to opioid or NSAID therapy. Gabapentin is not metabolized in humans but 40% is metabolized to N-methyl gabapentin in the liver in dogs. The parent compound and intermediate metabolite are excreted in the kidneys so dose adjustments might be needed in renal patients. The mean elimination half-life in dogs is two to four hours and the time to achieve steady-state concentration is less than a day.

Therapeutic range is reported at 4–16 μg/ml for seizure control. The dose can be gradually increased if necessary to a dose maximum of 1200 mg over three to four weeks to achieve and maintain clinical effects. Since self-mutilatory disorders may have a pain component either as a cause or maintaining factor, a treatment trial with gabapentin might be warranted.

Carbamazepine is a tricyclic compound, similar to imipramine in structure, that has been used as a mood stabilizer, anticonvulsant, and for neuropathic pain, specifically trigeminal neuritis in humans. Carbamazepine may also be useful in the treatment of compulsive disorders and aggression due to anxiety or frustration. In addition to the treatment of seizures in people, it is also used in the treatment of depression, mania, and for some explosive aggressive states (episodic dyscontrol), as well as aggression and other behavioral changes associated with temporal lobe epilepsy or other organic diseases. In animals, carbamazepine is slightly sedating, mildly anticholinergic, and does not cause significant muscle relaxation. In the European literature (see Ch. 21) it has been used in the treatment of canine aggression associated with social deprivation syndrome, in excitable, irritable, and aggressive forms of sociopathies toward people or other dogs. In cats, carbamazepine has been found to reduce some forms of fear-induced aggression, and may make individual cats more affectionate toward people. However, as with other drugs that reduce the inhibitory effects of fear, aggression toward other cats within the home is a potential adverse effect. In cases where psychomotor epilepsy might be a component of the problem, a trial with an anticonvulsant such as carbamazepine might also be warranted. The drug is monitored in people by maintaining therapeutic plasma ranges of 4–10 mg/ml. Both in people and in feline case studies, clinical response may be achieved with lower levels. Since the drug induces its own metabolism, reduction in blood levels may occur after a month of therapy. Side effects in people include ataxia, clonic/tonic convulsions, gastrointestinal upset, and locomotor difficulties. The drug is contraindicated in patients with known renal, hepatic, cardiovascular, or hematological disorders, and should not be used in pets kept for reproductive purposes. It has a short elimination half-life and dosing can be further complicated by the fact that the drug induces its own metabolism so that higher doses may be required to maintain effect over time. In humans, there is a risk for agranulocytosis and aplastic anemia, so that regular blood monitoring should be recommended. Other uses for gabapentin and carbamazepine for pain control are discussed in Chapter 9.

BETA-BLOCKERS

Since fear leads to the release of the neurotransmitter noradrenaline, beta-blockers such as propranolol have been used successfully to treat some forms of anxiety. By blocking beta-adrenergic activity, the physical symptoms of anxiety (rapid heart rate, increased respiratory rate, muscle tremors, palpitations, sweating, trembling, gastrointestinal upset) are decreased. Without these signals of fear, the fear response is diminished but there may only be mild improvement in psychological symptoms. Although they are seldom effective for generalized anxiety or panic situations, beta-blockers have been used successfully in people with situational or performance anxiety (e.g., stage fright), sometimes referred to as 'fight or flight' situations. They may also be useful in combination with anxiolytics medications for other forms of fear and anxiety.

Beta-blockers have been shown to suppress the offensive aggression of mice toward intruders. Propranolol may also act at central beta-adrenergic sites and may also inhibit aggression by elevating serotonin at the synaptic level. Since catecholamines are likely to lower the threshold for aggression, beta-blockers may be useful in reducing affective aggression, but this effect has not been validated in aggressive pets. Propranolol has been used in conjunction with benzodiazepines in people for social fears and phobias and in panic disorders that have not improved with benzodiazepines or antidepressants. It might also be combined with benzodiazepines, buspirone, SSRIs, or tricyclic antidepressants in dogs and cats for the treatment of fears, anxiety, and phobias (especially when there are strong somatic signs). Propranolol has also been combined with phenobarbital to control the behavioral signs in some canine cases of fears and phobias. Beta-blockers are contraindicated in pets with bradycardia, congestive heart failure, diabetes, or pulmonary diseases including asthma.

Since pindolol has more effect on serotonin receptors, it may have a central effect on aggression. Potential side effects of pindolol are panting, increased anxiety, and urinary incontinence. Studies in humans have shown an improved response to depression with pindolol plus fluoxetine vs fluoxetine alone. Pindolol is a mixed beta-agonist/antagonist. It may stimulate 5HT1A receptors, thereby increasing serotonin neuronal transmission at an earlier stage than would normally be observed with an SSRI alone. By blocking presynaptic autoreceptors, the initial down-regulation associated with reuptake inhibitors may be prevented. This results in augmentation and acceleration of the antidepressant effect of the SSRIs (i.e., accelerated antidepressant response). Propranolol has a short half-life in dogs, but longer-acting beta-blockers such as nadolol and atenolol do not cross the blood–brain barrier as readily and therefore would offer less central effect.

OTHER ANXIOLYTICS

Buspirone, an azapirone, is a selective anxiolytic that produces minimal side effects. It is a serotonin (5HT1A) receptor agonist, serving to enhance the neurotransmission of serotonin. It also acts as a dopamine (D2) antagonist. Its pharmacologically active metabolite, 1-pyrimidylpiperazine, is an a2-adrenoreceptor antagonist. It has been shown to be a relatively successful drug in controlling feline urine spraying. In one study, it was found to be effective in reducing feline urine marking in over 50% of cases, with less recurrence after withdrawal than drugs such as diazepam. The drug may be effective in the reduction of fearful conditions as well as the treatment of aggressive and compulsive disorders. Buspirone may be useful in reducing fear and building the confidence of an overly fearful pet, in its relationship with people or other pets. As with other anxiolytics, treatment with buspirone can lead to disinhibition and an increase in aggression. Buspirone is not indicated for the treatment of panic disorders and has not proven to be particularly effective in veterinary practice for pets with intense fears, anxiety, or phobias. In general it is considered a mild anxiolytic, which may 'take the edge off anxiety.' It may be useful in conjunction with SSRIs or clomipramine for the treatment of compulsive disorders, or even in combination with benzodiazepines for the treatment of some anxiety disorders. Buspirone produces no significant sedation or muscle relaxation and does not impair motor function, so that it is a good first choice for mild chronic fears and anxieties, which may have some similarity to generalized anxiety disorders or social phobias in humans. Since it does not lead to dependence, it is more likely that a pet can be withdrawn from buspirone (compared with a benzodiazepine) without recurrence of the problem. Major drawbacks of buspirone are its expense and the fact that one to four weeks may required to achieve clinical efficacy. It is also ineffective in cases where sedation, muscle relaxation, appetite stimulation, or an immediate anxiolytic effect are needed. Since it is dosed twice daily in cats, paroxetine or clomipramine might be more practical for owners of cats that are difficult to medicate.

Meprobamate was a favored anti-anxiety drug in the 1950s, but has since been replaced by more specific anxiolytics such as benzodiazepines and buspirone. It produces marked CNS depression and muscle relaxation, and at higher doses may impair learning. It may be useful in reducing aggression and anxiety, particularly when therapy with other anxiolytics produces excessive agitation or when more profound sedation is required. It is also useful in the treatment of insomnia in people. In addition to excessive drowsiness and ataxia, meprobamate can cause hypotension and drug dependence.

Clonidine is a noradrenergic agonist that stimulates central postsynaptic a2-receptors causing inhibition of vasomotor centers and decreased noradrenergic transmission. Although originally developed as an antihypertensive agent, it has been used in child psychiatry for the treatment of tics, Tourette's syndrome, ADHD, and aggression. Clonidine administration has been shown to inhibit firing of the locus ceruleus noradrenergic neurons in cats. Clonidine is sedating. In dogs, clonidine led to greatly increased non-REM sleep (43 times more potent than morphine), followed by a rebound waking. It is used for the treatment of hypertension but may have some behavioral effects on generalized anxiety, compulsive disorders, panic disorders, and phobias because of its effects on noradrenergic transmission. Other than hypotension, side effects in humans include sleep disturbances, excitation, and decreased concentration.

ANTIHISTAMINES

Antihistamines may be useful for the treatment of pruritus, self-trauma, and anxiety. Those antihistamines that have sedative CNS effects (hydroxyzine, chlorpheniramine, diphenhydramine, trimeprazine) may also be useful in situations of mild anxiety or overactivity, or to help induce sleep. Anxiety associated with car rides, excessive vocalization, and undesirable nighttime activity are conditions that may respond to antihistamine therapy. They may also be useful as a postoperative sedative, and for anxiety associated with pruritus. Since these antihistamines are anticholinergic, pet owners should be warned that they may cause a dry mouth and constipation, and are contraindicated in patients with glaucoma, urine retention, or hyperthyroidism. Cyproheptadine, an antihistamine with antiserotonergic effects, may also be an effective appetite stimulant in cats and dogs and may be useful for inducing sleep. It has also been used with variable success to treat urine spraying in cats. A number of the tricyclic antidepressants (discussed below) also have fairly strong antihistaminic effects. Therefore a drug such as doxepin might be useful for its combined mood elevating and antihistaminic effects when there is self-trauma.

SEROTONIN AGONISTS

The development of 5HT1A agonists such as eltoprazine held promise for the treatment of aggression. Early reports indicated decreased aggression in dogs and in a study of social hierarchy in young pigs, but plans for further development have been discontinued. Drugs that enhance serotonin transmission may reduce offensive aggression, while leaving defensive aggression, social, and exploratory behaviors intact. It does not sedate, nor lead to muscle relaxation. The partial 5HT1A/B agonist buspirone is discussed separately under other anxiolytics (above).

HORMONAL THERAPY

Synthetic progestins have been used for many years to treat feline inappropriate urination and some forms of anxiety and aggression. They are anti-androgenic, and cause non-specific depression of the CNS and an increase in appetite. However, because of their effects on the endocrine system, numerous unacceptable side effects may result. High doses or long-term use may lead to diabetes mellitus, adrenocortical suppression, bone marrow suppression, acromegaly, endometrial hyperplasia, pyometra, and mammary hyperplasia and carcinomas. Behavioral use of progestins should be avoided in intact females and, whenever possible, other drugs should be used first. When all else fails, progestins may be an effective treatment for controlling aggression (e.g., dominance aggression in dogs, territorial aggression in cats), and for cases of feline spraying, anxiety-motivated inappropriate urination, and psychogenic alopecia that are refractory to anti-anxiety agents. Progestins may also be the drug of choice for sexually dimorphic behaviors that do not respond to castration or when castration is contraindicated.

Since the presence of male hormones can lead to an increase in sexually dimorphic behaviors (such as mounting, mating, masturbation, roaming, urine marking, and perhaps some forms of aggression), there is some question as to whether drugs that might reduce the effects of androgens could also have an effect on behavior. Finasteride inhibits the conversion of testosterone into dihydrotestosterone so that both intra-prostatic and circulating DHT levels are reduced. However in clinical trials in males treated with finasteride for BPH there is little or no decline in libido and in canine studies there was no effect on serum testosterone. Delmadinone is an androgen antagonist that leads to suppression of secretory activity of the prostate gland but does not lead to lower serum DHT levels. Since neither of these drugs appear to lower circulating testosterone levels they are not likely to have any significant effect on reduction of androgen-influenced behaviors. Cyproterone acetate blocks the binding of dihydrotestosterone to the receptors in the prostate and decreases the production of LH so that testicular testosterone production is inhibited. It has been used for some androgen-influenced behavior problems and as a test of the effect that castration might achieve in a male dog. A dose of 3–5 mg/kg has been suggested. Leuprolide acetate and goserelin are gondandotropin-releasing hormone analogs which, after an initial short-term hormonal increase, lead to a suppression of ovarian and testicular steroid production (and likely adrenal sex steroid production) with chronic use. In effect, testosterone production is reduced to castrate levels so that these products may give a more true assessment of the effects of castration. Leuprolide has been used to treat adrenal disease in ferrets at a dose of 100 µg i.m. per month. A dose of 3.6 mg of depot goserelin has been shown to drastically reduce the blood levels of estradiol in females and testosterone in males after three weeks, and the duration of effect was three to five weeks. In female dogs with mammary cancer a dose of 60 µg/kg of depot goserelin every 21 days for 12 months decreased estradiol and progesterone levels, with no apparent toxic effects.

Diethylstilbestrol is used for the treatment of estrogen-responsive incontinence in spayed female dogs by increasing sphincter tone. Estrogens, however, can be toxic to the bone marrow and cause blood dyscrasias so that the lowest effective dose should be utilized and complete blood counts should be monitored regularly. Incontinence in neutered male dogs has been successfully treated with repository parenteral treatment of testosterone propionate, since most oral testosterone is rapidly broken down by the liver. The prostate should be regularly assessed in dogs undergoing testosterone therapy. Potential side effects are the development, aggravation, or recurrence of sexually dimorphic male behaviors. Testosterone and estrogen depletion may also be related to cognitive decline and possibly mood disorders (see Ch. 12 for details). It is as yet undetermined whether hormone replacement therapy might help to prevent or slow the progress of cognitive decline, or would lead to improvement of clinical signs. However, in old dogs with cognitive decline, estrogen-treated females made significantly fewer errors in size-reversal learning tasks but made more errors in spatial memory tasks.

DOPAMINE AGONISTS

Dopamine agonists such as bromocriptine directly stimulate dopaminergic postsynaptic receptors in the brain, which inhibits prolactin release from the anterior pituitary. In cats, bromocriptine has been reported to reduce urine spraying. Side effects include increased affection, prolapsed nictitating membranes, and inappetance for 24–48 hours. Oral tablets are available but exact dose rates have not been determined. It is thought that steady-state plasma levels are reached in 10 days and that the medication should be given twice daily for four to eight weeks. In humans the drug may cause dizziness, hypotension, and nausea (so it should be taken with food), and transient elevations in alanine aminotransferase (ALT), creatinine phosphokinase (CPK), blood urea nitrogen (BUN), aspartate aminotransferase (AST), and serum alkaline phosphatase (SAP). Bromocriptine may also be useful in the treatment of false pregnancy in dogs and in occasional cases of pituitary-dependent hyperadrenocorticism. Vomiting, diarrhea, hypotension (especially with the first dose), and behavior changes such as sedation and fatigue have been observed in dogs.

Cabergoline, which is not presently available in North America, is under investigation for the treatment of Parkinson's disease and prolactinomas of the pituitary gland in humans and may enhance sexual activity. It is a D2 receptor agonist that leads to decreased prolactin levels. It has been shown to reduce the signs of false pregnancy in dogs at a dose of 5 µg daily for five days in the food with a termination of the anestrus stage and an earlier return to proestrus.

ALPHA-ADRENERGICS

Alpha-adrenergics (sympathetic agonists) decrease incontinence by increasing urethral sphincter tone in cases of urethral incompetence. Once the pet regains urethral competence, the amount and frequency of administration should be decreased gradually to the lowest effective dose. Some pets become refractory to long-term use so that increased doses may ultimately be required. Phenylpropanolamine may also be helpful for excitement urination. Ephedrine may also be successful, although phenylpropanolamine is used more frequently since it is generally more effective and has fewer cardiovascular side effects. Phenylpropanolamine therapy has recently been removed from the human market because of the potential for hemorrhagic strokes. Side effects in pets might include bronchodilation, restlessness, hypertension, excitability, anxiety, panting, anorexia, irritability, tremors, and cardiac arrhythmias. These drugs are contraindicated in patients with glaucoma, prostatic hypertrophy, hyperthyroidism, diabetes mellitus, cardiovascular disorders, or hypertension. Antidepressants with anticholinergic and alpha-adrenergic effects, such as imipramine, may also be effective in the treatment of urethral incompetence.

ALPHA-ADRENERGIC ANTAGONISTS

Alpha-adrenergic antagonists inhibit peripheral vasoconstriction. A product called nicergoline has been released in the UK with claims of acting as a neuroprotective agent and increasing cerebral blood flow. It is recommended for dogs with age-related behavioral changes, decreased vigor, sleep disorders, and psychomotor disturbances. The product comes as a freeze-dried tablet; because of this format, the tablet cannot be broken for dosing small dogs. The company provides instructions for converting the product into a solution for dosing very small animals. Each tablet contains 5 mg nicergoline.

OPIATE ANTAGONISTS AND AGONISTS

Opiate peptides are released during stress and conflict. The activation of narcotic receptors may in themselves lead to some stereotypic behaviors. In addition, opioids activate the dopamine system, which may in turn lead to compulsive or stereotypic behaviors. Release of opioids may reinforce these behaviors. Endogenous opioids may also induce analgesia, reducing the pain that might otherwise inhibit self-mutilation. Thus, opiate (endorphin) receptor blockers may be effective in reducing some compulsive stereotypic behaviors, especially those that have been ongoing for a relatively short time. The resultant increase in pain perception may further reduce self-mutilation. Narcotic antagonists have been variably effective in the treatment of a number of compulsive and stereotypic disorders, such as self-mutilation, acral lick dermatitis, tail chasing, and flank sucking in Doberman Pinschers. Naltrexone can be given orally, but most other opiate antagonists or mixed agonists–antagonists are only available in injectible form. A trial with naltrexone would indicate its effectiveness, however, the drug may not be practical for long-term therapy because of its expense. It has also been found that supplying an exogenous source of opioids, such as hydrocodone, may be successful in the treatment of some self-mutilatory behaviors such as acral lick dermatitis.

LITHIUM SALTS

Lithium salts (lithium carbonate and lithium citrate) are used in the treatment of bipolar disorders and depression and explosive behavior disorders including aggression in people. Lithium may decrease the turnover of dopamine and reduce the functional activity of postsynaptic beta-adrenoreceptors. It may also enhance the effects of serotonin and increase acetylcholine synthesis. Lithium has been utilized for some forms of unpredictable severe aggression in dogs, but it is highly toxic and has a narrow window of efficacy. It therefore requires careful monitoring. If psychotic-type disorders truly exist in companion animals then lithium may be an appropriate treatment. In the European diagnoses (see Ch. 21), lithium has been used to treat a dysthymia of Cocker Spaniels associated with unipolar and bipolar disorders and possessive aggression. Lithium may be useful in combination with benzodiazepines or tricyclic antidepressants when these drugs alone have been unsuccessful in the treatment of stereotypic or compulsive behaviors. An ECG, blood profile, urinalysis, and thyroid level should be assessed prior to treatment and the drug should be avoided in patients with renal, cardiac, or thyroid disease. Therapeutic blood levels should be monitored and maintained in the range of 0.8–1.2 meq/l. Blood levels of lithium, kidney function, thyroid function, CBC, and EKGs should be monitored throughout the course of therapy. Potential side effects in humans include gastrointestinal upset, polyuria, weight gain, hypothyroidism, tremors, diabetes insipidus, and renal failure. Lithium toxicity can occur in humans if blood levels reach greater than 1.5 meq/l, so that levels should be maintained below this value if lithium is utilized in dogs and cats. In cats and dogs toxic signs include diarrhea, vomiting, hypotension, respiratory depression, and CNS effects including depression, muscle tremors, seizures, or coma.

MAO (MONOAMINE OXIDASE) INHIBITORS

Monoamine oxidase is an enzyme that metabolizes noradrenaline, dopamine, and serotonin. MAO inhibitors (e.g., phenelzine, isocarboxazid, tranylcypromine) inhibit both MAO A and MAO B and are irreversible in their actions. They cause elevations of the monoamine neurotransmitters, and are therefore used in the treatment of depression and phobic states in humans. Drugs such as phenelzine are an effective treatment for social phobias, anxiety, eating and panic disorders in humans. Therefore they may also be effective in some phobic and anxiety conditions in animals. However, they must be prescribed cautiously because they may have a number of side effects, including gastrointestinal upset, anticholinergic effects, insomnia, restlessness, sedation, and the potential for hypertensive crises. As with other antidepressants a therapeutic effect may not be achieved for up to four weeks.

Most MAO inhibitors non-selectively inhibit both MAO A and B, and have few animal applications. Since MOA inhibitors prevent the breakdown of adrenaline, noradrenaline, and serotonin, they are used to treat depression and some panic and phobic states in humans. They are less anticholinergic and less sedating than tricyclic antidepressants, but have the potential for greater side effects and may interact with a number of drugs that enhance the serotonin system (such as SSRIs and some TCAs), as well as foods that are rich in tyramine (such as cheese and wine) to precipitate a hypertensive crisis. Tyramine is normally inactivated by MAO in the gut. However, when non-selective irreversible MAO inhibitors are administered, tyramine may not be inactivated. This may lead to an increase in noradrenaline release leading to vasoconstriction and an increase in blood pressure. MAO inhibitors should not be taken concurrently and tyramine-containing compounds (e.g., cheese) must be avoided or decreased during MAO therapy. Adverse reactions include CNS stimulation, hepatotoxicity, dizziness, hypertension, or hypotension, dry mouth, blurred vision, and constipation. Newer selective reversible inhibitors of MAO such as meclobemide are far less likely to precipitate a hypertensive crisis and may therefore be a safer and more practical treatment option. However, they can lead to insomnia at night and daytime lethargy.

The drug selegiline (also known as l-deprenyl) selectively inhibits MAO B in the dog at therapeutic levels. Although no absolute increase in brain dopamine levels has been demonstrated in the dog, it may enhance dopamine transmission by inhibiting dopamine reuptake and by increasing phenylethylamine levels (which is a facilitator of dopamine activity). Selegiline may also enhance the release of norepinephrine. Selegiline also activates superoxide dismutase (which is elevated in the dog after selegiline therapy) and catalase, two enzymes which are responsible for removing free radicals. It may itself be a potent free radical scavenger. Because free radicals cause cell injury and may contribute to brain pathology and signs of aging, it has been hypothesized that selegiline decreases nerve damage and degeneration. Recent studies in several laboratories have confirmed that selegiline also exhibits 'rescue' of CNS and peripheral neurons damaged by trauma or neurotoxins. In fact, pretreatment with selegiline has been shown to prevent the damage caused by dopaminergic, serotonergic, and cholinergic toxins. Additional details on selegiline and its application for geriatric behavior problems are discussed in Chapter 12.

In both laboratory studies and field trials, selegiline has been found to improve cognitive function in aging dogs, and may be useful in the treatment of disrupted sleep–wake cycles, indifference to the environment, decreased responsiveness to commands, decreased attentiveness and activity, weakness or stiffness, and geriatric-onset housesoiling with no concurrent organic disease. Selegiline may also be effective in the treatment of some forms of pituitary-dependent hyperadrenocorticism (PDH), which may result from hypothalamic dopamine depletion. Dopamine inhibits the release of adrenocorticotropic hormone (ACTH), so that lack of dopamine would lead to oversecretion of ACTH. Administration of selegiline may promote normalization of dopamine levels, thus ameliorating clinical signs and returning balance of the hypothalamic–pituitary–adrenal (HPA) axis. Selegiline may also be effective in suppressing cataplexy in cases of canine narcolepsy. Selegiline is licensed in North America for the treatment of canine cognitive dysfunction and PDH. In Europe it is licensed for the treatment of emotional disorders as diagnosed in part by the EDED scale, which measures the combined effects of internal factors and response to external stimuli (see Fig. 21.3). Improvement has been reported in feeding, drinking, and sleeping disorders, physical signs such as tachycardia, diarrhea, and acral lick dermatitis, and to a lesser extent, learned and exploratory behavior. Syndromes based on the French diagnostic criteria that might be improved include the hypersensitivity–hyperactivity disorder, generalized phobic states, and emotional disorders with components of fear aggression, separation, and overattachment problems. To date, there have been no published studies on the efficacy of selegiline in geriatric cats, although there have been numerous reports of its efficacy for cognitive dysfunction and for emotional disorders in cats. Signs of cognitive dysfunction that might be improved include disorientation, increased anxiety, decreased responsiveness to owners and other stimuli, decreased nocturnal activity and vocalization, and decreased grooming and appetite. It has also been advocated by European behaviorists for the treatment of emotional disorders in cats including productive signs (such as aggression, insomnia, and bulimia) and deficit signs (such as anorexia and increased sleep). Improvement has been reported in cats with territorial aggression, fear or fear aggression, reduced appetite, compulsive licking, night waking, housesoiling and spraying, excessive vocalization, and overactivity. There was little effect on hyperattachment or predatory aggression, and no side effects were noted. A small study of four cats found no toxicity in cats at up to 10 mg/kg (10–20 times the typical clinical dose), with the only side effects being occasional vomition and excessive salivation at the highest dose.

In healthy laboratory dogs, spontaneous behavior was unaffected by once-daily oral doses below 3 mg/kg, while at higher doses there was stereotypical responding characterized by increased locomotion and decreased exploratory behavior (sniffing). These behavioral effects were thought to be due to increased levels of phenylethylamine resulting from inhibition of MAO B and/or dopaminergic enhancement by l-amphetamine metabolites of selegiline. It is important to note that the amphetamine that is a metabolite of selegiline is l-amphetamine and not d-amphetamine (which is a much more potent inducer of stereotypy). Gastrointestinal upset is occasionally seen, but usually improves when the drug is discontinued for a few days or may be avoided by using a lower starting dose. Hyperactivity and restlessness have also occasionally been reported. Toxicity has been reported on rare occasions in humans when selegiline is used concurrently with antidepressants, ephedrine, phenylpropanolamine, narcotics, or other MAO inhibitors (including amitraz). Therefore, these combinations should also be avoided in dogs.

CNS STIMULANTS

In some cases of overactivity disorders, learning deficits, and aggression in dogs, stimulants may have a paradoxical calming effect, in much the same way as they do for attention deficit disorders in humans. Of course these stimulants would generally have an activating effect and are therefore contraindicated in dogs that are displaying overactivity or aggression from other causes. Stimulants enhance the release of dopamine and block dopamine and norepinephrine re-uptake. This might then help to enhance inhibitory output from the frontal lobe to improve concentration and impulse control and decrease motor activity. Occasionally the less serotonergic antidepressants such as the tricyclic antidepressants or selegiline may also be useful in cases of ADHD. Most cases of hyper-activity are not due to any physiological disorders. In humans, attention deficit disorders (ADD) may or may not be associated with hyperactivity (ADHD). Attention deficit disorders in humans are associated with lack of impulse control, overactivity, and lack of attention, which interferes with the ability to learn. Hyperkinetic dogs have been reported to exhibit overactivity (barking, chewing, pacing), tachycardia, panting, salivation, lack of trainability, aggression, and failure to calm down in neutral environments. However, it has recently been speculated that dogs without hyperactivity that show signs of repetitive behaviors, increased aggressiveness or anxiety, poor learning or inattentiveness, and perhaps GI signs might also 'suffer' from ADD.

The diagnosis of hyperkinesis can be made by administering 0.2–0.5 mg/kg dextroamphetamine orally and then observing the dog every 30 minutes for one to two hours to determine if the dog's respiratory or heart rate decreases or the dog becomes calmer. Alternatively, methylphenidate can be prescribed for three days at 0.5 mg/kg in the morning and early afternoon. The target behaviors (repetitive behaviors, aggression, anxiety, overactivity, learning ability) and somatic signs (respiratory rate, heart rate, salivation) can then be assessed to determine if there has been any measurable improvement. If there is no improvement and there has been no aggravation of the condition, the dose can be increased by 0.25 mg/kg bid. After every three days, if there is improvement, the drug can be considered effective and the dose maintained. However, if there has been no improvement or aggravation of the condition the dose can be increased by another 0.25 mg/kg bid to a maximum daily dose of 2.0 mg/kg bid. In one European trial of dogs with signs of hypersensitivity–hyperactivity disorder (see Ch. 21 for details), about 55% of the dogs improved with methylphenidate therapy. Some of the dogs improved on fluvoxamine, selegiline, or sertraline therapy. CNS stimulants may also be indicated for narcolepsy.

ANTIDEPRESSANTS

Included in this category are the tricyclic antidepressants or TCAs (e.g., clomipramine, amitriptyline, doxepin, imipramine, and protriptyline), tetracyclic antidepressants such as mianserine, and the selective serotonin re-uptake inhibitors, SSRIs (e.g., fluoxetine, paroxetine, fluvoxamine, sertraline, and citalopram). Their primary function is as a stimulating or mood-elevating drug for the depressed human patient, who may have alterations in serotonin, norepinephrine, or to a lesser extent dopamine transmission. For depression in humans, the efficacy of SSRIs is similar to TCAs, however, the SSRIs may be better tolerated and have a lower dropout rate than tricyclic antidepressants such as amitriptyline and imipramine.

Since each antidepressant (or at least each class of antidepressant) may have markedly different effects on the neurotransmitters and receptors on which they may have an effect, the side effects and possible indications and applications may vary greatly between antidepressants. For example, the tricyclic antidepressants may have varying effects on the inhibition of re-uptake of serotonin and/or noradrenaline, as well as some effect on the histaminic, cholinergic, and alpha-adrenergic receptors. In general, blocking noradrenaline re-uptake should have an activating effect, while blocking serotonin re-uptake should have a calming effect. Antidepressants also produce varying degrees of sedation depending on the degree of anticholinergic, antihistaminic, and alpha-adrenergic blockade effects they produce. Alpha-adrenergic blockade may also lead to tachycardia, while cholinergic blockade may lead to a dry mouth, urine retention, constipation, or tachycardia. Doxepin and amitriptyline produce the strongest antihistaminic effects so that they may be particularly useful when sedative or antipruritic effects are desired. Of the tricyclic antidepressants, clomipramine is the most potent inhibitor of serotonin re-uptake relative to its effects on noradrenaline re-uptake. Clomipramine is metabolized to desmethylclomipramine, which inhibits to a lesser extent noradrenaline uptake.

Since clomipramine is licensed for use in dogs, its pharmacokinetics have been well documented and this work helps to establish a clear warning about psychotropic drug use in pets. As previously mentioned, one cannot assume that the metabolism and effects of an individual drug on a dog or cat will have the same effect as in humans. For example, when clomipramine is metabolized to desmethylclomipramine in dogs the ratio of clomipramine to desmethylclomipramine is higher (3:1) than it is in humans (1:2.5). Because of this lower desmethylclomipramine effect in dogs, less anticholinergic effects and less effect on noradrenaline transmission might also be expected. On the other hand, because of its effects on serotonin re-uptake, clomipramine may be effective in conditions where other TCAs might not, such as in the treatment of compulsive disorders. Selective serotonin re-uptake inhibitors (fluoxetine, sertraline, fluvoxamine, paroxetine, citalopram) primarily affect serotonin re-uptake, although fluoxetine and paroxetine might have a mild effect on noradrenaline re-uptake and sertraline might have a moderate effect on dopamine re-uptake. Antidepressants that inhibit noradrenaline uptake and have less effect on serotonin re-uptake, such as desipramine and protriptyline, may produce a more rapid response and might be better for pets that would benefit from mild stimulation. The anticholinergic and alpha-adrenergic effects of imipramine and amitriptyline may also be useful in the treatment of some forms of incontinence.

The primary mode of action of this category of psychotropic medications is to block 5HT or noradrenaline re-uptake into the presynaptic neuron, thereby increasing the concentration of the neurotransmitter into the synapse. They may take several weeks to achieve therapeutic effects. In humans, antidepressant response with fluoxetine is seen in about 55% of patients by two weeks, 80% of patients by four weeks, and 90% of patients by six weeks. Although it has been suggested that the time till efficacy may vary between tricyclics and SSRIs based on their half-lives and the neurotransmitters they affect, the time required to achieve the full effect, an alteration of postsynaptic receptor conformation through alteration of the cAMP pathway in the hippocampus as well as changes in serotonin transporters, would be approximately the same for all antidepressants. Initially, due to a blockade of the transporter, there is an accumulation of the neurotransmitter (serotonin or noradrenaline). The 5HT1A or noradrenaline (presynaptic) autoreceptors are stimulated, leading to a decreased firing of the central 5HT or noradrenergic neurons and a decrease in postsynaptic receptors (down-regulation). Therefore, at least initially, there is no marked increase in serotonin activity. Over a few weeks, the presynaptic receptors become desensitized, the presynaptic neuron resumes firing at a normal (or above normal) firing frequency (up-regulation), leading to increased serotonergic transmission. Long-term treatment leads to altered receptor function and structure through transcription and translation alterations in receptor proteins, a process that takes three to five weeks. Antidepressant administration leads to an increased production of the second messenger cAMP (cyclic adenosine monophosphate), increased activation of protein kinase A, and activation of the transcription factor cAMP response element binding protein (CREB). CREB activation leads to increases in the hippocampal growth factor BDNF (which is dramatically decreased in acute or chronic stress) and tyrosine kinases which stimulate mRNA transcription of new receptor proteins. It has been shown that BDNF is critical for the normal development and function of central 5HT neurons and for the elaboration of behaviors that depend on these nerve cells. The end result is that the postsynaptic neuron's metabolism and its response to the neurotransmitter (e.g., serotonin) are enhanced. Long-term potentiation of serotonin transmission has an inhibitory action on the locus ceruleus and a decrease in norepinephrine activity. Initial side effects of antidepressant therapy such as sedation, insomnia, decreased appetite, urine retention, or decreased energy level may resolve after about a week of treatment as the pet habituates to its effects.

In humans, antidepressants are utilized either alone or in combination for a variety of clinical disorders, many of which are extra-label uses. These include anxiety disorders, panic disorders, mood elevation, major depression, bipolar depression, dysthymia, anorexia nervosa, chronic bereavement, and impulsive or volatile forms of aggression as well as agoraphobia (SSRIs, imipramine), and social phobias (SSRIs, imipramine). In addition, antidepressants might be used for chronic pain disorders (amitriptyline, doxepin, desipramine, or perhaps SSRIs), obsessive–compulsive disorders (SSRIs or clomipramine), narcolepsy/cataplexy (imipramine, protriptyline and other antidepressants that suppress REM sleep), bulimia (SSRIs), premenstrual dysphoria (SSRIs, clomipramine), enuresis (imipramine, desipramine, nortriptyline, or amitriptyline), sleep walking and night terrors in children (TCAs), and for inducing sleep (amitriptyline, doxepin). In pets, antidepressants have been used successfully to treat a variety of conditions including compulsive disorders, urine marking, and some types of aggressive behavior. Antidepressants may also be successful in the treatment of chronic or recurrent fears and anxieties, but are seldom effective for acute anxieties (unless they are combined with other drugs such as beta-blockers and benzodiazepines), since they may take several weeks to reach therapeutic levels.

Antidepressants may have a number of applications in pet behavior therapy. One primary indication is for regulation of the behavior sequence. The drug may help the pet gain control of the initiation (beginning phase), termination, and intensity of the behavior. Phobias, generalized and chronic anxiety disorders, separation anxiety, panic, explosive or impulsive forms of aggression, compulsive disorders, painful disorders (such as idiopathic cystitis or self-traumatic disorders), and urine marking are just a few of the more commonly used applications where antidepressants might be considered alone or in combination with other therapeutic agents. For generalized and recurrent fears and anxieties, antidepressants may be preferable to anxiolytics since they are non-addicting, less sedating, and are unlikely to affect learning or training. However, for the immediate control of anxiety, phobias, and panic, benzodiazepines such as alprazolam or clonazepam may also be needed. These drugs could also be used concurrently or on an as-needed basis during antidepressant therapy.

Tricyclic antidepressants

Tricyclic antidepressants that might be considered most commonly for veterinary therapy would include clomipramine, amitriptyline, imipramine, and doxepin. Their primary therapeutic effect is to block re-uptake of noradrenaline and serotonin, and the extent to which each of these is affected is related to their differences in activity. Their effect on enhancing norepinephrine transmission in decreasing order of relative potency is desipramine, imipramine, amitriptyline, and clomipramine, while relative potencies for serotonin transmission are the opposite. They also have differing effects on muscarinic, adrenergic, and histaminic receptors, which would account for differing side effects. Most tricyclic antidepressants are well absorbed from the gastrointestinal tract and metabolized by the liver to an active intermediate metabolite, before excretion through the kidneys. Therefore they should be used cautiously in the elderly or when there is compromised hepatic metabolism. Since the drugs' effects on the brain last much longer than would be indicated by plasma levels, monitoring clinical efficacy through plasma levels is not generally useful, although there may be some correlation between plasma concentrations and adverse events.

Side effect profiles vary since their effects on neurotransmitters vary. Anticholinergic effects include dry mouth, constipation, urinary retention, and tachycardia, while antihistaminic effects might lead to sedation and hypotension, and alpha-adrenergic effects could lead to tachycardia and sedation. On the other hand, some side effects such as sedation or anticholinergic effects may be a potential benefit when sleep induction, sedation, or urine retention are desirable. TCAs may lead to inappetance and gastrointestinal upset. After several weeks, side effects may begin to taper off. Also, since there may be an initial period of down-regulation followed by increased serotonergic transmission and alteration of receptor conformation, there may be an initial alteration in behavior including restlessness, irritability, anxiety, or even increased aggression, which may not be indicative of the true end result. Antidepressants that activate noradrenergic systems, such as protriptyline, nortriptyline, and imipramine, may be more activating, have the potential for causing tremors and, in rare cases, an increase in anxiety or aggression.

Tricyclic antidepressants may lower the seizure threshold and may block sodium channels to the heart, leading to cardiac arrhythmias. However, in studies of pets with no pre-existing cardiac disease, tricyclic antidepressants such as clomipramine and amitriptyline had no effect on the EKG or cardiac function of dogs. TCAs are contraindicated in pets with pre-existing cardiac disease, seizures (doxepin, desipramine, or an SSRI might be safest if antidepressant therapy is necessary), glaucoma, or liver disease, and can interfere with the control of thyroid disease. Caution is needed when neuroleptics, cimetidine, and some SSRIs (except fluvoxamine) are used concurrently, since they can slow their metabolism leading to increased levels, while MAO inhibitors and antidepressants should not be used concurrently due to the potential for hypertension and serotonin syndrome.

Tricyclic antidepressants might be used in pets for the same problems as SSRIs but some (especially those that sedate) might be more effective at calming. In comparison, serotonin re-uptake inhibitors such as fluoxetine might be more likely to cause agitation and insomnia. Specific uses for TCAs might include generalized anxieties, separation anxiety, panic, phobias, urine marking in cats, and chronic anxieties with depressed mood as might arise in situations of chronic stress. Narcolepsy with

cataplexy may also be improved since tricyclic antidepressants suppress REM sleep. Since acetylcholine is a principal mediating neurotransmitter in predatory aggression, anticholinergic TCAs may be of some benefit in moderating or reducing predation. Although tricyclic antidepressants may also be useful at reducing aggression associated with anxiety or dyscontrol (impulsive, rage), a small study of the efficacy of clomipramine in dominance aggression in dogs found no improvement.

Clomipramine differs from the other tricyclic antidepressants because it is the most selective inhibitor of serotonin re-uptake. In fact, its indications and applications, in dogs and humans, more resemble those of the selective serotonin re-uptake inhibitors. Clomipramine is the only antidepressant presently licensed for use in pets, with label claims for dogs varying between countries, from generalized anxiety and separation anxiety to compulsive disorders. It may also be useful for panic, narcolepsy with cataplexy, neuropathic or chronic pain, and phobias (such as agoraphobia in humans). The only label claim for cats is in Australia, where it is licensed for urine marking. In toxicity studies, there has been no clinical effect on the EKG of healthy dogs. In a company-commissioned 28-day target safety study in which clomipramine was given to cats at up to 5 mg/kg daily, there was mild sedation and occasional pupillary dilation seen in the higher dose groups, and a slight decrease in food consumption. No other toxic effects were seen.

Other possible uses of tricyclic antidepressants in pets might include the following.

(a) **Imipramine**: for anxiety disorders, especially if there is a housesoiling component, enuresis, submissive or excitement elimination, incontinence, and narcolepsy. Other human uses for imipramine that might also be a consideration for dogs include school phobias and separation anxiety in children, anxiety and panic disorders including agoraphobia, chronic pain, bulimia, and attention deficit disorders with hyperactivity.

(b) **Amitriptyline**: for separation anxiety and generalized and chronic anxiety in dogs and cats, chronic or neuropathic pain and aggression associated with anxiety and panic. Because of its sedative, anti-anxiety, and antihistaminic effects as well as its potential for improvement of chronic pain, it may be particularly useful for some self-traumatic disorders such as the early stages of ALD-type lesions in dogs (e.g., displacement behaviors). In humans, amitriptyline is also used for insomnia and agoraphobia.

(c) **Nortriptyline**: a similar treatment profile to imipramine. It may be useful for enuresis and chronic pain and is preferred when anticholinergic effects and sedation need to be minimized. It may therefore be preferred for the elderly. It is the only TCA where serum levels can be monitored in people (50–150 ng/ml).

(d) **Doxepin**: for generalized anxiety and as an antihistamine. It may be particularly useful for some self-injurious behaviors such as early in the treatment of ALD. Doxepin is also used in humans to treat chronic pain and insomnia.

(e) **Protriptyline**: more activating and least sedating and might be used for cataplexy, narcolepsy, or hypersomnia.

(f) **Other antidepressant considerations**: more noradrenergic antidepressants such as nortriptyline, protriptyline, and imipramine might be preferable in pets that appear to have more negative, depressive, or dysthymic signs.

Atypical antidepressants

Mianserine is available in Europe but not in North America as an atypical antidepressant. It blocks presynaptic alpha-adrenoreceptors with little effect on serotonin transmission. Because of alpha-adrenergic and histaminic blockade, it is sedating and may lead to postural hypotension in people. It may be a useful adjunct for pain management and may be used to enhance the efficacy of fluoxetine therapy in depressed patients. It has been used in stage 2 hypersensitivity–hyperactivity disorders and reactive depression and phobias in dogs in Europe.

Selective serotonin re-uptake inhibitors

Selective serotonin re-uptake inhibitors, as the name implies, are for the most part selective in their blockade of the re-uptake of 5HT1A into the presynaptic neurons. Transporter and receptor conformation changes can take three to five weeks to take place. Therefore, six weeks or longer may be necessary to assess the therapeutic effects of these drugs. Abnormalities in central serotonin transmission in people may lead to anxiety and mood disorders, compulsive disorders, depression, and disturbances in eating and sleep. Selective serotonin re-uptake inhibitors may control or improve these conditions with little or no sedation and with no impairment of learning. In addition, since low 5HT turnover may be associated with irritability and impulsivity, serotonin re-uptake inhibitors have also been utilized in the treatment of some forms of aggression, especially those with an anxiety or panic component and those with episodes of impulsivity or dyscontrol (mental lapse aggression, rage syndrome). Doses for compulsive disorders (and bulimia in humans) are generally two to four times higher than the doses used for depression. Treatment of panic disorders may require an initial low dose to prevent exacerbation of anxiety, raised slowly over one to three weeks. In cats, selective serotonin re-uptake inhibitors may have some effect in the control of aggression that is associated with high levels of arousal. Although none of the SSRIs are presently licensed for pets, they may be effective in the treatment of chronic and generalized anxiety and panic disorders, phobias, generalized and chronic anxiety disorders, phobias, urine marking, and compulsive disorders. Published studies on the use of fluoxetine in pets have shown an improvement in owner-directed dominance aggression and acral lick dermatitis in dogs and an improvement in urine spraying in cats. Since the primary effect of clomipramine in pets is also the inhibition of serotonin re-uptake, it may be equally as effective as SSRIs in the treatment of many of these disorders. In rodent studies, sertraline, fluvoxamine, and fluoxetine inhibited some forms of aggressive behavior.

In comparison to TCAs, side effects from SSRIs are less common. They generally have less potential for cardiac effects including tachycardia and conduction disturbances. They may cause gastrointestinal signs such as anorexia, diarrhea, and nausea, and in some cases may lead to insomnia, agitation, tremors, or increased anxiety. There are also individual differences in effects amongst the SSRIs depending on the neurotransmitters they affect. Paroxetine may have anticholinergic effects including urine and stool retention, while fluvoxamine and paroxetine might be mildly calming. Antidepressants that increase serotonin may cause a serotonin syndrome, which in people is characterized by signs of nausea, confusion, hyperthermia, tremors, rigidity, seizures, coma, and death. However, these side effects are uncommon because, as the serotonin increases in the synaptic cleft, the increased activation of presynaptic autoreceptors leads to decreased firing of serotonin neurons (negative feedback). The net effect is an increase in serotonin availability, but the magnitude of the increase is limited by the decrease in serotonin release. The highest risk for serotonin syndrome is when antidepressants that inhibit serotonin re-uptake are combined with other drugs or supplements such as tryptophan or MAO inhibitors that also have the potential to increase serotonin.

Fluoxetine has a plasma half-life of approximately one day in dogs (compared with approximately two days in man), while its active metabolite norfluoxetine has a plasma half-life of approximately five days in dogs (nine days in humans). It is used in humans for depression, compulsive disorders, eating disorders, panic, phobias, and premenstrual dysphoria. Compared with other SSRIs, it is mildly activating, and may be helpful for overweight and hyperphagic patients. It has been used for the treatment of aggression, impulsiveness, and hyperactivity in dogs. On the other hand, it may cause insomnia and more agitation, trembling, or anorexia in comparison with other SSRI antidepressants. As a potent inhibitor of the

cytochrome P450 2D6 enzymes it may increase levels of TCAs and other drugs that are metabolized through this pathway, such as propranolol and neuroleptic agents (thereby increasing the risk of extrapyramidal signs). Through inhibition of the 3A4 enzyme there may be mild increases in the effects of benzodiazepines, buspirone, and carbamazepine.

Paroxetine has a much shorter half-life in humans (20 hours) and no active metabolites. It is used to treat depression and social phobias in humans and may have some anticholinergic effects including sedation, urine retention, and constipation. Its indications would be the same as other SSRIs in pets (aggression, urine marking, generalized anxiety, phobias, panic disorders, compulsive disorders). It may have the advantage of being somewhat more calming and therefore preferable for some anxiety disorders, but would not be indicated for hyperactivity disorders. It is less likely to lead to agitation and insomnia compared with fluoxetine and sertraline. Conversely, it may be more anticholinergic, leading to gastrointestinal upset, urine retention and, in particular, constipation. Paroxetine should be slowly withdrawn after therapy to avoid a rebound effect or increasing anxiety. As with fluoxetine it is a potent inhibitor of the 2D6 enzyme that may increase the level of TCAs and neuroleptics, but should have little or no effect on benzodiazepine doses.

Fluvoxamine is approved in humans for OCD but has similar antidepressant and mood-elevating effects as other SSRIs. It has a half-life of 15 hours in humans. Like paroxetine it might be mildly more calming than fluoxetine and sertraline, but does not have any significant anticholinergic effects. It is less likely to lead to anorexia and therefore may not be useful for hyperphagia, although it should still be effective for picas. It has been used in one small clinic study in Europe for impulsive, overactive, aggressive disorders and sleep disorders such as hyposomnia and insomnia with little or no effect on normal behaviors. Side effects might include nausea, vomiting, and sedation. Fluvoxamine might greatly decrease the clearance of benzodiazepines such as diazepam, clonazepam and alprazolam, propranolol, clomipramine, amitriptyline and imipramine, buspirone and theophylline, through its actions on P450 enzymes, 3A4, C19, and 1A2. Benzodiazepine and neuroleptic doses should be reduced by at least a third if these drugs are used concurrently with fluvoxamine.

Sertraline is another human antidepressant that has a half-life of 25 hours in man, but only five hours in dogs. Sertraline has an active metabolite that is 10 times less potent than its parent compound, which has little or no clinical significance. Sertraline has the lowest side effect profile in humans, and may cause mild somnolence rather than nervousness and anorexia. Side effects might include gastrointestinal upset and it might best be given with meals to increase absorption. Along with citalopram, sertraline has the least effect of the SSRIs on P450 enzyme systems, so that there are only mild concerns when using concurrently with other antidepressants or neuroleptics.

Citalopram is the newest licensed SSRI for depression in humans. It is the most selective inhibitor of serotonin re-uptake, and reaches a peak plasma level in four hours, with a half-life of 33 hours in humans and three and a half to eight hours in dogs, with no active intermedi-

ate metabolite. It has the highest safety margins against cardiotoxic effects compared with tricyclic antidepressants and selective re-uptake inhibitors in dogs and cats. In toxicology studies it is generally quite safe, but one study found that five of 10 dogs receiving 8 mg/kg per day died suddenly between 17 and 31 weeks following therapy. In one study of dogs with acral lick dermatitis, six of eight dogs improved on citalopram. In the initial stages of therapy with citalopram and perhaps other antidepressants there may be a temporary increase in aggression. In a study of the effect of citalopram on REM sleep in cats, citalopram increased deep slow wave sleep and decreased REM sleep. Like sertraline, citalopram had little effect on cytochrome P450 enzymes except a mild effect on 2D6 (Figs 6.5–6.7).

COMBINATION/AUGMENTATION THERAPY

Combining drugs might be the best way to achieve efficacy for some problems, based on human models and examples for psychotropic drug therapy. However, the drugs used for monotherapy are for the most part unlicensed and not entirely proven in veterinary medicine.

Cytochrome	Inhibitors	Potential interactions
1A2	Fluvoxamine++++	Tricyclic antidepressants including amitriptyline, clomipramine, and imipramine, neuroleptics including haloperidol, thioridazine, and clozapine
2C9	Fluoxetine+++ Fluvoxamine+\– Sertraline+\–	Piroxicam, warfarin
2D6	Fluoxetine++++ Paroxetine++++ Sertraline++ Citalopram++	TCAs Neuroleptics/antipsychotics including haloperidol, clozapine, respiridone, thioridazine – amphetamines Dextromethorphan Propranolol
2C19	Fluoxetine+++ Fluvoxamine++++	Amitriptyline, imipramine, diazepam, propranolol, omeprazole
3A4	Fluoxetine++ Fluvoxamine+++	TCAs, benzodiazepines including alprazolam, clonazepam, triazolam, buspirone, erythromycin, cisapride cortisol, cyclosporine diltiazem, estrogen, lidocaine, omeprazole, testosterone

++++ Greatest degree of inhibition, +++ moderate inhibition, ++ mild inhibition, +/– may lead to mild inhibition.

Figure 6.5 Effects of SSRIs on cytochrome P450 enzyme systems in humans.

Neurotransmitter deficiency	Clinical signs	SSRI
Serotonin	Depression, anxiety, panic, phobia, obsessive–compulsive, bulimia	Citalopram Fluoxetine Fluvoxamine Paroxetine Sertraline
Norepinephrine	Depression, decreased attention or concentration, decreased learning or memory, fatigue	Fluoxetine Paroxetine
Dopamine	Depression, decrease in attention, hypersomnia, decline in cognition, craving	Sertraline

Figure 6.6   Human applications for SSRI antidepressants.

Therefore, extreme caution and close monitoring must be exercised when using combination therapy. Specific drug combinations used in the French diagnostic system are covered in Chapter 21.

(a) Antidepressants may be effective in controlling panic attacks in humans. However, anxiolytics such as clonazepam, alprazolam, buspirone, or propranolol may also need to be added to more effectively reduce anxiety. A combination of sertraline and clonazepam has been shown to be effective in people. Concurrent therapy with benzodiazepines may be of particular importance during the initial stages of antidepressant therapy, since antidepressants take several weeks to be effective and may produce a transient restlessness and increase in anxiety (see below). In fact,

Most anticholinergic Amitriptyline*, imipramine, doxepin	**Moderately anticholinergic** Clomipramine, paroxetine nortriptyline, protriptyline	**Least anticholinergic** Fluoxetine, fluvoxamine, sertraline, citalopram
Most hypotensive Imipramine*, amitriptyline	**Moderately hypotensive** Clomipramine, doxepin, protriptyline	**Least hypotensive** Nortriptyline, fluoxetine, fluvoxamine, sertraline, citalopram, paroxetine
Most sedating Doxepin, amitriptyline	**Moderately sedating** Imipramine, clomipramine, nortriptyline, paroxetine, fluvoxamine	**Least sedating** Protriptyline, fluoxetine, citalopram, sertraline
Most antihistaminic Doxepin*, amitriptyline	**Moderately antihistaminic** Imipramine, protriptyline, clomipramine, nortriptyline	**Least antihistaminic** Fluoxetine, fluvoxamine, sertraline, citalopram, paroxetine
Most serotonergic Fluoxetine, fluvoxamine, paroxetine, sertraline, citalopram, clomipramine	**Moderately serotonergic** Imipramine, amitriptyline	**Least serotonergic** Protriptyline, nortriptyline, doxepin
Most noradrenergic Protriptyline*, nortriptyline	**Moderately noradrenergic** Amitriptyline, clomipramine, doxepin, imipramine	**Least noradrenergic** Clomipramine, fluoxetine
Most seizure potential Amitriptyline, clomipramine, imipramine, doxepin	**Moderate seizure potential** Protriptyline, nortriptyline	**Lowest seizure potential**** SSRIs

*Greatest effect.
**May be safest if there is a seizure focus but still a contraindication.

Figure 6.7   Comparative effects of antidepressants.

when an antidepressant such as fluvoxamine, fluoxetine, or imipramine is dispensed, a short course of a benzodiazepine such as alprazolam might be considered to overcome initial agitation or insomnia. Melatonin has also been combined with antidepressants for chronic anxiety and phobic disorders such as storm phobias. Tricyclic antidepressants and SSRIs (fluoxetine plus clomipramine or fluoxetine plus amitriptyline) can also be used to augment each other in compulsive, anxiety, and panic disorders. Since fluoxetine inhibits the metabolism of clomipramine, it increases its potency without increasing its dose. When combining a tricyclic antidepressant with fluoxetine or paroxetine, reduce the dose by 10–25%, and when combining with sertraline, reduce the dose by 50%.

(b) Clomipramine and SSRIs might be combined with buspirone, clonazepam, or pimozide for refractory obsessive–compulsive disorders. Lithium may enhance antidepressant therapy for compulsive disorders by enhancing pre-synaptic 5HT receptors that have been sensitized by antidepressant therapy.

(c) Pindolol and propranolol have been combined with SSRIs. They may take away the physiological signs of anxiety while the drug exerts its central effect, and may act to increase the availability of serotonin by preventing the initial down-regulation associated with antidepressant therapy.

(d) Benzodiazepines have been used in combination with antipsychotics to improve both positive and negative symptoms in people.

(e) Buspirone does not interact with other sedatives and therefore has been combined with beta-blockers, sedatives, antidepressants such as clomipramine and fluoxetine, or even benzodiazepines when additional anxiolytics effects are desired.

(f) In some cases, packaged drug combinations may even be available, such as chlordiazepoxide and amitriptyline, or chlordiazepoxide and clinidium (for stress colitis or irritable bowel).

FURTHER READING ON DRUG THERAPY

Albers LJ, Hahn RK, Reist C 2001–2002 Handbook of psychiatric drugs. Year 2001–2002 edn. Current Clinical Strategies, Laguna Hills, CA

Beaver BV 1994 The veterinarian's encyclopedia of animal behavior. Iowa State University Press, Ames, IA

Boeck V, Jorgensen A, Fredricson OK 1984 Comparative animal studies on cardiovascular toxicity of tri and tetracyclic antidepressants and citalopram; relation to drug plasma levels. Psychopharmacology (Berlin) 82(4):275–281

Brignac MM 1992 Hydrocodone treatment of acral lick dermatitis. Proceedings of the 2nd world congress of veterinary dermatology, Montreal

Brown SA 1988 Anticonvulsant therapy in small animals. Veterinary Clinics of North America, Small Animal Practice 18(6):1197–1214

Bruyette D, Ruehl WW, Smidberg TL 1995 Canine pituitary-dependent hyperadrenocorticism: a spontaneous animal model for neurodegenerative disorders and their treatment with l-deprenyl. Progress in Brain Research 106:207–215

Burghardt W 1996 Repetitive and self traumatic behaviors. Presentation to the American Veterinary Society of Animal Behavior specialty meeting AAHA, San Antonio

Center SA, Elston TH, Rowland PH et al 1996 Fulminant hepatic failure associated with oral administration of diazepam in 11 cats. Journal of the American Veterinary Medical Association 209(3):618–625

Cooper SJ, Hendrie CA 1994 Ethology and psychopharmacology. John Wiley, Chichester

Dehasse J 1999 Retrospective study on the use of Selgian [R] in cats. Presentation to the American Veterinary Society of Animal Behavior, New Orleans

Dehasse J 2001 The use of sertraline in dog behaviour medicine. In: Overall KL, Mills DS, Heath SE et al (eds) Proceedings of the third international congress on veterinary behavioural medicine. United Federation for Animal Welfare, Herts, UK, p 195–196

Dodman NH 1995 Pharmacological treatment of behavioral problems in cats. Veterinary Forum April:62–71

Dodman NH, Shuster L (eds) 1998 Psychopharmacology of animal behavior disorders. Blackwell Science, Oxford, p 332

Dodman NH, Shuster L 1994 Pharmacologic approaches to managing behavior problems in small animals. Veterinary Medicine 12:960–969

Dodman NH, Doneelly R, Shuster L et al 1996 Use of fluoxetine to treat dominance aggression in dogs. Journal of the American Veterinary Medical Association 209(9):1585–1587

Ferris CF, Melloni RH Jr, Koppel G et al 1997 Vasopressin/serotonin interactions in the anterior hypothalamus control aggressive behavior in golden hamsters. Journal of Neuroscience 17(11):4331–4340

Franz SC 1979 Enhancement of central norepinephrine and 5-hydroxytryptamine transmission by tricyclic antidepressants. Psychopharmacology (Berlin) 62(1):9–16

Fredricson OK 1982 Kinetics of citalopram in test animals; drug exposure in safety studies. Progress in Neuropsychopharmacology, Biology and Psychiatry 6(3):297–309

Fuller RW 1994 Uptake inhibitors increase extracellular serotonin concentration measured by brain microdialysis. Life Sciences 55(3):163–167

Goddard AW, Brouette T, Almai A et al 2001 Early coadministration of clonazepam with sertraline for panic disorder. Archives of General Psychiatry 58:681–686

Goldberger E, Rapaport JL 1991 Canine acral lick dermatitis: response to the antiobsessional drug clomipramine. Journal of the American Animal Hospital Association 27:179–182

Hart BL 1985 Behavioral indications for phenothiazine and benzodiazepine tranquilizers in dogs. Journal of the American Veterinary Medical Association 186(11):1175–1180

Hart BL, Eckstein RA, Powell KL et al 1993 Effectiveness of buspirone on urine spraying and inappropriate urination in cats. Journal of the American Veterinary Medical Association 203(2):254–258

Harvey MJA, Cauvin A, Dale M et al 1997 Effect and mechanisms of the antiprolactin drug cabergoline on pseudopregnancy in the bitch. Journal of Small Animal Practice 38:336–339

Hewson CJ, Luescher UA 1996 Compulsive disorders in dogs. In: Voith VL, Borchelt PL (eds) Readings in companion animal behavior. Veterinary Learning System, Trenton, NJ

Jones RD 1987 Use of thioridazine in the treatment of aberrant motor behavior in a dog. Journal of the American Veterinary Medical Association 191(1):89–90

Katsung BG 1995 Basic and clinical pharmacology, 6th edn. Appleton and Lange, Norwalk, CT, p 1–146

Keltner NL, Folks DG 1997 Psychotropic drugs, 2nd edn. Mosby, St Louis

Krawiec DR 1988 Urinary incontinence in dogs and cats. Modern Veterinary Practice 69(1):17–23

Kroll T, Houpt KA 2001 A comparison of cyproheptadine and clomipramine for the treatment of urine spraying in cats. In: Overall KL, Mills DS, Heath SE et al (eds) Proceedings of the third international congress on veterinary behavioural medicine. United Federation for Animal Welfare, Herts, UK, p 184–185

Landsberg GM 2001a Clomipramine – beyond separation anxiety. Journal of the American Animal Hospital Association 37:313–318

Landsberg GM 2001b Effects of clomipramine on cats presented for urine spraying. In: Overall KL, Mills DS, Heath SE et al (eds) Proceedings of the third international congress on veterinary behavioural medicine. United Federation for Animal Welfare, Herts, UK, p 186–189

Leonard BE 1997 Fundamentals of psychopharmacology, 2nd edn. John Wiley, Chichester

Levine ES, Litto WJ, Jacobs BL 1990 Activity of the cat locus ceruleus noradrenergic neurons during the defense reaction. Brain Research 531(1–12):189–195

Luescher UA 1993 Hyperkinesis in dogs: six case reports. Canadian Veterinary Journal 34:368–370

Lyons WE, Mamounas LA, Ricaurte GA et al 1999 Brain-derived neurotrophic factor-deficient mice develop aggressiveness and hyperphagia in conjunction with brain serotonergic abnormalities. Proceedings of the National Academy of Science USA 96(26):15239–15244

Marder AR 1991 Psychotropic drugs and behavioral therapy. Veterinary Clinics of North America, Small Animal Practice 21(2):329

Matsumoto M, Yoshioka M 2000 Possible involvement of serotonin receptors in anxiety disorders. Nippon Yakurigaku Zasshi 115(1):39–44

Maxmen JS, Ward NG 1995 Psychotropic drugs: fast facts, 2nd edn. WW Norton, New York

Milgram NW, Ivy GO, Head E et al 1993 The effect of l-deprenyl on behavior, cognitive function, and biogenic amines in the dog. Neurochemical Research 18(12):1211–1219

Nirenberg AA, Farabaugh AH, Alpert JE et al 2000 Timing of antidepressant response with fluoxetine treatment. American Journal of Psychiatry 157:1423–1428

O'Farrell V, Neville P 1994 Manual of feline behaviour. British Small Animal Veterinary Association, Cheltenham

Overall K 1997 Clinical behavioral medicine for small animals. Mosby, St Louis

Overall KL 1999 Behavior Q&A. Allow behavioral drugs ample time to take effect. Veterinary Medicine October:858–859

Perry P, Lund BC 1994 Clinical psychopharmacology seminar. Selective serotonin reuptake inhibitors. Virtual hospital. University of Iowa online continuing education for health care providers, December 2001. http://secundus.vh.org/providers/conferences/cps/13.html

Peterson ME, Kintzer PP 1994 Medical treatment of pituitary-dependent hyperadrenocorticism in dogs. Seminars in Veterinary Medicine and Surgery (Small Animal) 9(3):127–131

Pfeiffer E, Guy N, Cribb A 1999 Clomipramine-induced urinary retention in a cat. Canadian Veterinary Journal 40(4):265–267

Plumb DC 1995 Veterinary drug handbook, 2nd edn. Pharma Vet Publishing, White Bear Lake, MN

Pouchelon JL, Martel E, Champeroux P et al 2000 Effect of clomipramine on heart rate and rhythm in healthy dogs. American Journal of Veterinary Research 61:960–964

Pryor PA, Hart BL, Cliff KD et al 2001 Effects of a selective serotonin reuptake inhibitor on urine spraying in cats. Journal of the American Veterinary Medical Association 218(11):1557–1561

Ramboz S, Saudou F, Amara DA et al 1996 5-HT1B receptor knock out – behavioral consequences. Behavioral Brain Research 73(1&2):305–312

Reich M, Overall KL 2000 Electrocardiographic assessment of antianxiety medication in dogs and correlation with serum drug concentration. Journal of the American Veterinary Medical Association 216(10):1571–1575

Reisner IR 1994 Use of lithium for treatment of canine dominance-related aggression. Applied Animal Behavioral Science 39:183

Ruehl WW, Bruyette DS, DePaoli A et al 1995 Canine cognitive dysfunction as a model for human age-related cognitive decline, dementia and Alzheimer's disease: clinical presentation, cognitive testing, pathology and response to l-deprenyl therapy. Progress in Brain Research 106:217–225

Ruehl WW, Griffin D, Bouchard G et al 1996 Effects of l-deprenyl in cats in a one month dose escalation study. Veterinary Pathology 33(5):621

Sangdee C, Franz D 1979 Enhancement of central norepinephrine and 5-hydroxytryptamine transmission by tricyclic antidepressants: a comparison. Psychopharmacology (Berlin) 62(1):10–16

Saudou F, Amara DA, Dierich A et al 1994 Enhanced aggressive behavior in mice lacking 5-HT1B receptor. Science 265(5180):1875–1878

Schwartz S 1994 Carbamazepine in the control of aggressive behavior in cats. Journal of the American Animal Hospital Association 30:515–519

Sirinarumitr K, Johnston SD, Kustritz MVR et al 2001 Effects of finasteride on size of the prostate gland and semen quality in dogs with benign prostatic hypertrophy. JAVMA 218(6):1275–1280

Stein DJ, Mendelsohn I, Potocnik F et al 1998 Use of the selective serotonin reuptake inhibitor citalopram in a possible animal analogue of obsessive–compulsive disorder. Depression & Anxiety 8(1):29–42

Virga V, Houpt KA, Scarlett JM 2001 Efficacy of amitriptyline as a pharmacological adjunct to behavioral modification in the management of aggressive behaviors in dogs. Journal of the American Animal Hospital Association 37:325–330

White SD 1990 Naltrexone for treatment of acral lick dermatitis in dogs. Journal of the American Veterinary Medical Association 190:1073–1076

White MM, Neilson JC, Hart BL et al 1999 Effects of clomipramine hydrochloride on dominance-related aggression in dogs. JAVMA 215(9):1288–1291

Wiener JM 1996 Diagnosis and psychopharmacology of childhood and adolescent disorders, 2nd edn. John Wiley, New York

Wynchank D, Berk M 1998 Fluoxetine treatment of acral lick dermatitis in dogs; a placebo-controlled randomized double blind trial. Depression & Anxiety 8(1):21–23

Zito JM (ed) 1994 Psychotherapeutic drug manual, 3rd edn. John Wiley, New York

7

Complementary and alternative therapy for behavior problems

WHAT IS COMPLEMENTARY AND ALTERNATIVE VETERINARY MEDICINE (CAVM)?

The holistic approach to medicine is designed to examine the whole pet, including the clinical signs (both physical and behavioral), environment, and relationship with the owner to develop a lifestyle and treatment protocol based on the findings. Holistic thinking is centered on love, empathy, and respect, and treatment modalities utilize the most efficacious, least invasive, and least expensive and harmful path. However, this is not an approach that is unique to the field of complementary and alternative medicine, as this is how any caring and knowledgeable health care provider would practice. In the treatment of behavioral problems, an evaluation of all these factors is essential in making a diagnosis and developing an appropriate treatment plan. In addition, all aspects of veterinary medicine should be held to the same high standards. This includes documenting safety and efficacy for all therapies used.

Current examples of CAVM include such modalities as acupuncture/acutherapy/acupressure, nutraceutical therapy, phytotherapy (herbal medicine), chiropractic, homeopathy, aromatherapy, Bach flower remedies, energy therapy, low-energy photon therapy, magnetic field therapy, and orthomolecular therapy. Indepth discussions of these individual forms of therapy are well beyond the scope of this book.

IS ALTERNATIVE MEDICINE SAFER AND MORE EFFECTIVE?

In traditional medicine those therapeutic modalities that have not been tested or proven effective using established scientific principles are viewed cautiously or even skeptically. This seems prudent and does not imply that the therapy is not of value. Ideally, all medicaments and therapeutic modalities used in animals should be subject to the same stringent criteria for safety and effectiveness. In fact, if a drug or supplement has not been tested against placebo, has the potential for toxicity, or is used as an alternative to a proven effective drug, this may pose a greater risk to the pet and lead to higher expense for the owner (the antithesis of holistic practice). Over the years, new standards have been set for the safety and efficacy of drugs and supplements so that the unproven, ineffective, and perhaps even dangerous tonics and practices of the past have been replaced by medicaments and techniques that have proven to be effective. Yet, many of the alternative remedies have been revived from civilizations and centuries where knowledge of anatomy, physiology, cellular biology, genes and genetics, disease processes, pathogens, and even reproduction was virtually unknown.

This is by no means a condemnation of the many complementary modalities now available. In time, some will prove to be effective while others will prove to be ineffective or even harmful. Conventional practitioners must therefore remain cognizant of the potential benefits of complementary medical therapies, while complementary practitioners must validate the therapeutic effects of their treatment protocols. In the field of behavioral medicine, placebo effects of 50% or higher are not unusual, since measurement is generally subjective and other forms of owner intervention are likely to alter behavior. Therefore any supplement or medication, whether pharmaceutical, herbal, or homeopathic, that has not been subjected to an objective validated scoring system or has not been proven statistically superior to placebo should be considered untested or unproven with respect to efficacy. This has already sealed the fate of numerous highly promising drugs that did not meet safety or efficacy requirements when subjected to vigorous testing. Conversely, those treatment modalities that cannot be validated continue to thrive.

In behavioral medicine, the treatment program must include behavioral modification and environmental management techniques that identify and address both the underlying cause as well as perpetuating factors. Therefore, regardless of whether a drug or complementary form of treatment is utilized, a 'holistic' approach is needed to address all the issues that may have an impact on the pet's behavior (i.e., health, nutrition, environment, and behavioral management).

NATUROPATHIC THERAPY

Supplementation is a popular topic amongst dog owners, breeders, and veterinarians but there are many misconceptions and myths that need to be addressed and corrected. One of the reasons for supplementing diets is that the 'known requirements' are not necessarily the same as the 'actual requirements.' This was forcefully demonstrated to the cat food industry in 1975, when it was determined that cats require higher levels of taurine than were present in commercial diets at that time.

There is another use for supplements that is often forgotten in the debates between owners, breeders, pet food companies, and veterinarians – some dogs and cats respond to supplements even if there is no dietary deficiency. This is because some nutrients have positive pharmacologic benefits apart from their nutritional claims.

It is the concept of 'nutritional therapeutics' that often creates a brick wall between conventional medicine and those practitioners that seek out more natural alternatives. Of course, there need be no wall at all. There is more than enough room in health care for both perspectives. We are now 'rediscovering' some basic facts about nutritional therapy that today are making headlines – fiber can help prevent colon cancer; fresh vegetables can help prevent heart disease; St John's Wort may help treat mild depression. We sometimes forget that aspirin (acetylsalicylic acid) was originally derived from the bark of willow trees or that digitalis comes from the foxglove plant. Even the potent cancer drug taxol was first isolated from the Pacific Yew tree. In fact, many of the most popular drugs used today were originally isolated from nature rather than being created 'new' in a laboratory.

By law, in order to achieve licensing, veterinary drugs must be proven to be safe and efficacious by government agencies, such as the FDA-CVM in the United States and BVD in Canada. In Europe, the Food and Veterinary Office (FVO) was established in the Directorate-General for Consumer Policy and Consumer Health Protection in April 1997 as a commitment to European consumers that their health protection was of the highest priority. On October 5, 1999, President Prodi announced in the European parliament that food safety was a major priority and that a European Food Authority should be created to help achieve this objective. As a result of the White Paper on food safety (Brussels, 12.1.2000), a European Food Authority was proposed, whose responsibilities consisted of the preparation and provision of scientific advice, collection, and analysis of information, monitoring and surveillance, and the communication of all its findings to all interested parties. The White Paper outlined that the European Food Authority must function based on independence, excellence, and transparency.

In addition, toxicity, contraindications, drug interactions, and the potential for side effects must be established. Products that are sold as supplements or natural remedies, that do not make claims with respect to health or disease, can be sold in the absence of these same safeguards. However, when botanical and nutraceutical products are used as therapeutic agents, they are indeed being used as drugs, yet there are no regulations or assurances with regard to product quality, efficacy, tolerance, and safety

(PETS). In fact, in Canada, some compounds such as melatonin, tryptophan, and 5HT are not available because they have pharmaceutical indications but have not met the government standards for safety and efficacy that would be required of a drug.

Perhaps the biggest concern with botanicals and nutraceuticals is that there is no protection against substandard products. In addition, there is no standardization between competitive products, and there may even be variation between batches. The different species and different plant parts may vary considerably in their biochemistry and effectiveness, even varying on a seasonal basis. Only relatively recently have companies sought to standardize doses based on active ingredients for some of their products, and reflect this on the label. Yet independent studies continue to find great ranges in active ingredients from well below to well above the manufacturer claims. For example, in one study of glucosamine and chondroiton sulfate products, 84% of all tested products did not meet label claims, with contents ranging from 0 to 115%. Consumer Reports® found that the amount of key ingredients in saw palmetto, ginkgo biloba, echinacea, and ginseng varied greatly between brands and a Toronto Star study found that of three brands of garlic none met the label claims for allicin compounds, many ginseng compounds did not meet label claims for ginsenoside, and some feverfew compounds did not contain parthenolide at all. On the other hand, a recent Consumer Reports® did find consistency between brands of St John's Wort and Kava kava.

Toxic contaminants are another concern with these products. For example, eosinophilia-myalgia syndrome has been reported in humans due to contaminants in commercially available 5-hydroxytryptophan, which was being promoted for insomnia, depression, and headaches after tryptophan was banned. A number of Canadians developed nausea and vomiting when their dandelion root product was found to contain buckthorn bark. The California public health department found unlisted drugs or heavy metals in 32% of Asian patent medicines, Health Canada found unacceptable levels of mercury, strychnine, lead, and aristolochic acid (which may cause cancer and kidney failure) in a number of Chinese herbal products, and flurazepam and estazolam were isolated from one herbal sleep remedy. Another risk is that many people put a great deal of trust in these products because they are 'all natural,' yet their side effects, contraindications, and toxicity may exceed that of comparable drugs.

As mentioned, placebo control studies are generally lacking to prove the efficacy of many of these alternative products and therapies, and some recent studies are finding little therapeutic effect for herbal remedies such as ginseng. Perhaps what is most surprising is that a drug that has met the requirements for efficacy and safety by the FDA is then passed over in favor of a nutraceutical product that is untested and unregulated, just because it is labeled as 'natural.' Combination products with a variety of herbal extracts are also available, which may further cloud the true effectiveness of any one particular agent.

Finally, the issue of how to dose and how much to dose has yet to be established for most herbal medicinals. Literature on the use of these alternative medicines suggests that no standard method of dosing exists, that trial and error will be needed to find correct dosages, and that most dosages are based on the human dose (which is based on a 150 lb human male). Yet because of differences in absorption and metabolism between pets and people, this has not proven to be the case with many drugs. Even if a dose were to be established, the environment in which the plant grows, the part of the plant used, the age of the plant at harvest, handling after harvest, and the method of administration may all affect dose and efficacy. Also, since human medication may come in a variety of forms, creativity may be necessary to find a way to administer these herbs to animals.

Greater study on the pharmacognosy of these plants is needed, and the information made available to health care professionals. Expect that naturopathic remedies will eventually become mainstream medications once their active ingredients have been determined, and safe doses established and standardized. Complementary regimens will remain for those products with insufficient evidence to make label claims, or where patent protection is not available to permit profitable exploitation of the product.

HERBAL THERAPY (PHYTOTHERAPY) AND NEUTRACEUTICALS
Dosing

Doses for some products listed below have been suggested. Alternately, a calculation is made based on a percentage of the human dose. As absorption and metabolism may vary greatly between dogs, cats, and humans, this method of dose calculation may lead to inefficacy or additional potential for toxicity, so that close patient monitoring is essential. A dose can be calculated by taking the pet's weight, dividing by 150, and using this percentage of the human dose.

Cognitive enhancement

Ginkgo biloba trees produce a unique class of chemicals termed ginkgolides A, B, C, M, and J, as well as bilobalide, which alters a number of neurotransmitter systems in the brain, primarily increasing the activity of acetylcholine. There are also interactions with serotonin and norepinephrine, and ginkgo has been described as having antioxidant and neuroprotective effects as well. It may be effective at enhancing blood flow to the brain by promoting vasodilation and decreasing platelet aggregation. It has been used primarily for cognitive activation and is purported to improve memory loss, fatigue, anxiety, concentration, and depressed mood in the elderly. Although most human studies have been poorly designed, one recent multicenter study demonstrated significantly less decline in cognitive function of dementia patients with gingko therapy. It might be useful in the treatment of canine or feline cognitive dysfunction, but no efficacy data has been published. Ginkgo may affect coagulation so its use might be contraindicated with surgery or with other drugs that might affect clotting.

Phosphatidylserine is a membrane phospholipid that is purported to facilitate neuronal activities such as signal transduction, and it might help to maintain normal neurotransmitter levels (acetylcholine and dopamine). It might therefore be useful for improving signs of cognitive dysfunction, although no data has yet been published. A dose of 100–500 mg daily has been suggested in dogs.

Choline and phosphatidylcholine are precursors of acetylcholine (ACH) and, as such, may enhance ACH transmission, although there is no evidence to support their efficacy and no evidence that ACH enhancement would give benefit to senior pets.

Kava kava

Kava (the rhizome of the pepper plant *Piper methysticum*) has sometimes been hyped in the press as a natural alternative for benzodiazepines such as diazepam (Valium) and oxazepam (Serax). The active agents, known as kava-lactones (also known as kava-pyrones), interact with GABA receptors (as do the benzodiazepines) and might provide mild relief for anxiety. In humans, regular use can cause gastrointestinal disturbances, chronic use has caused rashes (kava dermatopathy), and combining kava with other anti-anxiety medications can be dangerous. Heavy consumption has been associated with increased concentrations of gamma-glutamyltransferase, suggesting potential hepatotoxicity. Although a few double-blind studies have shown an anxiolytic effect in humans, the studies were small. One six-week German study found kava to be equally effective as oxazepam in relieving anxiety. In humans, kava has been recommended as a muscle relaxant, sleep aid, and anxiolytic. In pets there have been no controlled studies, but it has been recommended for anxiety, as a sedative or muscle relaxant, or as a sleep aid, and for the treatment of psychogenic alopecia in the cat. Kava can be dosed on an as-needed basis. Kava kava has recently been removed from distribution in some countries because of potential hepatotoxic effects.

Passiflora extract

Passiflora incarnata (wild passionflower, maypop, apricot vine, granadilla, passion vine) is a climbing plant and the extract is prepared from the dried leaves, stems, and flowers. The main constituents of the extract are flavonoids (e.g., vitexin, isovitexin, apigenin, luteolin, isoorientin, schaftoside, isoschaftoside, and swertisin) and harman alkaloids that are sedating. Passion flower is available in a number of homeopathic remedies and has been used as a herbal remedy for its alleged sedative, hypnotic, antispasmodic, antineuralgic, and hypotensive action. There are no controlled studies to show its effectiveness, although it is authorized for the treatment of nervous unrest in Germany. In animals, *Passiflora* has been used as a sedative and anxiolytic, particularly for separation anxiety, although no controlled studies are available. It has been used empirically at 12 mg/kg bid.

St John's Wort

This substance has been recommended for anxiety and depression in humans. While early studies in Germany concluded that St John's Wort, *Hypericum perforatum*, was equally as effective as imipramine in trials on patients with mild depression, other studies have failed to consistently replicate these results. More recent studies suggest that this herbal remedy is no more effective than a placebo in treating major depression.

Other studies seem to suggest that St John's Wort might be an effective treatment for obsessive–compulsive disorder, similar to sertraline, a selective serotonin re-uptake inhibitor. One of the active ingredients is hypericin (and perhaps pseudohypericin), which inhibits monoamine oxidase (MAO) and can also produce phototoxic reactions in cells. Hyperforin, another constituent, blocks re-uptake of the neurotransmitters serotonin, norepinephrine, and dopamine, and prolongs the activity of these neurotransmitters. It is probably hyperforin, and not hypericin or pseudohypericin, that is responsible for most of the effects of St John's Wort.

The main cautions to the widespread use of St John's Wort in humans are dosage/purity issues and the risk of drug interactions. It appears likely that St John's Wort affects plasma concentrations of all drugs that are metabolized by the cytochrome P450 system. It may significantly affect blood concentrations of digoxin, warfarin, estrogen, cyclosporin, theophyllines, and protease inhibitors. St John's Wort should not be used concurrently with antidepressants.

There have been claims of its use in dogs and cats, but no controlled studies. If used, caution should be exerted because of the risk of photosensitivity, and there are the same drug contraindications as SSRIs. It has been suggested that St John's Wort is a broad-spectrum re-uptake inhibitor (serotonin, dopamine, and noradrenaline). It is said to sedate, reduce anxiety, improve mood and sleep, reduce inflammation (by inhibition of arachadonic acid eicosanoid metabolites), and may be useful in compulsive disorders. A dose of 10 mg/kg tid or 250–300 mg bid has been suggested for large breed dogs, and a dose of either 1/10th of the dog dose of anywhere from 25 to 75 mg bid to tid has been suggested for cats, but neither safety nor efficacy have been established. As with pharmaceutical antidepressants it has been suggested that it can take three weeks or longer for St John's Wort to achieve therapeutic success.

Valerian

Valerian, the herb derived from the roots of species *Valeriana officinalis* and *Valeriana wallichii*, has been used as a natural 'tranquilizer' and smooth muscle relaxant in animals, but controlled studies are not available. There are numerous potential active ingredients, including valerianic acid, isovalerianic acid, and valepotriates, but the mechanism of action is still incompletely understood. It is believed that the herb inhibits production of an enzyme that breaks down GABA, an inhibitory neurotransmitter. No toxicities have been reported, although it may be hepatotoxic in high doses or in combination with other products. Human studies have suggested that it can potentiate barbiturate-induced sleep. Similarly, its use should be avoided in animals to be anesthetized or in phenobarbital-controlled epileptics, and concurrent use with benzodiazepines should be avoided. In some human studies nocturnal waking and sleep quality was improved but placebo effects were high and several weeks were sometimes required to achieve success. In Germany it is approved as a calmative and sleep-promoting agent. Valerian is not meant to be used long term, but may have benefit as a treatment for helping pets sleep through the night, and for exposure to periodic stressors, such as travel, thunderstorm phobias, and acute anxiety.

Skullcap

Skullcap comes from the leaves of *Scutelleria laterifolia* and *Scutelleria baicalensis* and comes as a dried herb, liquid extract, or tincture. Its active component baicalin is purported to have anti-aggregant, anti-allergic, anticholinergic, anti-inflammatory, and antileukotrienic properties. In humans it has been recommended for the treatment of spasticity, movement disorders, and seizures, and as an adjunct to cancer therapy. In pets, it has been recommended as a sedative and a remedy for nervous tension.

There are no controlled studies to indicate any behavioral therapeutic effects in humans or pets. Side effects might include confusion, irregular heartbeats, and seizures in humans, and large doses can be toxic.

Catnip

Catnip or catmint produces an apparent euphoric or hallucinogenic reaction in some cats. It exerts its influence on the CNS through the olfactory bulb. The active ingredient in catnip (*Nepeta cataria*) is the essential oil nepatalactone, with the active ingredient being nepatelic acid. It is available as a leaf, but liquid and aerosol forms are also available. Catnip produces a pleasurable, estrus-type response in about 50–75% of cats. When cats sniff even a small amount of catnip, they may begin to head shake, lick, chew, or rub up against the catnip, and then begin to twitch, salivate, and roll on the ground, for up to 15 minutes. Catnip responsiveness is reported to be an autosomal dominant trait, with the response being exhibited by about eight weeks of age. It can be a useful reward or for counterconditioning in behavior modification programs, or to divert and distract cats in potentially problematic situations.

Hops

Hops have been used in people as a sedative-hypnotic, coming from the hop plant *Humlus lupulis*, a perennial vine. Although hop resin does not cause CNS depression, when stored it undergoes auto-oxidation to produce methylbutenol. It is often used as a tea but is occasionally smoked. It is also recommended for depression. It may be useful for anxiety or insomnia, but there are no studies in people or pets to determine dose, safety, or effectiveness to date. Side effects might include sedation, and allergic reactions including hives, wheezing, and malignant hyperthermia have been reported after ingestion of beer hops in dogs. Its use with anticholinergics, antidepressants, and antihistamines is not recommended.

Melatonin

Melatonin is an indolamine derivative of serotonin and is produced by the action of the enzymes N-acetyltransferase and hydroxyindole-O-methyltransferase, with the first step being rate limiting. It is also a dopamine inhibitor. Production is primarily within the pineal body and the hormone is secreted into the blood and into the cerebrospinal fluid, at high levels during the night and at low levels during the day. Specific receptors for melatonin are found in multiple brain areas, including the hypothalamus, cerebellum, and pineal body itself.

The hormone melatonin has a time-keeping function in many mammals and appears to adjust the timing of circadian rhythm information transmitted from the suprachiasmatic nucleus of the hypothalamus to entrain physiologic rhythms. A true physiologic role for melatonin in humans has yet to be clearly established, and plasma levels of melatonin can be low to undetectable even in presumably normal individuals. It has been reported to be useful for jet lag and sleep disorders in people. One recent study found that a dose of up to 5 mg in humans at the target bedtime (but not the 2 mg slow release product) was effective for overcoming jet lag, particularly for eastward flights of five time zones or more. Caution is recommended in people with epilepsy and those taking tranquilizers or benzodiazepines. Melatonin has also been used for seasonal affective disorders, childhood depression, and self-injurious behavior, but there are no controlled studies to show effectiveness in these conditions. Side effects in humans may include sleepiness, headaches, and gastrointestinal discomfort.

Recently, melatonin has been used to treat several poorly understood forms of alopecia in dogs, especially cyclic (seasonal) flank alopecia, several follicular dystrophies, and alopecia X. Melatonin has been used empirically at 1 mg for dogs less than 5 kg, 1.5 mg for dogs 5–12 kg, and 3–6 mg for large dogs up to three times daily. No controlled studies have been performed. It has also been used for anxiety and sleep disorders in cats at 0.5 mg for cats less than 5 kg, 1 mg for cats 5 kg and above, or at a dose of 200 µg per cat, raised in 200 µg increments to 1 mg per cat if not sufficiently effective.

Melatonin has also been used in the treatment of a number of canine fears and phobias. In one case report, melatonin was used in dogs in the treatment of extreme fear and thunder phobia, in conjunction with amitriptyline in a dog that did not want to leave the house, and the author also reported effective control of other fireworks and thunder phobias with melatonin at 0.1 mg/kg q 24 h (up to tid), in conjunction with behavioral therapy.

SAM-e

SAM-e (S-adenosylmethionine) is a synthetic form of a metabolite of methionine and adenosine triphosphate (ATP). This essential metabolite initiates three major biochemical pathways – transmethylation, transsulfuration, and aminopropylation. It is a methyl donor, which means that it donates carbon methyl groups to other molecules in the body. It may help to maintain the function of certain neurotransmitters in the brain, including dopamine and serotonin. It may be useful in promoting liver function, joint mobility, and to elevate mood in depressive states in humans. A deficiency may result when decreased production of the enzyme SAM-e synthetase develops, whether from disease or the effects of aging. Supplementation with SAM-e is preferable, since administration of its precursor, methionine, may have side effects, and won't work if there is a concurrent SAM-e

synthetase deficiency. SAM-e is a precursor in the production of hepatic glutathione, which is important for protection of free radical injury. It may also help protect the liver from the adverse effects of prednisolone. Although most studies have been small or used injectable forms of SAM-e, there is some evidence that it is effective in the treatment of mild to severe depression when compared with imipramine. As with other antidepressants, it can take three weeks or longer for SAM-e to be effective. Although there are no reported contraindications or side effects other than stomach upset, insomnia, or an increase in euphoric state, it may increase the effects of other antidepressants. There are no reports of its use in pets for behavioral disorders. It is used primarily in animals with acute and chronic liver disease, diabetes mellitus, hyperadrenocortism, and pancreatitis.

TRYPTOPHAN

Tryptophan is a precursor in the production of serotonin, and lower levels of tryptophan in the diet have been associated with a fall in serotonin levels that might be associated with impulsivity, sleep disturbances, and mood and memory alterations. Therefore, it has been suggested that tryptophan supplementation might be effective in enhancing mood and memory and treating impulsive behavior. Although there has been toxicity reported with tryptophan and 5HT supplementation, no clinical benefits have been reported in pets, except for one study where a low-protein diet and tryptophan supplementation were combined (see Ch. 8 for details). In a study of silver foxes it was found that tryptophan supplementation reduced fear and enhanced exporation in the female silver fox.

Eosinophilia-myalgia syndrome has been reported in humans due to contaminants in commercially available 5-hydroxytryptophan. In addition, ingestion of toxic doses of 5-hydroxytryptophan has been reported in dogs, with signs resembling serotonin syndrome (seizures, tremors, depression, hyperthermia, gastrointestinal upset) which, at doses of 23 mg/kg and higher, in some cases lead to death.

ANTIOXIDANTS

For discussion on the effects of antioxidant supplements on behavior, see Chapters 8 and 12.

Essential fatty acids

Docosahexanoic acid (DHA) and eicosapentanoic acid (EPA), both found in marine oils, are known to reach high concentrations in the brain, where they contribute to neuronal cell membrane plasticity and health. They may be of benefit in maintaining neuronal health in senior pets and may even have an anti-inflammatory effect (in fact, fatty acids are supplemented in the new Hill's b/d™ diet). In addition, they may have an effect on other behavioral conditions since they have been advocated for learning deficits and attention deficit disorders in children, schizophrenia, and a variety of mood disorders. However, to date, there is no data to support their efficacy in the treatment of canine and feline behavior problems.

HOMEOPATHY

The basic principles of modern homeopathy were developed by an Austrian Medical Doctor, Samuel Hahnemann, in the mid-1800s. Homeopathy works on the principle of like cures like. Hahnemann purportedly based this system on the fact that quinine (used to treat malaria at the time) can produce malaria-like symptoms when given in overdose. The theory is that a product that would produce the same behavioral or physical symptoms in

a healthy individual in large amounts can cure a patient's symptoms in small amounts. The homeopathic remedy is prepared by repeatedly diluting the substance to render it non-toxic, while retaining its biologic value. In fact, each successive dilution is typically one part in 100, so that homeopathic potency is measured in centesimal Hahnemannienne. Between each dilution, the remedy is shaken vigorously. So, for example, a remedy that has had six successive dilutions (1 in 100) would be recorded as 6c (6cH in some countries) and would signify that the original substance has been diluted $1/1\,000\,000\,000\,000$. If the dilutions had been one in 10, the potency is shown as 6x or D6. Although the amount of substance may be undetectable after dilution, the remedy is said to contain the vibrational energy essences that match the patterns present in the ailing patient. These remedies may be made from plants, minerals, drugs, or animal substances. Although there is no scientific evidence to support any claims of efficacy, the extreme dilution of the ingredients is likely to render them entirely safe. The major difference between homeopathy and all other allopathic forms of therapy has to do with dose-related claims. In allopathic medicine, whether traditional Western medicine or naturopathic therapy, ingredients given in more concentrated forms and dosages have proportionally more effect. In homeopathy, the remedies are believed to get stronger the more they are diluted and the less active ingredient provided. Thus, in homeopathy, a remedy of 30c is considered stronger than one of 6c, even though it is diluted to one part in 10^{60}!

A variety of homeopathic remedies have been suggested in the treatment of behavior problems. In theory, these would be specifically designed by a homeopathic practitioner for the needs of the individual pet (e.g., ignatia or pulsatilla for separation anxiety, *Belladonna* or *Nux vomica* for aggression, *Calcarea phosphorica* for pica, *Aconitum napellus* for thunderstorm phobias, phosphorus for low generalized anxiety, etc.).

Calms Forte™ is a combination homeopathic remedy that has been recommended as an alternative to psychotropic drugs in the treatment of nervous tension and insomnia.

BACH FLOWER REMEDIES

A physician, Edward Bach, developed Bach flower remedies in the 1930s. They are intended to improve the emotional state of the human or pet, using minute dilutions of therapeutic plant essences. There are 38 essences, and up to five can be combined at once to meet all of the animal's physical and behavioral needs. Each remedy is purported to correct a specific emotional upset, such as fear, pain, resentment, and possessiveness. Accordingly, these remedies require that the practitioner/dispenser assess the pet's disturbed emotional state, such as timidity, jealousy, or despondency. Up to 12 remedies have been suggested for separation behaviors and up to 13 for fear and anxiety. The use of the appropriate combination of remedies involves determining how the animal reacts to certain stimuli and then targeting the treatment to the particular pet's needs (e.g., difficult if left alone vs panics if left alone). In addition to the lack of data to substantiate the efficacy of any of these remedies, the ability to categorize a pet's emotional state at so fine a level seems entirely subjective and arbitrary even for the most skilled of behaviorists. Other combinations have been purported to control urine-spraying, aggression between pets, carsickness, stress-induced cystitis, fear, and grieving. Rescue Remedy™ is a combination of five of Bach's flower essences that is recommended for an immediate or acute treatment of stressful and anxious events. It is intended to comfort and counter panic.

Despite the lack of any data to support the efficacy of these products, they continue to gain popularity.

ACUPUNCTURE

Acupuncture involves piercing the skin with slender needles at predetermined acupuncture points, and then the manipulation of these points by needling, injection, ultrasound, laser, magnetic induction, or electrical stimulation. Acupuncture is said to stimulate the vital force (Qi) within the animal to bring about homeostasis and healing. Clinical abnormalities (disease, pain, behavior problems) are believed to be brought on by imbalances within the individual. This renders the individual susceptible to the effects of external influences such as pathogens and environmental toxins. Needling of acupuncture points is intended to bring about balance along the lines of energy called meridians. It is said to lead to alteration in neurotransmitter pathways. Brain mapping studies have revealed correlation between acupuncture point stimulation and cortical activation. Although the primary indication for acupuncture would likely be pain management (see Ch. 9 for details), it has also been purported to be effective in the treatment of respiratory, neurological, and gastrointestinal conditions, and behavior problems such as aggression, anxiety, behavioral anorexia, depression (especially with respect to grief), and compulsive disorders such as compulsive overgrooming in cats and acral lick dermatitis in dogs. It is purported to affect the serotonin system, and be a faster and more effective form of therapy (three 15-minute treatments over three to four weeks). There are no controlled studies to show improvement of behavior problems with acupuncture.

THERAPEUTIC TOUCH

TTEAM was originally developed by Linda Tellington Jones as a method of modifying behavior in horses to help them focus and learn. This was eventually modified to apply to all animals, and the physical manipulation technique known as TTOUCH or Tellington Touch was introduced. TTEAM is intended to foster special connections between people and pets, and although there are numerous anecdotal reports of its effectiveness, there is no experimental data to support such effectiveness. Because of the relationship between body and mind, physical improvements have also been reported.

TTOUCH is a form of manipulation of the skin, as opposed to massage, which manipulates the muscles. It is intended to stimulate the nervous system (by activating different types of brain waves), using circular motions with the hands. In the veterinary hospital, the technique is purported to decrease pain and restore intestinal function following surgery, or to relax the fearful pet. Wands (feathers) can be used to start, beginning with the least threatening area of the body, and this can then progress to direct manipulation when (if) the fear subsides and the pet becomes approachable.

While handling exercises, massage therapy, and relaxation exercises can be beneficial to the pet and its relationship with its owner, it is uncertain whether the specific exercises associated with TTOUCH have any added benefits.

MAGNETIC FIELD THERAPY

In this form of therapy, magnets are used to alter the energy fields of the individual. They can be applied directly to the individual, or used as bedding or sleeping mats. Their primary indications are purported to be improvement of circulation and pain management. However, there are also claims that magnetic therapy can improve anxiety, stress, clinical depression, attention deficit disorder, and attention deficit hyperactivity disorder. There is no known mechanism of action, although transcranial stimulation is said to enhance serotonin metabolism. Magnets have also been used at acupuncture stress points. There are no studies to show improvement of behavior with magnetic field therapy in humans or pets.

VETERINARY CHIROPRACTIC

Chiropractic manipulation is intended to correct vertebral subluxations that may affect the innate vital force of the individual. Correcting the subluxation allows the force to fully express itself, thereby bringing about healing. Not only is manipulation intended to correct mechanical imbalances related to the neuromuscular consequences of subluxation, but it is also purported to improve a variety of physiologic conditions from diabetes to cancer as well as a variety of behavioral conditions. No known studies have demonstrated that chiropractic is effective in the management of behavior problems in dogs and cats.

AROMATHERAPY

Aromatherapy uses volatile oils to bring about psychologic or physiologic response. Oils can be administered by nebulization, topical application, and occasionally orally. Essential oils are obtained from the flowers, buds, fruits, leaves, bark, roots, or seeds of plants. Although organic, pesticide-free plants are recommended, synthetic oils are also sometimes used. Direct therapeutic effects of aromatized oils have not been documented.

In behavior therapy, pairing neutral stimuli (including a scent) with a reflexive emotional response can lead to the development of conditioned stimuli. The odor (conditioned stimulus) can then evoke a variety of emotional responses that may be used to calm an anxious pet, or conversely may lead to anxiety if the odor has been paired with a painful or unpleasant stimulus. Since dogs have such a sensitive sense of smell, odors may become conditioned stimuli for a number of different responses.

PHEROMONE THERAPY

Pheromones are substances that regulate behavior by olfactory means. They are an important aspect of social and sexual communication between members of a species. Appeasing pheromones, produced by the mother in the first few days after birth, play an important role in the attraction and attachment of newborn to mother. Synthetically produced appeasing hormones appear to have a relaxing effect for both young and adults of a species.

Pheromones are detected in the vomeronasal (VNO) or Jacobson's organ. In most species, this organ is enclosed within a capsule formed by the vomer bone (or cartilage), found along each side of the nasal septum. The cavity is lined with a chemosensory epithelium that includes bipolar receptor neurons. Large blood vessels run alongside the VNO, and access to stimulus molecules causes a vascular pumping effect such that stimuli are drawn through the duct into the lumen of the organ. To introduce the pheromone into the vomeronasal organ, many animals use an act known as flehmen, in which the lips are curled back and the tongue moves the odors along. Flehmen is exhibited in cats, but in dogs a combination of tongue lapping and panting is used to introduce the pheromones into the vomeronasal organ. In cats, the VNO duct opens into the nasopalatine (NP) canal, which connects the nose with the mouth. The VNO seems to be exquisitely sensitive to pheromones, but may respond to other substances presented in higher concentrations. The VNO receptor neurons have axons that leave the VNO capsule, extending dorsally across the nasal septum and beneath the olfactory mucosa, and carry signals to the accessory olfactory bulb. Axons then relay the information to the amygdala and from there the VNO system projects directly to the preoptic area and to the hypothalamus.

A number of synthetic forms of these pheromones are currently under development, and a few have now been introduced for companion animal behavior therapy. Five pheromones (F1 to F5) have been shown to have clinical effects in cats and two have been commercially produced, the F3 pheromone Feliway™ and the F4 pheromone Felifriend™.

Feliway™ is a synthetic analog of the F3 fraction of the feline facial pheromone that has been developed to reduce urine spraying in cats. Since urine spraying may be a response to anxiety or conflict, Feliway™ is designed to stop the spraying and direct the cat toward a more affiliative form of marking, cheek gland bunting. In a number of studies, Feliway™ led to a reduction in spraying in anywhere from 74 to 97% of cases, but less than 50% may show complete resolution. In a recent study, Feliway™ was shown to improve grooming and food interest in hospitalized cats, and food intake was increased when cats were housed in their own carrier and Feliway™ was applied. Feliway™ has also been reported to be effective in reactive, territorial forms of scratching. Feliway™ may be useful in acclimating cats to new environments and in the reduction of both the somatic stress responses and anxiety-related behaviors associated with transportation (car travel). Feliway™ may also have a mild calming effect during intravenous catheterization, especially when combined with acepromazine. The product is available as a spray, as well as a heat-activated, electric room diffuser.

Another synthetic feline facial pheromone containing the F4 analog, Felifriend™, has been developed in Europe but is not yet available in North America. The natural pheromone is reported to be associated with familiarization and allomarking in cats. Preliminary studies indicate that it might be useful for introducing a new cat to a resident cat and in the introduction of cats to dogs, new people into a household, or other potentially fear-inducing situations such as veterinary visits. At present the product is only available in France, Belgium, and Japan in a spray designed to be applied to the individual to whom fear is being exhibited.

A dog appeasing pheromone (D.A.P.™) is now available as a 'plug-in' room-diffusing spray, which is a synthetic version of the bitch's mammary tissue pheromones. Its primary indication is to reduce anxiety when

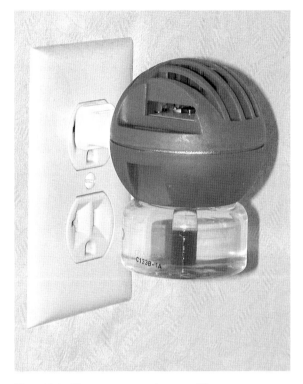

Figure 7.1 Pheromone spray in room diffuser.

introducing a puppy to a new home. It may also be useful for reducing anxiety associated with changes in the pet's schedule or environment, noise phobias, and in the treatment of separation anxiety (Fig. 7.1). Another product in development is a dog collar impregnated with D.A.P.™, which may help to reduce anxiety both inside and outside the home.

REFERENCES

Adebowale A, Cox D, Liang Z et al 2000 Analysis of glucosamine and chondroiton sulfate content in marketed products and the Caco-2 permeability of chondroitin sulfate raw materials. Journal of the American Nutraceutical Association 3(1):37–44

Allen JM 2001 Herbal medicines and dietary supplements. Skeptical Inquirer 25(1):36–46

Allison RW, Lassen ED, Burkhard MJ et al 2000 Effect of a bioflavonoid dietary supplement on acetaminophen-induced oxidative injury to feline erythrocytes. Journal of the American Veterinary Medical Association 217(8):1157–1161

Aronson L 1999 Animal behavior case of the month. Journal of the American Veterinary Medical Association 215(1):22–24

Barber J 2000 Magnetic therapy for animals. Interdisciplinary Forum for Applied Animal Behavior, Austin, TX

Bauer JE 2001 Evaluation of nutraceuticals, dietary supplements, and functional food ingredients for companion animals. Journal of the American Veterinary Medical Association 218(11):1755–1760

Beaubrin G, Grey GG 2000 A review of herbal medicines for psychiatric disorders. Psychiatric Services 51:1130–1134

Fadda F 2000 Tryptophan-free diets: a physiological tool to study brain serotonin function. News in Physiological Science 15:260–264

Fernstrom MH, Ferntrom JD 1995 Brain tryptophan concentrations and serotonin synthesis remain responsive to food consumption after the ingestion of sequential meals. American Journal of Clinical Nutrition 61(2):312–319

Gaultier E, Pageat P, Tessier Y 1998 Effect of a feline appeasing pheromone analogue on manifestations of stress in cats during transport. In: Proceedings of the

32nd congress of the International Society for Applied Ethology, Clermont-Ferrand, France

Griffiths CA, Steigerwald ES, Buffington CA 2000 Effects of a synthetic facial pheromone on behavior of cats. Journal of the American Veterinary Medical Association 217(8):1154–1156

Gwaltney-Brant SM, Albertson JC, Khan SA 1999 5-Hydroxytrytophan toxicosis in dogs: 21 cases (1989–1999). Journal of the American Veterinary Medical Association 216(12):1937–1940

Hersheimer A, Petrie KJ 2001 Melatonin for prevention and treatment of jet lag (Cochrane Review). In: The Cochrane Library 1

Hornfeldt CS 1994 *Nepeta cataria* (catnip) 'poisoning' in cats. Veterinary Practice Staff 6(5):1, 7

Hunthausen W 2000 Evaluating a feline facial pheromone analogue to control urine spraying. Veterinary Medicine 95(2):151–155

Klarskov K, Johnson KL, Benson LM et al 1999 Eosinophilia-myalgia syndrome case associated contaminants in commercially available 5-hydroxytrytophan. Advances in Experimental Medical Biology 467:461–468

Kronen PW, Ludders JW, Erb HN 2000 The F-3 fraction of feline facial pheromones calms cats prior to intravenous catheterization. In: Proceedings of the 7th World Congress of Veterinary Anesthesia, Berne

Lieberman HR, Caballero B, Finer N 1986 The composition of lunch determines afternoon plasma tryptophan ratios in humans. Journal of Neural Transmission 65(3&4):211–217

Mercer JR, Silva SVPS. In: Burger IH, Rivers JPW (eds) Nutrition of the dog and cat. Waltham symposium number 7. Cambridge University Press, p 207–227

Milgram NW, Estrada J, Ikeda-Douglas C et al 2000 Landmark discrimination learning in aged dogs is improved by treatment with an antioxidant diet. Society of Neuroscience Abstracts 26(1):531

Milgram NW, Head E, Cotman CW et al 2001 Age dependent cognitive dysfunction in canines: dietary intervention. In: Overall KL, Mills DS, Heath SE et al (eds) Proceedings of the third international congress on veterinary behavioral medicine. Universities Federation for Animal Welfare, Wheathampsead, UK, p 53–57

Pageat P 1996 Functions and use of the facial pheromones in the treatment of urine marking in the cat. In: Proceedings and abstracts, XXIst congress of the World Small Animal Veterinary Association, Jerusalem

Pageat P 1997 Usefulness of F3 synthetic pheromone (Feliway) in preventing behaviour problems in cats during holidays. ESVCE Newsletter 3(4/5):31–32

Schoen AM, Wynn SG 1998 Complementary and alternative veterinary medicine. Principles and practice. Mosby, St Louis

Scott S 1999/2000 Acupuncture and its role in behaviour therapy. Companion Animal Behavior Therapy Study Group Newsletter Winter: 7

Wulff-Tilford ML, Tilford GL 1999 All you ever wanted to know about herbs for pets. BowTie Press, Irvine, CA

Wynn SG 1999 Emerging therapeutics. Using herbs and nutraceutical supplements for animals. AAHA Press, Lakewood, CO

8

Feeding and diet-related problems

THE PHYSIOLOGICAL INFLUENCE OF DIET ON BEHAVIOR

There has long been a perceived relationship between diet and behavior, but few scientific studies have been conducted to provide any meaningful conclusions. The term animal psychodietetics has been advanced to describe the relation between nutrition and behavioral changes. It is important to realize that nutrients can impact upon the behavioral process in a number of intriguing ways. Since synthesis of neurotransmitters depends on the availability of circulating precursors (tryptophan for serotonin, choline for acetylcholine, and tyrosine for catecholamines), diet is likely to affect the availability of these precursors. However, the amount of nutrient ingested, its level in the brain, and its effect on nerve transmission are not linearly correlated. For example, the conversion of tryptophan to serotonin appears to be affected by the amount of carbohydrate in the diet (i.e., increasing serotonin release with increased carbohydrate) and the synthesis of serotonin might then decrease the amount of carbohydrate the animal wants to eat.

In addition, the innate feeding instincts of dogs and cats include hunting and all aspects of prey stalking, chasing, and the kill. Scavenging is also a normal canine behavior. These activities utilize energy and occupy time in the animal's day. Dogs and cats kept as house pets and fed a highly palatable processed and concentrated food once or twice a day may be receiving a complete nutritious daily ration, but there may be behavioral consequences of this type of feeding regimen. Behavior therapy for many problems should include ways to make the pet work or play for its food, or make the pet's feeding and chew times last longer. Although feeding live prey or dead carcasses is impractical, providing toys and feeders that require manipulation to release the food, utilizing search games where the pet has to find its food, training the pet to receive food as a reward for tasks and tricks, or freezing food can increase the time and work required to obtain food rewards.

It is not unreasonable to assume that some dogs and cats might have behavioral problems related to their diet, and that a change in diet might be a consideration when pets display abnormal behavior patterns such as aggression, or difficulty in trainability.

Although premium commercial diets may be formulated by veterinary nutritionists to very exacting specifications, supplemented to meet all of the pet's needs, and may have a fixed ingredient formula designed specifically for each life stage, this is not the case for most pet foods. Many commercial diets are high in calories and may have poorly digestible ingredients, which may lead to inadequate or imbalanced levels of vitamins and minerals. In addition, protein levels in some pet foods may be unnecessarily high for the pet's needs. It has also been suggested that additives, flavorings, preservatives, and other processing enhancements may potentially have adverse effects on health or behavior in some animals, although there is little evidence to document this assertion. In fact, for the most part, these additives increase the nutritional balance, palatability, and safety of pet foods.

While it is possible to have adverse food reactions that result only in behavioral changes, in most cases one would expect more diverse signs (e.g., dermatologic, neurologic, or gastrointestinal) if there were an adverse reaction to dietary ingredients. An elimination diet (i.e., one that did not contain the suspected offending ingredients) could be used to test this hypothesis.

However, pet owners cannot merely change to an alternative diet to test their suspicions, since this may not eliminate the offending ingredient, especially if it has been added prior to being obtained by the manufacturer. For instance, ethoxyquin is a common pet food preservative and has attracted a lot of attention (from breeders especially) as a potential cause for a variety of poorly defined conditions. Testing the hypothesis by feeding a diet that purports to have 'no ethoxyquin added' might seem like a reasonable step, yet might not actually address the concern. For example, if the pet food company bought their meat from a distributor that had already preserved it with ethoxyquin, they are well within their rights to advertise that they didn't 'add' ethoxyquin; however, it does not mean that the diet is ethoxyquin-free. In these instances, it is often best to have owners prepare meals from grocery sources, where they can carefully control preservatives, flavorings, and supplements.

Protein, carbohydrate, and tryptophan

Most concerns of behavior specialists focus on the role of protein in behavior problems. Both the quantity of protein and its quality and extent of processing have recently become suspect. It has been suggested that high-meat diets may possibly result in lowered levels of the neurotransmitter serotonin in the brain, because of the high level of amino acids competing with tryptophan (from which serotonin is formed) for the carrier that transports amino acids across the blood–brain barrier. Low serotonin levels have been associated with aggression in some animals. Therefore, it has been suggested that a reduction in protein or supplementation with tryptophan (a serotonin precursor) might lead to a reduction in aggression. Another suggestion is that a reduction in carbohydrate content and increased protein may lead to a decrease in excitability and overactivity. In humans, eating protein-rich meals after an overnight fast leads to a reduction in plasma tryptophan, while high-carbohydrate meals increase tryptophan.

Tryptophan-free diets lead to a reduction in serotonin synthesis in humans and laboratory animals. In rats, a carbohydrate meal fed after a fast led to a rise in tryptophan, but tryptophan was not elevated if the carbohydrate diet was fed within two hours of a protein meal. Studies that measured serotonin metabolites in the CSF after ingestion of diets with a variety of protein levels in dogs have found no differences regardless of diet fed.

In a recent canine study, the level of protein (high vs low) in the diet or addition of l-tryptophan had no effect on fearfulness or hyperactivity. Low-protein diets (approximately 18% of dry matter) with tryptophan supplementation were shown to lower territoriality scores, while high-protein diets without tryptophan supplementation were most likely to lead to dominance aggression. Therefore, addition of tryptophan and lowering of protein in the diet may also reduce dominance aggression. Supplementation with 2 mg/kg of 5-hydroxytryptophan might be considered, but controlled trials have not yet been performed. In a previous study dealing with dogs, low-protein diets were found to reduce territoriality in a small population of dogs, but this was not reproduced in the most recent study. Other forms of aggression were unaffected.

Carbohydrate levels are another area of interest. It is believed that when high-carbohydrate diets are fed, tryptophan reaches the brain in higher amounts and results in the production of serotonin. This may have a calming effect on the animal, making it less aggressive. However, if the increase in carbohydrates is accomplished by decreasing protein in the diet, then this may be a contributing factor. Supplementing the diet with vitamin B_6 (pyridoxine) might also be beneficial, because this aids in the production of serotonin. An almost contradictory approach suggests feeding low-carbohydrate diets (e.g., 12% carbohydrate with the balance made up equally of protein and fat) to calm overly excitable animals.

Another concern, often posed by dog trainers, is that training problems are more common in dogs fed dry food than those fed a canned ration. If training problems related to dry rations do exist, they are more likely to be related to preservatives than low moisture content, but there is no data to suggest that this is in fact the case. Since canned food is heat-sterilized before packaging, preservatives are not needed. In dry foods, expected to last for months on store shelves without being refrigerated, many chemicals, especially antioxidants and flavor enhancers, must be added to the foods to keep them edible.

Only recently has any scientific research been directed in this area, so little is actually known about the influence of various components of the diet on behavior. It remains a very intriguing area of applied animal behavior.

ANTIOXIDANT-SUPPLEMENTED DIETS

A recent development in canine preventive health care is a senior diet supplemented with antioxidants, mitochondrial cofactors, and essential fatty acids, which has been shown to improve the performance of a number of cognitive tasks when compared with older dogs on a non-supplemented diet. While a variety of 'antioxidant' diets have recently been developed, controlled laboratory testing on Hill's canine b/d® diet showed that dogs over seven years of age fed the supplemented diet performed better on a variety of memory and learning tasks than dogs that did not receive the supplemented diet. Docosahexanoic acid (DHA) and eicosapentanoic acid (EPA), both found in marine oils, are known to reach high concentrations in the brain, where they contribute to neuronal cell membrane plasticity and health. The diet is supplemented with antioxidants including ascorbic acid (vitamin C), vitamin E, and beta-carotene, which help to maintain oxidative protection. The addition of lipoic acid and l-carnitine is intended to enhance mitochondrial function and decrease free radical production. More details on this diet and its use in canine geriatric cognitive dysfunction can be found in Chapter 12.

No such diet has been tested on cats, but it is not unreasonable to expect that oxidative stress and the accumulation of toxic free radicals may also have a similar effect on aging, the brain, and behavior in cats. Therefore, decreasing oxidative stress and increasing free radical clearance should also be considered in senior cats.

THE USE OF NATURAL SUPPLEMENTS FOR BEHAVIOR THERAPY

Supplements that might be useful in the treatment of behavior problems are discussed in the section on alternative therapy in Chapter 7.

DIAGNOSIS OF DIET-RELATED BEHAVIOR PROBLEMS

The hypothesis of high-protein or preservative-rich diets contributing to behavior problems can be tested by feeding a high-quality but low-protein diet and watching for changes. Prior to placing a pet on a protein-restricted diet, it is essential that there are no abnormalities on physical examination and that routine blood and urine tests are normal. By using a homemade novel protein diet, preservatives and additives can be avoided and the single protein source may help to identify pets with adverse food reactions (although a trial for dietary intolerance may require up to eight weeks).

When feeding a homemade diet, the protein sources that are suitable include boiled chicken, lamb, fish, or rabbit combined with boiled white rice or mashed potatoes. This also limits problems that might occur from high-cereal diets (e.g., exorphines), milk proteins (e.g., casomorphine), and preservatives. The meal should be mixed as one part meat to four parts carbohydrate and fed in the same amount as the regular diet. Only fresh water should be provided during the trial, preferably bottled to control local water supply contaminants. No supplements, treats, or snacks should be given. This diet is not nutritionally balanced but that should make little difference for the seven to 10 days in which the trial is being conducted.

If there is a response to the diet trial, it will then be necessary to determine whether specific ingredients in the food (allergens, additives, preservatives) or the relative content of ingredients (protein vs carbohydrate) are implicated in the changes in behavior. Therefore, the next step in a homemade diet trial is to challenge the pet with potential offenders. The first test would be to increase the protein component of the diet (50:50) to see if there is a behavioral change. If so, this helps confirm the diagnosis and that it is the protein component that is contributory. At this point a careful reassessment for medical problems such as hepatic encephalopathy might be warranted. If the behavior problem does not recur with the increase in protein, new protein sources, vegetables, treats, and commercial foods can be reintroduced slowly to determine the role of specific ingredients, additives, and preservatives in the problem.

Other options would be to test the dog's response to commercial diets such as (a) a reduced-protein canned diet (e.g., prescription formulas designed for renal disease), which would provide a balanced restricted protein diet with no preservatives or (b) a hydrolyzed protein or novel protein diet over eight weeks to test for a food sensitivity/intolerance.

MANAGEMENT OF DIET-RELATED BEHAVIOR PROBLEMS

For animals that respond to a homemade low-protein preservative-free diet, there are many options available. Regular use of a homemade diet should be discouraged unless a completely balanced ration can be formulated. Low-protein diets are commercially available (such as those prescribed for kidney disease) and are the most convenient option. If owners are selecting their own foods from a pet supply outlet, they must look for diets with high-quality protein in moderate amounts and an easily digested carbohydrate source. Start with canned diets, which tend to have few if any preservatives. Dry foods have the most preservatives. If the condition worsens when the pet is put on to a commercial ration, there are likely to be more problems than just protein content to consider.

For dogs with reactions to preservatives, canned foods are an option and there are also preservative-free diets commercially available. Both of these are usually acceptable, but current regulations make it almost impossible to be assured that there are actually no preservatives in preservative-free diets. Manufacturers only need to list on the label those preservatives that they add during ration preparation. There is no guarantee that the manufacturer did not purchase the raw ingredients already preserved. If the pet improves when placed on a homemade diet, then the role of additives might be considered. When commercial diets cannot be used, homemade diets remain a final option. At this point, it is worth having a diet recipe prepared by a nutritionist to ensure that nutritional requirements will be met. Alternatively, computer software is available so that customized diets can be formulated by practitioners.

PREVENTION OF DIET-RELATED BEHAVIOR PROBLEMS

Since most diet-induced behavior problems are idiosyncratic, it is often not possible to predict and prevent most cases. There are some general guidelines, however, that might be helpful. Clients do not need to feed their dogs high-protein diets. The average house pet consumes a diet that contains much more protein than is needed for amino acid requirements. The result is a loss of expensive protein in the feces and urine, or a conversion of the excess energy into fat. Neither of these makes sense.

It is possible that some pets have reactions to preservatives (e.g., ethoxyquin, butylated hydroxyanisole (BHA), butylated hydroxytoluene (BHT), etc.), but that most of these reactions are idiosyncratic or subclinical. This is no different from acknowledging that some people cannot tolerate monosodium glutamate (MSG) in Chinese food, or sulfites at a salad bar. The difference between people and pets is that people dine on these foods occasionally, whereas pets consume commercial diets for their entire lives, day after day. If people consumed MSG with every meal, every day, we might find that

more people 'cross the threshold' and develop clinical problems. We should strive, then, to provide pets with wholesome diets that do not require extensive preservation. Canned diets contain the least amount of preservatives. Home-delivered, preservative-free, home-prepared, and frozen pet foods are all options with which the veterinarian should be familiar.

There is some anecdotal evidence that behavior problems due to some dietary ingredients may be familial. Some breeds seem to react to preservatives (e.g., Cavalier King Charles Spaniel), some to exorphines (Golden Retrievers), and others to serotonin-influencing factors of different meat proteins. Research remains to be done to confirm these possibilities. Neutering animals with these dietary idiosyncrasies will lessen the contribution of any hereditary factors to the breed gene pool.

Case example

Willard, a two-year-old male Doberman Pinscher, was presented with an owner's complaint of 'weird' behavior. Apparently, Willard would have episodes when he was hyperactive, combined with periods when he slept a lot. When he was hyperactive, he would run in circles in the back garden until he was exhausted. If he was confined indoors, he would press his head against his owners and would not leave them alone. They had tried punishing him with harsh words and locking him in the laundry room, but to no avail. They first noticed the problem at about eight months of age, and felt that it was getting worse.

At the time of his behavioral consultation, Willard was his placid self and demonstrated no evidence of hyperactivity. There were no abnormal findings on clinical examination. The owners felt that he may be worse in the evenings, but they had difficulty pinpointing any pattern to his hyperactivity. Willard was fed ad libitum. The differential diagnoses included toxicity (including food reactions, hepatic encephalopathy, and copper-induced hepatopathy), forms of epilepsy, and even a variant of normal behavior. Laboratory testing included a hematological profile, urinalysis, and biochemical pro-file that included bile acids (fasting and two-hour postprandial), ammonia, serum alkaline phosphatase, glucose, cholesterol, urea, creati-nine, and serum alanine aminotransferase.

The results of laboratory testing were not con-clusive. There were moderate elevations of serum bile acids with mild hyperammonemia and hypoglycemia. Ammonium biurate crystals were only infrequently observed in the urine. Radiographs did not demonstrate a significantly smaller liver than anticipated. In consultation with the owner, it was decided that the case did not warrant liver biopsy and quantitative determination of hepatic copper levels. The ten-tative working diagnosis was possible hepatic encephalopathy. A low-protein diet challenge was suggested, in which Willard was fed a low-protein homemade diet using chicken and rice with four small meals being fed daily, rather than the ad libitum feeding to which Willard was accustomed.

After five days on the homemade low-protein diet, the owners felt there was a marked improvement in Willard's behavior. He still had lots of energy but they did not notice any bizarre behaviors. The owners were advised to feed a high-quality but low-protein commercial ration. After two months on this diet, they reported few episodes of hyperactivity. They were happy with the results and chose not to pursue a specific diagnosis with further tests.

OBESITY

Obesity is the most common nutritional disor-der in North America, outnumbering all defi-ciency syndromes combined. A sad statistic is that over 25% of dogs in North America are overweight. It is likely that obese pets do not live as long as those of normal weight. They suffer more from heart problems; they fatigue easily, and are at increased risk of developing diabetes mellitus. Obese pets also have a decreased resistance to infection and are more prone to anesthetic complications should sur-gery ever be necessary. Links with many other clinical problems have been suggested

but have yet to be clearly demonstrated. Today, more than ever, pets are being 'killed with kindness' as their owners allow them to become obese.

Obesity becomes more common as pets get older. Females are more prone to obesity than males, and neutered pets are more likely to become obese than intact pets. Unfortunately, people who are obese themselves are much more likely to have obese pets, attesting to the significance of environmental factors in pro-moting obesity. Genetic factors are also contrib-utory. Labrador Retrievers, Cocker Spaniels, Collies, Dachshunds, Beagles, Basset Hounds, Shetland Sheepdogs, and some terriers are more prone to obesity than other breeds. Some breeds, most notably the German Shepherd Dog, Boxer, Whippet and, Greyhound, actually have a lower incidence of obesity than other breeds. Although genetics plays a role, clearly the most important factors leading to obesity are providing pets with excessive calories and inadequate physical activity. Obesity is rarely seen in wild animals and only infrequently seen in working dogs. It is the household pet, rarely exercised, confined to the home, and fed a high-quality diet, that is most prone to obesity.

The pet food industry markets diets with the consumer in mind and provides very palatable, high-calorie diets. The supplement market con-tributes biscuit treats and fatty acid supplements that are usually calorie-dense. The owner, with a firm emotional bond to the pet, wants to provide a healthy, tasty meal that the pet will devour and ask for more. The veterinarian, in the posi-tion of health-concerned middleperson, must counsel the owner about what is really in the best interests of the pet.

Diagnosis and prognosis

Pets are considered obese when they are 20% more than their ideal weight. This can be done by comparing the weight with compiled charts or approximated by visual inspection (fat cover-ing of ribs) and palpation. What is often more critical is to determine the reason for the obesity.

In most cases, the owners would rather believe the pet has a medical problem (hypothyroidism is a favorite), rather than consider that they are the most important cause. All obese pets should have a thorough physical examination and laboratory profile (complete blood count, serum alanine transferase (ALT), amylase/lipase, alkaline phosphatase, thyroid profile, urinalysis, cholesterol, creatinine, glucose, insulin), but most cases are due to owner feeding practices.

Owners often find it difficult to believe they are overfeeding their pets. Feeding practices may further complicate matters. The food may be left available to the pet all day, so that feeding can continue all day. Snacks are an important addition to the feeding routine even though most 'treats' contain 60 kcal or more apiece. Coat-care supplements of fatty acids are also calorie-dense. Therefore, veterinarians counseling owners of obese pets must be prepared to determine the animal's caloric needs, all calorie contributors in the pet's diet, and the amount of calorie-burning activities in the pet's lifestyle. Most owners can manage the problem more effectively when they can see, in black and white, where the problem lies. In these cases, the prognosis is good. A poor prognosis is given when owners refuse to admit there is a problem or blame the situation on others.

Management

Obesity can be dealt with intelligently and effectively if pet owners are willing to pay attention to the facts. Owners must be committed to helping their pets lose weight and must realize that the pets will be healthier and happier if they make the effort. All weight reduction programs should be performed under the supervision of a veterinarian to reduce the risk of complications from obesity or from weight loss.

There are a variety of weight reduction diets, each marketed to reduce the intake of calories while maintaining optimum nutrition. In dogs, there is some evidence that pets might be more satiated with increased fiber in the diet, but the owners will need to deal with the increased stool volume. Extra caution must be taken to restrict calories more gradually and to monitor food intake when beginning a weight reduction program in cats to prevent hepatic lipidosis. Decreasing intake in calories through diet, restricting treats, and increasing calorie utilization through increased activity and exercise are the basics of any weight loss program. However, behavioral management may be the true key to success.

Regularly scheduled meals and snacks often reduce the client's tendency to overfeed the pet. Making them count calories also makes them more likely to comply with a weight reduction program. Several behavioral modification programs help to reinforce the concepts needed in successful dieting. Clients should be cautioned that when they give in to begging, they only reinforce that behavior and make weight loss even more difficult. Stimulus control modification is used to regulate the cues that trigger feeding; in other words, certain stimuli may have inadvertently become paired with feeding and these need to be carefully managed. Such stimuli might include the owner's arrival home (the dog anticipates a treat), entering the kitchen, opening cupboards, drawers, or the refrigerator, or even just sitting in the kitchen. Avoiding these cues, moving food treats to a different cupboard, and changing routines can therefore be an important aspect of behavioral therapy. Another alternative is to insist that the dog performs an appropriate command each time it approaches and begins to beg (e.g., 'down-stay'), and to gradually extend the down-stay with each subsequent approach. As a reward the pet can then receive a patting session, a play session, a chew toy, or a walk. This technique does little to decrease approach and begging, but does help the owners gain control over the situation. The pet gains no calories from its demands and begging, and the owners learn that there are other rewards that can be just as fulfilling to the pet. Clients must not associate feeding with 'quality time' for their pet. Thus, the pet should only be given food in its bowl and be fed in only one location. This helps deter the animal from seeking meals and treats elsewhere, and from begging.

Once the weight has been safely lost, it is important not to resort to the old behaviors that resulted in obesity to begin with. It is usually recommended that the calorie content of the diet be left at 90% of requirements rather than 100%, because snacks are bound to creep back into the diet at some point.

Prevention

Obesity is the number one nutritional problem affecting dogs and cats and it is a health concern that is entirely preventable. Pets count on their owners for their health care needs, and calorie restriction rather than caloric excess should be the operative concept. Caloric restriction not only prevents obesity, but may lower the risk of musculoskeletal problems and cancer. Unfortunately, weight loss in pets is no easier for most owners than their own diet needs. Proper nutrition requires a basic philosophical change so owners understand the difference between optimal nutrition and overnutrition.

Case example

Brandy, a 19-kg, six-year-old English Cocker Spaniel, was seen during a routine annual examination. The owners were not sure why Brandy was overweight because he only ate one cup of food twice daily, just as recommended by the pet food manufacturer. They thought that perhaps he might have problems with his metabolism because he also was not very 'spunky,' and that it might have something to do with the fact that he was neutered before one year of age.

The physical examination of Brandy was unremarkable other than his obvious weight problem. A worksheet was used to determine 'everything' that Brandy ate on a typical day as well as his usual exercise schedule. Both of the owners worked and Brandy was left alone most of the day. They left food available for him at all times but some of it was still in his bowl when they got home at night. He got three cereal bis-

cuit snacks in the morning when they left for work, three when they returned, and three before bedtime. He also got table scraps occasionally, but not consistently and not in large quantities.

The owners were not convinced that Brandy was being overfed, but agreed to explore the situation with us further. Routine hematological and biochemical tests (including a thyroid profile of free and total levels) were normal or negative. The owners were then given these facts: Brandy should be receiving about 850 kcal daily based on an ideal weight of about 14 kg. The biscuit treats were 90% dry matter (3.60 kcal/g DM) and 25 g each. His nine treats a day amounted to 810 kcal, almost a whole day's caloric requirements! The dry food being fed contained 3.67 kcal/g DM and was 90% dry matter. Further mathematics was unnecessary to convince the owners of Brandy's caloric excess.

The plan was to give Brandy only one treat twice a day, following each of his two meals. Brandy required 850 kcal per day but we decided to create a caloric deficit of 250 calories/day so there could be a safe weight loss of about 250 g per week. Taking into account the owners' wishes, the diet was formulated to account for both pet food and biscuit treats. Therefore, Brandy would be getting 600 kcal per day, 162 kcal from his biscuit treats. The owners did the math too so they could see that Brandy should receive only 438 kcal per day from his dog food, split between two meals. Knowing the caloric density and dry matter of the food (see above), this means that Brandy should receive about 132.5 g of food a day, or 67 g with each meal. The owners were informed about specially formulated weight loss diets but decided they could follow this regimen. They were also going to play fetch with him for 10 minutes each morning before they went to work and take him for a one-mile walk each evening.

On re-examination 12 weeks later, Brandy was a svelte 16 kg and much more energetic. The owners did have some difficulty sticking to the regime and augmented his diet with carrots and popcorn. Brandy really liked the carrots and sometimes preferred them to the cereal treats. They did miss some walks and did not always have time for fetch but, overall, they were fairly consistent. We decided that Brandy could go on a maintenance diet of 90% of his requirements (about 765 kcal/day) while getting only one biscuit treat daily. This meant that Brandy could get about 207 g of food daily, rather than 132.5 g. The owners were happy with the compromise.

PICA

Pica is an abnormal craving or appetite for ingesting non-food substances. While young animals will chew on a wide variety of substances, the items are rarely ingested. Starch and soil eating has been documented in humans on severely deficient diets. The cause of pica in pets is unknown. Pica can be a dangerous condition, as well as a nuisance. Some forms of pica, such as the wool eating of cats, 'barbering,' or rock chewing, and soil eating in dogs, may be compulsive disorders.

Fabric eating can be seen as part of the compulsive wool-sucking syndrome exhibited by some cats. The problem seems to appear most frequently in oriental breeds, but can be manifested in cats of mixed origin. Many causes have been suggested for this problem, including heredity, early weaning, stress, malfunction of the neural control of appetitive behavior, separation anxiety, and persistence of infant kitten oral behavior. Woolen items are most commonly chosen, but affected cats may well chew on any type of available fabric including cotton, silk, and synthetics. The behavior is most likely to begin during the first year of life and may resolve on its own during early adulthood (see Chs 10, 15, and 16 for a more detailed description of this topic).

Diagnosis and prognosis

Pica is diagnosed by observing the abnormal behavior. There are no specific laboratory tests that might provide additional insight, but a full medical workup is essential, particularly in those cases that are of adult or geriatric onset and where there are no discernible behavioral causes. Medical conditions that lead to nutritional deficiencies or electrolyte imbalances, gastrointestinal disturbances, conditions that lead to polyphagia, and CNS disturbances should all be ruled out. The prognosis is variable, depending on the individual and the material consumed.

Management

By keeping the ingested objects away from the pet, providing appropriate chew toys, or changing the diet to a dry, bulky, nutritionally balanced food, the problem may be corrected. Depending on the pet's level of motivation to chew, taste aversion or booby traps can be used to keep the pet away from selected areas or items. Underlying problems that may fuel the behavior, such as stress or separation anxiety, should be corrected.

Clomipramine or a selective serotonin reuptake inhibitor (such as fluoxetine) may be helpful when the pica is compulsive, such as seen in feline wool-sucking/chewing problems.

Case example

Rama was a 12-year-old neutered male Siamese cat with a penchant for climbing underneath one particular sofa, tearing holes in the covering, and consuming the stuffing. There were several other pieces of furniture that held no interest for Rama.

The physical examination of Rama was routine. He was a very healthy specimen with no clinical abnormalities. Routine laboratory workup included fecal assessment, hematology, biochemistry, serum T_4, and viral profiles for feline leukemia virus and feline immunodeficiency virus. No abnormalities were detected on any of the tests.

The first approach involved providing additional oral stimulation and alternative outlets for play and investigation. The owners switched Rama to a dry high-fiber cat food, and provided additional play sessions and cat toys. Although Rama's destructiveness may have decreased, he continued to return to the sofa to chew. Next, the owners attempted booby-trapping the couch with taste aversives and motion-activated alarms, but Rama always managed eventually to get beneath the couch to eat the stuffing. When the owners made a barricade around the base of the couch completely denying access, Rama proceeded to dig between the cushions and tried to chew into the stuffing from the top. Remote punishment with a water rifle was also attempted, but Rama continued to return to the area in the owner's absence. Frustrated, the owners finally got rid of the couch. Although they were cautioned that Rama might turn his attention and energy to another piece of furniture, this did not happen. The ultimate cause of the pica was not determined, but the increase in environmental stimulation and removal of the target of Rama's chewing had successfully resolved the issue.

COPROPHAGIA

Coprophagia is an ingestive behavior involving the consumption of feces. It is not uncommon in the canine population but is rare in the feline population. Dogs may selectively ingest their own feces, feces of other dogs, feline feces, ungulate feces, other mammalian feces, or may consume any type of feces that is available. Whereas adult bitches will consume the feces of their puppies, all other forms of coprophagia might be considered abnormal. The problem tends to be seen more frequently in puppies, but most eventually outgrow it. Puppies may indulge in coprophagia as harmless investigative or playful behavior, and owners must be cautious not to inadvertently reinforce the behavior by giving the puppy additional attention when it consumes feces. Pets that are underfed or placed on an overly restricted diet may have a voracious appetite, which may also include coprophagia. Pets that have been overfed, and those with gastrointestinal conditions such as malabsorption or trypsin deficiencies, may have higher amounts of undigested ingredients remaining in the feces. These feces might then be palatable enough to appeal to some dogs.

Similarly horse and cat feces can be particularly appealing to some dogs. It is commonly thought that inadequate exercise and environmental stimulation may make a dog more likely to consume its own feces.

Diagnosis

The ultimate cause of coprophagia in adult dogs has always been elusive. Some feel that the problem is behavioral, while others are convinced there is an organic reason. One of the most important aspects of diagnosis, and determining what diagnostic tests might be required, is the medical history:

1. What stools are being ingested (own stools, or those of another dog in the home, other animals, all dogs).
2. Signalment: age of onset, sex, neuter status, stage of estrous cycle.
3. Diet, including any recent change in diet and any caloric restriction recently implemented.
4. Medical health – especially as it pertains to appetite, weight, metabolic rate, and digestion.
5. Concurrent medication including those that might have an effect on appetite.
6. Stool consistency, volume, appearance, frequency, and any evidence of tenesmus.

Soft stools, incomplete digestion of food within the stools, evidence of steatorrhea, increased stool frequency or volume, or a voracious appetite might indicate a problem with maldigestion or malabsorption. Other gastrointestinal disturbances such as inflammatory bowel disease, systemic health problems including renal failure and endocrinopathies, medications such as glucocorticoids, central nervous system diseases, or any disease process that causes polyphagia might lead to picas and coprophagia. Calorie-restricted diets, especially those that are not balanced or do not adequately satiate the dog, may also lead to picas including coprophagia. Recent research has suggested that there may indeed be a medical component to the problem in some cases. In a small study of nine coprophagic dogs conducted by two of the authors (G.L., L.A.), all had at least one laboratory abnormality that could explain the problem. The laboratory profile included a complete blood count, complete biochemical profile, amylase, lipase, trypsin-like immunoreactivity (TLI), vitamin B_{12}, folate, fecal fat, fecal trypsin, fecal muscle fiber, trace minerals (including zinc, selenium, copper, iron, magnesium, and boron), and fecal sedimentation. Most had borderline to low TLI, while others had abnormalities in folate, cobalamin, or other nutrients. None of the dogs had internal parasites (determined by fecal sedimentation) or abnormal fecal fat or trypsin levels. In addition, four of the nine dogs showed some benefit when supplemented with a plant-based enzyme supplement. The appropriate diagnostic tests will therefore need to be based on the physical examination and medical history, but some blood and urine tests and a fecal analysis will be the minimum requirement for most cases.

If no medical cause can be identified, then the behavioral history should be closely assessed including:

- Description of the problem including when and where the coprophagia takes place.
- Owner's response and attempts at correction to date.
- Any changes in household, diet, health prior to onset of problem.
- Other signs of pica or oral behavioral disorders.
- Other behavior problems or behavioral pathology related to changes in appetite, sleep, stereotypies, etc.
- Housetraining status including where and when the pet eliminates.
- Other pets and their relationships.
- Housing including daily schedule for play, exercise, attention, training, and elimination.

Management

If the cause of the coprophagia cannot be determined, environmental modifications are the best chance for therapeutic success. Denying access to feces is the first step. The yard should be cleaned regularly so that there are no feces available to the dog. For the dog that eats its own feces, it should be possible to take the dog out to eliminate and upon completion teach him to immediately come to the owners and sit for a favored reward while the owner cleans up the stool. Only after elimination is complete should the owner consider allowing the dog to remain outdoors unsupervised. For dogs that eat other dogs' stools, the dog should be walked on a leash and head halter and given a stern, verbal correction and a quick pull on the leash when it attempts to sniff or ingest other feces. The pet must be under constant supervision while outdoors. Tossing a shake can near the pet or using a remote activated citronella collar every time it attempts to consume feces, or painting aversive tasting (odorless) substances on the underside of feces, may occasionally be effective. However, if the feces are not consistently coated with the deterrent or the pet is not constantly supervised, the behavior (which is self-rewarding in the coprophagic dog) will persist. In addition, most dogs are likely to detect which stools are pretreated based on odor. Although generally impractical, placing a nauseant in the stool (e.g., LiCl) is the only deterrent likely to be permanently effective.

Dietary changes are successful with some but not all coprophagic dogs. Some dogs are less likely to be coprophagic when a more highly digestible diet is fed or when meat tenderizers or proteolytic enzyme supplements are added to the meal. Most dogs appear to prefer ingesting well-formed or even frozen feces, so adding fiber or vegetable oil to the diet might result in a less-formed and less-appealing stool. Adding a variety of concoctions to the diet has been advocated, but there seems to be no consensus that they work on a regular basis. The exception seems to be plant-based enzyme supplements, but this needs to be evaluated in more dogs before firm conclusions can be made. Products used for reducing stool appeal must be appetizing or tasteless when initially consumed but suitably aversive when they are degraded in the intestinal tract and appear in the stool.

Coprophagia has always been a difficult condition to treat. However, new studies suggest that veterinarians should always conduct a thorough medical and laboratory investigation before dismissing coprophagia as a behavioral problem.

Case example

Ginger was a seven-year-old apricot Poodle with a history of coprophagia spanning many years. The owner had been unable to curb the habit, despite scolding Ginger and adding various noxious agents (such as cayenne pepper) to the feces in the back yard. At first Ginger was repulsed by the agents, but after a while it seemed that Ginger had actually developed a taste for them. Otherwise, the owner felt that Ginger was a perfect pet.

Physical examination was unremarkable. Laboratory evaluation consisted of routine hematology and biochemistry, fecal sedimentation (rather than flotation), TLI, vitamin B_{12}, folate and fecal trypsin, muscle fiber and fat. There were some striated muscle fibers evident in the feces and the TLI was marginal but not in the diagnostic range for exocrine pancreatic insufficiency. It was concluded that there might be a marginal pancreatic enzyme insufficiency as part of the problem.

Treatment consisted of environmental, behavioral, and dietary modification. The owner was advised to accompany Ginger outdoors so that there was no opportunity to find stools except when the owner was supervising. Ginger was fitted with a remote citronella collar and was walked on a long extendable leash and head halter. As soon as Ginger eliminated she was taught to return to the owner's side and sit for a food reward while the owner cleaned up the feces. While on leash, if Ginger began to mouth the stools of other dogs, she was immediately interrupted. If she began to explore other dogs' stools while off leash the remote citronella collar effectively interrupted the behavior. The diet was changed to a low-fiber highly digestible ration, which was topdressed with a plant-based enzyme supplemental (containing bromelain, papain, and phytase). Re-evaluation eight weeks later revealed a dog that was much improved. Although Ginger still occasionally ate feces, it was not with the same relish that she once possessed. Six months later, the owner reported that Ginger rarely if ever consumed feces.

THE 'FUSSY' OR 'PICKY' EATER

Both dogs and cats can be finicky when it comes to diet preference. In most cases, the problem stems from previous feeding experiences or heritable responses to feeding situations, although underlying medical problems can contribute. Occasionally, the pet will be reluctant to eat a commercial diet because it has learned that if it waits long enough it will receive more palatable food from the owner.

The causes of most true feeding idiosyncrasies are unknown at this time. It is known that odor, taste, texture, and temperature can be adjusted to tempt the problem feeder to eat, and that novel foods may increase appetite.

Diagnosis and prognosis

The diagnosis is usually straightforward but there are some caveats. If the owner complains of a finicky pet, or one that occasionally 'skips' meals, attain an accurate weight of that animal to determine if it is in the normal range. In many cases, these so-called 'finicky' eaters are of normal weight (or even overweight) and do manage to consume all the calories needed on a daily basis. Some dogs may even skip an occasional day with no ill effects. This appears to be a normal mechanism for maintaining optimal weight. It is important to rule out the possibility that the pet is obtaining food elsewhere, either from a neighbor or by hunting. Make sure to inquire about treats. It is not unusual for biscuit treats to contribute 50–100 kcal apiece; this can account for a substantial portion of daily requirements.

For pets that are labeled 'fussy' or 'picky' and are underweight, a complete history and thorough medical evaluation needs to be obtained to consider underlying disease processes.

Pancreatic, dental, gastrointestinal, kidney, and liver disease can all account for 'dietary discrimination.'

Management

All pets with underlying medical problems need to have them addressed. One of the most insidious causes of dietary discrimination is dental disease. Routine dental care is imperative but often underutilized in practice. It has been estimated that over 85% of dogs and cats have periodontal disease by four years of age. It can be inferred from that, that many dogs and cats may have dental pain and discomfort that could interfere with feedings. It is critical that all medical problems be appropriately addressed.

For those healthy animals that continue to turn up their noses at mealtime, there are some alternatives. The first step is to limit the use of treats and table scraps and see if the owner is pleased with the change. If not, be prepared to calculate the caloric needs of the animal (tables available in nutrition texts) based on its age, weight, and health status and determine the caloric load of the diet being fed. Most commercial diets, especially the gourmet cat foods and the super-premium dog foods, are exceptionally calorie-rich. Because of this, less needs to be fed. Owners often have a preconceived notion of how much their pet should be eating, and it may be completely unrealistic. They tend to try more and more expensive diets (providing more and more calories) and wonder why their pets are getting worse (i.e., eating less). Sometimes, switching to a food that is less calorie-dense will solve the problem because the pet consumes more to achieve its daily caloric needs. Rewards (such as flavored treats and play) can be given each time the pet voluntarily eats its designated food.

Things you can do for the 'picky' eater

- Moisten the food with warm water if you are using dry food. This tends to make hard foods tastier and more chewy.

- Most dogs prefer the flavors of beef, chicken, pork, or lamb rather than vegetable protein such as soy, corn, and wheat. Choose a food that provides these more desirable ingredients. Cats prefer beef, chicken, fish, and pork; select these ingredients for finicky cats.
- Heating the food in an oven or microwave can enhance the flavor.
- Add flavor enhancers to the diet, such as liver or poultry broths or bouillon cubes.
- Consider adding very small amounts of cooked garlic to the food. Use small amounts of cooked garlic cloves, not garlic oil. Don't overdo it! Excess garlic can be toxic to both dogs and cats.
- Add fresh fruit purées as a dressing on the food. Mashed apple or banana are good choices to try first. If necessary, the same effect can be gained by adding small amounts of artificial sweeteners such as aspartame. Go light on raisins and grapes, since toxicities have been reported in dogs fed large amounts.
- Add some freshly cooked food (e.g., hamburger, liver, chicken) to the diet to encourage the 'picky' pet to eat. Slowly wean them off the fresh-cooked food on to the commercial ration.
- Try a super-premium dog food or gourmet cat food that provides increased levels of protein and fat. Pets need to eat less of these foods to achieve their daily requirements. Owners must be aware that this will not make them less finicky, only assure that even a little bit of food will provide maximal caloric intake.
- Add small amounts of commercial cat food to the dog food diet. Cat food has many more flavor enhancers, and is high in fat, high in protein, and loaded with B vitamins. Many dogs find it very appealing.
- Limit treats. The picky pet may be filling up on treats instead of eating its meals.
- If the pet is finicky because a new diet is being introduced, add small amounts of the new diet to the previous diet, then gradually increase the proportion of the new diet.

- Feed small amounts at a time and introduce other foods gradually to foods that are eaten.
- In hospitalized cats, providing the cat with its own carrier and synthetic facial pheromone may increase food intake.
- Avoid hovering over the pet, being too pushy, or trying to coax too much.
- Provide adequate amounts of daily exercise.

*Adapted from Ackerman L 1996 What every dog owner, breeder and trainer should know about nutrition. Alpine Publications.

Prevention

Normal, healthy pets rarely try to starve themselves. Most finicky pets actually receive adequate nutrition on a daily basis. Owners should receive veterinary counseling about how much their pet should be eating, based on the food being fed. This requires the veterinarian to be able to determine the caloric needs of the pet, and the caloric density of the food and any treats or table scraps being fed. Everything should be added into the equation.

To help deter pets from becoming 'picky' eaters, they should receive a variety of different food sources so they can develop their 'tastes' while still young. This may significantly impact on food preferences later in life.

Case example

Kwai-Chang was a three-year-old, 7-kg Pekinese. His owner was concerned because he almost never completely ate his dinner. She was worried that he might starve to death without her intervention. She was not sure how much he was eating because she fed him dry food by hand. She guessed he was only eating 15–20 pieces of this and only if she handfed him. He wouldn't touch the dry food if it just sat in his bowl. Some days he would only eat his treats and never touch his dry food. She also gave him one fatty acid capsule daily for an undetermined skin ailment.

On physical examination, Kwai-Chang was a healthy and happy Pekinese and not considered underweight. The owner was perplexed as to how he could not be losing weight on such a meager diet. Together we determined that Kwai-Chang had a daily requirement of about 600 kcal. On average, the owner gave him about six small treats daily, more when he would not eat any of his dinner. Each of the small biscuit treats was about 60 kcal, so six were contributing a total of about 360 kcal to his daily caloric intake. The calories in the fatty acid supplement could not be determined from the label and necessitated contacting the company directly. The caloric contribution from each fatty acid capsule was determined to be 10 kcal.

The goal was to lessen the number of treats given daily, substituting a balanced ration. The owner was certain that this could not be done. We decided to commence feeding Kwai-Chang a commercial dry cat food, enough to provide 600 kcal/day. The owner was cautioned not to give any treats to the dog or she would be sabotaging our efforts. She agreed that she would not feed any treats as long as Kwai-Chang ate the food within the first 48 hours. The owner called the next day to say that Kwai-Chang liked the new food but still pestered her for treats. The owner was instructed to ignore the begging as the behavior was merely being rewarded by intermittently providing food or attention. Stimuli, situations, and routines that might lead to begging were identified so that begging would be diminished (see obesity management above for details). Since the owners were unwilling to put up with the persistent demands and could not control Kwai-Chang sufficiently to stop the begging, it was decided to use substitute rewards such as toys and play. It was explained that these would also serve to reward the begging but at least Kwai-Chang would learn not to expect food. Each time Kwai-Chang approached they were instructed to have him perform a short 'down-stay' and then go and get a favorite toy and begin a play session. Kwai-Chang's begging quickly diminished, although he still approached for attention and play. The owners were also instructed on methods of stimulus control (see obesity section above). Four weeks later Kwai-Chang was still 7 kg and healthy and the owner was convinced he was eating much more than he ever had. She wanted to give him treats again, so three high-fiber low-calorie treats per day (20 kcal each) were added to the daily ration. The owner was instructed, however, to provide the treats only as training rewards and never to give them on demand. Over the next three months, the owner was able to wean Kwai-Chang entirely off the cat food diet, and onto a palatable canine diet. Six months later, Kwai-Chang was 7.5 kg and healthy, and the

owner reported that he had a 'normal' appetite; she was very proud that her 'intervention' had saved Kwai-Chang from starvation.

Appetite stimulants

Drugs such as the antiserotenergic antihistamine, cyproheptadine, and benzodiazepines such as diazepam, oxazepam, or flurazepam may be useful as appetite stimulants on a short-term basis.

FURTHER READING

Ackerman L 1993a Adverse reactions to foods. Journal of Veterinary Allergy and Clinical Immunology 1(1):18–22

Ackerman L 1993b Effects of an enzyme supplement (Prozyme) on selected nutrient levels in dogs. Journal of Veterinary Allergy and Clinical Immunology 2(1):25–29

Ackerman L 1993c Enzyme therapy in veterinary practice. Advances in Nutrition 1(3):9–11

Annunziata C, Shell L, Thatcher C et al 1996 Effects of a low protein diet on levels of serotonin in canine cerebrospinal fluid. Behavioral Abstract in American Veterinary Society Animal Behavior Newsletter 18(2):3

Aschheim E 1993 Dietary control of psychosis. Medical Hypotheses 41:327–328

Ballarini G 1990 Animal psychodietetics. Journal of Small Animal Practice 31(10):523–532

Blackshaw JK 1991 Management of orally based problems and aggression in cats. Australian Veterinary Practitioner 21:122–124

Brown RG 1989 Dealing with canine obesity. Canadian Veterinary Journal 30:973–975

Buffington CAT 1994 Management of obesity – the clinical nutritionist's experience. International Journal of Obesity 18(Suppl 1):S29–S35

Butterwick RF, Wills JM, Sloth C et al 1994 A study of obese cats on a calorie-controlled weight-reduction programme. Veterinary Record 134(15):372–377

Christensen L, Redig C 1993 Effects of meal consumption on mood. Behavioral Neuroscience 107(2):346–353

Davenport GM, Kelley RL, Altom EK et al 2001 Effect of diet on hunting performance of English pointers. Veterinary Therapeutics 2(1):10–23

DeNapoli JS, Dodman NH, Shuster L et al 2000 Effect of dietary protein content and tryptophan supplementation on dominance aggression, territorial aggression, and hyperactivity in dogs. Journal of the American Veterinary Medical Association 217(4):504–508

Diez M, Leemans M, Houins G et al 1995 Specific-purpose food in companion animals. The new directives of the European Community and practical use in the treatment

of obesity. Annales de Médecine Vétérinaire 139(6):395–399

Dodman NH, Reisner I, Shuster L et al 1996 Effect of dietary protein content on behaviour in dogs. Journal of the American Veterinary Medical Association 208(3):376–379

Edney ATB, Smith PM 1986 Study of obesity in dogs visiting veterinary practices in the United Kingdom. Veterinary Record 118:391–396

Fernstrom JD 1994 Dietary amino acids and brain function. Journal of the American Dietetic Association 94(1):71–77

Fernstron MH, Fernstrom JD 1995 Brain tryptophan concentrations and serotonin synthesis remain responsive to food consumption after the ingestion of sequential meals. American Journal of Clinical Nutrition 61(2):312–219

Gentry SJ 1993 Results of the clinical use of a standardized weight-loss program in dogs and cats. Journal of the American Animal Hospital Association 29(4):369–375

Griffith CA, Steigerwald ES, Buffington CAT 2000 Effects of a synthetic facial pheromone on behavior of cats. Journal of the American Veterinary Medical Association 217(8):1154–1156

Halliwell REW 1992 Comparative aspects of food intolerance. Veterinary Medicine September:893–899

Houpt KA 1993 Pharmacology and behaviour. In: Animal behaviour. The TG Hungerford refresher course for veterinarians. Postgraduate Committee in Veterinary Science, University of Sydney, Sydney, Australia, July, p 51–59

Kallfelz FA, Dzanis DA 1989 Overnutrition: an epidemic problem in pet animal practice? Veterinary Clinics of North America 19(3):433–445

Legrand Defretin V 1994 Energy requirements of cats and dogs – what goes wrong. International Journal of Obesity 18(Suppl 1):S8–S13

Lieberman HR, Caballero B, Finer N 1986 The composition of lunch determines afternoon plasma tryptophan concentrations in humans. Journal of Neural Transmission 65(3&4):211–217

Markwell PJ, Edney ATB 1996 The obese patient. In: Kelly N, Wills JM (eds) Manual of companion animal nutrition and feeding. BSAVA Publications, Cheltenham, p 109–116

Markwell PJ, Butterwick RF, Wills JM et al 1994 Clinical studies in the management of obesity in dogs and cats. International Journal of Obesity 18(Suppl 1):S39–S43

Mugford RA 1987 The influence of nutrition on canine behaviour. Journal of Small Animal Practice 28(11):1046–1055

Neville PF, Bradshaw JW 1994 Fabric eating in cats. Veterinary Practice Staff 6(5):26–30

Norris MP, Beaver BV 1993 Application of behaviour therapy techniques to the treatment of obesity in companion animals. Journal of the American Veterinary Medical Association 202(5):728–730

Quandt C 1994 Anorexia and obesity – nonorganic causes and their control. Praktische Tierarzt 75:109–110

Robinson I 1992 A taste for survival. In: Waltham feline medicine symposium. Waltham, Kal Kan Foods, Vernon, CA, p 55–64

Scarlett JM, Donoghue S, Saidla J et al 1994 Overweight cats – prevalence and risk factors. International Journal of Obesity 18(Suppl 1):S22–S28

Schoenthaler SJ, Moody JM, Pankow LD 1991 Applied nutrition and behaviour. Journal of Applied Nutrition 43(1):31–39

Wallin MS, Rissanen AM 1994 Food and mood: relationship between food, serotonin and affective disorders. Acta Psychiatrica Scandinavica 89(Suppl 377):36–40

Wurtman RJ 1983 Food consumption, neurotransmitter synthesis, and human behaviour. Experientia Supplement 44:356–369

9

Pain assessment, pain management, sedation, and anesthesia

One might wonder why the topic of pain management would appear in a text on veterinary behavior. First and foremost, the issue of humane care and the alleviation of pain and suffering should be a critical issue in any discussion of pet care. Specifically, however, pain assessment, response to pain medications, and the overall well-being of the pet depend heavily on the measurement and assessment of the pet's behavior. Pain and discomfort can lead to numerous behavioral signs including fear, withdrawal, retreat, vocalization, and aggression. Effective pain control and management is an integral part of relieving these signs.

Neuropathic pain (pain arising from nerve injury) may present with sudden, intense, or unusual behavioral changes (such as self-injurious behaviors, postural or gait changes, or vocalization), which may not respond to treatment with traditional pain medications such as NSAIDs or opioids. In fact, neuropathic as well as some chronic painful conditions may respond better to drugs that are traditionally associated with behavioral and neurological medicine, such as tranquilizers, anticonvulsants, and antidepressants.

BEHAVIORAL ASSESSMENT OF PAIN

There have been numerous studies on the assessment of pain in companion animals and the effectiveness of pain medications. Although results have been variable between studies and there may be significant variability between observers, there is fairly strong evidence that subjective pain scores from trained observers are sufficiently accurate to determine the need for pain management, especially with respect to acute pain such as from trauma or surgical procedures. In fact, behavioral responses to palpation, activity, mental status, posture, and vocalization have been shown to be reliable indicators of pain and the response to analgesics by dogs and cats during the postoperative period. Quantitative behavioral measurements have been shown to be an effective way to evaluate pain and response to analgesia after surgery. More objective physiologic measurements on the other hand, including heart rate, respiratory rate, blood pressure, plasma cortisol, and beta-endorphin concentrations, may not be significantly different when comparing controls with those undergoing surgery.

Using behavioral measurements the following information has been obtained:

- After elective orthopedic surgery, ketoprofen alone had a greater level and longer duration of analgesia action than dogs given butorphanol or oxymorphone alone.
- A single postoperative injection after ovariohysterectomy in a cat of either ketoprofen, buprenorphine, or pethidine led to lower pain scores with the least need for interventional analgesia in the ketoprofen-treated cats.
- Butorphanol injections for the day of surgery and the first full day after, or a transdermal fentanyl patch applied eight hours prior to declawing (and for two days after), led to significant improvement in appetite and pain scores over controls.
- Carprofen, ketoprofen, meloxicam, and tolfenamic acid provided good postoperative analgesia following ovariohysterectomy in cats for up to 18 hours when treated with a single dose at extubation, although rescue interventional analgesia was required for one of 10 cats in each of the tolfenamic acid, ketoprofen, and meloxicam groups.

- Ketoprofen and tolfenamic acid, along with amitriptyline and pentosan polysulfate, have been suggested as potential therapy for recurrent idiopathic cystitis in cats.

Pain assessment scale for surgical and medical patients

There is a great deal of individual variation in the pet's reactivity to painful stimuli, the pet's response to pain, and the pet's baseline behavior with the observer. In addition, pack animals and those that are potential prey may mask signs of illness and discomfort. Dogs may continue to wag their tails and cats may continue to purr even though they may be experiencing severe pain. Therefore, a safe general rule of thumb for pain management is that pets likely feel pain in much the same situations as would a person. In addition, if the pet exhibits tachycardia or tachypnea, pain medication should be given to a level that will reduce the heart and respiratory rate toward normal.

In both dogs and cats, signs of distress, agonistic body postures and expressions, and avoidance or escape attempts might be indicative of pain, especially when compared with expressive behaviors and postures such as attention soliciting, whining, or purring and head rubbing, which might be indicative of pain relief. On the other hand, changes in behavior such as vocalization and aggression are not specific to pain and may be associated with many other stimuli as well as drugs used for anesthesia and premedication (e.g., noise sensitivity, excitement on induction, or recovery). Therefore pain-scoring systems that rely solely on agitation, movement, and vocalization alone have been shown to be unreliable.

Some method of evaluating pain in hospitalized pets should be implemented in each veterinary clinic so that postoperative, ongoing pain management can be modified to suit the needs of each pet on a case-by-case basis. Pets that might be experiencing pain should be monitored regularly for a change in condition. Improvement or deterioration in categories should be compared when determining response to pain medication or the need for additional medication. However, there may be great variability in pain assessment scores between observers, so that a standardized scoring system between hospitals, staff, and studies may not be possible (such as the one in Fig. 9.1). Pain scores range from 0 (no pain) to 5 (severe/maximal pain).

Pain assessment for caregivers at home

Radiographic, neurologic, and physical examination by the veterinarian are important components of the initial assessment and follow up. But when pets are being cared for in the home, pain will need to be assessed by the owner. Since signs of pain may be subtle, any change in the pet's behavior, physical health (e.g., mobility), or response to pain therapy should be reported.

(1) *General*: Any change in behavior, whether desirable or undesirable, could be indicative of pain or disease. For example, a pet could become more affectionate and 'clingy' or less interactive and irritable, or either increasingly or decreasingly vocal.

(2) *Physical health*: Changes in physical health or the pet's medical condition may be indicative of pain. These might include change in appetite or drinking, a change in volume or frequency of urine or stool output, straining during elimination, panting, change in gait, change in posture whether standing or at rest, decreased exercise tolerance, weakness, stiffness, incoordination, or discomfort when touching or manipulating an area of the body.

(3) *Behavior*: With pain, there might be a change in behavior, either an increase or decrease from baseline (i.e., what is normal for the pet). Owners should monitor for, and report, a change in responsiveness to stimuli, change in interactions with owners, increased irritability, fear, anxiety, apathy, depression, waking at nights, restless

Score	Description
0	No pain. Relaxed. Normal gait, greeting, and play. No apparent pain on palpation. Lies down and sleeps comfortably. Normal heart rate and respiration unless excited or anxious. Normal appetite and grooming. Normally attentive to environment
1	Mild. May be mildly affected gait, mild abnormal stance, or mild limping if limb injury. May sleep normally but dreaming (REM pattern) may not be present. May be mild reaction to palpation of area. Attentive to stimuli but may be mildly distracted. Not depressed
2	Movement becoming more restricted. If limb injury may stand with toe on ground and gait may be altered (lame). Abdomen may be tucked. May lick or chew surgical/painful area. Orients to site of surgery or injury. Mild objection to palpation. Quiet attitude – may be uncomfortable when trying to rest and not lying in a curled up position. May be depressed and less responsive to stimuli
3	Movement restricted. May stretch legs, arch, or guard abdomen. May be partial weight bearing at rest or movement if limb injury. May be slow to rise. May vocalize, lick, withdraw, or attempt to bite when surgical or painful site palpated. Restless, agitated, may tremble, head may be down and tail may be tucked between legs. May not sleep well. May be less responsive to caregiver. May be excessively quiet or may occasionally vocalize. Heart rate may be increased and respiration increased or shallow. Pupils may be dilated. Appetite may be decreased
4	Movement severely restricted. Body posture arched, extended, or tucked. Movement slow or jerky. No weight bearing at rest or when moving if injured limb. May avoid, vocalize, or attempt to bite if moved or manipulated. Guarding of painful area. May chew, bite, or lick area. Depressed with little interest in surroundings but will respond to a direct voice. May groan, whine, or show facial expressions of distress. May 'scream' when touched or approached. May defecate or urinate without moving. May not move due to pain. Hypertension, tachycardia, and possibly tachypnea
5	Severe (excruciating pain). Tense, writhing, shivering, or no movement (partially comatose). No weight bearing and may refuse to stand or walk. May be unsolicited howling. Fixed stare – may not respond to any stimuli. Pain elicited whenever patient touched. May be hyperesthesia and hyperalgesia. Breathing may be labored

Figure 9.1   Pain assessment scoring for hospitalized pets.

sleep, vocalization, repetitive behaviors such as excessive licking, decreased grooming, or self care, change in elimination habits.

(4) *Response to therapy*: If the pet has been placed on medication in an attempt to relieve pain, any improvement should be noted and reported.

MANAGING PAIN

Prior to exposure to noxious stimuli (e.g., surgery), pre-emptive pain management should be instituted. Pre- and perioperative analgesia are the most effective means of minimizing postoperative pain and improving outcome. Balanced analgesia that involves the combination of two or more classes of analgesic drugs is generally most effective. For example, the use of NSAIDs or local anesthesia can inhibit transduction at the site of injury, a local nerve block can be used to prevent transmission of the nerve impulse, and pain 'modulation' pathways in the spinal cord.

The simplified assumption that a pet under sufficient depth of anesthesia will not perceive pain is no longer valid. Although anesthetics inhibit the perception of pain, anesthetic recovery can be improved, and the need for postoperative pain medications reduced, by blocking *transduction* at the site of injury, blocking the *transmission* of pain, and enhancing spinal *modulation* to prevent noxious stimuli from sensitizing the nervous system. An understanding of the potential for pain with each procedure and the drug regime that might best prevent this pain is therefore an important aspect of humane care.

Pain pathways and pain management

By understanding how pain is perceived, a combination of pharmaceutical agents can be used to remove pain or reduce its intensity.

- The pain pathway begins at the nociceptive receptors in the sensory nerve endings.

Transduction can be prevented by the use of local anesthesia at the site of pain perception. Non-steroidal anti-inflammatory drugs and intra-articular opioids can also diminish transduction by decreasing inflammatory elements such as prostaglandins at the site of injury.

- Transmission of pain can be prevented by blockade of peripheral nerves and nerve plexuses, with local anesthetic infiltration or by epidural injection.
- Modulation of pain within the spinal cord can be augmented by opioids, NSAIDs, or alpha 2 adrenergic agonists.
- The perception of pain can be modulated by general anesthesia, systemic opioids, and alpha 2 agonists.
- Other forms of pain management that do not involve drug therapy may also need to be considered. Decreasing mobility of the affected area, support, cold or heat packs, physical therapy such as massage or stretching, and the prevention of further trauma or damage to the area by bandaging or using an Elizabethan collar may all be useful.

Types of pain

Pain can be either physiologic or pathologic. Physiologic pain arises from heat, cold, or pressure and leads to protective behavioral responses. Pathologic pain can arise from inflammation (burning, freezing, trauma/injury, surgery, hypoxia) or neuropathic processes (nerve injury). Most physiologic and pathologic pain improves with therapy with traditional analgesics such as NSAIDs and opioids alone or in combination with local anesthetics, benzodiazepines, general anesthesia, or alpha 2 agonists. However, some chronic painful conditions and neuropathic pain may be more responsive to non-traditional forms of pain management such as anticonvulsants (e.g., carbamazepine and gabapentin) and tricyclic antidepressants such as amitriptyline, nortriptyline, and desipramine.

Drugs for pain control and behavioral management

Tranquilizers

The primary purpose of tranquilizers, both pre- and postsurgically, is to relieve anxiety, quiet the patient sufficiently for transport and restraint, prevent self-trauma and excessive activity post-surgically, and to prevent emesis. Pheno-thiazines are dopamine antagonists, and can cause a decrease in arterial blood pressure and a decrease in the seizure threshold, while having minimal effect on anxiety. However, the use of phenothiazines prior to anesthesia can help to ease induction, reduce the dose of anesthesia required, decrease emesis, and ease the recovery. Benzodiazepines, on the other hand, reduce anxi-ety and act as a muscle relaxant and anticonvul-sant, while causing minimal respiratory and cardiac depression.

Opioid agonist–antagonists

Opioids are analgesics that do not affect con-sciousness except when used at the high end of the dose range. The opioid receptors responsible for analgesia are mostly mu receptors and to a lesser extent kappa. Sigma receptors produce dysphoria and hallucinations but not analgesia. Opioids may be agonists, agonist–antagonists, or antagonists. They act to inhibit pain transmis-sion in the dorsal horn, inhibit somatosensory afferents at supraspinal levels, and activate des-cending inhibitory pathways.

Morphine, oxymorphone, fentanyl, and hydro-morphone are narcotic agonists. Morphine is the prototype opioid agonist which targets primarily mu and to a lesser extent kappa receptors. Its major effect is analgesia. It produces a marked increase in 5HT synthesis. Its action is probably in the nucleus raphe magnus-spinal system. It depresses the medullary respiratory, cough, and vasomotor centers and stimulates the vomit-ing center. It stimulates the sphincters of the gas-trointestinal tract so that it may be constipating, although it also increases intestinal peristalsis and immediate defecation. Its duration of effect for pain control is approximately two to six hours.

Oxymorphone and hydromorphone are app-roximately 10 times more potent than morphine and last approximately four to six hours. Both are primarily mu agonists. However, unlike morphine, neither is thought to release hista-mine when given i.v. When oxymorphone (0.2 mg/kg) is combined with a tranquilizer such as acepromazine (0.1–0.2 mg/kg), it may induce neuroleptoanalgesia that is sufficient for anesthesia induction or restraint for diagnostic procedures.

Fentanyl is a synthetic opioid with a potency 100 times that of morphine. It is available for humans as a transdermal patch, which has been used successfully for both dogs and cats. In dogs the 50 µg/hr patch provides analgesia for about 72 hours, but will need to be applied 12 to 24 hours in advance to achieve its maximal level of analgesia, and may last up to 24 hours after the patch is removed. In cats, the 25 µg/hr patch is usually effective for 60 hours or longer and achieves maximal effect within six to 24 hours of application. For smaller animals the seal of the patch can be folded back before applying to the skin so that only part of the fen-tanyl is released.

When using fentanyl patches for postopera-tive pain control, there may be some variability in effect between pets since these patches have been designed for absorption through human skin, and require good adherence for proper absorption (skin to patch contact). Therefore, management should be constantly monitored to ensure that it is adequate.

Butorphanol and buprenorphine are opioids with agonist–antagonist properties, while nalox-one is an opioid antagonist. Buprenorphine is useful for feline pain control, especially with buccal application of an oral liquid formulation. If oxymorphone is administered preoperatively, its sedative effects might be reversed postopera-tively with naloxone while maintaining or even enhancing postoperative analgesia.

Alpha 2 agonists

Xylazine and medetomidine are alpha 2 agonists that induce sedation and analgesia at recommended doses. Alpha 2 agonists likely exert their analgesic action through similar modulatory pathways as opioids, so the combined effects of opioids and alpha 2 agonists may be additive or synergistic. In addition they inhibit norepinephrine release in the locus ceruleus, thalamus, and cerebral cortex, leading to sedation that further decreases pain perception. Alpha 2 antagonists are commonly used alone, or in combination with benzodiazepines or opioids such as butorphanol as pre-anesthetic agents. They may produce sufficient sedation and analgesia to allow for diagnostic procedures, minor surgical procedures that might be performed under local anesthesia, and for dogs that are difficult to restrain or too fractious to handle. Alpha 2 agonists should be used with caution or avoided in pets that are elderly or those with cardiovascular compromise. Anticholinergics such as glycopyrrolate or atropine can be given to prevent against bradycardia, and the medetomidine antagonist atipamazole can be given to hasten recovery or to reverse the cardiovascular, respiratory, or sedative effects.

Non-steroidal anti-inflammatory drugs

NSAIDs are anti-inflammatory drugs that inhibit cyclooxygenase. Cyclooxygenase activity leads to the production of prostaglandins, which are important mediators of inflammation but are also responsible for protection of the gastrointestinal tract as well as maintenance of renal blood flow during states of hypotension. Potential side effects include gastric ulceration, nephrotoxicity, and diminished hemostasis. Since NSAIDs inhibit cyclooxygenase they act to block prostaglandin synthesis. There are at least two forms of cyclooxygenase (COX). Inflammatory prostaglandins are derived primarily from COX-2, although COX-1 may play a lesser role in some inflammatory conditions. COX-2-mediated prostaglandins also play a role in healing and in homeostasis with the kid-

ney. Prostaglandins responsible for homeostatic mechanisms in the gastrointestinal tract are derived primarily from COX-1. Therefore drugs that are more selective for COX-2 inhibition may have less potential for gastrointestinal side effects. In one study, administration of carprofen, etodolac, and placebo to healthy dogs caused less gastrointestinal ulceration than buffered aspirin. Tolfenamic acid, meloxicam, deracoxib, carprofen, and etodolac are more selective for COX-2 inhibition in comparison with ketoprofen and aspirin.

Meloxicam is a COX-2 selective NSAID, approved for dogs in Canada and Europe. There are no hepatic or renal contraindications and there is minimal antithromboxane activity. It is dosed at 0.2 mg/kg the first day followed by 0.1 mg/kg daily. Pain control can be maintained for up to 24 hours.

Carprofen is a COX-2 preferential NSAID, approved for dogs. In Europe, it is also approved for a single perioperative injection in cats, which may control pain for up to 30 hours. Nephrotoxicity and hemostatic deficiencies are not a concern, although there have been rare cases of hepatotoxicity in dogs. It is dosed at 4.4 mg/kg daily and has recently been licensed for control of postoperative pain.

Ketoprofen inhibits both COX-1 and COX-2 and is approved for use in dogs and cats in Europe and Canada. Side effects include the potential for decreased hemostasis and increased risk for gastrointestinal ulceration in comparison with NSAIDs that are more selective for COX-2. It has been shown to provide excellent postoperative analgesia for up to 24 hours. It is dosed at 2 mg/kg the first day, followed by 1 mg/kg daily.

Etodolac preferentially inhibits COX-2 and is approved in the United States for management of pain associated with osteoarthritis at a dose of 10 to 15 mg/kg daily. It may also be useful for other chronic painful conditions. The primary side effects are gastrointestinal, but at a rate significantly less than aspirin.

Tolfenamic acid is approved for cats and dogs in Europe and Canada for controlling both acute and chronic pain at a dose of 4 mg/kg for three to four days followed by three to four days off. It preferentially inhibits COX-2 and should be used cautiously postsurgically because of its antithromboxane effects.

Deracoxib, the only coxib-class drug approved for dogs, has just recently been released in the US. Coxib-class drugs are the most selective for COX-2 inhibition. The dose for acute pain management is 3–4 mg/kg daily and for chronic pain it is 1–2 mg/kg daily.

Adjunctive analgesics

In humans, some forms of neuropathic pain (e.g., diabetic neuropathy, trigeminal neuritis) and other chronic painful conditions such as lower back pain may not respond to NSAIDs and opioids, and may be more responsive to drugs that have been licensed for other applications. These include tricyclic antidepressants, such as amitriptyline, imipramine, and desipramine, which may perhaps act by serotonergic and noradrenergic-mediated enhancement of descending inhibitory pathways, anticonvulsants, such as gabapentin, and NMDA receptor antagonists, such as ketamine and dextromethorphan. Although NSAIDs alone or in conjunction with opioids may be effective for neuropathic pain, these adjunctive forms of pain management are increasingly becoming a first line of therapy. On the other hand, they have little to no effect on nociceptive pain. Nociceptive pain is pain resulting from stimulation of peripheral nerve endings, while neuropathic pain is pain that is initiated by a lesion or dysfunction of the nervous system. Peripheral neuropathic pain is generated through a focal inflammatory process rather than axonal destruction.

There is increasing evidence that some of these adjunctive forms of pain management may also be useful in cases of neuropathic pain and other chronic painful conditions that are not sufficiently improved with traditional analgesics. Therefore practitioners should consider these alternative agents in (a) painful conditions that are refractory to traditional analgesics, (b) medical conditions such as idiopathic cystitis where other forms of pain management have not traditionally been effective, (c) suspected cases of neuropathic pain, and (d) as a diagnostic aid and potential treatment for self-mutilatory disorders such as cats that attack and injure their tails or incessant scratching of the face and neck.

Tricyclic antidepressants

In addition to their antidepressant or behavioral effects, amitriptyline, nortriptyline, and desipramine also appear to have analgesic effects that may be particularly useful in the treatment of neuropathic pain as well as headaches, lower back pain, and cancer-related pain. In humans, they have been used alone or as adjunctive therapy to treat the pain associated with diabetic neuropathy, central poststroke pain, pain associated with migraine headaches, cancer-related neuropathic pain, and postherpetic neuralgia. The behavioral effects of antidepressants may also be useful if there is a concomitant anxiety or depressive component. Tricyclic antidepressants may control peripheral neuropathic pain by acting as sodium channel blockers. They may have an inhibitory effect on nociceptive pathways by blocking the re-uptake of serotonin and norepinephrine. However, inhibition of serotonin re-uptake is not likely a primary factor in pain control since selective serotonin re-uptake inhibitors are not generally effective, although one recent study found similar efficacy with fluoxetine and amitriptyline for lower back pain. Tricyclic antidepressants (TCAs) also potentiate the analgesic effects of opioids. In humans, a response to therapy is generally seen in three to 10 days.

In pets, amitriptyline, imipramine, or nortriptyline might be considered for the control of neuropathic pain, such as might be associated with spinal injuries and cancer that is refractory to traditional analgesics. TCAs have been suggested as a treatment for cats with idiopathic cystitis because of their effects on both pain (may prevent the degranulation of mast cells in the bladder wall, which in turn decreases the release of substance P) and behavior, and might be considered for suspected neuropathies (e.g., facial mutilation).

Selective serotonin re-uptake inhibitors and clomipramine may also be effective in some cases of chronic pain.

Anticonvulsant therapy

Antiepileptic drugs are used in treatment regimes for human neuropathic pain and might also be useful for pain management in pets. Their mechanism of action is unknown but is likely similar to the antiepileptic mechanisms of each drug. Most of the drugs in this category, as well as tricyclic antidepressants, have some ability to block sodium channels. Although carbamazepine and clonazepam may be effective, gabapentin may be a better alternative because it has fewer side effects and fewer drug interactions.

There may be some subtle differences between the pain management afforded by antidepressants, which are reported to be more effective for continuous burning pain, and anticonvulsants, which are more effective for lancinating pain. First-generation anticonvulsants such as carbamazepine and perhaps clonazepam have previously been the drugs of choice for lancinating pain. However, they showed limited efficacy and the potential for numerous side effects and drug interactions with carbamazepine. Second-generation anticonvulsants such as gabapentin have fewer side effects and fewer drug interactions and may be more effective in the treatments of shooting, burning, and throbbing pain.

Gabapentin is an analog of GABA (for further drug information, see Ch. 6). It is an anticonvulsant that may also be effective in humans for anxiety and dementia as well as refractory panic disorder, generalized anxiety disorder, obsessive–compulsive disorders, and orthostatic tremors. In humans it has also been used as monotherapy or as an add on to opioids or NSAIDs for the control of a variety of neuropathic and refractory chronic painful conditions including trigeminal neuralgia, postherpetic neuralgia, central poststroke pain, and neuropathic cancer pain.

In veterinary patients, gabapentin has been reported to be effective in patients with pre-sumed neuropathic pain associated with vertebral fracture, and has been suggested as either a treatment or diagnostic aid for cats with self-mutilation of the tail or of the head and face. Gabapentin may also be effective in dogs for neuropathic pain and a therapeutic trial might be considered for refractory cases of self-mutilatory disorders. If therapy is effective at achieving pain management, the dose should be gradually lowered until the lowest effective dose is determined.

Carbamazepine is similar to imipramine in structure and has been used as a mood stabilizer, anticonvulsant, and for neuropathic pain, specifically trigeminal neuritis in humans, and may also have some behavioral effects (see Ch. 6 for details). Dosing can be further complicated by the fact that the drug induces its own metabolism, so that higher doses may be required to maintain effect over time.

Ketamine

Low-dose ketamine, an NMDA receptor antagonist, may prevent and reverse windup, the neuronal hyperexcitability that occurs following constant stimulation of pain receptors. A continuous rate infusion of 2 µg/kg/min is used, with an initial bolus of 0.5 mg/kg if needed. For CRI analgesia, ketamine should be combined with a sedative or opioid (at lowered doses due to synergistic effects). The spinal cord modulatory effects of ketamine may be effective in the treatment of neuropathic pain.

Alternative forms of pain therapy

Although generally beyond the scope of discussion of a behavioral text, there are also a number of other forms of pain management that do not utilize pharmacologic agents. These might include acupuncture, herbal, nutraceutical, vitamin, and mineral preparations, homeopathic therapy, aromatherapy, and a variety of forms of massage and touch therapy. Many of these therapeutic modalities are also purported to be effective in behavior therapy (see alternative medication section – Ch. 8).

Acupuncture

Neuroanatomic acupuncture is used in the treatment of pain and neurologic impairment, and may exert its effects by restoring neural regulation, reducing inflammation, optimizing endogenous pain control, and resolving somatic dysfunction. Percutaneous electrical nerve stimulation (PENS) is a form of acupuncture in which there is stimulation of peripheral nerves, nerve roots, and the autonomic system in accordance with the myotomal, sclerotomal, and dermatomal distribution of pain.

The following information was contributed by Kate Gentry DVM, Certified Veterinary Acupuncturist:

When practiced properly by well-trained veterinarians, acupuncture techniques can provide very profound and useful analgesia in small animal patients. While most often used for chronic pain amelioration or palliative therapy, acupuncture produces very good pain control in many acute pain situations including trauma, intraoperative, and immediate postoperative situations. The fact that acupuncture alone has been used in place of anesthesia in some instances speaks to the effectiveness of this method when used properly. It is also useful to note that the dosages of some anesthetics and analgesics can be significantly decreased when acupuncture is used as an adjunct for anesthesia and pain control.

Acupuncture is also useful in painful situations such as acute trauma and shock when some analgesics may cause difficulty in patient evaluation or may have undesirable side effects. Acupuncture is also extremely useful in calming the patient in such circumstances. Many of our patients are very frightened and stressed in hospital surroundings, despite our best efforts on their behalf. Relieving tension, fear, and anxiety greatly facilitates our treatment results and raises pain thresholds.

The most common uses for acupuncture for 'acute' problems are trauma, dental pain, and surgery, any orthopedic surgery (especially in the immediate postoperative period), cesarean pain, and abdominal and sternotomy incisional pain. Acute intervertebral disc pain can also be decreased. Some of these situations respond better to electroacupuncture than simple needling or aquapuncture techniques. Many problems require a combination of meridian, distal, and local point treatment in order to provide the best analgesia and facilitate healing. Each case involves an individual and should be treated as such. This is why it is so important to use a qualified veterinary acupuncturist rather than relying on 'trigger-point' techniques.

While it is beyond the scope of this book to explain exactly how acupuncture works in pain control, acupuncture exerts its effects by influencing all of the following parameters of pain:

- Peripheral nervous system via several specific nerve fiber types, including both sensory and motor fibers.
- Central nervous system pain pathways that are very complex and include nociceptive, neuropathic, idiopathic, and psychogenic aspects of pain. Acupuncture is quite effective in calming patients as well, thus allowing the practitioner to better assess a diseased state. A great deal of 'pain' that we see in our patients is often a misinterpretation of the 'fight-or-flight' response.
- Somatovisceral pathways in which peripheral pain causes secondary visceral pain. There is also strong evidence that acupuncture addresses a reversal of this pathway, known as the 'viscerocutaneous reflex,' whereby diseased organs refer pain to acupuncture points. This is a partial explanation of the effectiveness of diagnostic acupuncture when using peripheral points to aid in the diagnosis of underlying organ pathology.
- Neurotransmitters, which affect pain perception via the release of endorphins, encephalins, serotonin, dynorphin (an extremely powerful opiate with 200 times the analgesic effect of morphine), and catecholamines.

• Local reaction to needle insertion, which includes the release of histamine, leukotrienes, bradykinin, prostaglandins, and acetylcholine. Also considered here are agents such as eosinophils, antibody production, and an amplification of the vasoactive phase, all of which act to mediate tissue damage and facilitate tissue repair. Thus the reduction of pain is also a factor of immunological mechanisms stimulated by acupuncture.

As one can see, there is no one mechanism that can explain all of the many facets in which acupuncture exerts its effects in pain management. New research and data acquisition is constantly being conducted, updated, and published. As our scientific methods improve, we will no doubt see increased emphasis placed upon the incorporation of acupuncture as an integral part of our pain control treatment plans.

Compulsive disorders and neuropathic pain

There are a number of self-injurious and self-mutilatory behavioral conditions in dogs and cats that might be either (a) induced by medical causes or (b) a compulsive disorder arising out of conflict. These include tail chasing and attacking (which can lead to sufficient damage to require surgical intervention), scratching of the face and neck, and self-trauma directed at other body parts including acral lick dermatitis. Traditionally, these cases have been worked up as dermatologic, painful, and neurologic diseases and diagnosed as a compulsive disorder if underlying medical causes have been ruled out and the behavioral definition of compulsive disorders has been met. However, there may be sufficient similarity to some of the neuropathic pain conditions in humans to first warrant a therapeutic trial with gabapentin, carbamazepine, clonazepam, or amitriptyline. In humans with trigeminal neuritis, stabbing, shooting, or electric shock-type pain may arise in the region of the mandibular and maxillary nerves, predominantly in adults over the age of 40, possibly due to chronic facial demyelination. Although this type of pain may be poorly responsive to traditional analgesics, the condition can often be successfully controlled, with carbamazepine, clonazepam, or gabapentin.

FURTHER READING

Cambridge AJ, Tobias KM, Newberry RC et al 2000 Subjective and objective measurements of postoperative pain in cats. Journal of the American Veterinary Medical Association 217(5):685–690

Carroll GL, Howe LB, Slater MR et al 1998 Evaluation of analgesia provided by postoperative administration of butorphinol to cats undergoing onychectomy. Journal of the American Veterinary Medical Association 213(2):246–250

Dowling PM 2000 Potential therapies for recurrent idiopathic cystitis in cats. Veterinary Medicine 95(7):512–515

Firth AM, Haldane SL 1999 Development of a scale to evaluate postoperative pain in dogs. Journal of the American Veterinary Medical Association 214(5):651–659

Franks JN, Boothe HW, Taylor L et al 2000 Evaluation of transdermal fentanyl patches for analgesia in cat undergoing onychectomy. Journal of the American Veterinary Medical Association 217(7):1013–1019

Gaynor J 2001 Pain scoring and other means of evaluation. Veterinary Forum October: 45–47

Grisnaux E, Pibarot P, Dupuis J et al 1999 Comparison of ketoprofen and carprofen administered prior to orthopedic surgery for the control of postoperative pain in dogs. Journal of the American Veterinary Medical Association 215:1105–1110

Guay DRP 2001 Adjunctive agents in the management of chronic pain. Pharmacotherapy 21(9):1070–1081

Hansen B 2001 The use of NSAIDs in pain management. Veterinary Forum October:48–51

Hansen BD, Hardie EM, Carroll GS 1997a Physiological measurements after ovariohysterectomy in dogs: what's normal. Applied Animal Behavioral Science 51:101–109

Hardie EM, Hansen BD, Carroll GS 1997b Behaviour after hysterectomy in the dog: what's normal. Applied Animal Behavioral Science 51:111–128

Holton LL, Scott EM, Nolan AM et al 1998 Comparison of three methods used for assessment of pain in dogs.

Journal of the American Veterinary Medical Association 212(1):61–66

Jones CJ, Budsberg SC 2000 Physiologic characteristics and clinical importance of the cyclooxygenase isoforms of dogs and cats. Journal of the American Veterinary Medical Association 217(5):721–729

Mathews KA 2000 Pain assessment and general approach to management. Veterinary Clinics of North America, Small Animal Practice 30(4):729–755

Mathews K 2001 Dealing with pain in the clinic. Veterinary Forum November:41–47

Mathews KA, Pettifer C, Foster R et al 1999 A comparison of the safety and efficacy of meloxicam to ketoprofen to butorphinol for control of postoperative pain associated with soft tissue surgery in dogs. In: Proceedings of the symposium on recent advances in non-steroidal anti-inflammatory therapy in small animals, Paris, p 67

Muir WW, Woolf CJ 2001 Mechanisms of pain and their therapeutic implications. JAVMA 219(10):1346–1356

Papich M 2001 What does cox selectivity mean? Veterinary Forum November:39–41

Pibarot P, Dupuis J, Grisneaux E et al 1997 Comparison of ketoprofen, oxymorphone hydrochloride, and butorphinol in the treatment of postoperative pain in dogs. Journal of the American Veterinary Medical Association 211(4):438–444

Reimer ME, Johnston SA, Lieb MS et al 1999 The gastrointestinal effects of buffered aspirin, carprofen and etodolac in healthy dogs. Journal of Veterinary International Medicine 13(5):472–477

Robertson SA, Taylor PM, Bloomfield M et al 2001 Systemic uptake of buprenorphine after buccal administration in cats. Meeting, American College of Veterinary Anesthesiologists

Schoen A 2001 Veterinary acupuncture – ancient art to modern medicine, 2nd edn. Mosby, St Louis

Schreiber S, Vinokur S, Shavelzon V et al 2001 A randomized trial of fluoxetine versus amitriptyline in musculo-skeletal pain. Israeli Journal of Psychiatry and Related Sciences 38(2):88–94

Schwerdtner I, Thalhammer JG 1999 Do expressive behavioral indicators in cats undergoing orthopedic surgery relate to postoperative pain? In: Proceedings of satellite symposium of the 9th world congress on pain management, Vienna, Austria

Shafford HI, Lascelles BDX, Hellyer PW 2001 Preemptive analgesia: managing pain before it begins. Veterinary Medicine June:478–491

Slingsby LS, Waterman-Pearson AE 1998 Comparison of pethidine, buprenorphine and ketoprofen for postoperative analgesia after ovariohysterectomy in the cat. Veterinary Records 143(7):185–189

Slingsby LS, Waterman-Pearson AE 2000 Postoperative analgesia in the cat after ovariohysterectomy by use of carprofen, ketoprofen, meloxicam or tolfenamic acid. Journal of Small Animal Practice 41(10):447–450

Thurmon JC, Tranquilli WJ, Benson GJ (eds) 1996 Lumb and Jones' veterinary anesthesia, 3rd edn. Williams and Wilkins, Baltimore, p 183–210

Yoshida T, Tanaka C, Umeda M et al 1995 Non-invasive measurement of brain activity using functional MRI toward the study of brain response to acupuncture stimulation. American Journal of Chinese Medicine 23:319–325

10

Stereotypic and compulsive disorders

INTRODUCTION

In this chapter we review some intriguing abnormal behaviors of pets. These abnormal behaviors fall into two major categories: pathophysiological (i.e., resulting from a physical or medical problem) and experiential (arising from exposure or lack of exposure to environmental and social interactions). Pathophysiological examples have been dealt with in numerous sections throughout this book. These might include genetic physical problems (such as hip dysplasia, deafness, or hydrocephalus), or genetic behavioral or physiological problems (such as narcolepsy, or nervousness in Pointers) or acquired problems (such as rabies, nutritional deficiencies, or toxins). Disease processes and their effects on behavior are discussed in more detail in other sections of the book, especially as they apply to the aging process (see Chs 12, 21).

Because of genetic, medical, hormonal, nutritional, and physical differences, and the effects of early learning and experience, two pets exposed to the same external stimuli may have different levels of motivation or varying levels of arousal. How an animal copes or responds to this arousal is also dependent on these internal factors and mechanisms. Situations that might lead to stress or arousal include the pet's physical or social environment, the availability of resources, and the availability of appropriate releasing stimuli for species-typical behaviors (e.g., chew toys, scratching posts). De-arousal is achieved by satisfying the pet's desires through the performance of normal species-typical behaviors.

Experiential abnormal behavior might arise during development (e.g., inadequate socialization), may be reactive (resulting from factors in the environment or management of the pet), or may be conditioned through reinforcement. Reactive abnormal behavior generally results from conflict brought about by the pet's level of arousal and the inability to perform an appropriate behavior to reduce arousal. The motivation to perform a particular behavior is brought about by any combination of intrinsic or extrinsic factors. To achieve de-arousal the pet may respond by engaging in a normal response with respect to the stimulus (e.g., scratching, urine marking, retreat, aggression). However, when there are no appropriate behaviors to achieve de-arousal the pet may redirect its behavior toward a less suitable target, may engage in vacuum activities, may display displacement activities (normal behaviors out of context), or may redirect its behavior to an alternate target (redirected behavior). There may be a genetic component to the type of displacement or vacuum activity an individual pet displays, as breed predispositions have been identified (Fig. 10.1). Stereotypic behavior has been shown to have a strong genetic component and minimal effects of social influence in some species such as mice.

Some specialty disciplines, especially neurology, dermatology, and nutrition, have recognized the significance of behavioral manifestations in a variety of conditions. In dermatology, for instance, there is growing interest in psychodermatology, which is also referred to as psychocutaneous medicine and dermato-psychosomatics. An exploratory model called the neuro-immuno-cutaneous-endocrine (NICE) network envisions these apparently unrelated systems as being linked by peptides, proteins, cytokines, and hormones. The term animal psychodietetics has been advanced to describe the relation between nutrition and behavioral changes, and there are now even commercial diets available that purport to specifically support the brain's nutritional needs. There is little doubt that even more conditions will be recognized as sharing a behavioral component, and a variety of different and complementary treatment options will likely become available.

COMPULSIVE DISORDERS

Compulsive disorders in dogs and cats have also been referred to as stereotypies and obsessive–compulsive disorders (OCD), and may be difficult to differentiate from neurological conditions including seizure foci. They may be similar to the stereotypies described in other species, such as the repetitive or ritualized pacing seen in zoo animals or cribbing in horses. These are

Disorder	Breed
Tail chasing	Australian Cattle Dog
	German Shepherd
	English Bull Terrier
Spinning	English Bull Terrier
Flank sucking	Doberman Pinscher
Self-injurious behavior, acral lick dermatitis	Large breed dogs
Rock chewing, eating	Labrador Retriever
Checking hind end	Miniature Schnauzer
Sticking head under objects and freezing	English Bull Terrier
Fly snapping	King Charles Cavalier Spaniel
	Bernese Mountain Dog
Wool sucking	Siamese/Burmese (cats)

Figure 10.1 Breed predilection for displacement and compulsive disorders (adapted from Andrew Luescher).

thought to arise as a response to conflict related to confinement or husbandry practices. Stereotypic behaviors are described as being repetitive, constant, and serving no apparent purpose. This may be an accurate description for some of the canine and feline behaviors such as floor scratching, pacing, and wool sucking. However, this does not describe all of the compulsive disorders seen in dogs and cats, since some of these behaviors involve no repetition (e.g., freezing, staring), and there can be variability in their expression. In humans, the term OCD is used to describe a group of behaviors with repetitive motor features such as trichotillomania (hair pulling). Obsessions are intrusive thoughts that are often related to checking (e.g., repeatedly checking to see if a stove has been turned off or a security system turned on to the extent that it becomes difficult to leave the home) or concern for contamination (e.g., excessive washing). Because of similarities in some of the signs in pets and humans, and the fact that serotonin re-uptake inhibitors are effective for both, it has been proposed that the term OCD be used to describe the syndrome in pets. However, since it is unknown whether animals have obsessive thoughts, many behaviorists prefer the term compulsive disorder (Fig. 10.2).

A definition of compulsive disorders proposed by Hewson and Luescher (1996) is 'behaviors that are usually brought on by conflict, but that are subsequently shown outside of the original context. The behaviors might share a similar pathophysiology (e.g., changes in serotonin, dopamine and beta-endorphin levels or metabolism). Compulsive behaviors seem abnormal because they are displayed out of context and are often repetitive, exaggerated or sustained.'

Causes of compulsive disorders

Compulsive disorders initially arise from behavioral arousal, stress, conflict, and frustration, which can lead to anxiety or displacement beha-

Compulsive disorders in dogs	Compulsive disorders in cats
Locomotor	
Spinning or tail chasing	Skin ripple/agitation/running, feline hyperesthesia
Stereotypic pacing/circling/jumping	Circling
Fixation – staring/barking/freezing/scratching	Freezing
Chasing lights, reflections, shadows	Excessive/intense chasing of imaginary objects
Barking – intense/rhythmic/difficult to interrupt	Excessive vocalization/howling
Head bob/tremor/head shaking	
Attacking food bowl, attacking inanimate objects	
Apparent hallucinatory	
Air biting or fly-snapping	Staring at shadows/walls
Staring, freezing, startle	Startle
Star/sky gazing	Avoiding imaginary objects
Self-injurious or self-directed	
Tail attacking, mutilation, growl/attack legs or rear	Tail attacking, mutilation, growl/attack legs or rear
Face rubbing/scratching	Face scratching/rubbing
Acral lick dermatitis – licking/chewing/barbering	Chewing/licking/barbering/overgrooming
Nail biting	Nail biting
Flank sucking	Hyperesthesia?
Checking rear	
Oral	
Sucking/licking	Wool sucking
Pica, rock chewing	Pica
Polydypsia/polyphagia	Polydypsia/polyphagia
Licking of objects/owners	Licking of objects/owners
Also may include self-directed oral behaviors (see above)	Also may include self-directed oral behaviors (see above)

Figure 10.2 Expression of compulsive disorders in dogs and cats.

viors. Understimulation or lack of appropriate outlets for the pet's innate needs may also lead to anxiety-induced, displacement, or vacuum activities. Over time, the consequences of these behaviors (medical, learned, conditioned), alterations in neurotransmitters, and genetic predisposing factors may result in a progression to a compulsive behavior. It is also possible that medical causes could be initiating factors.

There may be a common pathophysiology for all compulsive disorders, but it is also possible that the neurotransmitters involved may vary between presenting complaints, or that there may be changing involvement as the problem progresses. In time, as our ability to diagnose and treat becomes increasingly sophisticated, other medical, neurological, or dermatologic causes may be identified.

There appear to be at least two different mechanisms by which compulsive disorders arise. Locomotory compulsive disorders such as tail chasing or jumping in place tend to develop in situations of stress, anxiety, conflict, or frustration. They tend to be displayed most commonly in situations of high arousal, and are often so intense that it may be difficult to interrupt the behavior. By contrast, oral (e.g., wool sucking) and self-directed compulsive behaviors (such as flank sucking and acral lick dermatitis) may develop more acutely without any obvious conflict, and are most likely to be displayed in situations of minimal stimulation. In fact, it has been suggested that they may even help to calm the pet. They may be a form of vacuum activity (innate behaviors with no available outlet). Self-directed forms of oral compulsive disorders may be perpetuated by endorphin release. Behaviors that appear to have a hallucinatory component may also represent another category of compulsive disorders. As research into animal behavior advances and new drug options become available, it may become increasingly necessary to differentiate between these different causes. However, at present a similar treatment program (drugs that inhibit serotonin re-uptake combined with behavioral and environmental management) appears to be equally effective for most forms of compulsive disorders.

Although compulsive disorders are usually associated with states of anxiety and may affect health (weight loss, self-trauma), there may be no apparent effect on mental or physical well-being. It is possible that in some cases the stereotypy may serve as a coping mechanism, leading to a reduction in arousal. Dogs and cats that perform oral compulsive behaviors may appear to 'settle down;' veal calves that tongue roll develop less stomach ulcers than herd mates who do not tongue roll. However, in a study of pigs with compulsive disorders, there was no measurable improvement in cortisol, heart rate, or endorphin levels.

Behavioral pathogenesis of compulsive disorders

If a pet experiences stress, anxiety, arousal, conflict, or frustration, the resultant behavior might be an appropriate response to the stimulus, or alternatively, a redirected or displacement behavior might be exhibited (Fig. 10.3). Possible behavioral etiologies for a compulsive disorder might include:

- Insufficient stimulation.
- Alterations in schedule or routine.
- Inconsistent or improper training (i.e., inappropriate use or timing of punishment and rewards).
- Anxiety-inducing situations – fear, anxiety, conflicting signals, inconsistency, inappropriate punishment.
- Household changes (moving, renovations).
- Addition or departure of family members or other pets from the home.
- Introduction of new pets or family members.
- Alterations in health or behavior of a family member (e.g., physical illness, baby becoming a toddler).
- Intense or recurrent situations of fear or anxiety.
- Other situations of conflict (e.g., punishment during play).
- Other situations of frustration (e.g., blocking access to stimuli). For example, a barricade

Conflict-induced behaviors	Conflict occurs when the pet is motivated to perform two opposing behaviors (e.g., approach and withdrawal). Because the pet is unable to display the two opposing behaviors simultaneously, and if the pet is sufficiently aroused that it cannot inhibit its response, a displacement behavior may be exhibited
Frustration-induced behaviors	Frustration refers to a situation in which the pet is motivated to perform a behavior but is not able to do so (e.g., prevented from chasing). The barrier may be physical (as when access to the stimulus is blocked) or behavioral (the pet suppresses its response because of the possible consequences). The resultant behavior could be a displacement behavior or a redirected behavior
Displacement behavior	A displacement behavior is a normal behavior shown at an inappropriate time, appearing out of context for the occasion (e.g., spinning, tail chasing). Displacement behaviors may also be observed in situations of arousal when there is no appropriate outlet for de-arousal. Examples of displacement behaviors include yawning, eating, vocalization, grooming
Redirected behavior	When an animal is motivated to perform an activity (e.g., territorial protection, fear aggression, marking) but is unable to gain access to the principal target (see frustration above), the behavior may be directed at an alternative target (e.g., the owner, another pet, or an object)
Vacuum activity	When the pet is highly motivated to perform an instinctive behavior but there is no available outlet, a vacuum activity may be exhibited (flank sucking, licking, etc.). These activities have no apparent useful purpose
Stereotypies	Stereotypies are defined as unvarying, repetitive behavior patterns that have no obvious goal or function. Stereotypic behaviors may be displacement or compulsive behaviors, such as tail chasing. They may also be due to physiological changes such as neurological disorder (circling, head bobbing)

Figure 10.3 Behaviors associated with the development and expression of compulsive disorders.

that prevents a dog from greeting or social contact.

The displacement or anxiety behavior may then be reinforced, either by the 'self-enjoyment' of engaging in the response, the success of the response by negative reinforcement (i.e., a threat is withdrawn), or by positive reinforcement (e.g., attention, toy, treat). Also, the consequences of the behavior may add to the pet's anxiety if the owner is upset or anxious. Some owners may attempt to punish the undesirable behavior, which could serve as reinforcement (attention) if the attempt at punishment is mild, a source of anxiety, or a further source of conflict. If the situations of conflict or frustration persist or recur, the behavior may generalize to other situations in which the pet is anxious or aroused. Over time, as the number and type of situations in which the behavior is elicited increases, the threshold for exhibiting the behavior decreases, and the behavior becomes compulsive. At this point, the behavior may be observed at times when there is minimal to no anxiety or conflict. A behavior may be termed compulsive when it has no

apparent goal, the onset is emancipated from the original stimulus or context in which it was observed, the behavior is repetitive, exaggerated, sustained, or intense, and it may be difficult to interrupt or may not stop spontaneously. This lack of control of the initiation, expression, or termination of the behavior may improve with drugs that inhibit serotonin re-uptake. In severe cases, the threshold may be so low that the compulsive behavior may be exhibited at all times except when the pet is engaged in some other behavior 'of need' (e.g., eating, drinking, sleeping, fear/defense, play). Genetic factors may predispose certain breeds, lines, or individuals to develop compulsive disorders and determine how they are expressed.

Medical pathogenesis of compulsive disorders

Medical problems such as head shaking, circling, or self-directed chewing or licking may also be the initiating factors in establishing a behavior pattern that becomes compulsive. The consequences of the behavior may further perpetuate the problem, including (a) secondary infection, inflammation, pain, or pruritus arising from licking or chewing, (b) owner responses that lead to reinforcement such as providing a treat, toy, or attention (including some attempts at punishment), (c) owner responses that increase the level of anxiety or conflict (punishment, inconsistent responses), or (d) neurotransmitter alterations, including endorphin release, which may serve to reinforce the behavior.

Pathophysiology of compulsive disorders

The pathophysiology of CD is not well understood. Beta-endorphins, dopamine, and serotonin have all been implicated, primarily based on response to therapy. High doses of dopaminergic drugs such as amphetamines and apomorphine can induce stereotypies and dopamine antagonists such as haloperidol and thoridiazine may result in suppression of stereotypies. Selegiline (dopa regulator) is also occasionally effective (e.g., for overgrooming).

Another possibility is that compulsive disorders are mediated through opioid receptors, since opioid antagonists such as naltrexone have been successful at reducing stereotypies in dogs, sows, and horses. In addition, drugs that supply an exogenous source of opiates, such as hydrocodone, have also been reported to be effective in the treatment of acral lick dermatitis. It was suggested that endorphin release was serving as an internal mechanism for reinforcement, and that they might play a role in the early development of compulsive disorders (especially those that are self-directed). However, studies to date have not identified any increase in blood endorphin levels.

Abnormal serotonin transmission has also been suggested to be a mechanism by which stereotypies are induced. Based on human models for the treatment of obsessive–compulsive disorders, drugs that inhibit serotonin re-uptake (e.g., clomipramine, fluoxetine, fluvoxamine) have been shown to be most effective in the treatment of canine and feline compulsive disorders. Serotonin involvement has also been documented in a study of voles with stereotypies.

In time, it is likely that the specific neuropathological mechanisms for each compulsive behavior will be determined, as well as whether different presentations have different neurotransmitter involvement, and perhaps even the genetic basis for the striking breed predilection of some of these disorders. In fact, some European behaviorists believe that stereotypies arise in a number of behavioral conditions and that the other clinical signs associated with the stereotypy should be used as diagnostic criteria and in deciding what treatment to use. They define stereotypies as having no obvious function, not having a normal stop (e.g., excessive, persistent), seeming to have no internal regulation and to interfere with normal behavioral function. In addition to stereotypic or compulsive disorders, the following classifications have been proposed by European behaviorists including Patrick Pageat and Joel Dehasse:

- *Hypersensitivity–overactivity disorder*: the puppy does not show any bite control and there is hypervigilance to routine, everyday stimuli. There may be less sleep but there is no alteration in the sleep cycle. Selegiline, fluvoxamine, and fluoxetine may improve these conditions. (Authors' note: this does not refer to immunologic hypersensitivity, but rather to a behavioral tendency.)
- *Hyperactivity disorder* (also referred to as hyperkinesis or ADHD): motor activity is in excess and not responsive to correction, redirection, or restraint. There may be an increased basal heart rate and respiratory rate. These dogs seldom stay still, sleep less than most dogs, and do not undergo normal habituation to stimuli. These dogs may be responsive to methylphenidate, dextroamphetamine, or in some cases fluvoxamine, fluoxetine, imipramine, or amitriptyline.
- *Permanent anxiety disorder*: these dogs are constantly in a state of inhibition, prone to

displacement activities (which may become stereotypic self-injurious behaviors), and have an absence of self-defense. Selegiline, clomipramine, or an SSRI may improve this condition.

- *Deritualization anxiety disorder*: this disorder begins after a change in the social group (in an adult dog), and there is a lack of social contact and permanent social withdrawal. Communication-related stereotypies may arise (e.g., vocalization) and the dog may be overly defensive of body contact. Selegiline may improve this condition.
- *Unipolar disorder*: this develops in adult dogs. They may be cyclically hypervigilant, overexcitable, agitated, and unable to stop behavioral sequences and have hyposomnia. They may exhibit stereotypies, ingest their food quickly with regurgitation and reingestion, develop a fixed gaze toward objects, and have irritable or possessive aggression. Selegiline may improve this condition.
- *Dissociative disorder*: this arises between five months and five years. The dog becomes increasingly less receptive to the environment, and may have motor stereotypies (such as circling) with hallucinatory events. The dog may appear stunned or dazed at times. There is dilation of the brain ventricles, peaks on the EEG occipital region, and sometimes demodicosis. When there is a stereotypic component these dogs may respond to risperidone, which blocks receptors for both serotonin and dopamine. The dose is 0.5 to 1.0 mg per square meter. If there is a hallucinatory component, an SSRI may be effective.

General approach to diagnosis

The first step in diagnosis is to identify troublesome clinical signs and determine whether they might be consistent with the diagnosis of a compulsive disorder. A physical examination and a baseline set of diagnostic tests are essential. Although a complete blood count, urinalysis, biochemical panel (for instance, assessing kidney function, liver function, glucose, protein, etc.), and endocrine screen (thyroid and adrenal profile) might be a minimum requirement for all compulsive disorders, the clinical presentation may dictate the need for additional tests. For example, a neurological or ophthalmologic assessment and associated tests might be indicated for hallucinatory-type signs such as snapping at imaginary objects; a complete dermatologic assessment would be necessary for self-directed chewing or licking; a modified water deprivation test may be needed to rule out psychogenic causes of polydipsia; while ultrasonography or specialized gastrointestinal diagnostics such as contrast studies or scoping may be indicated for picas and coprophagia. When inflammation, pain, and infection are present, these can either be a cause of the clinical signs, or a secondary or concurrent factor in a compulsive disorder. The diagnosis of compulsive disorders can only be made once all other possible causes of the clinical signs have been ruled out. In some cases, a therapeutic response trial may also be an important part of the diagnostic workup.

Although the physical examination, laboratory tests, and observation of the pet may provide valuable diagnostic information, the pet may not display the behavior in the veterinarian's presence, so that a video recording of the behavior may be a valuable diagnostic tool.

If all possible medical causes have been ruled out, controlled, or resolved, and the problem persists, then the history and video are needed to further work up the cases so that an accurate behavioral diagnosis can be made (anxiety or conflict-induced, conditioned or reinforced, compulsive) and an appropriate treatment plan implemented. The history should evaluate the details of the problem itself, as well as any other behavioral signs that might indicate the stereotypy is part of a larger problem. The history must include information about:

- The pet, including the signalment, personality, developmental history, training, and any other concurrent behavior or health problems.

- The family, including other pets and their relationships, the pet's daily schedule, the environment, and the problem.
- The problem itself, how and when it started, how it has progressed or changed, when, where, and how often the problem occurs, any stimuli or events that precede the problem, the owner's response, and a detailed description (including video if available) of the problem itself.
- Concurrent behavioral problems and somatic signs that might indicate the stereotypy is a component of another problem (e.g., cognitive dysfunction, an attention deficit hyperactivity disorder).

Differential diagnoses

Compulsive disorders must be differentiated from medical problems and any other behavior problems that could be causing the clinical signs.

If the signs arise only in response to identifiable situations of anxiety and conflict, then the problem may not yet be compulsive and treatment should be focused on ensuring a desirable response to the stimuli. When the abnormal behaviors are exhibited only in the owner's presence, it is possible that the owner's responses to the behavior are a primary factor in development and maintenance of the problem (conditioned, reinforced, causing conflict). Other possible differentials are the repetitive, hallucinatory, fixated, or stereotypic behaviors that are seen in hypersensitivity, hyperactivity, anxiety, unipolar, and dissociative behaviors discussed earlier (European diagnoses).

Neurological diseases and diseases of the special senses

Many of the 'hallucinatory' signs, as well as the locomotor and self-injurious compulsive disorders, must be differentiated from neurological conditions of the central nervous system, disorders of the special senses, and neuropathic pain syndromes.

Seizure foci differ from compulsive disorders in that seizures arise independent of any specific stimuli or events, do not appear with any degree of regularity or predictability, cannot be interrupted, may have a recognizable pre- and/or postictal phase, and often improve with anticonvulsant therapy. In one study of tail chasing, along with other behavior problems, such as irrational fear and unprovoked aggression in Bull Terriers, an abnormal EEG was found in seven dogs (no control dogs), while seven of eight dogs had hydrocephalus (two of three controls). Treatment with phenobarbital was effective in five of seven dogs. In compulsive disorders, most pets are aware of their surroundings and appear normal as soon as they are interrupted. Neurological disorders such as hydrocephalus, brain tumors, or vestibular disease that might lead to circling, head bobbing, tremors, or repetitive pacing will often have a deficit in balance, or other neurologic components such as a head tilt, nystagmus, strabismus, or an alteration in personality or mentation. If a neurological disorder is suspected, then additional neurological tests such as imaging or CSF studies would be indicated.

Sensory disorders could induce hallucinatory-type behaviors such as snapping at or attacking imaginary or inanimate objects, freezing and staring, chasing shadows, lights, and reflections, head bobbing, and star or sky gazing. In addition, self-injurious behavior such as tail attacking, and intense chewing, licking, or scratching of the face, feet, neck, sides, flanks, or rear could be induced by pain. Although response to NSAIDs, opioids, or anti-inflammatory drugs should rule out pain as a possible diagnosis, neuropathic pain may not respond to traditional analgesics and the use of tricyclic antidepressants such as amitriptyline or anticonvulsants such as gabapentin or carbamazepine might be more effective for ruling out a painful etiology (see Ch. 9 for more details).

Dermatologic differentials

Perhaps the most extensive diagnostics are needed for self-directed and self-injurious behaviors (such as acral lick dermatitis in dogs and compulsive overgrooming in cats), to rule out all possible traumatic, inflammatory, infectious, parasitic, immunologic, and neoplastic causes. In addition to a physical examination and diagnostic tests (e.g., trichogram, biopsy, microbial culture, skin scraping, fungal culture), therapeutic trials may be necessary to rule out potential causes such as parasitic hypersensitivity, atopy, food allergies, and neuropathic pain.

On another note, the relationship between behavior and allergy may be more complicated than at first glance. In many cases of urticaria in humans, an allergic cause cannot be found and stress is a presumptive diagnosis. In addition, it has been reported that stress has a negative impact on cutaneous permeability barrier function (i.e., increased permeability) and that co-administration of tranquilizers blocks this dysfunction. Therefore, if percutaneous absorption of allergens leads to pruritus in the atopic patient, could stress predispose the patient to developing atopy? If this is indeed true then preventing stress or controlling the underlying stress with behavior therapy or drugs may in turn help control the underlying allergy.

While a medical or painful condition could cause all of the clinical signs of self-injurious behavior, medical treatment might not entirely resolve the signs if there is a concurrent compulsive disorder. In fact, since self-injurious behavior and the owner's attempts to treat the problem are likely to cause or aggravate anxiety and conflict, both conditions could very well coexist.

Picas, polydipsia, licking, sucking, and chewing of inanimate objects

Gastrointestinal disorders, dental, and oral disease, primary CNS disturbances such as brain tumors or hydrocephalus, electrolyte imbalances, metabolic diseases, and toxins such as lead can induce licking, sucking, chewing, and picas of inanimate objects, licking of owners, and air licking. Picas may also be caused by excessive restriction of calories (i.e., weight loss diets) and any medical condition that could cause

polyphagia. Similarly numerous medical conditions from Cushing's disease to diabetes insipidus might induce polydipsia. Licking, chewing, polyphagia, polydipsia, and picas can also be a side effect of drug therapy. In geriatric pets, repetitive behaviors including licking, chewing, and picas might be associated with brain aging and cognitive dysfunction (see Ch. 12).

Treatment of compulsive disorders – behavioral approach

Since compulsive disorders may initially arise from either anxiety or medical problems, these conditions must first be addressed. However, once the underlying cause is treated and all reinforcing factors have been removed, behaviors that are truly compulsive will often persist. For some problems, such as flank sucking in Doberman Pinschers, or the Golden Retriever that carries towels in its mouth, the problem may be sufficiently benign that treatment may not be necessary. In fact, treatment may only be necessary if the behavior poses health risks to the animal or is sufficiently annoying to the owner. For some pets, the behavior may be the most practical and acceptable outlet for reducing stress or resolving underlying conflict.

In some cases, the initiating factors for the stress or anxiety may still be present and will continue to perpetuate (or reinitiate) the problem until they are identified and resolved. In addition, any medical problems that may have developed secondary to the chewing or licking (e.g., pain, inflammation, infection) may have to be treated concurrently.

For most compulsive disorders, the treatment program includes a more intense and structured program of interaction and stimulation for the pet, and modifications to the pet's environment. The goal is to avoid situations of conflict and anxiety, and to motivate the pet to perform acceptable activities that are enjoyable to the pet, and incompatible with the undesirable. An environment that is predictable, highly stimulating, and in which the owners are consistent in their training, commands, and interactions is least likely to be stressful. Overall, the pet should receive regular interactive activities with its owners and other pets, and enough acceptable ways to occupy its time when on its own that the balance of the day is spent settled and sleeping.

For dogs, stimulation and physical activity might be increased by providing additional training sessions (perhaps with the use of a clicker to ensure a reward-based program), additional play and exercise sessions, and flyball or agility training. In addition, the dog will need to be provided with toys and other activities or outlets for play and exploration to keep it occupied and contented when the owners are not around and the pet is not asleep. If the dog is sufficiently food-motivated, toys that require manipulation to release food, toys that are stuffed or coated with food, and food or treats that have been frozen can provide extended interest and play. Dogs that are more motivated by chewing should be provided with durable and appealing chew toys, while those that prefer to explore could be given a variety of novel toys (with or without food) strategically placed throughout the home. Occasionally, the introduction of another pet can provide additional social companionship and a playmate for the pet when the owner is not available. Some dogs may even be interested in videos. A valuable training technique for dogs is to train a 'settle' or 'soft' command to quiet and relax the pet when it is excessively aroused, or is about to be left alone (Fig. 5.13 – handout #23 on the CD). Cues that are associated with a calm, relaxed part of the day, such as a video, music, or favorite blanket, may help to relax the dog and some dogs may be more relaxed if they are provided with their own bed or den. Head halter training can provide additional control and may be a more successful way to train and calm the dog.

For cats, interactive sessions with the owners and some stimulating toys and activities to occupy the cat should reduce the time spent in compulsive activities. Some cats will be contented and distracted simply by providing additional opportunities to explore. A comfortable area to view the indoor environment (e.g., bedding, a high perch, or activity center) or the out-side world (e.g., through a window) may be beneficial. A cat video might even help. If the cat's favored forms of play are to chase and pounce, then the owners should interact by providing moving targets with a wand or dangling toys. With the appropriate rewards, time, and patience, cats can also be trained to respond to basic commands such as come, sit, and dance. In addition, toys that can be chased or batted can be left available for self-play when the owner is not around. Cats may also be attracted to new areas to explore (e.g., boxes, paper bags, perches, new toys) and might be particularly interested in investigating toys or posts and play areas that can be scratched, or fresh herbs for chewing. Feral cats spend a considerable amount of time searching for food. Owners can hide some dry food and special food treats in the environment so that the cat has to actively find and work for its food. Offering live prey would also be a logical but generally impractical suggestion, although it might be practical to freeze food, or hide it within toys that require manipulation such as batting, rolling, or even scratching to deliver the food. Occasionally, the introduction of another pet can provide additional social companionship and an outlet for play, but could also result in increased anxiety.

Compulsive disorders that are displayed when the owner is present must be replaced with an acceptable alternative response (see Fig. 3.26, handout #22 on the CD, on reward-based training and response substitution). This requires supervision, identification of stimuli and situations where the problem might arise, and a pet that has been well trained through positive reinforcement so that it is quickly responsive to a command that will distract and settle it (see Fig. 5.13, settle handout #23 on the CD). With good observation and history, many owners can identify when and where the problem is likely to arise, so that the behavior can be interrupted as soon as it starts. At this point, through commands, settle down exercises, and play, the owner should be able to have the pet engaged in an acceptable response. Sometimes a disruption device such as a whistle, squeaker, water spray, citronella spray, remote citronella collar, shake can, or ultrasonic device may be helpful. Alternatively, a long leash left attached (during supervision) may be useful for quickly interrupting the compulsive behavior as it starts. Punishment, whether verbal or physical, should be avoided as it may further increase anxiety and conflict. Positive attention, such as talking soothingly to the pet or giving it something it wants, during the performance of the behavior should also be avoided. If the pet continues to exhibit the compulsive behavior, some means of prevention may be needed. Cage confinement or Elizabethan collars might be useful, but these products alone merely prevent the expression of the problem and can further aggravate the pet's anxiety. Diagnostic and treatment considerations for specific problems are discussed below. For a client handout treatment summary see Figure 10.4.

Drug therapy

Drug therapy for compulsive disorders may be needed concurrent with the behavioral and environmental techniques to achieve the highest level of improvement. Drugs that affect serotonin transmission (in particular clomipramine, a tricyclic antidepressant, and the selective serotonin re-uptake inhibitors) appear to be most successful for compulsive disorders in humans and pets. Improvement rather than complete control or resolution is most likely to be achieved with drug therapy (Fig. 10.5).

Medication is usually prescribed for eight to 12 weeks before deciding whether the full effects are beneficial, and some patients may require an increased dose. If the problem improves, then medication should be continued for at least six months, but may have to be continued lifelong.

A number of drugs have been utilized in human medicine for the treatment of obsessive-compulsive disorders such as the SSRIs paroxetine, fluoxetine, sertraline, fluvoxamine, and citalopram, as well as the tricyclic antidepressant clomipramine. Other tricyclic antidepressants are not sufficiently selective for serotonin to be effective. Except for clomipramine, none of these drugs have yet been licensed

for companion animal use. Regular physical examinations and blood profiles should be performed prior to drug use and at six- to 12-month intervals if the pets are maintained on drugs for long-term use.

Clomipramine is a tricyclic (cyclic or heterocyclic) antidepressant, licensed for the treatment of canine separation anxiety in the United States, but is also licensed for the treatment of canine compulsive disorders in Canada, Australia, and Europe. Selective serotonin re-uptake inhibitors (SSRIs) may also be effective in the treatment of compulsive disorders. Compared with tricyclic antidepressants, SSRIs cause little or no hypotension, have negligible anticholinergic effects (with the exception of paroxetine), and cause less sedation and fewer cardiac conduction disturbances. They may occasionally lead to increased restlessness, agitation, insomnia, weight loss, and gastrointestinal upset in humans. Studies have shown the effectiveness of clomipramine in canine compulsive disorders, including spinning, tail chasing, and acral lick dermatitis, and in feline compulsive disorders such as psychogenic alopecia (or overgrooming) and excessive vocalization. Clomipramine is the most selective inhibitor of serotonin re-uptake of all the tricyclic antidepressants. The side effects and contraindications for clomipramine are discussed in Chapter 6. Tricyclics other than clomipramine, or merely anxiolytic drugs such as benzodiazepines, are highly unlikely to have an effect on compulsive disorders. Clinical trials on cases of acral lick dermatitis have been performed for clomipramine, fluoxetine, and sertraline and a series of case studies showed some improvement in tail chasing in terriers. In one study, citalopram was successful in the treatment of six of nine dogs with acral lick dermatitis and in general has little to no cardiotoxic effects in most dogs and cats. However, there have been anecdotal reports of aggression during the first week or two prior to regulation, and in an initial study five of 10 dogs receiving 8 mg/kg per day died between four and seven months from the onset of therapy.

STEREOTYPIC AND COMPULSIVE DISORDERS

1. Compulsive disorders often arise from situations of conflict or anxiety. If the source of the conflict can be identified in the initial stages, it may be possible to resolve the problem without drugs. This might be accomplished by finding all situations where the problem occurs and either avoiding the situation entirely or teaching the pet to display a different, more acceptable behavior.

2. Medical problems might actually be the underlying reason that a pet exhibits a particular behavior. Therefore, before diagnosing a compulsive disorder, all possible medical problems must be considered. In addition, once a medical problem causes a pet to begin exhibiting a behavior (e.g., licking, chewing) it can become compulsive.

3. Over time, the constant repetition of the problem and your response to the dog may lead to a change in neurotransmitters in the brain so that the behavior may begin to appear more frequently or in more situations than before. Sometimes it becomes exaggerated or so intense that it may be hard to interrupt. At this point, the behavior may have become compulsive and may require a combination of behavior management, changes to the household, and drugs to improve or control the problem. In addition, if the initial conflict and anxiety are not identified and controlled, the problem will not be entirely resolved.

4. Determine whether your response may in any way be contributing to the problem. If you are trying to stop your pet either by patting or offering a treat, then this serves to reward the behavior. Similarly, punishment may merely serve as a form of attention. If you raise the level of punishment or show any anxiety or upset in your response to the dog, then you will likely add to your pet's anxiety and conflict.

5. If you observe the pet displaying the undesirable behavior, be calm, interrupt it without saying anything or looking at it, and redirect its behavior to another activity (play, exercise, toys stuffed with food). Your goal is to train the dog to exhibit an acceptable alternative response while remaining calm and consistent and then reward! This can be accomplished by:

   a) Using a physical control device such as a leash and head halter or an interruption device such as a water spray, shake can, ultrasonic device, or remote citronella spray to stop the undesirable behavior. Then reward the desirable response.

   b) Training the pet to perform an acceptable response through command training (e.g., settle, down). Use the command as soon as the behavior starts (or can be anticipated) and then reward the desired response.

   c) Walking away or ignoring the pet. Once the behavior stops, look for a desirable behavior to reinforce.

6. Environmental changes can cause some pets to become more anxious. Returning to a more acceptable environment for the pet may improve the problem. Increasing the pet's interest in exploring and playing may reduce the level of anxiety and the performance of the undesirable behaviors.

   a) Cats: give your cat some new places to perch, some new areas to climb or scratch, or some bags or boxes to explore. Sometimes cats will show interest in the TV or a video. Toys that hang, dangle, or can be batted are attractive to many cats. There are now toys where food can be stuffed inside, that the cat manipulates by scratching, chewing, rolling to get the food out. Some cats are attracted to kitty herb gardens.

   b) Dogs: most dogs are attracted to toys that contain food and those that can be chewed. A variety of chew and play toys for dogs have been developed that can be coated, filled, or stuffed with food to attract and distract the dog for long periods of time. Freezing food and treats after inserting them in the toys can increase the duration of time spent chewing. Dogs that enjoy investigating and exploring may be better distracted by games where they have to search to find new toys and treats. Videos designed for dogs to view may be of interest to some dogs.

7. Interactive play provides social contact, attention, and more physical activity for the pet. Exercises, play, and working sessions for dogs might include walks, jogging, swimming, agility, fetch, flyball, or other chase-related games (soccer, football, Frisbee, hockey). Cats are more likely to be stimulated by toys that can be batted, chased, or pounced upon. Toys that can be dangled in front of the cat to chase or can be rolled across the floor often work best. Games with food as a reward may also help maintain interest. Training sessions can be

Figure 10.4   Client handout for compulsive disorders (handout #4 – printable from the CD).

an effective form of attention, mental stimulation, and positive social interaction for both dogs and cats. Sometimes obtaining another pet, or providing play sessions with other pets, can help reduce the time spent engaging in compulsive disorders.

8. The goal of training, exercise, play, exploration, feeding, and social interactions is to help calm the pet so that it is either relaxed, settled and sleeping, or displaying appropriate acceptable behaviors (rather than displaying compulsive behaviors). Helping your pet develop a comfortable resting area and setting up some cues and situations that help to relax the dog can further reduce compulsive displays. A favored blanket, a TV or CD, or a special odor might be associated with these relaxation sessions and times. A settle down command for dogs (see settle handout) can be particularly useful. A diet change or natural supplement may help to calm the pet or reduce anxiety.

9. It may be necessary to temporarily block the performance of the behavior (e.g., Elizabethan collar, bandaging, sedative, leash control) so that repetition of the behavior does not cause further injury or damage.

10. Medical drug therapy: if there is a medical component to the problem, then drugs to resolve infection, pain, or inflammation may be needed.

11. Behavioral drug therapy: drugs that help return the serotonin system back to a more normal state of function are usually needed for compulsive disorders. Sometimes drugs that reduce anxiety can be useful as well.

Figure 10.4 (*continued*)

Antidepressants should be maintained at the same dose before considering a higher dose or switching to a different medication. If the owner achieves satisfactory control with drug therapy, then the drug can be weaned by approximately 25% every two to four weeks to determine the lowest effective dose. Slow weaning is also preferable to prevent the possibility of a rebound effect.

In European studies, selegiline has also been used successfully in some forms of stereotypic behavior in dogs in cases related to 'emotional disorders' (chronic anxiety with physical signs such as gastrointestinal upset, alterations in drinking or appetite, or alterations in sleep–wake cycles). It may also be effective for repetitive and stereotypic behaviors associated with cognitive dysfunction syndrome. In a retrospective study on the use of selegiline in cats, 10 of 12 cats with stereotypic self-licking improved.

When drugs that inhibit serotonin re-uptake are not effective, then the diagnosis should be reconsidered or alternative drugs (or additional drugs) might be considered. Although there is no strong evidence for the use of any of the following drug regimes, they might be a consideration when the potential benefits outweigh any potential risk. Unfortunately, the risk of using a drug that has not been studied in dogs or assessed in combination with other drugs is entirely unknown.

Opioid antagonists have been reported to be effective in the treatment of compulsive disorders, but they have not proven to be practical in the treatment of clinical cases, since most are injectible agents and the half-lives are extremely short. In addition, they seem to be most effective early in the development of compulsive disorders.

Dopamine antagonists such as thoridiazine and haloperidol might, in theory, be useful in the treatment of some compulsive disorders, but have a higher risk of adverse effects, especially extrapyramidal effects. Although there is at least one report of a reduction of aberrant motor behavior in dogs (tail mutilation, aggression, vocalization, air biting), the effects may be due to a general suppression of all motor output (Parkinsonian catalepsy).

Hydrocodone has been reported to be effective in one small study of dogs with acral lick dermatitis, perhaps because of its effect on pain, or perhaps as an exogenous source of opioids that might counter any benefit of opioid release gained from the performance of the compulsive disorder.

Drug class	Drug	Dog	Cat
Tricyclic antidepressants			
	Clomipramine	2–3 mg/kg bid	0.5–1 mg/kg q 24h
	Doxepin	0.5–1.0 mg/kg bid or 3–5 mg/kg q 8–12h	0.5–1.0 mg/kg q 12–24h
	Amitriptyline	1–4 mg/kg PO bid	5–10 mg/cat q 24h
Selective serotonin re-uptake inhibitors			
	Fluoxetine	1–2 mg/kg sid (used up to 4 mg/kg per day in Europe)	0.5 mg/kg sid
	Fluvoxamine	0.5–2 mg/kg bid (used up to 8 mg/kg per day in Europe)	0.5–1 mg/kg q 24h
	Paroxetine	1 mg/kg q 24h (used up to 5 mg/kg per day in Europe)	0.5 mg/kg sid
	Sertraline	2–5 mg/kg divided bid	
Opiate agonists and antagonists			
	Hydrocodone	0.25 mg/kg q 8h	0.25–1 mg/kg q 8–12h
	Naltrexone	2.2 mg/kg PO sid/bid	2.2 mg/kg q 24h
Monoamine oxidase inhibitor			
	Selegiline	0.5–1 mg/kg q 24h	0.5–1 mg/kg q 24h
Antipsychotics (neuroleptics)			
	Thioridazine	1–2 mg/kg bid	
	Haloperidol	0.5–4 mg/dog sid/bid	
	Pimozide	1–10 mg daily	
Atypical antipsychotics			
	Risperidone	0.5–1 mg/m^2	

Figure 10.5 Drug therapy for compulsive disorders.

Prognosis

With a combination of drugs and behavior therapy, about two-thirds of compulsive disorders can be well controlled. Most cases will require long-term attention to the pet's training and environment, as well as perhaps drugs. Cases that are refractory are often due to poor owner compliance, as well as those with longer duration.

SPECIFIC COMPULSIVE DISORDERS AND THEIR TREATMENT

Acral lick dermatitis (lick granuloma)

Acral lick dermatitis is a distinct clinical entity in which dogs lick at one or more of their limbs, often causing significant damage. Although there may be a somewhat different etiology, some dogs may compulsively lick or chew other parts of the body (perhaps at the site of previous injury or inflammation). It is not unusual to find the area denuded of skin, and it may be raw and weeping, or thickened and granulomatous. There may be one or more possible initiating factors, with dermatological, behavioral, and neurological etiologies all being possibilities. Large breeds such as Doberman Pinschers, Great Danes, German Shepherd Dogs, Labrador Retrievers, Golden Retrievers, and Irish Setters are most commonly affected. Males are affected twice as often as females. Dogs with acral lick dermatitis may also have some degree of sensory neuropathy. Lack of stimulation is frequently cited as an underlying cause, but the licking may also be a displacement behavior, arising out of situations of conflict, frustration, or anxiety. Underlying anatomical abnormalities (e.g., arthritis, fracture, neural entrapment), or infectious or inflammatory causes, may be contributory.

Regardless of the initiating cause, damage is then done to the skin, which potentiates the sensation and persistent licking. Affected dogs begin licking at a site, removing hair, causing inflammation, and finally removing layers of the skin, sometimes down to the bone. The area becomes raw and weeping, and the chronic trauma itself becomes irritating, further stimulating the dog to lick and chew (Fig. 10.6).

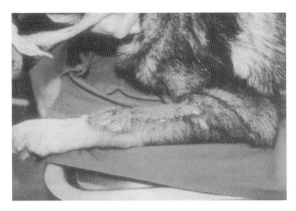

Figure 10.6 Acral lick dermatitis: self-trauma to the foreleg of a dog. Reprinted with permission from Ackerman L 1989 Practical canine dermatology. American Veterinary Publications. Photo courtesy of Lowell Ackerman.

Diagnosis and prognosis

The underlying etiology cannot always be confirmed by clinical signs alone. Differential diagnoses include: stress or conflict, neoplasia (e.g., mast-cell tumor), parasitism (e.g., demodicosis), mycotic dermatitis, pyoderma, trauma (e.g., fracture, neural injury, prior wound, foreign body), focal allergic manifestation (e.g., id reaction, contact eruption, adverse food reaction, atopy), and acral mutilation syndrome. Bacterial and fungal cultures, skin scrapings, cytological examination, and biopsies should be performed to rule out organic causes. Radiography of the affected limb is recommended, and periosteal reactions of underlying bone are commonly seen. In most cases, a fair to guarded prognosis is given to dogs with acral lick dermatitis. However with persistence, time, and effort, the underlying cause might be able to be identified, and the prognosis improved by concurrently treating all underlying and potentiating factors.

Treatment

With true behavioral acral lick dermatitis, treatment must be directed at both the psychological impairment and the skin disorder. Therefore, even if an underlying behavioral problem can be diagnosed and treated with behavioral management and drug therapy, concurrent treatment of the skin condition is essential. Medical therapy might consist of treatment with long-term antibiotics, anti-inflammatory agents, and denying access to the area until the lesion begins to heal. In fact, if the underlying anxiety has been previously resolved, then medical therapy alone may prove to be effective. Behavioral management might include the diagnosis and treatment of those situations and stimuli that lead to conflict, stress, or anxiety, as well as drug therapy with clomipramine or selective serotonin reuptake inhibitors. In general, several months of therapy are likely to be needed before the lesions (and the compulsive licking) are resolved. At that point, if the underlying problems have been resolved, the lesions may not recur when the drug is withdrawn.

Any situation leading to conflict may be an inciting factor for acral lick dermatitis in dogs that are genetically predisposed to developing these problems. In time, as with other compulsive disorders, the problem may become generalized to other situations, even those in which the pet's level of stress, anxiety, or conflict is relatively low. When the licking occurs in the owner's presence, those stimuli that directly precede the licking, as well as the owner's response, should be closely scrutinized. Stimuli or situations that might cause the problem might then be identified and modified or eliminated, and owner responses that might be reinforcing or aggravating the problem can be corrected. If the licking cannot be entirely resolved, then response substitution is generally the most practical means of improving the problem. If the times and situations in which the dog might lick can be anticipated, it should be possible to train and reinforce an alternative acceptable behavior. Alternatively, distraction or disruptive devices (e.g., audible and ultrasonic alarms, remote citronella spray, a leash and head halter) can be used to interrupt the licking so that an alternative response can be achieved and reinforced.

Increasing play and exercise before departures and increased environmental stimulation (objects to chew and tear apart, toys and boxes with food hidden inside, providing food in a variety of locations or with a timed feeder, getting another pet, day care) may be useful for keeping the pet occupied and distracted (see separation anxiety and destructive chewing in Chs 11 and 15). Although aversive techniques are seldom practical or effective, treatment with remote control shock collars and bandaging the area and applying 'hot' or 'bitter' sprays have been successful. The key to therapy is that the aversion must be strong enough to deter the behavior, and that the pet receives the aversive stimulus contingent on every event until the behavior ceases. Whenever the aversive treatment cannot be effectively applied, an Elizabethan collar should be used to prevent access to the area. Care should be taken when considering the use of aversive stimuli in treating this condition because some cases may take a turn for the worse with this approach.

Pharmacological intervention is often required as an adjunct to most treatment programs for compulsive disorders. Clomipramine, a tricyclic antidepressant, or an SSRI such as fluoxetine, are generally the most effective, but will need to be combined with appropriate environmental and behavioral therapy. Alternatively, doxepin or amitriptyline, both tricyclic antidepressants, might be useful both for their behavioral as well as their antihistaminic effects; however, they do not generally have sufficient effect on serotonin re-uptake to be as effective as clomipramine and the SSRIs. Equally important is to help resolve any concurrent or secondary medical problems that might be present. Deep pyoderma may be a frequent sequel to a long-standing problem, and therefore a lengthy course of an appropriate antibiotic may lead to significant improvement, while drugs to control pain and inflammation may also provide effective relief. Bactericidal antibiotics (such as cephalosporins, potentiated penicillins, and trimethoprim-potentiated sulfonamides) are recommended for a minimum of six weeks to treat secondary infections, which can contribute to perpetuation or recurrence of lesions. Corticosteroids injected into the lesion or applied topically with a penetrating agent, such as dimethyl sulfoxide (DMSO), have been quite successful, but the potential dangers of long-term corticosteroid use must be considered. One of the most popular topical remedies has been adding 3 ml of flunixin meglumide (Banamine) to an 8-ml container of fluocinolone and DMSO (Synotic); the mixture is applied once to twice daily. Because of the potential risk of applying potent corticosteroids in DMSO long term, attempts have also been made to use safer products, such as equal parts DMSO and solutions containing 1% hydrocortisone (e.g., HydroPlus). Another topical combination product is formulated by mixing one part capsaicin 0.25% (HEET) to two parts Bitter Apple (isopropyl alcohol, water, bitter extract). All of these topical remedies are best used in combination with a long-term bactericidal antibiotic regimen, and a behavioral drug, such as clomipramine.

Pentoxifylline has also been used in veterinary dermatology for a variety of purposes, including vasculitides, atopy, dermatomyositis, as well as adjunctive therapy for acral lick dermatitis. Although it is in the class of drugs known as methylxanthines, it does not have significant bronchodilating effects. Its primary mode of action is to reduce blood viscosity, by improving red blood cell membranes, inhibiting microvascular constriction, and decreasing red blood cell and platelet aggregation. It may have immunomodulatory effects (inhibition of cytokines and tumor necrosis factor alpha, increased B and T-cell activation), as well as a beneficial effect on wound healing. A dose of 15 mg/kg tid has been recommended.

Hydrocodone has been shown to be effective in some cases, perhaps to reduce pain and discomfort or perhaps to supply an exogenous source of opiates so that the dog's 'need' is satisfied. In some cases, especially those compulsive disorders of early onset, opiate antagonists such as naltrexone or naloxone may be effective, but these have not proven to be a practical treatment regime. Haloperidol at perhaps 1–2 mg/kg bid has also been suggested to augment other pharmacologic therapy in refractory cases, but is rarely used in dogs.

Other therapeutic regimes that have also been used with variable success include cryosurgery, radiation therapy, excisional therapy, laser surgery, acupuncture, and injections of cobra antivenin. In a study using radiation therapy, a successful clinical response was seen in six of 17 cases (35%). In another 24% (four cases), there was resolution but with eventual recurrence. Total radiation dosage was within the range of 625–4500 cGy, delivered in fractions of 261–1000 cGy, and administered at three, four, or seven-day intervals. Thus, radiation therapy might be considered in cases that do not respond to other treatment modalities.

It is sometimes necessary to use bandaging or Elizabethan collars to deny access to the lesions for the first few weeks of therapy. On the other hand, these techniques could lead to increased anxiety, thereby compounding the problem.

Prevention

Acral lick dermatitis may be impractical to prevent since it can arise from many different underlying causes, both behavioral and medical. Since insufficient stimulation may be a predisposing factor, providing an environment with a favored resting area, a variety of appealing play toys whenever the pet is left alone, consistent training, and sufficient play and exercise may go a long way in reducing the possibility of the dog developing ALD. In addition, to prevent an emerging problem from becoming compulsive, it is essential that the owner identify and report the signs immediately, so that behavioral modification can be implemented. At this point, the problem may be anxiety-induced, so that identifying and resolving the underlying cause(s) of the anxiety and increasing stimulation and distractions may prove to be effective without the need for any drug therapy.

Owners of dogs that have been treated for acral lick dermatitis should be counseled about controlling stress in the pet's life. Consideration should be given to the prophylactic use of psychoactive medication, exercise, and environmental stimulation when highly stressful situations cannot be avoided.

Case examples

Case 1 Midnight, a four-year-old, spayed female Labrador Retriever cross, was presented for a 2-cm thickened ulcerated lesion on the left foreleg. The owner had had a baby two months prior to the onset of the problem. The owner reported that the pet had started intermittently licking the area four months before. There was no history of trauma. During the past month the licking had been constant. Yelling at the pet was only successful in distracting it temporarily. Prior to the middle of the pregnancy, the owner and the dog often jogged together and spent a lot of time in the park. The pet had had little training and had always been a bit unruly. Since the baby was born, the unruliness had been a major problem and the owner frequently found herself scolding the pet. A thorough medical workup uncovered no other problems. The underlying problem was conflict due to major changes in the dog's daily life, and a change in the relationship with the owner.

The wife and husband were encouraged to alternate in taking the pet on at least one long walk each day, and hire a dog walking service to provide a second long daily walk. The owners were taught how to teach the dog to sit, lie down, and stay on command, so that it could be given commands that would keep it out of the way when needed and prevent unruly behavior. Food lure training using an upbeat tone was stressed. This gave the owners a way of controlling the pet and preventing undesirable behavior, so that scolding decreased. The owners were told to develop a set of rules for how they expected the pet to behave and to reinforce desired behavior consistently and avoid reinforcing undesired behavior. Cephalexin was prescribed for six weeks and the lesion was bandaged lightly and sprayed with a bitter spray when the owners were not available to supervise.

Six weeks later the dog was re-examined: the lesions were well on their way to healing. The owners felt that there was considerable improvement, but that the dog still licked the area occasionally, although not as often as before. A solution of topical fluocinolone and DMSO was dispensed, to be applied to the area as 5 drops bid for the next 10 days. Antibiotics were continued for another four weeks. It was suggested that a bitter topical solution be applied to the area for another three weeks after that. The rationale was that the behavior may have been ingrained enough that the dog was licking out of habit. A re-evaluation one month later revealed a dog that was essentially normal, and all therapy was discontinued. A follow-up six months later showed the condition was still in remission.

Case 2   Chloe, a six-year-old, spayed female English Springer Spaniel, presented with an erosive, nodular lesion on the left hind leg of three months' duration. The owner believed that Chloe was happy and well adjusted, and had too busy a life to be bored. A hemogram and biochemical profile were unremarkable and biopsies taken from the lesion for histopathologic assessment revealed a granulomatous reaction around a fragment of plant material, believed to be a thorn. A good prognosis was given and Chloe was discharged on cephalexin 22 mg/kg bid. Sutures were removed at 10 days and a recheck examination was scheduled for one month later.

At the recheck visit, Chloe was her typical happy self, but there was now an erosive-ulcerative lesion extending from the biopsy site proximally, which Chloe apparently had been licking at rather extensively. At this point, the main differential diagnoses were acral lick dermatitis at a site of previous trauma, or the potential that a microbial infection (e.g., sporotrichosis, phaeohyphomycosis) may have been introduced with the thorn. Repeat biopsies revealed changes most consistent with acral lick dermatitis and no evidence of infectious agents.

At this point, treatment was initiated with clomipramine at 3 mg/kg bid, the antibiotic was continued, and the owner was requested to apply a combination product of Bitter Apple (2/3) and capsaicin (HEET) (1/3). An Elizabethan collar was applied for the first 10 days to deny Chloe access. The owner telephoned a few days later that Chloe was visibly upset with wearing the Elizabethan collar and she was instructed to remove it. Chloe was rechecked two weeks later and seemed to be leaving the leg alone; it was healing nicely. Two weeks after that, the leg was almost completely healed and the clomipramine dose was reduced to 2 mg/kg bid. Two weeks after that, the leg was completely healed; the antibiotic was discontinued, as was the topical solution. The dose of clomipramine was reduced to 1.5 mg/kg bid.

Approximately one week after discontinuing everything, the owner telephoned to say that Chloe was starting to lick at the leg again. Clomipramine was re-instituted at 2 mg/kg bid for four weeks and the topical solution was used for 10 days and then discontinued. After the four weeks, the clomipramine dosage was reduced to 1.5 mg/kg bid for another four weeks, then 1 mg/kg bid for yet another four weeks. At the end of that time, all therapy was once again discontinued. This time the condition remained in remission and did not require further therapy.

Psychogenic polydipsia

Increased drinking and urinating are generally due to medical problems. As with most behavioral disorders, a behavioral cause should only be considered when all other causes have been considered. However, if no abnormalities are identified on blood or urine tests, the water intake is excessive and the urine is not sufficiently concentrated, then a behavioral or psychogenic cause might be possible. One possible pathogenesis of stress-induced polydipsia would be the overproduction of cortisol that is associated with chronic stress or anxiety disorders.

If all laboratory results are within normal limits and the urine is not concentrating, then diabetes insipidus and renal medullary washout must also be ruled out. The owner should measure water intake for two to three days and then start DDAVP by applying 2 drops of the intranasal solution into the conjunctiva for five to seven days. If the water intake is decreased dramatically or the urine concentration increases by greater than 50%, then a diagnosis of diabetes insipidus can be made. If the response is not significant, the test may need to be repeated using gradual water reduction beginning about three days prior to the test. On the first day 120 ml/kg/day should be the maximum water intake, two days before water should be limited to 90 ml/kg/day, and then 60–80 ml/kg/day on the day before the test.

Dogs with psychogenic polydipsia should be able to concentrate their urine when water is deprived, but the test is potentially dangerous if there has been medullary washout and the test is done too quickly. A gradual water deprivation test can be excessively time consuming. Five days before the test the water is limited to a maximum of 120 ml/kg/day, and this is reduced to 90 ml/kg/day two days before the test, then 60 ml/kg/day on the day of the test. At this point some dogs with psychogenic polydipsia will be able to concentrate, but others will have to be deprived to a point of dehydration before they will concentrate.

Treatment

For pets with psychogenic polydipsia, sources of conflict and anxiety must be identified and reduced. Stimulation in the form of increased social play, training, and exercise sessions as well as the addition of numerous self-play activities such as manipulation toys and chews (low salt) should be added. If the pet's increased drinking occurs primarily when the owners are at home, the stimuli and events that precede the drinking and the owner's response should be assessed and modified. Overall water intake should be controlled by the owners and provided on a regular basis throughout the day to meet the dog's daily requirements. Access to puddles of water and open toilets should be prevented. Ice cubes, toys filled with frozen fruit drinks, frozen food treats, dripping taps, water bottles, and self-watering devices may be helpful to slow the intake. Drugs for anxiety such as buspirone or antidepressants such as SSRIs for compulsive disorders might also be useful

adjuncts to therapy. Anticholinergic drugs should be avoided since they can decrease salivary secretion, dry mucous membranes, and increase thirst.

Flank sucking

Flank sucking represents a poorly understood condition in which a dog nurses a patch of skin on its flank. The dog will hold a section of flank skin in its mouth and hold the position, resulting in changes as simple as a dampened, ruffled haircoat to more severe changes including raw, open sores. The Doberman Pinscher is the breed most commonly affected and the trait has been followed through certain bloodlines, suggesting a hereditary component. The cause has not been determined but the problem may occur more frequently when the dog is under stress. In time the condition often becomes compulsive (to a point where some dogs perform the behavior whenever they are not sleeping or engaged in some other activity). Psychomotor epilepsy is another suggested cause.

Diagnosis and prognosis

Flank sucking is an exclusion diagnosis so a thorough medical evaluation is warranted before this label is applied. A minimum database should include multiple skin scrapings, fungal culture, fecal evaluation, and impression cytology. Biopsies of affected areas and radiographic studies are extremely helpful at eliminating the possibility of other contributing medical causes. Flank sucking becomes the operative diagnosis when no physiological reasons can be found for the behavior.

Management

Too few reports of cases of flank sucking have been published to be able to make generalizations about treatment. In many cases the sucking does not cause significant lesions or damage, and does not interfere with the apparent health or behavioral welfare of the pet. In these cases, the flank sucking, although compulsive, may be an acceptable 'coping' mechanism. When the behavior does cause physical damage or becomes so compulsive as to contribute to other behavior problems (decreased eating, poorly responsive or aggressive toward owners when approached during sucking), then treatment is necessary (Fig. 10.7). In these cases behavioral modification and medical intervention may be useful. It has also been proposed that flank sucking is a manifestation of psychomotor epilepsy. Accordingly, it has been treated in some instances with medications such as phenobarbital and potassium bromide.

Prevention

Until more is known about the causes of flank sucking, prevention remains an elusive goal. Since the condition is most commonly reported in Doberman Pinschers, affected dogs should not be used in breeding programs.

Case example

Bart, a two-year-old intact male Doberman Pinscher, was presented for sucking on the skin in the flank area. The problem had started six months previously and occurred most fre-

quently in the early evening. The owner was concerned that some local discomfort was causing the behavior and would gently talk to the pet as she inspected the skin in the area that was being sucked. Differential diagnoses included flank sucking, demodicosis, dermatophytosis, and foreign body reaction (including injection site granuloma). Skin scrapings and fungal culture were both negative, although a contaminant growth of *Alternaria* was found on the dermatophyte test medium. Foreign body reaction could not be eliminated from our considerations without a biopsy, which the owner was reluctant to permit. It was decided that the problem would be pursued on a behavioral basis and that further diagnostic work would be done if this failed to resolve the situation.

Bart was fitted with an Elizabethan collar to prevent sucking when the owner was not able to observe and correct it. Each time she had to leave the dog alone, he was provided with a dental rope toy coated with a small amount of peanut butter, and a rubber toy with a piece of meat tucked inside. The owner started a vigorous exercise program with the dog just prior to the time at which the sucking usually occurred. She was told not to say anything to Bart when she noticed him sucking. Whenever the dog

Step	Comments
Reduce stress	• Reduce sources of anxiety within the environment – desensitize and countercondition to stimuli
Increase interactive activity and stimulation – provide structured routine	• Training, play, exercise initiated on a regular and consistent basis from the owner – develop a healthy and stable social relationship with the owner in control
Distraction – provide alternative outlets	• Food-laden toys, alternative devices or objects for chewing, and activities (find the food)
Deny access to behavior if excessive damage or anxiety	• E collar or bitter sprays
Response substitution	• Train to perform acceptable alternative behavior
Positive reinforcement-based training	• Train to settle/relax on command – train to go to a settle down area – use a head halter if needed for additional control
Interrupt (do not punish)	• If dog observed in behavior, interrupt it with an ultrasonic device, remote citronella, water device, or by pull of a leash (if leash and head halter left attached)
Drug therapy	• Clomipramine or SSRI – additional medication for pain, inflammation, or infection if self-injurious • Phenobarbital or potassium bromide if suspected cause is psychomotor epilepsy

Figure 10.7   Management of flank-sucking dogs.

started sucking, the owner was instructed to blow a whistle to distract him, wait 10 seconds or longer (but before the sucking resumed), and then play with him, review obedience, or take him for a long walk.

Bart improved markedly but the owner reported that whenever she was lax in the exercise program, the problem started to recur. Given the options of additional testing and drug therapies, she elected to persevere and see that Bart received the exercise he apparently needed.

Tail chasing in dogs

Compulsive tail chasing is not an uncommon behavior in dogs. In addition to a compulsive disorder, it may be due to a displacement behavior (i.e., in response to conflict or frustration), an epileptic episodic behavior, a neuropathological disorder, a psychotic or hallucinatory disorder, or acrodermatitis. Some cases, such as those seen in Bull Terriers, may exhibit a more intense spinning or whirling behavior, which may be refractory to behavior modification techniques. Other concurrent behavior problems, such as aggression, have been reported in 'spinning' Bull Terriers. In some cases, the problem may have started as play behavior that was reinforced by the owner by either offering a treat or toy or by trying to disrupt the behavior with insufficient levels of punishment. If the owner displays anxiety or uses excessive punishment, additional conflict may arise.

Diagnosis and prognosis

The diagnosis is based on the findings of a dog with tail chasing behavior and no evidence of a medical problem. The minimum database should consist of a complete blood count, biochemical profile, urinalysis, fecal evaluation and, when possible, an electroencephalogram (EEG). The tail should be carefully evaluated for any evidence of foreign body penetration, trauma, or inflammation. Any deviations to the tail or pain on palpation are good reasons to consider radiographic studies. The prognosis is good for those behaviors that have been reinforced and conditioned but will otherwise be guarded to poor, unless an effective drug can be found to resolve the condition.

Management

Management of this problem must be based on treatment of the potential causes and contributing factors to the problem. Tail chasing behavior that has been inadvertently reinforced can be treated by removing all attention and rewards when the behavior begins. Interrupting the behavior with distraction, aversive devices, or a halter and leash might also be successful. Identifying those stimuli that initiate the behavior and either avoiding these stimuli or desensitizing and counterconditioning the dog to these stimuli might also be effective (see treatment for acral lick dermatitis above for more details). When the behavior cannot be interrupted, when the behavior occurs independent of specific stimuli, or when the specific stimuli cannot be avoided or controlled through desensitization and counterconditioning, drug therapy is likely to be required (Fig. 10.8). Compulsive disorders may be responsive to treatment with clomipramine or selective serotonin re-uptake inhibitors in addition to the environmental and behavioral management discussed above. European behaviorists have reported some success with selegiline in spinning English Bull Terriers or with respiridone when the 'hallucinations' are severe (per Patrick Pageat).

If the condition is responsive to narcotic antagonists (e.g., naltrexone), then endogenous opioid release is likely to be at least one of the mechanisms involved. Since narcotic antagonists are inconvenient to administer long term, and are also expensive, combinations of pentazocine and naloxone may be used instead. It is also possible that narcotic therapy (hydrocodone) may be useful in these cases. Epileptic conditions may respond to phenobarbital or potassium bromide therapy. For tail mutilation, see self-injurious behavior below.

Clomipramine	2–3 mg/kg bid
Fluoxetine	1–4 mg/kg bid
Paroxetine	1 mg/kg q 24h (up to 5 mg/kg)
Fluvoxamine	0.5 to 2 mg/kg bid
Sertraline	2–5 mg/kg divided bid
Carbamazepine	4–20 mg/kg divided bid/tid
Doxepin (anxiety/antihistamine)	0.5–5 mg/kg bid/tid
Amitriptyline (anxiety/antihistamine/pain)	2–4 mg/kg bid
Naltrexone	2.2 mg/kg sid
Phenobarbital	2–3 mg/kg bid
Gabapentin	5 mg/kg tid

Figure 10.8 Drug treatment for tail chasing and self-mutilation in dogs.

Prevention

Until the cause of compulsive tail chasing is better understood, there are no clear-cut ways of preventing it. Owners must be advised as to how attention and rewards contribute to behavior problems, so that these factors can be prevented. Appropriate selection and use of distraction and agents to interrupt the problem might also be successful. Since there seems to be some breed predilection, at least for Bull Terriers, there may be a genetic component to the problem. Thus, affected dogs and their siblings should not be used in breeding programs.

Case example

Rocky was a three-year-old male neutered Lhasa Apso who barked incessantly and chased his tail whenever the owner entered the home. The problem began about one year ago during a time when Rocky had a lapse in housetraining and for several weeks in a row the owner frequently punished Rocky upon arriving home and finding a mess in the house. The pet would start to approach the owner, then back away and run in circles while barking. The owners admitted that at the start they had found the tail chasing 'funny' and 'cute' and had encouraged the behavior. When the behavior became incessant, the owner then attempted to calm Rocky down by patting or lifting him, but recently had resorted to stopping the behavior by feeding Rocky as soon as the behavior started.

The barking and tail chasing initially developed as a result of anxiety. The pet was caught in an approach–avoidance conflict, wanting to greet the owner, but fearful of being punished. The owner's attention rewarded the behavior and it became a conditioned response. A reinforcement of basic obedience commands and a session at obedience school were recommended to gain more control over Rocky. Interruption of the behavior with a startle device was suggested and, provided the dog responded by stopping his barking and circling, the owner could reward Rocky with a favorite treat such as a piece of freeze-dried liver. In the interim, the owners were advised to ignore Rocky completely at homecomings until he calmed down. After a few weeks of success with obedience training the owners began to apply the retraining techniques. At first a shake can was thrown on the floor when they entered, but although Rocky was deterred for a few seconds he would not respond to the command and reward cue so that he soon habituated to the shake can. The owners were therefore advised to try entering the home through their side door (which would provide a slightly different set of cues), and Rocky was fitted with a citronella spray anti-bark collar. As soon as the owner entered and barking began, the citronella collar was activated and Rocky would shake his head and retreat. Although the collar did not have any direct effect on the circling, it effectively interrupted both behaviors. The owners would then call Rocky to come and sit and provide the food reward, and the conditioned circling and barking behaviors were permanently subdued. The owners decided to leave the citronella collar on whenever they were out, and were aware that all barking was eliminated (the type that disturbed the neighbors as well as the territorial barking) while Rocky was wearing the collar.

Feline psychogenic alopecia

Cats are normally fastidious groomers and as much as 30–50% of their time awake is spent performing some type of grooming behavior. Alopecia can result when cats overgroom and remove fur, usually over their topline. The diagnosis of psychogenic alopecia is reserved for those cases in which there is no underlying dermatological or physiological condition. Elimination of such dermatological or physiological conditions requires a complete workup, which should include a complete physical examination, as well as skin scrapings, fungal culture, biopsy, complete blood cell counts, elimination diets, parasiticide response trials, endocrine function tests, and evaluation for allergies. In our practice, numerous patients initially referred to the behavior service for psychogenic alopecia have been found to have underlying medical problems that were causing the alopecia. In fact, a majority of these cases had a medical cause (Figs 10.9, 10.10).

It is thought that feline psychogenic alopecia may be a displacement activity resulting from conflict or frustration, which in time might become compulsive. Anxiety, lack of stimulation, and the desire for human contact can result in excessive grooming. Changes in the owner's schedule resulting in separation anxiety, inappropriate punishment, and new people or animals in the environment may all be potential causes of this type of problem. A study that examined grooming time in relation to stress and drugs that increase or decrease dopamine levels found that grooming was significantly increased after an injection of apomorphine and decreased following an injection of haloperidol. The results support the concept that stress is able to induce excessive grooming and

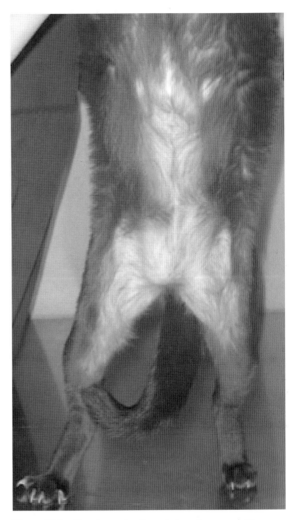

Figure 10.9 Psychogenic alopecia in a four-year-old Burmese cat.

emphasizes the role of dopamine in relation to stress.

Diagnosis and prognosis

The first diagnostic step is physical examination to assess the pattern of distribution of hair loss, whether there are any primary skin lesions or evidence of parasites, and to determine if there is any evidence of underlying illness. Blood and urine tests, skin scraping, dermatophyte culture, and trichogram are important components of the

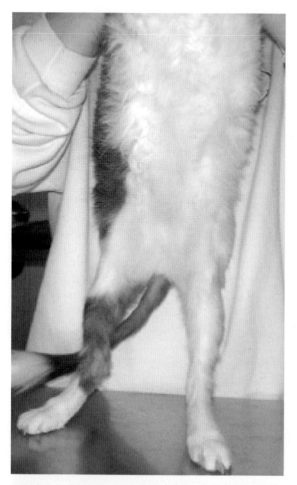

Figure 10.10 Tyson – a seven-year-old neutered male with food allergy and atopy.

many cats are secretive groomers and owners may report that they never see their cat lick or chew. The other clinical clue is that a cat with psychogenic alopecia will only have hair loss on those parts of the body that can be reached with the tongue. In contradistinction to conditions such as dermatophytosis and allergy, in cats with psychogenic alopecia the top of the head and back of the neck will be spared of hair loss, except in those cases where scratching is considered to be a component of the problem.

Parasites can cause a hypersensitivity reaction leading to pruritus and hair loss, yet no parasites may be observed. Therefore a therapeutic response trial would be an important component of the workup to rule out mites and fleas as a possible cause. Adverse food reactions may also cause pruritus and hair loss. In cats with food allergies there may be little or no improvement with corticosteroid therapy, and it may take up to eight weeks for cats on a therapeutic trial to improve. Therefore the exclusive use of either a novel protein or hydrolyzed protein (low-allergen) diet should be part of the diagnostic workup.

Many cats with presumed psychogenic tendencies have been shown to have atopy. This finding is also supported by the breed predisposition toward Siamese, Abyssinians, and Himalayans. Thus, apparent overgrooming can result from the pruritus of an allergic skin condition and there need not be concurrent primary dermatological lesions. Feline inhalant allergies are most appropriately diagnosed by intradermal allergy testing; blood tests do have value, but depend on the quality of the laboratory performing the test. Complete remission with corticosteroid therapy (typically injectible methylprednisolone acetate), while not diagnostic of any specific medical condition, may help to rule out a behavioral cause. Therapy often includes antihistamines (chlorpheniramine, clemastine, or cetirizine), fatty acids (combinations of cis-linoleic acid, gamma-linolenic acid, and eicosapentanoic acid), and immunotherapy.

In a small group of 16 cats referred to our facility with a history and clinical signs consistent with psychogenic alopecia, after an exten-

initial workup, and while a biopsy might also be a consideration, it is unlikely to be of diagnostic importance unless primary lesions are evident. On examination, it is important to determine whether the fur is being removed by excessive grooming and that the hairs are not being shed. This can be quickly and effectively confirmed by a trichogram in which hairs are plucked, placed on a microscope slide, and viewed microscopically. Whereas endocrine conditions have hairs with telogen bulbs predominating, fur that has been removed by licking shows evidence of shear. This confirms only that the alopecia is due to excessive grooming, not the ultimate cause. This alone can be valuable, because

sive workup only four showed any evidence of a behavioral component and two of these patients had concurrent medical causes for the self-trauma. Of the remaining 12 cases, two were atopic, two had adverse food reactions, one had parasitic hypersensitivity, and the remaining seven had both atopy and an adverse food reaction. The rest had various combinations of concurrent atopy, adverse food reactions, and parasitic hypersensitivity. In these cases it is assumed that an erroneous diagnosis of psychogenic alopecia was made because the diagnostic protocols eliminated one etiology at a time, and the patient continued to self-traumatize because a concurrent cause of pruritus persisted. On the other hand, the relationship between behavior and allergy may be more complicated than at first glance. As mentioned earlier in this chapter, a link was found in humans between stress and an increase in epidermal permeability. Therefore, if percutaneous absorption of allergens leads to pruritus in the atopic patient, stress might predispose the patient to developing atopy.

Management

Since anxiety and conflict have likely been initiating factors, any possible sources of anxiety must be identified and resolved. Behavioral and environmental management techniques to reduce conflict between cats in the household, helping the cat adapt to household changes, and improving relationships between the cat and family members (or other relevant environmental changes) can be combined with Feliway™ and anxiolytic medications (buspirone, benzodiazepines, tricyclic antidepressants) to reduce underlying anxiety. Although it is uncertain whether cats suffer from true separation anxiety, the techniques used for reducing destructive behavior and increasing environmental stimulation (play centers, chew toys, food or catnip-packed toys, videos, increased interactive play) can all be tried if the behavior tends to occur in the owner's absence (see feline destructive behavior in Ch. 16). Gradually helping the cat adapt to long owner absences by providing a number of short departures of varying

lengths may help. Reducing access to any stimuli that might cause anxiety may be the most practical suggestion for some problems.

For compulsive disorders, clomipramine or one of the selective serotonin re-uptake inhibitors should be used in combination with behavior therapy. In addition, if there is a pruritic component, concurrent medical therapy may be needed. Response to medication varies greatly between individuals and some cats will not respond to any of these drugs. The owner should be counseled to avoid inadvertently reinforcing the behavior by giving the cat attention when it is grooming. Well-timed distractions, unassociated with the owner, are more beneficial than aversive stimuli in stopping the performance of the behavior. Increased self-play and interactive play should also help to reduce the time spent on overgrooming.

Prevention

Reducing stress in the cat's life and using anxiolytic medication prior to and during stressful situations for the cat with a history of psychogenic alopecia may prevent further problems. Owners of cats that have been treated for psychogenic alopecia should be counseled about controlling stress in the cat's life. Consideration should be given to prophylactic use of psychoactive medication, exercise, and environmental stimulation when highly stressful situations cannot be avoided.

Case examples

Case 1 Thai, a nine-year-old neutered female Siamese cat, was presented for symmetrical alopecia along the sides and dorsum of the lumbar area. The owner had noticed little change in the cat's grooming behavior, but it had been hiding quite a lot since a new roommate and his dog moved into the apartment two weeks ago. A complete medical/dermatological workup revealed no underlying medical etiology.

Since the problem appeared to be anxiety-induced, Thai was given 5 mg amitriptyline sid and confined to a quiet area of the apartment for the initial two weeks. During that time, the owner set about doing a number of things with the cat that would distract it from the dog. New toys were purchased, a 'kitty garden' of sprouting wheat was provided, and a chair was moved to a window so the cat could look outside. The owner had daily play sessions with the cat and used food rewards to teach it to come when he whistled. Obedience training was recommended for the dog so that sit-stays could be used to control its behavior when the cat was present. After two weeks, a baby gate was placed in the doorway to the cat's confinement room. This allowed the cat to see the dog and move about in its room without being bothered by the dog. It also allowed the dog to habituate to the cat, so it didn't get excited every time it saw it. After four more weeks, the owner held exercises during which the dog would be on a leash responding to sit-stays for its owner, 6 m (20 ft) away from the door to the cat's room. While standing next to the gate, the cat's owner would whistle and call the cat for a treat. Gradually, the cat was called through the gate into the main room. High resting areas were provided for the cat, so that when it started spending more time in the main room, it could rest in a safe area. As the cat showed less anxiety, hair regrowth was noted. Once the cat started spending an appreciable amount of time in the living areas of the apartment, it was gradually weaned off the amitriptyline.

Case 2 Lucy was a four-year-old spayed female Burmese cat who had a two-year history of hair loss along the belly and the posterior surfaces of all four legs. She also had a history of intermittent vomiting once or twice weekly that had been attributed by the referring veterinarian to the excessive licking and swallowing of hair. After an extensive diagnostic workup and minimal response to treatment trials she was referred to our behavioral service but was first 'rerouted' to our staff dermatologist.

The owner agreed to take part in a clinical trial in which a systematic approach to diagnostics would be followed. The blood and urine tests were normal, no abnormalities were seen on physical examination, and the trichogram revealed that the hair had been broken from lick-ing. A skin biopsy showed no evidence of any underlying cause (mild inflammation due to licking) and the dermatophyte culture and skin scrapings were negative. A parasiticide response trial was unsuccessful so that both mites and fleas were eliminated as possible causative factors. After an eight-week trial of a hydrolyzed protein diet, Lucy was at least 50% improved. The food was continued and a corticosteroid-response trial (20 mg of methylprednisolone acetate SQ) did not lead to any further improvement of the hair loss, but the vomiting ceased entirely (and a presumptive diagnosis of inflammatory bowel disease was made) (see Fig. 10.9).

Lucy was maintained on oral prednisone therapy, which helped to control the signs of inflammatory bowel disease as well as the hydrolyzed protein diet, and was then placed on fluoxetine at 2.5 mg daily along with a program of increased interactive play, short training sessions, and some boxes and paper bags with small pieces of lamb as treats to encourage investigation and play. Most of the remaining alopecia and any evidence of excessive grooming were resolved, and after six months a novel protein (lamb-based) diet, daily prednisone, and alternate-day fluoxetine therapy were able to achieve long-term maintenance.

Feline hyperesthesia

Feline hyperesthesia is a poorly understood condition that has also been referred to as rippling or rolling skin syndrome, twitchy skin syndrome, atypical neurodermatitis, neuritis, and feline neurodermatitis. The expression of clinical signs can be variable, perhaps indicating somewhat different etiologies. Once the behavioral signs begin, the cat may be difficult to interrupt or distract, and redirected aggression might be a possible consequence. Most cats begin with rippling of the skin and muscle spasms or twitching along the thoracolumbar region. This may be accompanied by vocalization, an arched back, exaggerated tail movement, and agitation. These signs may be induced by simply rubbing or scratching along the back in some cats. In others the signs may occur spontaneously.

Drug	Dosage
Clomipramine	0.3–0.5 mg/kg sid
Fluoxetine	0.5–1 mg/kg q 24h
Fluvoxamine	0.5–1 mg/kg q 24h
Paroxetine	0.5 mg/kg sid
Amitriptyline	1–2 mg/kg q 24h
Oxazepam	0.2–0.5 mg/kg q 12–24h up to 2.5 mg/kg
Phenobarbital	2–3 mg/kg PO q 12–24h
Selegiline	0.5–1 mg/kg q 24h
Chlorpheniramine maleate	1–2 mg/cat bid/tid
Doxepin	0.5–1 mg/kg q 12–24h
Megoestrol acetate	2.5–10 mg/cat q 24h
Gabapentin (neuropathic pain)	2.5 mg/kg bid
Carbamazepine (neuropathic pain)	25 mg bid

Figure 10.11 Feline drug doses for psychogenic alopecia, hyperesthesia, and self-mutilation.

Feline hyperesthesia may also be associated with more exaggerated signs including running, jumping, or self-directed aggression (biting, chewing, intense grooming). Some cats may appear to startle, hallucinate, and dash away, and may even defecate as they run away.

In most cases, an anxiety-induced displacement behavior or compulsive disorder is likely the cause, but a number of dermatologic, medical, and painful conditions have also been speculated to be possible etiologies (or contributing factors). Petit mal seizures, spinal lesions, dermatologic conditions such as food allergy, and systemic diseases such as toxoplasmosis or hyperthyroidism should all be considered. More recently, a vacuolar myopathy, similar to inclusion body myositis in humans, has been identified in the epaxial muscles of five affected cats (March et al 1999).

Diagnosis and prognosis

The diagnostic workup will need to focus on both the medical and behavioral factors that might cause or contribute to the development of feline hyperesthesia. Medical differentials that might cause or contribute to hyperesthesia include dermatologic conditions such as parasitic hypersensitivity (e.g., flea bite dermatitis), food allergy, atopy, or any condition that might cause pain or irritation in the lumbar or perineal regions, such as intervertebral disk dis-

ease, FLUTD, anal sacculits, trauma, neoplasia, or myositis. Any disease process that affects the central nervous system, and those that alter the pet's behavior or reactivity to stimuli, need to be diagnosed or ruled out as possible contributing factors (e.g., seizure focus, FIV, FeLV, toxoplasmosis, etc.).

The signs of hyperesthesia may be considered a normal response to physical stimulation and arousal in some cats. However, since this condition may arise at any age, it is most likely that conflict and anxiety are at least in part responsible for the development of the clinical signs and that in some cats the problem may progress to a compulsive disorder with little or no identifiable stimuli preceding the behavior. The history may reveal factors in the environmental or social relationships (between the cat and humans, cats or other pets) that can be leading to anxiety and stress.

Management

At present it is not known whether hyperesthesia represents a distinct syndrome or the common endpoint of many different conditions. Any medical problems that cause or contribute to pain, discomfort, or irritation must be diagnosed and treated. After ruling out or controlling any underlying medical problems, therapeutic drug trials may be needed to rule out dermatologic causes (e.g., parasiticide trial, food trial), neurological causes (e.g., phenobarbital trial), inflammatory conditions (e.g., corticosteroid trial), or painful conditions (e.g., opioid, analgesic, or gabapentin trial). For a suspected diagnosis of inclusion body myositis, a therapeutic trial with acetyl-L-Carnitine 50 mg/kg every 12 hours, CoEnzyme Q10 1 mg/kg once daily, riboflavin 50 mg once daily, and vitamin E 20 IU/kg once daily has been suggested.

Behavioral management requires the identification and control of those stimuli that lead to the behavior. Avoiding or minimizing these stimuli, or using desensitizing and counterconditioning techniques so that the cat learns to 'tolerate' these stimuli, may be successful at reducing the cat's level of arousal. Increasing stimulation in the cat's environment (see discussion of other compulsive disorders) as well as drug therapy with clomipramine or an SSRI may be effective.

Prevention

Until more is known about feline hyperesthesia, it is unlikely that we can effectively prevent the condition, except to avoid or desensitize the cat to those stimuli that cause arousal.

Case example

Rip was a three-year-old neutered male Burmese cross that the owners claimed had always been sensitive about being stroked or groomed along his hind end. From the time he was obtained at four months of age, any time Rip was petted or brushed over his dorsal lumbar region, his skin would ripple, he would vocalize, and within a minute or two he would run away and begin to groom himself. However, over the past few months, any time the owners attempted any grooming or physical contact distal to his shoulders, Rip would immediately howl, his skin would ripple, his pupils would dilate, and he would run away and begin to lick around the perineal region. This behavior was also observed a few times each week when there was no approach or contact by the owners.

On examination, Rip was physically restrained by being wrapped in a large blanket. With his head covered he allowed visual examination of the skin but as soon as his lumbar region was touched, he howled, the skin rippled, and he made frantic attempts to escape. There were no physical abnormalities noted except for a small amount of hair loss in the perineal region. A blood profile, CBC, and urinalysis were drawn and revealed no abnormalities. Rip was then admitted for examination under anesthesia. No fleas or flea dirt were noted and there were no physical abnormalities except for moderately enlarged and impacted anal sacs, which were thoroughly flushed. Rip was sent home with two weeks of a trimethoprim-potentiated sulfonamide combination, but there was no apparent improvement in signs. It was suspected that Rip had always had a mild displacement behavior, but the pain and irritability associated with the anal sacculitis had aggravated the condition and he had now developed a conditioned response with both medical and behavioral components. A dietary exclusion trial, a parasiticide response trial, and a corticosteroid trial also led to no significant improvement.

Rip was placed on 2.5 mg clomipramine daily, and the owners were given a desensitization and counterconditioning program, which incorporated hand-feeding of all food and treats, and increasing levels of contact during these feeding times. At first, contact was limited to touching the back just distal to the shoulder region, but in time the owner moved farther back and increased to a slightly stronger level of petting. An increase in manipulation play toys as well as increased owner-initiated play was also introduced. Over a period of four weeks the owner was gently stroking the hind end successfully (with mild skin rippling and vocalization). However, when the clomipramine dose was reduced the vocalization and rippling dramatically increased. The cat was re-admitted for examination and although the anal sacs were only minimally distended, they were removed prophylactically. The cat was subsequently maintained on 2.5 mg of clomipramine daily.

Wool sucking and pica in cats

Compulsive disorders may be ingestive, which in cats may involve sucking or picas. Although nutritional deficiencies, metabolic disease, gastrointestinal disturbances, CNS disturbances, or an extremely restrictive diet might contribute to picas, many cats begin to suck or ingest non-food items for entirely behavioral reasons. There may be conflict or underlying anxiety that is an inciting factor, but like other oral compulsive disorders, lack of stimulation along with genetic predisposing factors may be the cause. In a European study of 152 cats exhibiting pica, most were Burmese or Siamese. The most common materials were wool (93%), cotton (64%), synthetic fabrics (53%), rubber or plastic (22%), and paper or cardboard (8%) (Bradshaw et al 1997). Many cats that begin as wool chewers may progress to other targets. Pica most commonly occurred either about two months after rehoming or between six and 18 months (i.e., at the time of sexual or territorial maturity). However, there was no effect of neutering on reducing the problem.

Prevention, booby traps, and taste deterrents may stop the chewing and sucking of household objects, but do not resolve the problem. Over time, denying access to the favored target without providing alternative outlets for the behavior may lead to the development of new preferences. Providing alternative oral stimulation in the form of bulky, dry, or chewy foods might satisfy the desires of some cats. Increased fiber in the diet or providing opportunities to chew on dog chew toys, dental diets, or even meat and gristle that are attached to bones may satisfy the need of some cats. It has also been suggested that a woolen or sheepskin garment be made available to the cat. Since picas may also arise as a displacement behavior from anxiety and conflict, any source of household conflict should be identified and resolved. Some of these cases may be compulsive disorders so that therapy with clomipramine, paroxetine, or fluoxetine at 0.5 mg/kg daily may need to be considered.

Self-injurious behavior of dogs and cats

In some cases the stereotypic or repetitive behaviors, such as scratching of the face and neck or tail chasing with mutilation, may lead to varying degrees of self-trauma and injury. These cases may be a component of compulsive disorders, sequelae to compulsive or displacement behaviors, or an entirely separate entity arising from pain. As in the discussion of compulsive disorders, underlying medical causes (dermatologic, neurologic, metabolic) must first be ruled out. In addition, secondary medical factors such as concurrent infections must also be considered and treated. A displacement behavior arising from conflict or a compulsive disorder are both considerations for diagnosis and treatment.

However, when the self-trauma leads to injury, a painful component may be the cause or a perpetuating factor. Surgery to amputate a damaged tail tip, or to excise damaged tissue, may be necessary to aid healing, but is unlikely to lead to an improvement in the underlying condition. In some cases, a trial with an opioid or NSAID might be effective. However, for neuropathic pain, anticonvulsants such as gabapentin, or a tricyclic antidepressant such as amitriptyline, might be more effective (see Ch. 9).

Miscellaneous compulsive and stereotypic disorders

There are a number of additional problems that have been described in dogs and cats that might arise in situations of conflict, anxiety, or stress. These behaviors may then become more frequent or repetitive and be initiated by numerous other stimuli, which were not associated with the original conflict or displacement behavior. In dogs, these might include checking, pacing, circling, digging, phantom chewing, incessant or rhythmic barking, fly snapping or chasing unseen objects, freezing and staring, polydipsia, sucking, licking, or chewing on objects (or owners), and other forms of self-mutilation. In cats, hunting and pouncing at unseen prey, running and chasing, paw shaking, freezing, excessive vocalization, and self-directed aggression such as tail chasing or foot chewing may all be manifestations of displacement or compulsive disorders. In each case, it is essential to diagnose, rule out, or treat any medical condition that might contribute to the problem. In addition, medical problems might arise as a result of the chewing, digging, or licking, and these have to be treated as part of the therapy (as in acral lick dermatitis, tail chewing, or 'gum' chewing). If the problem persists after all medical problems are diagnosed, treated, or ruled out, behavioral modification, environmental manipulation, and drug therapy may also be indicated.

FURTHER READING

Ackerman L 1989a Practical feline dermatology, 2nd edn. American Veterinary Publications, Goleta, CA

Ackerman L 1989b Practical canine dermatology, 3rd edn. American Veterinary Publications, Goleta, CA

Ackerman L 2000 The genetic connection. AAHA Press, Lakewood, CO

Blackshaw JK, Sutton RH, Boyhan MA 1994 Tail chasing or circling behaviour in dogs. Canine Practice 19(3):7–11

Bradshaw JWS, Neville PF, Sawyer D 1997 Factors affecting pica in the domestic cat. Journal of Applied Animal Behavioral Science 52:373–379

Brignac MM 1992 Hydrocodone treatment of acral lick dermatitis. In: Proceedings of the 2nd annual world congress of veterinary dermatology, Montreal

Brown SA, Crowell-Davis S, Malcolm T et al 1987 Naloxone-responsive compulsive tail chasing in a dog. Journal of the American Veterinary Medical Association 190(7):884–886

Dehasse J 1998 Clinical management of stereotypies in dogs. Presented to the AVSAB annual conference, AVMA

Dehasse J 1999 Retrospective study on the use of Selgian in cats. Presentation to the American Veterinary Society of Animal Behavior annual meeting

Dodman NH, Shuster L, White SD et al 1988 Use of narcotic antagonists to modify stereotypic self-licking, self-chewing, and scratching behaviour in dogs. Journal of the American Veterinary Medical Association 193(7):815–819

Dodman NH, Bronson R, Gliatto J 1993 Tail chasing in a bull terrier. Journal of the American Veterinary Medical Association 202(5):758–760

Dodman NH, Knowles KE, Shuster L et al 1996 Behavioral changes associated with complex partial seizures in Bull Terriers. Journal of the American Veterinary Medical Association 208:688–691

Eckstein RA, Hart BL 1996 Treatment of acral lick dermatitis by behavior modification using electronic stimulation. Journal of the American Animal Hospital Association 32:225–230

Fox MW 1965 Environmental factors influencing stereotyped and allelomimetic behaviour in animals. Laboratory Animal Care 15:66–67

Fredricson OK 1982 Kinetics of citalopram in test animals; drug exposure in safety studies. Progress in Neuropsychopharmacology, Biology and Psychiatry 6(3):297–309

Garg A, Chren MM, Sands LP et al 2001 Psychological stress perturbs epidermal permeability barrier homeostasis: implications for the pathogenesis of stress associated skin disorders. Archives of Dermatology 137:78–82

Goldberger E, Rapoport JL 1991 Canine acral lick dermatitis: response to the anti-obsessional drug clomipramine. Journal of the American Animal Hospital Association 27:179–182

Hart BL 1976 The role of grooming activity. Feline Practice 6:14

Hartgraves SL, Randall PK 1986 Dopamine agonist-induced stereotypic grooming and self-mutilation following striatal dopamine depletion. Psychopharmacology 90:358–363

Hawkins J 1992 Gum-chewer syndrome: self-inflicted sublingual and self-inflicted buccal trauma. Compendium for Continuing Education for Practicing Veterinarians 14(2):219–222

Hewson CJ, Luescher UA 1996 Compulsive disorders in dogs. In: Voith VL, Borchelt PL (eds) Readings in companion animal behavior. Veterinary Learning Systems, Trenton, NJ, p 153–158

Hewson CJ, Luescher UA, Parent JM et al 1998 Efficacy of clomipramine in the treatment of canine compulsive disorder. Journal of the American Veterinary Medical Association 213(12):1760–1765

Iglauer F, Rasim R 1993 Treatment of psychogenic feather picking in birds with a dopamine antagonist. Journal of Small Animal Practice 34:564–566

Jones RD 1987 Use of thioridazine in the treatment of aberrant motor behavior in a dog. Journal of the American Veterinary Medical Association 191(1):89–90

Kennes D, Odberg FO, Bouquet Y et al 1988 Changes in naloxone and haloperidol effects during the development of captivity induced jumping stereotypy in bank voles. Journal of Pharmacology 153:19–24

Luescher UA 1998 Pharmacologic treatment of compulsive disorder. In: Dodman NH, Shuster L (eds) Psychopharmacology of animal behavior disorders. Blackwell Science, Malden, MA, p 203–221

Luescher UA 2000 Compulsive behavior in companion animal behavior problems. In: Houpt KA (ed) Recent advances in companion animal behavior problems. International Veterinary Information Service (www.ivis.org)

Manteca X 1994 Fly snapping syndrome in dogs. Veterinary Quarterly 16(Suppl 1):S49

March P, Fischer JR, Potthoff A et al 1999 Electromyographic and histological abnormalities in epaxial muscles of cats with feline hyperesthesia syndrome. In: Proceedings of the 17th ACVIM, Chicago, IL

Marks SL, Merchant S, Foil C 2001 Pentoxyfylline: wonder drug? Journal of the American Animal Hospital Association 37:218–219

Mason JD 1991 Stereotypies: a critical review. Animal Behaviour 41:1015–1037

McKeown D, Luescher A, Machum M 1988 Coprophagia: food for thought. Canadian Veterinary Journal 29(10):849–850

Moon-Fanelli AA, Dodman NH 1998 Description and development of compulsive tail chasing in terriers and response to clomipramine treatment. Journal of the American Veterinary Medical Association 212(8):1252–1257

Nesbitt GH, Ackerman LJ 1998 Dermatology for the small animal practitioner. Veterinary Learning Systems, Trenton, NJ

Overall KL 1992 Recognition, diagnosis, and management of obsessive–compulsive disorders. Canine Practice 17(2):40–41, 17(3):25–27, 17(4):39–43

Overall KL 1994 Use of clomipramine to treat ritualistic stereotypic motor behaviour in three dogs. Journal of the American Veterinary Medical Association 205(12):1733–1741

Overall KL 1997 Clinical behavioral medicine for small animals. Mosby, St Louis

Pobel T, Caudrillier M 1997 Evaluation of selegiline hydrochloride in treating behavioural disorders of emotional origin in dogs. Companion Animal Behavior Study Group. In: Proceedings of the first international conference on veterinary behavioural medicine, Universities Federation for Animal Welfare, Potters Bar, UK

Rapaport JL, Ryland DH, Kriete M 1992 Drug treatment of canine acral lick, an animal model of obsessive–compulsive disorder. Archives of General Psychiatry 49:517–521

Rivers B, Walter PA, McKeever PJ 1993 Treatment of canine acral lick dermatitis with radiation therapy: 17 cases (1979–1991). Journal of the American Animal Hospital Association 29:541–546

Rushen J, Schouten W, de Pasille WAMB et al 1990 Are stereotypies in pigs a coping mechanism? In: Proceedings of the Society for Veterinary Ethology, Montecatini Terme, Pistoia, Italy, p 4

Sawyer LS, Moon-Fanelli AA, Dodman NH 1999 Psychogenic alopecia in cats: 11 cases (1993–1996). Journal of the American Veterinary Medical Association 214(1):71–74

Schwaibold U, Pillay N 2001 Stereotypic behaviour is genetically transmitted in the African striped mouse Rhabdomys pumilio. Applied Animal Behavioral Science 74:273–280

Schwartz S 1993 Naltrexone-induced pruritus in a dog with tail-chasing behaviour. Journal of the American Veterinary Medical Association 202(2):278–280

Scott DW, Miller WH, Griffin CE 2001 Small animal dermatology, 6th edn. WB Saunders, Toronto, p 1069

Seksel K, Lindeman MJ 1998 Use of clomipramine in the treatment of anxiety-related and obsessive–compulsive disorders in cats. Australian Veterinary Journal 76(5):317–321

Shell LG 1994 Feline hyperesthesia syndrome. Feline Practice 6:10

Stein DJ, Hollander E 1992 Dermatology and conditions related to obsessive–compulsive disorder. Journal of the American Academy of Dermatology 26:237–242

Stein DJ, Mendelsohn I, Potocnik F et al 1998 Use of the selective serotonin reuptake inhibitor citalopram in a possible animal analogue of obsessive–compulsive disorder. Depression & Anxiety 8(1):39–42

Tuttle J 1980 Feline hyperesthesia syndrome. Journal of the American Veterinary Medical Association 176:47

Tuttle JL, Parker AJ 1980 Diagnosing, treating feline hyperesthesia syndrome. DVM 11:72

Virga V 1999 It's more than skin deep – behavioral dermatology: self-injurious, compulsive and related behaviors. In: 15th proceedings of AAVD/ACVD meeting, p 13–24

Voith VL, Marder AR 1988 Feline behavioural disorders. In: Morgan R (ed) Handbook of small animal practice. Churchill Livingstone, New York, p 1045–1051

Walton DK 1986 Psychodermatoses. In: Kirk RW (ed) Current veterinary therapy. IX. Small animal practice. WB Saunders, Philadelphia, PA

Willemse T, Spruijt BM 1995 Preliminary evidence for dopaminergic involvement in stress-induced excessive grooming in cats. Neuroscience Research Communications 17(3):203–208

Wynchank D, Berk M 1998 Fluoxetine treatment of acral lick dermatitis in dogs: a placebo-controlled randomized double blind trial. Depression & Anxiety 8(1):21–23

Young MS, Manning TO 1984 Psychogenic dermatoses. Dermatological Reports 3:1

11

Fears and phobias

THE FEAR RESPONSE

The fear response is a rather complex physiologic response involving a variety of areas of the brain. When a threatening or fear-evoking situation is perceived, an animal must react instinctively to survive: it either readies for confrontation or runs away. This sudden stress response is accompanied by an almost instantaneous surge in heart rate, blood pressure, respiratory rate, and metabolism, which are essential for a life-saving, rapid reaction. These physiological changes occur in part by activation of the locus ceruleus, a nucleus in the brain stem. It acts like the alarm system for the brain, triggering a response that prepares the animal to deal with a threatening situation. The locus ceruleus is the principal noradrenergic area of the brain, and the origin of most of the brain's norepinephrine pathways. Noradrenergic neurons, using norepinephrine as their communicating neurotransmitter, project from the locus ceruleus along discrete pathways to the cerebral cortex, limbic system, and the spinal cord, as well as other areas. Experimental stimulation of this area will trigger a fear response, and ablation of the area will mute the fear response. A physiologic explanation for panic attacks suggests an overactivity in this area of the brain, leading to these episodes.

It is suspected that the amygdala recognizes the alarm from the locus ceruleus and instantly calls up the memories of past events that were

227

fear evoking. The amygdala is a small almond-shaped structure deep inside the brain. It appears to be the central site for fear conditioning. Upon receiving nerve signals indicating a threat, the amygdala sends out neurosignals that result in autonomic arousal (increased heart rate and blood pressure), diminished pain sensation, enhanced startle reflex, stimulation of the hypothalamic–pituitary–adrenocortical axis (accompanied by the release of stress hormones), and defensive behavior. These physiological changes are associated with the emotion of fear.

The amygdala receives sensory input from the thalamus, a way station for incoming sensory information. This can occur via a direct connection between the two structures or indirectly from the thalamus through the auditory portion of the sensory cortex. The direct connecting tract does not communicate detailed information about the stimulus, but is very fast, an important consideration for an animal facing life-threatening danger. The indirect tract involves an area of the cortex that interprets sensory inputs and then sends relevant signals on to the amygdala. The indirect tract through the sensory cortex takes more time but allows for a more refined interpretation of input signals.

Within the amygdala is the lateral nucleus, which is important for fear conditioning. In this process, an individual learns to fear a neutral stimulus that has been paired within a primary fear-evoking stimulus. In humans, fear conditioning is thought to play a role in the development of such anxiety disorders as post-traumatic stress disorder, phobias, and panic disorder. Another important area of the amygdala is the central nucleus. This area is responsible for releasing signals that trigger a 'fight or flight' response.

Within the amygdala is a rich network of internal synapses, which provide communication between the various areas of this structure. These interior tracts may retain the response to the frightening stimulus even after fear conditioning has occurred. Because of this, an individual with an exceptionally strong fear of a certain stimulus or situation may go through

behavioral treatment that appears successful, but have the phobia return during a very stressful situation. It is suspected that the communication pathways that lead from the thalamus to the amygdala and those between the thalamus and the sensory cortex return to normal, but the amygdala's internal circuits do not.

The hippocampus is another major nucleus of the limbic system and is involved in memory storage. It has anatomical connections with the amygdala and hypothalamus. Neuroimaging studies have found a reduction in the size of the hippocampus in humans with post-traumatic stress disorder. The reduced volume is apparently due to the atrophy of dendrites in a select area of the hippocampus. It has also been discovered that atrophy in the same hippocampal region occurs in animals exposed to chronic psychosocial stress. The atrophy is thought to be due to stress-induced increases in glucocorticoids. The individual is thought to be less able to draw on memory to evaluate the nature of the stressor when the hippocampal function is compromised.

Dysregulation of these fear pathways appears to be important in manifestation of the symptoms associated with phobias and anxiety disorders. This dysregulation involves alterations in the activity of a number of neurotransmitters (including serotonin, norepinephrine, gamma-aminobutyric acid). These neurochemical systems are tightly integrated, such that changes in one system readily elicit changes in another. Of these neurotransmitters, serotonin and GABA are inhibitory and typically quiet the stress response. These neurotransmitters have become important targets for therapeutic agents.

Problems involving excessive fear responses may be due to inherited behavioral tendencies, inadequate early environmental experiences, inadequate early socialization, a learned aversion due to an unpleasant experience, medical or behavioral pathology, or a combination of these factors (Fig. 11.1). Dogs and cats that have not been sufficiently socialized to members of their species as well as other species during the critical period of socialization may develop fears that are particularly difficult to correct at a

FEAR	
Determinants of fear	
Genetics	• Unconditioned stimuli for fear such as predators, environmental danger, novel situations, and social threats • Temperament
Environmental experiences	• Inadequate socialization • Sensory isolation during development • Traumatic/aversive experiences (conditioning) • Consequences/learning (reinforcement by owner or learning to escape fear-provoking stimuli)
Components of fear	
Physiology	• Activation of autonomic and neuroendocrine systems with influence on the cardiovascular system, pupils, piloerection, and glucose metabolism
Behavior	• The type of fearful behavior that is exhibited is determined by genetics (species, breed, individual), experience, type and intensity of stimulus, and presence/absence of conspecifics • The function of fearful behavior is to remove the stimulus (threats) or remove the animal from the stimulus (escape behavior)
Emotion	• Although it has not been scientifically proven to exist in animals, observations of the behavior of fearful dogs and cats suggest that they experience this emotion

Figure 11.1 The nature of fear.

later age. The result can be the same for individuals that miss experiences with varied environmental stimuli during the early months of life.

When dogs and cats are exposed to new stimuli, the outcome will depend in part on the pet's sociability (genetics, stage of development), previous experience with similar stimuli, and the emotional or medical condition of the pet at the time of exposure. If the outcome is positive then the dog may exhibit eager anticipation with further exposure. If the stimulus has no consequence, the pet may ignore the stimulus with further exposure. However, pets that have an unpleasant experience, or perceive that the stimulus might be harmful, will avoid or become increasingly wary or fearful of the stimulus. An intensely unpleasant or aversive event can lead to an intensely fearful and lasting 'memory' of the stimulus (one-event learning). Although the pet may only become fearful of specific stimuli (discrimination) such as a noise (e.g., gun fire), place (e.g., veterinary clinic), or person (e.g., neighbor's child), some pets may generalize to many similar stimuli (e.g., all novel noises or all unfamiliar children). In addition, the pet may become fearful of events that preceded the unpleasant situation (e.g., the car ride that precedes the veterinary visit). Dogs that are highly

aroused cannot make conscious decisions and are likely to respond with an automatic fight or flight response when exposed to a potentially aversive or noxious stimulus. High states of anxiety place the dog in a state of hypervigilance, where fear responses are automatic, and preclude the possibility of any cognitive response to the stimulus. Therefore, only if the pet's level of arousal is sufficiently reduced can it review options and make conscious decisions as to whether a stimulus is positive, fearful, or of no consequence. Arousal can be reduced by ensuring that the pet is calm through training by using products for control such as head halters, by selecting an appropriate environment for exposure, and through selection and control of appropriate stimuli for retraining. Drug therapy may also be useful for highly aroused pets that cannot be effectively settled through training alone.

Regardless of the cause, each fear-eliciting event that does not ultimately have a positive outcome is likely to further aggravate the problem. Since the goal of retraining and correction is to change the association with the stimulus to one that is positive, any response on the part of the owner, or the stimulus that might lead to a negative or unpleasant consequence, will further increase the fear and anxiety. Therefore punishment and other aversive correction techniques must be entirely avoided, and the stimuli should be controlled and non-threatening during retraining. In addition, if the owner displays any emotions of anger or anxiety, this too is likely to increase the pet's anxiety. Every exposure to the fearful event or stimulus that does not yield a positive outcome may further aggravate the problem. Also, if the pet escapes from the situation or a threatening display leads to retreat of the stimulus, then the behavior has been negatively reinforced because the threatening stimulus has been removed. An owner's attempts to calm and reassure the fearful dog may also serve to reinforce the fearful displays. The consultant must examine the owner's response to the fearful pet to identify and eliminate any potentiating factors. In treating a fear-related problem, it is often just as important to tell the family what not to do, as it is to tell them what to do.

For successful resolution of the problem, owners must be counseled to use appropriate behavioral modification methods. Behavior modification techniques that may be utilized include flooding, habituation, systematic desensitization, counterconditioning, shaping, positive reinforcement, and techniques that teach the pet an alternate acceptable response that can be reinforced (response substitution, differential reinforcement). The first step is to identify and control every stimulus or situation that might evoke fear until the program is successfully completed. If a situation arises during the conditioning program that might trigger an aggressive response, it is important that the pet is well controlled so that injuries are unlikely. For example, if the pet is in a crate, on a leash, or wearing a muzzle or head halter, aggression can usually be prevented, and escape can be thwarted.

BASIC BEHAVIORAL MODIFICATION AND THE FEARFUL PET

Some of the techniques covered in Chapter 5 are particularly relevant to managing fears and phobias. These include flooding, habituation, systematic desensitization, counterconditioning, shaping, response substitution, and positive reinforcement. They can be used individually or together in behavioral modification therapy (Fig. 11.2).

Reducing or eliminating fearful behavior requires identification of all stimuli that might cause fear, and avoiding exposure to these stimuli until the pet responds effectively to the owner's commands in a variety of neutral, non-threatening situations. By pairing a tone, clicker, or visual cue with each food reward, these new cues can become a powerful reward or distraction for further training. A leash attached to a head halter system may be helpful for some owners that have difficulty gaining control and getting the pet to respond to commands.

DESENSITIZATION, COUNTERCONDITIONING, AND CONTROLLED EXPOSURE TECHNIQUES

It can be helpful to begin by teaching the pet to sit-stay or down-stay for something special. Rewards should be highly motivating to the pet (food, favorite toy), and should be withheld at all other times except for training sessions. Once the pet has been effectively trained to respond to obedience commands, the owner can begin to expose the pet to controlled levels of the fearful stimuli.

For desensitization, the pet is trained to perform the behavior for a very highly favored reinforcer while exposed to a level of the stimulus that is below the level that will evoke a fear response. Rewards are given only if the pet responds to the commands without showing any fear. Gradually, the pet is exposed to progressively stronger levels of stimuli, and rewards are given for sequentially closer stages approaching the desired behavior. In time, the pet should perform the desired behavior in the presence of the full stimulus. Should the threshold for fear be surpassed at any point in the desensitization program, so that the pet exhibits a strong fear response, the owner should return

Step	Comments
Identify all fear-provoking stimuli	• All stimuli that might evoke fearful responses must be identified to determine the focus for desensitization and counterconditioning exercises
Identify the threshold for the fear response	• The amount, intensity, or proximity of the fear-provoking stimulus that is required to elicit signs of fear should be established in order to set a sub-threshold starting point for behavioral modification
Control the pet's environment	• Prevent exposure to fear-provoking stimuli or situations that occur outside training sessions
Control the pet's response	• The pet must not be allowed to escape or to harm itself or others during behavioral modification. Accomplishing this might include the use of a crate, muzzle, or halter. Use of any of these devices is only appropriate if they do not result in increasing the pet's fear. Before retraining can begin the owner must be able to calm and settle the pet in the absence of any fear-evoking stimuli. See handout #23 (Fig. 5.13) for training dogs to settle
Modify the behavior	• For dogs, it is helpful to use highly motivating rewards such as food, social attention, or a favorite toy to reward 'sit-stay' or 'down-stay' or other settle commands prior to exposure. Then, the command can be used to settle and calm the pet when low-level exposure to the fear-evoking stimulus is begun. Cats can be rewarded with food, patted, played with, or groomed during exposure depending on what the individual prefers
	• When the pet responds immediately and positively to commands, begin desensitization by exposing the pet to a stimulus intensity just below the threshold that would evoke fear. Reinforcements are associated with exposure to the stimulus as soon as the pet shows no fear
	• Gradually increase the intensity of the stimulus
	• Controlled flooding with a stimulus intensity above the threshold for a fearful response can be used for pets with mild problems and good owner control – as soon as the pet settles, reinforcement is given
	• A control device such as a head halter or a disruption device such as a citronella spray may initially be an effective way to get the pet's attention and settle it down so that the reward can be given and the positive association accomplished
Calm the dog – change the fear response to one that is positive	• In order to achieve a positive association with the stimulus the owner must remain calm and in control. Any anxiety on the owner's part as well as most forms of punishment (from raised voice to physical techniques) will further increase the pet's anxiety. In addition, the stimulus for retraining should be non-threatening to the pet as a fearful or aggressive person or pet will further add to the pet's anxiety
Avoid reinforcing or punishing fearful displays	• If the pet is consoled when it is acting fearfully, the fear-related behavior may be reinforced
	• If the pet is punished, the state of fearful arousal may increase during subsequent exposures to fear-eliciting stimuli

Figure 11.2 Behavioral modification techniques used for fearful behaviors.

to an earlier level of training and proceed in smaller increments. By withholding rewards except for training sessions, the pet should learn to associate positive experiences with the formerly fearful stimuli.

If the pet's problem is mild and the owner has good control, controlled flooding techniques (continuous exposure to stimuli above the threshold that elicits fear) may be faster than and as effective as desensitization for reducing fear. The stimulus should be presented at a reduced level, just sufficient to bring about a minimal fear or anxiety response. A leash and head halter can be helpful for some owners and pets in providing increased control and ensuring compliance. The pet should be exposed to the stimulus until it shows no sign of fear. Once all signs of fear subside and the pet responds to the owner's commands, rewards should be given. The strength of the stimulus can gradually be increased for each succeeding training session until the pet will accept exposure to the stimulus at full intensity without exhibiting any fear (Fig. 11.3).

BEHAVIOR MODIFICATION FOR FEARS AND PHOBIAS TOWARD NOISES, LOCATIONS, AND OBJECTS IN DOGS (INANIMATE STIMULI)

There are many different stimuli that can frighten your dog. This handout is designed to develop a program for improving or resolving fear to inanimate stimuli such as places, noises, or objects. When the fear is excessive or exaggerated, your dog may be exhibiting a panic response in which case drug therapy might be useful in combination with the behavior techniques below. Fear can be generalized so that it occurs as a response to a variety of noises or locations, or whenever it is confronted with something new or novel, or it may be a specific fear or phobia such as thunderstorms or a specific location (e.g., tile floors).

Treatment of fear

In simple terms, the pet must be exposed to the fearful stimulus until it sees that there is nothing to fear and settles down. If the association with the stimulus can be turned into one that is positive, the pet may actually develop a positive attitude when exposed to the stimulus.

Desensitization is used in combination with counterconditioning to change a pet's attitude or 'feeling' about the stimulus from one that is negative to one that is positive. Desensitization involves controlled exposure to situations or stimuli that are weaker or milder than will cause fear. Counterconditioning is then used to change the dog's response to the stimulus (noise, location, object) by associating the dog's favored rewards with the stimulus. The dog is then gradually introduced to similar but progressively more intense stimuli paired together with the presentation of the favored reward. If an inappropriate response (fear, escape attempts, aggression) is exhibited then an attempt should be made to interrupt the situation and calm the dog, at which point a reward can be given for success.

Response substitution is used to train the dog to perform or display a new acceptable response (e.g., sit, settle) each time it is exposed to the stimulus. Again, rather than attempting to overcome an intense response, the training should be set up to expose the dog with stimuli of reduced intensity to ensure a successful outcome. A head halter and leash can be used to ensure success and both the release (negative reinforcement) and positive reinforcement can be used to mark and reinforce an acceptable relaxed response.

Owner responses such as a raised voice, anxiety, fear, or punishment will only serve to heighten the pet's fear or anxiety. Similarly, an overly intense exposure to the stimulus will further aggravate anxiety. Be certain to retrain only with calm, controlled stimuli. The goal of training is to reinforce appropriate, desirable responses. Therefore, it is critical that rewards are not given and that the stimulus and the dog are not removed from the situation until the dog is calm and settled.

Steps for treating a pet that is fearful of inanimate objects and sounds

1. Identify all stimuli and situations that cause the pet to be fearful. Remember that there can be multiple stimuli that add to the fearful response so that each stimulus should be identified separately. For example, a pet that is fearful of a vacuum cleaner might be afraid of the sound or sight of the vacuum cleaner, the person using the vacuum cleaner, and the locations in which it is used. Pets fearful of thunder may also react to the rain, the flashes of lightening, increasing darkness, and even the drop in barometric pressure or static electric charges associated with the storm.
2. Do your best to prevent your dog from experiencing the stimuli except during the retraining sessions. This may be difficult for certain stimuli such as thunderstorms so that the options may be to use sedatives or confinement areas where your dog can avoid the stimuli (e.g., a room with no windows, minimal noise from the outside, and music for distraction).
3. Train the dog to relax or settle on command, in the absence of any fear-evoking stimuli (see our handout on settle training). Begin in an environment where the dog is calm, focused, and has minimal distractions. Gradually proceed to progressively more difficult and distracting locations and situations. The initial conditioning should be done by family members with whom the pet is calmest, most controlled, and responsive. For some dogs, using a head halter improves the speed and safety of training. Once the dog will reliably settle, focus on the family member, and accept rewards in a variety of environments then training can progress to more fear and anxiety-evoking situations.

Figure 11.3   Behavior modification for fear and phobias toward noises, locations, and objects in dogs – inanimate stimuli (client handout #8 – printable from the CD).

Steps for treating a pet that is fearful of inanimate objects and sounds (*continued*)

4. For storm and fireworks phobias it can be extremely useful to train the pet to settle or go to a location where the dog feels comfortable and secure, and where the auditory and visual stimuli can be minimized, such as a crate with a blanket or cardboard appliance box as cover. In addition, positive cues can be implemented that further calm and distract the dog. This can be accomplished by pairing a CD, video, white noise, or even a towel or blanket that has the owner's scent with each positive settle training session.

5. Each stimulus that leads to fear must be identified and placed along a gradient. The gradients must be set up so that initial exposures are mild. Each stimulus must be muted or minimized and presented in a controlled manner. It will be necessary to find some means of reproducing the stimuli so that they can be muted or minimized and presented in a controlled manner along a gradient of increasingly stronger stimuli. A tape recording, video, or CD might be a good starting point for retraining to the sound of the stimulus. Location and the person handling and training might also be factors that could be controlled to reduce the fearful response. For example, if a pet is afraid of the sound of the vacuum, the sight of the vacuum, the movement of the vacuum, the person using the vacuum, and the location of exposure, then these may all need to be controlled and introduced separately.

6. Determine the pet's most favored rewards (reinforcer assessment) and save these for the retraining and conditioning sessions. For some pets, food is the strongest reinforcer, while others may be more responsive to a favored play toy or social contact. The reward is presented to the pet along each step of the gradient for non-fearful responses, such as a relaxed sit. The trainer should use a quiet, relaxed, upbeat tone of voice.

7. Advance along the gradients very slowly. If you happen to proceed through a step too quickly and the pet responds fearfully, everyone should relax, look away from the pet, and ignore it. Once the fear response has ceased for five seconds or more, the stimulus can be reintroduced at a slightly lower level and desensitization and counterconditioning proceed.

8. Once each stimulus has been controlled and presented along a gradient of increasingly stronger stimuli and the pet acts calmly and shows no anxiety in the presence of any of the single stimuli, the separate elements can then be combined and gradually introduced as a group (e.g., the vacuum running, with a person moving it toward the pet).

Considerations

If the stimulus evokes anxiety from the beginning of the training session and the dog cannot be calmed or the pet is not responsive to commands, then either the stimulus is not sufficiently muted, the dog is not sufficiently trained or controlled, or the reward is not sufficiently motivating. It may be necessary to redesign a proper stimulus gradient so that a slower, more cautious approach can be taken. Command–reward training should be reviewed in the absence of any stimuli. A leash and head halter may need to be considered. Stronger reinforcers should be used or feeding time can be delayed to increase the pet's appetite.

Remaining calm is important for everyone. Any anxiety displayed by the owner or person doing the training as well as any anxiety or fear associated with exposure to the stimulus may further increase the pet's anxiety. Punishments and harsh corrections should also be avoided.

Figure 11.3 (*continued*)

FEAR OF PEOPLE

Some pets show fear toward a particular person, all unfamiliar people, or a type of person (child, baby, man in uniform, man with beard – Fig. 11.4). Depending on how a pet was socialized when it was young and the experiences it has with people at any time during its life, it may be fearful of individuals with whom it is not familiar or with those it associates with an aversive experience.

Diagnosis and prognosis

The fearful response may be aggression toward the stimulus or cowering, shaking, freezing, or escape. Signs of conflict that suggest a pet is becoming uncomfortable in a situation include

> **Any of the following groups may evoke a fear response if the pet has had little exposure to them:**
> - Babies, children, elderly
> - People in uniform
> - People whose appearance differs from family members (color, height, facial hair)
> - Disabled individuals
> - Men or women, depending on circumstances

Figure 11.4

displacement behaviors such as yawning, licking, or scratching. Changes in appearance associated with fear include: tail held low or tucked, ears held back, avoidance of eye contact, lowered body position, leaning away, lateral recumbency, and submissive urination. In most fearful situations, the animal will attempt to perform behaviors that help it avoid interaction with the fear-evoking stimulus or increase the distance between it and the stimulus. Innate behavior patterns, learning, and conditioning determine whether the animal will freeze, flee, or fight. The situation can prove dangerous if the fear response involves aggression, especially when the animal has no avenue for escape.

The prognosis is somewhat variable but is considered good for most cases if the duration is short, the pet was adequately socialized to people, the problem started during adulthood, and the owner can exert control over situations during which the pet interacts with people. The prognosis is poor for pets that have shown fear of people as well as other environmental stimuli from an early age without ever being exposed to anything considered aversive in relationship to people or other stimuli, and that live in environments where control of fear-eliciting stimuli or situations is difficult.

Management

A variety of techniques can be utilized for the treatment of fear (Figs 11.2, 11.3, 11.6, 11.7–11.9). Regardless of the method used, successful treatment requires that the owner identify all fear-evoking stimuli so that they can be reintroduced to the pet under controlled situations. Over time, the goal is to teach the pet to associate the sti-

muli with desirable events. It is important for owners to be aware that reassuring or rewarding the pet when it is exhibiting fear-related behaviors may reinforce the behaviors, while punishment (as well as any anxiety on the part of the owner) is likely to increase anxiety and also aggravate the problem.

For each fearful stimulus the owner should develop a gradient or hierarchy of stimuli from the least fearful to the greatest. Controlling the appearance or presentation of the fear-eliciting stimuli (Figs 11.3–11.5) and the distance between them and the pet are just two means for developing this gradient. The conditioning should take place in a friendly, non-threatening environment, where the pet can easily be controlled. For some pets, it might be helpful to hold the first session on neutral territory such as at the neighborhood park. The goal is to associate the potentially fearful stimulus with a favored treat (or other highly positive stimulus), so that the association is changed into an emotional state that is positive (counterconditioning). The key to success is that the stimuli can be controlled and presented along a gradient from the mildest (which should cause no fearful response) to the greatest (desensitization). If the pet begins to show anxiety and the response turns into one that is acceptable, such as sit (e.g., using a command, disruption device, or head halter), then this desirable, alternative, competing response should be reinforced with one of the pet's favored reinforcers (response substitution, differential reinforcement) (see Ch. 5 for definitions and details). During exposure techniques, the pet must be well controlled. A leash, head halter, or crate might also be useful for aggressive pets or pets that might attempt to escape.

For fear of people, training should begin with a person with only slightly similar characteristics to the type of person that elicits the fear response. For example, if the pet is afraid of children under five years of age, it should first be desensitized to approach and handling by teenagers. The pet can also be desensitized to the sounds of children playing by exposing it to tape recordings before actually beginning conditioning sessions with children. Pets that are

Dog that is afraid of men

Gradient of stimuli
- Familiar women — LESS FEARFUL
- Unfamiliar women
- Familiar boys
- Unfamiliar boys
- Familiar men
- Unfamiliar men — MORE FEARFUL

Figure 11.5 Example of a gradient of stimuli for a dog that is fearful of unfamiliar men.

afraid of men with beards should first be conditioned to approach and handling from men without beards, or even to a member of the family wearing a beard. Carrying a doll wrapped in a blanket and playing a recording of a baby can be a first step in teaching a pet to be less anxious around babies.

At first, the strangers should ignore the pet, and the owners can give treats if no fear is exhibited at a safe distance. Next, the treats can be given by the stranger but only if the pet approaches voluntarily in a non-fearful manner. Although the pet should not be pressed to endure an uncomfortable situation, it can be counterproductive if the visitor leaves before the pet calms down. Fearful dogs may cower and retreat but some may attack. Therefore the owner should proceed cautiously and slowly during subsequent sessions to ensure safe and successful retraining. While a head halter and leash works best for controlling a dog's response, a leash and basket-type muzzle may

be a better means of ensuring safety. For cats, an open carrying cage or a body harness and leash can help to ensure control and safety, as well as prevent escape.

Before bringing strangers into the home for conditioning exercises, the owner should first desensitize the pet to arrival cues. Begin by desensitizing it to sounds at the door by having family members ring the bell or knock at the door and enter. The bell should be rung repeatedly in close succession until the pet habituates and all undesirable or fearful responses cease. Each time the bell rings or the person knocks and the pet shows no undesirable response, it should be given a very tasty food reward or favorite toy. Next, invite people to visit that the pet knows and around whom it feels the most comfortable. Have the pet on a leash at a safe distance away from the door. When the visitor enters, he should ignore the dog and avoid making eye contact. If the pet shows no signs of fear, it should be asked to sit for a tasty food reward. Once indoors, the visitors should ignore the pet and provide attention only if it approaches in a friendly, non-fearful manner. The distance between the visitor and the pet can be decreased and approaches can be facilitated by casually flipping small pieces of meat toward the pet. Extending a hand with food instead of flipping it is more likely to inhibit approach behavior and should initially be avoided. Next, proceed to other people that the pet has previously met and finally to strangers. If the pet is most afraid of adult men, then this set of exercises should first involve unfamiliar

STIMULUS GRADIENT FOR DOG THAT IS AFRAID OF MEN IN UNIFORMS

1. Female owner wears uniform and approaches
2. Second owner or handler gives command and rewards with treat or toy
3. Female owner in uniform gives command and rewards with treat or toy
4. Repeat with male owner in uniform
5. Repeat with familiar women in uniform
6. Repeat with unfamiliar women or boys in uniform
7. Repeat with familiar men in uniform
8. Repeat with unfamiliar men with no uniform
9. Repeat with unfamiliar men in uniform (slower progression would be possible by beginning desensitization to people wearing a portion of the uniform, before the full uniform is applied)

Figure 11.6 An example of a hierarchy or gradient for desensitization of a dog that is fearful of men in uniforms.

Step	Comments
Identify stimuli and thresholds	• It is important to identify specific stimuli that cause the pet to be fearful so that behavioral modification can be wholly effective. For example, the pet may not be afraid of all men, just those with beards • The distance between the pet and strangers, as well as the type of behavior by strangers that triggers fear, should be identified
Establish a gradient of stimuli	• If the distance at which the pet recognizes a person is 15 m and the distance at which it begins to show signs of fear is 8 m, exposure should start between these two extremes • The pet with a fear of small children might first be introduced to older children. Pets that are fearful of babies can be exposed to blankets with a baby's scent and a low-volume tape recording of the baby. Pets afraid of men with beards might be introduced to men with moustaches only, or a family member wearing a fake beard. Similarly, pets afraid of unfamiliar men in uniforms or hats may first be approached by family members or women in uniforms or hats
Desensitization and counterconditioning	• Select a quiet location with few distractions where the pet is most comfortable for training. Make sure the pet is controlled and cannot harm itself or others • Exposure starts with the pet under full control and at a distance from a stranger where it recognizes the person but at which it shows no signs of fear. Associate favored rewards with the presence of the stimulus • Use reinforcer assessment to determine the pet's favored rewards so that these can be saved and used for these counterconditioning sessions • Very slowly decrease the distance between the pet and the person • The pet is gradually exposed to people with slightly different characteristics in a variety of situations
Response substitution & differential reinforcement	• Develop a stimulus gradient as with desensitization above • Insure that the pet and the stimulus are well controlled so that an appropriate acceptable response can be achieved • Using a previously trained command, e.g., sit, focus (a food lure can also be utilized), an acceptable response which is incompatible with the undesirable response must be achieved • Favored reinforcers are then given to mark and positively reinforce the correct response • Use reinforcer assessment to determine the pet's favored rewards so that these can be saved and used for these counterconditioning sessions • A head halter allows for additional safety and control to achieve the desirable response in a more immediate manner. An immediate release when the appropriate response is achieved also provides a form of negative reinforcement • Disruptive devices such as air horns, squeaky toys, or citronella sprays may also be useful for interrupting the undesirable response so that the desirable response can be reinforced • Very slowly decrease the distance between the pet and the person • The pet is gradually exposed to people with slightly different characteristics in a variety of situations
Flooding	• If the owner has good control of the pet and the fear is mild, the pet can be treated using controlled flooding during which it is exposed to a level of the stimulus that is just above the fear threshold. The pet is continually kept in the presence of the stimulus until it becomes calm • Once the pet shows no sign of fear, rewards should be given and the training session may be ended • Confinement crates and head halters are good accompaniments. Use of any of these devices is only appropriate if it does not result in increasing the pet's fear
Drugs and pheromones	• Feliway™ and D.A.P.™ diffuser sprays may be useful for reducing anxiety in the indoor environment. Felifriend™, which is presently available only in Europe, may help to reduce interspecific and intraspecific fears and anxiety (see Ch. 7) • Drugs are generally not effective when the fear is toward a specific stimulus as these dogs and cats will still be fearful of that stimulus even after drugs are administered. In addition anxiolytic drugs may disinhibit and lead to increased aggression. On the other hand for mild fears and anxiety buspirone might be effective, while for more generalized anxiety, states of panic, or responses that appear impulsive or excessive (e.g., long refractory period) tricyclic antidepressants such as clomipramine or amitriptyline or SSRIs such as paroxetine or fluoxetine might be useful

Figure 11.7 Steps in the management of pets with fear of people.

| Drugs and pheromones (*continued*) | • For pathological states that might be associated with anxiety and aggression, see the discussion of the European approach in Chapters 4 and 21
• Alternative therapy and dietary adjustments might occasionally be useful (see Chs 7 and 8)
• Drug desensitization might be another option (see Chs 5 and 6 for details). Benzodiazepines such as alprazolam might be utilized before an exposure session. If the desired response can be achieved for three or more consecutive sessions then the drug might be reduced by 25% and the program repeated until the pet can be retrained without medication. Alternately the benzodiazepine might be used on an ongoing basis (e.g., clorazepate tid and reduced by 25% weekly if the pet has improved) |

Figure 11.7 (*continued*)

women followed by exercises with unfamiliar young adult men, and finally adult men. The owner should save all rewards that are especially valued for training sessions, so that the pet learns to really look forward to the presence of visitors or strangers.

Some pets do better if the greeting is delayed. In this case, the pet is confined before the visitor comes to the home. Upon arrival, the visitor is taken to the far end of the largest room in the home and asked to sit. The owner gives the visitor a bowl containing small pieces of meat and instructs the person to sit quietly, avoid eye contact with the pet, and completely ignore it when it is brought into the room. After a short period, a family member goes to fetch the pet from the confinement area. The pet is asked to sit for a tasty treat and a leash (and head halter if needed) is placed on the pet. The pet is led to the room, but is asked to sit for a tasty treat every three to five feet along the way. The owner enters the room with the pet and sits about six to eight feet away. The visitor initially ignores the pet, flips food to it, and proceeds as described in the previous paragraph.

When the pet's fear abates to the point that it is relaxed and safe to allow certain visitors to pet it, it is helpful to put in place the '*Sit for a treat before petting*' rule. Visitors are told that they may only touch the pet if they ask the pet to sit and give it a treat that it eats first. This does several things that help make the situation safe. If, for some reason, the pet is too anxious to eat, and might bite, the interaction will not progress to physical interaction. Having the pet defer to the person by responding to a command inhibits

aggressive tendencies. Giving a treat reminds the pet that it is good to have this person around, so it shouldn't do anything that might send the source of the treats away. And lastly, since the person is required to get the pet's attention before reaching for it, it prevents the pet from being caught by surprise and snapping defensively (Figs 11.8, 11.9).

Prevention

Fear of people can often be prevented by proper and sufficient socialization. The young animal should be exposed to a wide variety of people during its socialization period in the early months of life, taking care that it is not so overwhelmed as to become fearful. Treats, play, and upbeat social interaction will facilitate socialization. The veterinarian should be instrumental in reinforcing these notions for all owners.

Case examples

Case 1 Chimo, a two-year-old entire female American Eskimo Dog, became panicked whenever someone on in-line skates approached during a walk.

The owner was instructed to review the dog's obedience training, using small tidbits of meat for rewards. The meat was only given during training sessions and each time it was given, the owner said 'It's OK' to condition a happy, food-anticipatory response whenever the words were said. As the dog became fearful when it was within 12 m of skaters, the owner was instructed to walk the pet and take it to between

BEHAVIOR MODIFICATION FOR FEAR OF PEOPLE OR PETS IN DOGS (ANIMATE STIMULI)

There are many different stimuli that can frighten your dog or lead to an aggressive response. Although fear can lead to avoidance and escape attempts, the dog that is defensive or aggressive when it is frightened can pose a serious danger. This handout is designed to develop a program for improving or resolving fear of animate stimuli, such as people and other animals. Fear can be generalized to all people or animals of a certain type (e.g., children, strange dogs) but can also be quite specific so that fear may only be exhibited with specific people (e.g., delivery men with beards) or in specific situations.

Treatment of fear

In simple terms, the pet must be repeatedly exposed to the fearful stimulus until it sees that there is nothing to fear and settles down. If the association with the stimulus can be turned into one that is positive, the pet may actually develop a positive attitude when exposed to the stimulus.

Desensitization is used in combination with counterconditioning to change a pet's attitude or 'feeling' about the stimulus from one that is negative to one that is positive. Desensitization involves controlled exposure to situations or stimuli that are weaker or milder than will cause fear. Counterconditioning is then used to change the dog's response to the stimulus (person, other animal) by associating the dog's favored rewards with the stimulus. The dog is then gradually introduced to similar but progressively more intense stimuli paired together with the presentation of the favored reward. If an inappropriate response (fear, aggression, attempts at retreat) is exhibited, then an attempt should be made to interrupt the situation and calm the dog, at which point a reward can be given for success.

Response substitution is used to train the dog to perform or display a new acceptable response (e.g., sit) each time it is exposed to the stimulus. Again, rather than attempting to overcome an intense response, the training should be set up to expose the dog with stimuli of reduced intensity to ensure a successful outcome. A head halter and leash can be used to ensure success and both the release (negative reinforcement) and positive reinforcement can be used to mark and reinforce an acceptable relaxed response.

Owner responses such as a raised voice, anxiety, fear, or punishment will only serve to heighten the pet's fear or anxiety. Similarly, a fearful, anxious, or threatening stimulus to the dog will further aggravate anxiety. Be certain to retrain only with calm, controlled stimuli. The goal of training is to reinforce appropriate, desirable responses. Therefore, it is critical that rewards are not given and that the stimulus and the dog are not removed from the situation until the dog is calm and settled.

Steps for treating a pet that is afraid of animate stimuli (people, other animals)

1. Identify all stimuli and situations that cause the pet to be fearful (e.g., tall men, loud women, young children playing).
2. Prevent the dog from experiencing the stimuli except during retraining sessions.
3. If there is aggression associated with the fear, then your dog should be trained to wear a head halter or basket muzzle so that safety during exposure exercises can be ensured.
4. Train the dog to relax or settle on command in the absence of any fear-evoking stimuli (see our handout on Settle training). Train only in locations where the dog is calm, focused, and has minimal distractions. The initial training should be done by family members with whom the pet is calmest, most controlled, and responsive. The head halter can be used to ensure immediate success.
5. Once the dog will reliably settle, focus on the family member, and accept rewards in a variety of environments, then training can progress to stimulus exposure, desensitization, and counterconditioning and response substitution.
6. Often, a familiar dog or a familiar person can be used as the initial training stimulus to ensure that the dog will show a relaxed and positive response in the problem environment (e.g., greeting other dogs on the street, greeting strangers at the door).

Figure 11.8   Behavior modification for dogs that are afraid of people or pets (client handout #9 – printable from the CD).

Steps for treating a pet that is afraid of animate stimuli (people, other animals) (*continued*)

7. Reinforcer selection: for both counterconditioning and response substitution, the dog's favored rewards should be used. You should make a list of all the rewards your dog may enjoy and save the top few for training. In fact, to increase the motivational value of the rewards, you should deprive the dog of these favored rewards except for these training sessions.

8. You will need to develop a gradient for introduction to the fearful stimulus so that initial exposures are mild. Setting up sessions with good stimulus control can be difficult and take a great degree of forethought but is essential for successful counterconditioning and response substitution training.

    (a) First, make a list of all the stimuli that might incite fear or anxiety. Stimuli may be visual, auditory, tactile, olfactory, and on rare occasions associated with taste. There may be multiple stimuli to which you will have to desensitize and countercondition. For example, a dog that shows a fear response to children on bicycles riding past the front of the home may show anxiety related to the bicycles, the children, the actions, the sounds, the location, and the owner's response.

    (b) Once each stimulus is identified, a means of controlling the stimuli along a gradient of increasingly stronger stimuli must be developed. A gradient can be designed using distance (from far enough away to cause minimal response and gradually closer), similarity (e.g., from least similar age or size to most similar), activity level (from no movement to high activity), or location (from most calm and controllable location to most difficult or distracted), and with different handlers (from trainer to family member with least control)

    (c) To ensure minimal fear with the initial exposure, be certain to begin at a time and location where the pet is calmest and train with the family member or trainer who can best calm the dog.

    (d) Advance along the gradients very slowly. If you happen to proceed through a step too quickly and the pet responds fearfully, relax, and settle down the pet. By using a leash and head halter, it is often possible to calm and distract the dog with a pull upward to get eye contact with the owner and a gradual release. Once the fear response has ceased for five seconds or more, move the person or animal back about five feet. Then, have the person or animal advance one foot, give the pet a reinforcer, and stop the session for one to 24 hours depending on the magnitude of the fear response.

    (e) The favored reward is paired with success and calmness at each new step along the gradient. Always end each session on a positive note and start at that level or below with subsequent sessions.

Fear/anxiety toward people

For aggression toward people, stimuli to consider that might lead to anxiety include visual cues such as physical characteristics (e.g., sex, age, race, dress, infirmities), attitude and actions, olfactory cues (odor), and auditory cues. As people begin to interact with your dog, tactile cues may also be a factor to consider so progress slowly with each new stimulus.

Fear/anxiety toward other animals

For aggression toward other animals, stimuli to consider that might lead to anxiety include visual cues such as physical characteristics (e.g., species, breed/color, size, age), postures, facial expressions and actions, olfactory cues (odors, pheromones), and auditory cues (e.g., growl). As the other animal begins to interact with your dog, tactile cues may also be a factor to consider, so progress slowly with each new stimulus.

Handler/location cues: as mentioned, the cues and responses of the owner as well as the location or situation in which the exposure takes place might also have an impact on whether the pet is more or less likely to be anxious. Use a person who is confident, calm, and in good control to begin training sessions and use a location where success is most likely.

Example

A dog might be most fearful and show aggression toward young boys at a distance of 15 m or less while playing in front of the house. Four gradients could be used for the boys: distance between the dog and the stimulus, appearance of the stimulus, location of the stimulus, and actions of the stimulus. Along the distance gradient, the

(*continued*)

Figure 11.8   (*continued*)

Example (*continued*)
exposure sessions would start at 15 m (i.e., beyond that which would evoke the fear response) and progress toward the dog. The appearance gradient might progress from adults to teenagers to familiar boys to unfamiliar boys. The activity gradient might begin with the stimulus standing quietly and progress gradually toward more intense play, and a location gradient might begin with desensitization and counterconditioning away from home before moving to your own property.

In this example, if the fear was toward boys on bicycles or roller blades, then desensitization and counterconditioning with the bicycle or roller blades will also be necessary. One method might be to use a family member for training the dog to have a positive association with the bicycle and then riding the bicycle, before combining the two stimuli (unfamiliar children and bicycle riding).

Figure 11.8 (*continued*)

15 and 22 m of a skater, say 'It's OK,' ask the pet to 'sit-stay' for food, and then walk off in a different direction to look for another skater to repeat the exercise. Gradually, the exercises were performed closer to the skaters. Finally, skaters were asked to toss food to the pet as they skated by. Within 10 days, Chimo showed no fear of the skaters, approached them voluntarily, and would even sit in anticipation of a food reward.

Case 2 Norm, a three-year-old male neutered domestic short-haired cat, displayed fear aggression toward a teenage member of the household. Whenever he approached, the cat scampered away or would lash out aggressively. Attempts to hold the cat down, pat it, and provide food only served to heighten the escape attempts and aggression.

Controlled flooding and habituation techniques using a cage were implemented while exposing the cat to the teenager. The first step in exposure training was to place the cat in a crate in a room with the teenager present. The cat was to be ignored, and the teenager was to go about his daily routines in the presence of the cat. The cat was offered a portion of its daily allotment of food only when the son was close by. Each training session was terminated and the cat released only when its fear subsided. Food and affection were completely withheld by all family members except during training sessions. After a few training sessions, the cat showed no fear when the

teenager entered the room and would eat food if provided by the owners. At this point the family was instructed that all food and treats should be given only by the teenager. He was to carry favored treats with him and offer them through the bars of the cage. In time, the cat would voluntarily take food from the teenager through the bars of the cage. Since no other family members were allowed to feed or pat the cat, it soon learned to approach the teenager to solicit food and affection. Amitriptyline at 5 mg once daily was used for the first few weeks of the exposure technique, and was then successfully reduced and terminated over the next month. After a total of two months, the cat showed no fear of the teenager and even eagerly approached him for play sessions.

PETS AND CHILDREN

New or expectant parents typically have three major concerns: (1) How to prevent pet behavior problems from occurring after the baby arrives; (2) How to introduce the baby to the pet; and (3) How to keep the child safe around the family pet, as well as other animals. Pet owners often assume that jealousy is the cause of problem behaviors associated with the arrival of a new child into the home, but this is not really the case. Most problems result from the anxiety caused by significant alterations in the pet's environment and the way the family interacts

DESENSITIZATION AND COUNTERCONDITIONING FOR FEAR IN CATS

This approach is useful for training cats to handle situations that they find fearful. In simple terms, your cat must be exposed to the fearful stimulus until it sees that there is nothing to fear and settles down. If the association with the stimulus can be turned into one that is positive, your cat should gradually develop a positive attitude when exposed to the stimulus.

Desensitization is used in combination with counterconditioning to change a pet's attitude or 'feeling' about the stimulus from one that is negative to one that is positive. Desensitization involves controlled exposure to situations or stimuli that might cause fear at levels that are minimal enough that your cat will adapt. Counterconditioning is then used to change the cat's response to the stimulus (e.g., person, other animal, etc.) by associating the cat's favored rewards with a mild form of the stimulus. The cat is then gradually introduced to similar but progressively more intense stimuli paired together with the presentation of the favored reward.

Response substitution is used to train the cat to perform or display an acceptable response (play, food acquisition) each time it is exposed to the stimulus. Rather than attempting to overcome an intense response, the training should be set up to expose the cat to stimuli of reduced intensity to ensure a successful outcome. Desirable responses should be reinforced while attempts at escape should be prevented and any fearful response should be interrupted (e.g., with a leash and harness or a disruption device such as compressed air). If the cat's attention can be successfully diverted, the appropriate response can then be rewarded.

Owner responses such as anxiety, fear, a raised voice, or any form of punishment will only serve to heighten the pet's fear or anxiety. Similarly a fear or anxiety-inducing stimulus presented to your cat will further aggravate anxiety; be certain to retrain only with calm, controlled stimuli. The goal of training is to reinforce appropriate, desirable responses. Therefore, it is critical that rewards are not given while the cat is displaying an inappropriate response. In addition, neither your cat nor the stimulus should be removed until the cat is settled. Of course, if there is any chance of injury then quickly and safely removing the cat from the situation will have to take priority.

Treatment
1. Safety first: because a fearful cat can quickly become aggressive, precautions must be taken before beginning a treatment program for fear aggressive cats. Ideally, exposure to stimuli should be sufficiently positive and gradual so that no fear is exhibited. The cat should be entirely separated from the fearful stimulus except during retraining sessions. If necessary, a restraint device such as a leash and harness works well for some cats so that they can be interrupted from a distance and moved into a separate room until they calm down. Other options include using a large blanket to cover and wrap the cat and carrying it to a separate room until it calms down. Some cats may be successfully interrupted with a spray from a water rifle, citronella product, canister of compressed air, or with a noise device.
2. Stimulus identification: each and every fear-eliciting stimulus must be identified, including people or animals, and in what situations fear is likely to arise. For some cats, fear may be generalized so that all strangers or other animals lead to fear and anxiety, while for some cats the fear may be only to specific stimuli such as a particular family member or other pet in the home.
3. Stimulus control: some method of controlling exposure to the stimulus must then be devised, so that a safe and effective desensitization program can be implemented. Avoiding interactions with the stimulus is the safest approach, but improvement cannot be made without exposure to the stimulus. Using a leash and harness, a crate or separation across a doorway can be used to initiate exposure exercises with animate stimuli (e.g., people, other cats) while videos or audiotapes might be useful for auditory stimuli.
4. Stimulus gradient: each stimulus will need to be presented along a gradient from low (least fear evoking) to high (most fear evoking). To develop a gradient you will need to determine which situations, people, places, or animals are most likely to evoke fear, as well as how to minimize and control these stimuli for retraining. For example, a cat that is fearful of strangers may be most fearful of the approach of young children, and least fearful of adult visitors that ignore the cat.

Figure 11.9 Desensitization and counterconditioning for cats that are afraid of people or other cats (client handout #10 – printable from the CD).

Treatment (*continued*)

5. Reinforcer selection and assessment: for most cats, special food or treats are likely to be of highest appeal, so that these reinforcers should be identified and saved exclusively for desensitization, counterconditioning, and reward training. By depriving your cat of these rewards until the training session, the reward may then be a strong enough motivator to overcome low levels of fear when exposed to the stimulus. Favored toys, catnip, and even short periods of affection may also be effective for counterconditioning, if they are saved exclusively for the exposure sessions.

6. Pretraining: using a 'learn to earn' type program, many cats can be trained to have a positive and predictable response to commands or phrases. In this program, prior to giving the cat any reward or anything of value, the cat must first exhibit an appropriate response. A few basic phrases or commands, such as 'come' or 'feeding,' 'play time' or 'go to your room,' could be learned by the cat if the commands are always followed by a reward. In addition, a positive association needs to be made with any new control technique. If the cat is to wear a harness or be locked into a new confinement area, food, treats, or play should be provided.

7. Other techniques for reducing anxiety: the use of pheromones and drug therapy may also be useful at reducing anxiety so that the behavioral retraining program can have faster or better results.

8. Desensitize and countercondition.

   (a) You must begin with safe and effective control of both your cat as well as the fearful stimuli. For fear toward a particular person, the person should be situated at sufficient distance to avoid further aggravation of the fear, but with fear toward another cat, additional control mechanisms may be required for each cat. Although sufficient distance and counterconditioning with highly motivating rewards may be successful, it may be necessary to implement better physical restraint to ensure success. This can be accomplished with a body harness and leash or a crate for one or both cats. Sometimes your cat and the stimulus (other cat, people) can be separated by confinement behind a common solid door (until the cat adapts to the odor and sounds of the stimulus) or across a glass or screen door, which would allow for safe visual exposure as well.

   (b) The next step would be to gradually reduce the distance when the cat is calm and takes the rewards in the presence of a minimized stimulus. If barriers have been used, the goal is to gradually get the cat into the same room with the stimulus (person, pet) at sufficient distance that the cat will take the food or treat.

   (c) If the cat exhibits any fear at any step in the desensitization program, you are progressing too quickly. Go back to the step that was successful and repeat it a few times before progressing again. Always end on a positive note.

   (d) Habituation and flooding: if the cat is restrained (e.g., leash and harness) or in a crate and shows mild fear but cannot escape, it may be possible to continue low-level exposure to the stimulus (e.g., the person or other cat ignores the cat). Food treats can be intermittently offered when the cat is sufficiently settled (habituates) or is sufficiently distracted to take the treat.

Fear of people: desensitization and counterconditioning

1. Remember that the goal of training is for the cat to learn to make positive associations with the stimulus. Therefore each step should end on a positive note, with the cat receiving a reward before proceeding to the next level. Conversely, there should be no negative interactions so that if there is any need for interrupting an undesirable behavior (e.g., getting the cat off a counter), this should only be done by a person the cat is already comfortable with using a disruption device (and not verbal or physical punishment).

2. Start by exposing the cat to the person at sufficient enough distance that there is no fear and your cat eats the food or treats. Another alternative is to keep your cat on a leash and halter, in a crate, or across a doorway (preferably glass or screened) in an adjacent room, with constant low-level exposure to the person and when the cat habituates (shows no fear) offer it a favored treat or food reward. If the cat is fearful of a particular person or type of person (unfamiliar child), the training can begin with milder stimuli, such as a calm teenager or a familiar child that causes no fear.

(continued)

Figure 11.9 (*continued*)

Fear of people: desensitization and counterconditioning (*continued*)

3. The stimulus intensity is gradually increased. The person may move a little closer at this or at future training sessions, but do not progress further until your cat takes the reward and is calm. Next, the goal will be for the person to give or offer the reward to the cat, or to throw it near the cat so that it approaches to take the reward. It might be helpful to think of the cat that cautiously approaches a child in a high chair (and therefore cannot approach the cat) because food is being dropped on the floor. Each further exposure should always be positive.

Fear of other cats: desensitization and counterconditioning

1. Introduction of a new cat into the household or reintroducing a cat in the home to one that it fears must be done slowly and cautiously so that each association with the other cat has a positive outcome.

2. To begin, the cats must be safely controlled so that no setbacks or injuries can occur. Using distance, a body harness on one or both cats, crates for one or both cats, or the cats on opposite sides of a common doorway, the fearful cat (or cats) must eat and be calm before progressing. On rare occasions, if the odor of one cat is sufficient to incite fear in the other cat, it may be helpful to offer food or treats while grooming each cat with a brush or towel that has been used on the other cat.

3. At this point, if both cats have been in crates, the more fearful cat may be allowed out, and the food, treats, toys, or catnip should be given progressively closer to the other cat's crate. If the cats have been eating on opposite sides of a solid door, a screen or glass door could be used next, or the door kept ajar about 2 cm during feeding. When both cats can be placed out of the crates in the same room together while eating at a sufficient distance to avoid fear, a leash and harness on one or both cats may be necessary to avoid injury and setbacks. If one or both cats do not eat, separate them and do not give any food until the next feeding session. If the cats eat at that time, repeat the same distance at the next feeding. If things go well the next time, the dishes can be moved a little closer together.

4. Progress slowly! Allowing either cat to interact in a fearful or aggressive manner sets the program back. The cats must remain separated except for times such as feeding when the cats are distracted, occupied, and engaged in an enjoyable act. In other words, good things are associated with the presence of the other cat. Another technique that may help is to rub the cats with towels and switch from one cat to the other to mix their scents.

5. If the boldness or aggression of one cat is leading to the fear of another, then placing a bell on the aggressor, supervising and inhibiting any inappropriate behavior of the aggressor, or drugs for the aggressor may be useful.

Once the desensitization and counterconditioning progresses to a state where the two cats are completely reintroduced, providing sufficient climbing and perching areas, or a cat door that can only be accessed by the fearful cat, may further improve the long-term outcome.

Figure 11.9 (*continued*)

with the pet. Changes in feeding, exercise, and play schedules; changes in what the pet is allowed to do; changes in how the pet gets attention; and inconsistencies in the way the owner interacts with the pet can all lead to problems. Preparing the family pet for the new baby includes taking steps to ensure that the changes are gradual and not overwhelming for the pet, and reviewing household rules so that the family has the control needed to direct the pet into desired behaviors.

Although most families take a positive relationship between children and pets for granted, things are not always idyllic. Pets don't innately know how to behave around children, and children don't come into this world with the knowledge of what to do or not to do when it comes to interacting with animals. While most dogs and cats accept the new arrival, some do not. The dogs that are most likely to have social problems are the ones that have had little contact or a previous unpleasant experience with babies or children, and have had little training. Genetics also plays a role in the dog's sociability, predatory instincts, and temperament, which may have an impact on how the dog interacts with children. Cats can be unpredictable around children, from avoidance to intense interest. Fortunately, most problems can readily be avoided with some forethought and training.

Dogs and children

Preparing puppies for children

Preparation for a good relationship between the pet and children begins when the dog is a puppy. To accomplish this, there should be frequent opportunities for the young pup to meet children during its early months of life. The puppy should be introduced to the children when they are calm and treats should be used to facilitate the introductions. Another concept the young pup needs to learn is that being touched can be pleasant and should not be feared. These early interactions help prevent the development of fear, avoidance behavior, and aggression toward children when the pet is older.

All family members should make a point of gently handling the pet and touching it in all the ways that a child might touch it. Frequently touching the tail, ears, and body, as well as gently tugging on the collar and hair, will make the pet less likely to be upset when a child does this later in life. Any type of physical punishment, painful punishment, or threats with a hand should be avoided. If the pet associates hand movement with discomfort, it might bite when the child moves a hand toward it. All pets must learn that the human hand is friendly and not to be feared.

Some dogs show aggression when approached while they eat. This behavior can be avoided by teaching the young pup that it is good to have company when it eats. A family member should occasionally sit on the floor with the puppy while it eats. During this time, the pet can be gently touched all over. Pieces of kibble should be picked from the bowl and hand fed to the pup. The bowl should periodically be picked up for a second and placed back on the floor. If the family member occasionally slips a piece of meat or a chunk of canned food into the bowl while the pet is eating its dry food, it will look forward to having humans nearby at dinnertime. By doing these exercises, the pup will learn that there is no risk that humans will steal its food, but the meal actually improves when humans are nearby.

Preparing the adult dog for the new baby

The first thing to consider is the dog's temperament. All types of aggression should be considered potentially dangerous. Determine if the dog growls or snaps when touched, disturbed while eating, playing with toys, or resting. If the dog exhibits any type of aggression, including aggression toward other animals or people outside the family, this should be resolved before the baby arrives. Even if the dog gets along well with children, the child that inadvertently gets too close to the dog that exhibits territorial aggression may get injured.

As soon as the mother learns of her pregnancy, some thought should be given to preparing the dog for the inevitable changes that occur when a new baby joins the family. It is very important that the dog be under reliable verbal control. If the pet will readily respond to 'sit,' 'down,' 'stay,' and 'settle,' then the owner will have the tools with which to control the dog and decrease the incidence of undesirable behaviors that may result in punishment, confinement, and increased anxiety. It is very important to have the pet under reliable verbal control. An unruly, active dog can be as much of a threat to the baby as an aggressive dog. The more happy situations that occur involving the pet and the baby, the more likely that the relationship will be positive and that 'an unpleasant association' will not develop.

Another important consideration is the pet's daily schedule, as well as the type and amount of interactions with family members the pet is currently used to getting. Once the baby arrives, this may be dramatically changed. The goal is to make the changes gradual and less noticeable to the pet. Feeding, exercise, and play schedules should be gradually adjusted to one that will fit the family's situation once the baby is home.

Since the needs of a new baby are very time consuming, there will no doubt be a reduction in the amount of physical attention that can be given to the dog. The amount should be gradually decreased until you arrive at an amount that can be maintained. How the attention is given is also very important. If your pet is used to getting attention whenever he nudges or licks, he will be very confused when he suddenly can't get what he wants on demand. A good way to handle this is to ignore pushy behaviors and give attention only when the pet is leaving you alone or as a reward for responding to one of your commands ('shake,' 'sit,' 'down'). Other things that will need to be worked on are those behaviors that are permitted now, but won't be permitted when the baby is at home. Jumping up on family members, lying on furniture, climbing onto your lap, or excessive barking are behaviors that often must be changed.

The dog can also be prepared for the homecoming by doing exercises that prepare it for the new noises and smells that coincide with the baby's arrival. If the dog gets upset when it hears strange sounds, a recording can be made of baby noises (cooing, crying, screaming, etc.). If the recording causes any signs of anxiety it should then be used for a desensitization and counterconditioning program. The recording should first be played at sufficiently low volume that the dog shows no anxiety, while jovially requesting obedience commands for tasty food treats. Very gradually the volume can be increased as the weeks go by until the pet seems comfortable with these noises at high volumes. Have the owners do this exercise at least 15 minutes per day. To prepare the pet for the new smells that will arrive with the baby, have the owners take something home from the hospital, such as a towel or blanket with the baby's scent. The dog should be commanded to sit and the object presented. Have the owner say the baby's name in an upbeat tone and give it lots of praise. On occasion, some dogs will be made anxious by the owner constantly carrying or nursing the new baby. Testing the dog by carrying around and fussing with a doll (especially one that actually moves

and makes crying sounds) can be useful. If there is any anxiety, a positive association should be made with this doll using favored food rewards, affection, or a favored play toy (see Fig. 11.8, handout #9 on the CD, and Appendix C, Fig. 10, handout #17 on the CD).

When the baby comes home

Since the dog has not seen his mistress for several days, there will probably be a great deal of excited greeting behavior when the mother arrives with the baby. Therefore, if someone else carries the baby into the home, the mother can greet the dog without worrying that he might accidentally scratch the baby. It is important to set the dog up to succeed by anticipating problems and taking steps to prevent them whenever possible. By taking this approach, scolding, punishment, and anxious feelings associated with the presence of the baby can be prevented.

The owners should wait until the excitement has died down and the pet is calm before introducing the dog to the baby. That may be later in the same day or could be several weeks afterward. The dog should slowly be brought to meet the baby. Careful judgment must be exercised in deciding when to allow the dog close enough to sniff. If there is a chance the dog might jump, use a leash. If more control is needed, a head halter and leash can be utilized. (If there is <u>any</u> likelihood that the dog might bite, consider using a muzzle. Lightweight, basket wire or plastic muzzles are well tolerated by many dogs.) If it can be predicted that a head halter or muzzle is likely to be utilized, it would be best for the owners to accustom the dog to wearing these before the arrival of the baby. The owners should <u>NEVER</u> (no matter how sweet, trustworthy, or friendly the pet appears) allow an unsupervised dog around the baby.

It is especially important to be vigilant when the baby is crying, kicking, or waving its arms. This could cause a curious dog to jump up and scratch or otherwise injure the infant. During these times, it is wise to put the pet in a 'down-stay' away from the baby, put it in another room with a very special chew toy, or confine it to the yard. The owners should immediately seek additional guidance if the pet exhibits any predatory behavior (stalking, strong focus, odd whining, unusual interest) around the baby.

Whenever the dog is in the room with the baby, the family should act very happy and praise all acceptable behaviors (e.g., not jumping, being calm, responding to commands, being relaxed when the baby cries, etc.). The idea is to promote desirable behaviors and to make the dog look forward to the baby's presence because it is associated with a lot of positive attention. This association can be made more dramatic by reducing the amount of attention or treats the dog gets when the baby is not around. In this way, the dog learns that the presence of the baby is associated with positive events, and the absence of the baby is not. The biggest mistake owners make when they try to shape their dog's behavior is to concentrate on telling the dog what is wrong, while neglecting to tell it what is right. It doesn't work any better with dogs than it does with children. A good exercise to bring about the association of good feelings for the baby is for one parent to sit in a room and hold the baby, while the other adult asks the pet to respond to commands for tasty food treats. Commands should be given in a very happy tone and lots of praise should accompany the food treats. The exercises should then gradually be moved closer and closer to the baby.

As children grow up

As the baby continues to grow and mature, the dog may be exposed to a variety of new stimuli from crawling to toddling to walking and even trying to approach or take things away from the dog. Even if the dog has adapted nicely to a particular stage in the child's life, owners must always be prepared for a change in the relationship between the child and pet. Interactions between dogs and young children should always be supervised. The spontaneous, active behavior of children is exciting for most dogs, and easily elicits rough play from them. Encouraging the child to give tasty food rewards to the pet for responding to 'sit' commands is a simple way to teach the pup to keep its paws on the ground and expect good things whenever it is around children.

An important thing to remember is that children are great imitators. Members of the family must not do anything to the pet that they do not want the child to do. This includes physical punishment, teasing, and rough play. Children don't innately know how to interact with animals, so they must be taught how to approach, handle, and play with the pet. For example, fetch is a great game for the child and dog to share with each other. While some dogs will tolerate any type of normal physical contact, the child will be safer if taught to avoid making contact around the eyes, ears, and head, and to pat the dog along its side. Hugging and getting face-to-face is not well tolerated by some dogs and is also best avoided. If the dog is small, the child will also need to learn the proper way to comfortably pick the dog up.

Children should have some control over the pet and this can begin at a relatively early age. Once the child is talking, a family member can hold the child in the lap and teach the pet to sit when the child gives a command. This can be done by coaching the child to say the command word at the same time as the adult. Gradually, the adult can begin whispering the word so the child gives the command alone. This can be repeated with other commands. When the child is old enough, he or she can request deference from the dog before giving it things that it wants (toys, treats, play) by asking it to respond to a command first. Non-aggressive pets can be taught to look forward to having the child present while they eat by doing a safe, easy exercise such as carrying the child over to the pet while it eats and holding it a safe distance above the pet. As the pet eats, the child can drop small pieces of meat into the bowl or on the floor next to the bowl.

Children must also learn some rules about other pets. The most important rule is that the child must NEVER pet another family's pet or give it food unless an adult gives permission. Dogs on a leash, by food, by toys, sleeping, tied down, or running loose should never be approached. All family members must also follow these rules for them to work, as children are imitators. Children must be taught about avoiding a pet that is exhibiting potentially dangerous behavior. Aggressive behavior is fairly obvious to most children, but few children know that fearful animals should also be avoided. The owners should review aggressive postures with their child (growling, loud barking, hair standing on end) and fearful behaviors (trembling, crouching, ears down, tail tucked) so that the child learns to avoid these animals. If the child is approached by a dog that is acting aggressively, he or she should stand very still like a tree, say nothing, hold the arms against the body, and avoid eye contact with the dog. If the child is on the ground or knocked down, he should curl into a tight ball, cover the ears with his fists, and remain still and quiet until the animal moves far away. The necessary responses are contrary to what most children will do when threatened. Children should also be instructed what to do if a bite occurs. They should try to remember where the bite occurred, what the dog looked like, where it went following the bite, and to report the bite to an adult immediately.

Cats and children

How the cat responds to a new baby or to children will be directly related to previous experiences with babies, children, and strangers, and the cat's genetic temperament. Some cats will adapt quickly to children and new babies by either ignoring them, or eventually seeking them out for investigation or social contact (e.g., bunting or cheek rubbing), while others may immediately be inquisitive, playful, and affectionate. While investigation, seeking affection, and social contact may be desirable, these behaviors must be well supervised since they can still lead to injury to the child, or inappropriate responses from the child to the pet. On the other hand, some cats may be particularly fearful, which could lead to avoidance, decreased social interactions with owners or other pets, or aggression.

There are three basic considerations for helping cats to best adapt to new babies or children. The first is to adapt the cat's schedule, owner interactions, and environment slowly so that it is prepared for the arrival of the new baby. The second is for the owners to supervise all interactions with the cat and the baby to ensure safety, and so that positive interactions can be rewarded. The third is to help the child adapt to the needs of the cat so as to prevent the development of behavior problems.

Adapting the home in advance

Some cats can become stressed and anxious when there are changes to their daily routine, social interactions, or environment. The cat's response may be a change in behavior or attitude with respect to humans or other cats (increased fear and avoidance or increased irritability and aggression), urine or stool marking of the environment, or displacement behaviors such as overgrooming with hair loss (psychogenic alopecia). There may also be an impact on the cat's physical health, such as a change in appetite (whether markedly decreased or increased), activity level (increase or decrease), sleep–wake cycles, or organ dysfunction. Owners should consider how the daily schedule, social interactions, and household will need to be changed when the new baby arrives and begin to slowly adapt the cat to these changes in advance of the new arrival. Wherever possible the changes should not only be made slowly, but should be associated with positive events and interactions such as food treats, affection, and play. For example, if the cat initiates play by chasing and play attacking moving objects, the owners should initiate and provide play sessions and play toys to meet the cat's needs and discourage the cat-initiated play. If there are rooms, counters, and areas of the house that will be made out of bounds for the cat when the child arrives, then the owners should begin in advance to keep the cat out of these areas, and teach the cat where it is allowed to sleep, play, and explore. It may also be advisable to obtain and set up new furniture in advance of the baby's arrival, as some cats can be particularly sensitive or reactive to new structures and new odors brought into their homes.

Some cats may get upset when they hear strange sounds. For these cats, a recording can be made of baby noises (cooing, crying, screaming, etc.). The recording should be played at a level that is low enough to cause no anxiety while offering tasty food treats, play, or catnip toys. The volume should be gradually increased over several weeks until the cat seems comfortable with these noises at high volumes. To prepare the pet for the new smells that will arrive with the baby, a towel or blanket with the baby's scent can be brought home from the hospital. The cat should then be taught to associate the object with food or petting. On occasion, some cats may become anxious or overly investigative when the owner carries, changes, or nurses the new baby. Testing the cat by carrying around and fussing with a doll (especially one that actually moves and makes crying sounds) can be useful. If there is any anxiety, a positive association should be made with this doll using favored play toys, treats, or food rewards before the baby arrives (see Fig. 11.9, handout #10 on the CD, and Appendix C, Fig. 11, handout #16 on the CD). If there is concern that additional safe control will be required to supervise and introduce the cat and baby, then training the cat to wear a body harness can be extremely useful.

When the baby arrives

The simplest rule to help with the arrival of the baby is for all interactions with the cat and the baby to be supervised, so that any potential problems (whether fearful, overly aggressive, overly affectionate, or overly playful) can be identified. Then, with the aid of a behavior consultant, the particular concerns can be addressed. At all other times, such as when the baby is sleeping or playing in its playpen, access to the baby should be prevented. Even an affectionate cat could choose to lie down next to the young baby, and this might be particularly dan-

gerous for babies that cannot yet raise their heads or turn over. When the cat and child are together, all positive and appropriate interactions should be reinforced and desirable responses gradually shaped. It can be particularly helpful to identify all things positive to the cat (food, affection, play, catnip, treats) and provide them when the baby and cat are together, while reducing their availability when the baby is not around. If the cat reacts fearfully, or unpredictably, or there is a potential danger or risk to the new child, then a body harness can be used to help control the introductions. If there are any changes in the cat's general demeanor, health, activity level, feeding, drinking, and elimination, these are signs that should be reported to the clinic as these changes may not pose a risk for the child, but they may indicate that the cat is not coping well with the new arrival. Occasionally, Feliway^{TM} or even anxiolytic drugs may help the cat to adapt if it is excessively anxious, although there is also the possibility that these drugs will lead to disinhibition and an increase in aggression.

As children grow up

As the child grows and becomes more mobile and interactive, the relationship between the cat and child may change. At both extremes, increasing fear and anxiety and overexuberant playful behavior could be problematic. As always, supervision to assess the cat's response to the child and the child's interactions with the cat is the best way to ensure that desirable responses are reinforced and any undesirable responses are identified. If problems do arise, preventing interactions may be the safest plan, but a program of careful and entirely positive reintroduction is generally required to improve the relationship (see Fig. 11.9, handout #10 on the CD, and Appendix C, Fig. 11, handout #16 on the CD).

Zoonoses

It is rare for cats and dogs to spread disease to humans, but it can occur. The number one health risk is from the physical injuries caused by bites and scratches, so that injury prevention and safety are the overriding concern. Owners should be advised that keeping pets vaccinated, in good health, and free from parasites (including fecal analysis once or twice a year) is generally all that is required to prevent most zoonotic diseases. Dermatologic (skin) conditions should be evaluated to determine that there are no parasites (fleas, mites) or fungal infections (ringworm). If there is any gastrointestinal upset, the dog's stools should be thoroughly assessed for internal parasites or potentially zoonotic bacteria. Conversely, if one or more family members develops skin lesions or a gastrointestinal disorder, the pet should be checked to make certain that there is no shared (zoonotic) disease process. The yard should be kept free of stools by cleaning up after each elimination, and family members should wash thoroughly after playing in the yard, or cleaning up the pet's stools. It is also advisable to avoid allowing the pet to lick the face of children (especially around the mouth or eyes) and to teach the children to wash thoroughly after play sessions. Any bite or scratch, no matter how minor, should be thoroughly cleaned and disinfected and wounds that break the skin or appear to become infected should be reported to a medical authority.

This information is available in Appendix C, Figs 10 and 11, handouts #16 and #17 on the CD.

FEAR OF ANIMALS

Depending on how a pet was socialized and what types of experiences it had when it was young, it may be fearful of members of the same or of other species. Lack of contact or experience with other animals of the same or other species during the socialization period can result in a pet that is fearful of other animals. This can be dangerous if the fearful pet responds with aggression. Therefore, steps should be taken to overcome the fear of a stimulus (e.g., introducing a new puppy or kitten to another pet) as soon as it is identified (Fig. 11.10). Early intervention with desensitization and counter-

conditioning can usually rectify the problem (see Fig. 3.10).

On occasion, a single traumatic event that is associated with another animal can lead to fear of that animal. This seems to be more likely to occur in cats. For example, if one cat in the household hears a sudden, frightening noise while it is resting and looks up to see another pet nearby it may associate the frightening event with that pet and hiss at or avoid it whenever it is nearby. Owners that try to suppress behaviors directed toward other pets (overexuberance, lunging) by using harsh punishment techniques may cause or further aggravate fearful behaviors.

Diagnosis and prognosis

Exposure to an individual animal or a certain species consistently elicits signs of fear. Fear may result in aggression by some pets, while others respond by cowering, remaining motionless, or attempting to escape. These behaviors may be associated with trembling, hypersalivation, elimination, or dilated pupils.

Pets that have exhibited a strong fear response from a very early age (eight weeks or younger) with no suspected exposure to traumatic environmental events may be very difficult to treat successfully. The prognosis is good for cases in which the pet was adequately socialized to animals, the problem started during adulthood, the problem has existed for a short duration, and the owner can exert control over situations during which the pet interacts with other animals.

Management

Successful treatment requires that the owners first identify all stimuli or situations that elicit a fear response. Next, the owner must take steps to expose the pet to these stimuli or situations under controlled circumstances (Fig. 11.11). This is accomplished by employing desensitization and counterconditioning exercises during which the pet receives something highly desirable for being non-anxious in the presence of weak or distant fear-evoking stimuli or response

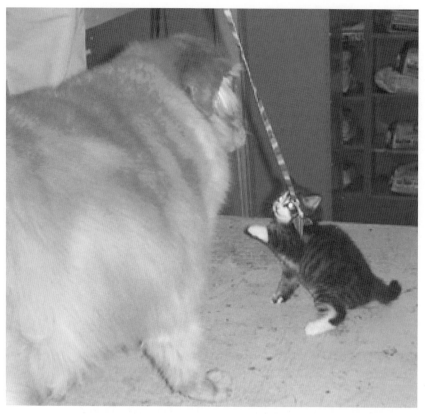

Figure 11.10   When introducing a new kitten to a household there may initially be fear of unfamiliar people and animals (such as the household dog).

substitution techniques where the dog is taught to display an acceptable response in the presence of the stimulus. Begin in a neutral environment with a well-socialized, -behaved, -trained, and -controlled animal as the stimulus. There should be sufficient distance between the animals so that both are relaxed. The starting distance should be an interval at which the pet can recognize the other animal, but not close enough to it that any fear is elicited. The fearful pet should receive something it values (food, play, grooming, social attention) for exhibiting no fear in the presence of the fear-provoking stimulus. As the session progresses, the distance between the animals is gradually reduced. It is often helpful to keep one or both pets on a leash and head halter. Muzzles may be needed for some situations to ensure safety. For cats, it is often best to have both pets in crates or on a

leash and harness until the fear response is sufficiently decreased. To enhance the value of the reinforcer, ensure that all special rewards are saved for training sessions. In time, the pet will learn to associate the presence of other animals with positive experiences (Fig. 11.12).

It is important that the owners are aware of when rewards are appropriate and when they are contraindicated. Rewarding, reassuring, or consoling the pet when it is fearful may reinforce fear-related behaviors. Punishment should not be used in fearful situations and can actually make the problem worse, and anxiety or frustration on the part of the owner may further add to the pet's anxiety. Inhibited nipping by a pet that is mildly nervous when another dog approaches may escalate to more serious displays of aggression if it learns to expect a beating as the outcome of interactions with other animals.

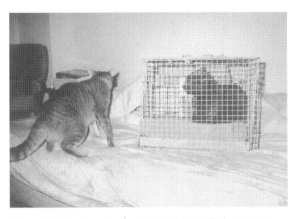

Figure 11.11   Using habituation and controlled exposure (flooding) techniques to reduce fear.

Prevention

Fear of animals can be a relatively easy problem to prevent. Proper socialization is critical for this purpose. The young animal should be exposed to as many different, well-behaved animals as possible during its socialization period. Adequate supervision and control are important when introducing the pet to other animals in order to ensure that the interaction is amicable. The veterinarian should be instrumental in reinforcing these notions in all owners and recommending appropriate social activities such as puppy classes and early obedience training, especially if the animal is the only pet in the home. Continued ongoing positive exposure to other pets should be continued into adulthood.

Case example

Tom, a two-year-old male cat, was recently adopted from a shelter by a family with a six-year-old female Labrador Retriever. The dog showed no desire to interact with the cat and ignored it for the most part. Whenever the dog entered the room the cat's eyes would dilate, it would hiss, show piloerection, and quickly run away.

The owners initially separated the pets at all times except during training sessions. Twice daily, the dog received a long walk to ensure it would be quiet while working with the cat. During the desensitization and counterconditioning sessions, the dog was attended by a family member and fed at one end of a large room to keep it distracted. At the same time, the cat was brought to the opposite end of the room and fed pieces of chicken and tuna while it was in a crate. During the next stage, the cat was fed in the same area but out of the crate, while it was controlled with a halter and leash. For the course of the remaining sessions, both pets were kept on leashes. Gradually, the pets were moved closer during the sessions. Eventually, the cat was allowed free roam in the house. High resting areas were made available to the cat. In order to continue to associate pleasant experiences with the presence of the dog, the owners were instructed to call the cat and give it a treat whenever the dog entered the room or moved about in the room.

NOISE PHOBIAS

Noise phobias are common in animals. Some examples of fear-evoking noise stimuli are thunder, gunshots, and fireworks.

Diagnosis and prognosis

The diagnosis of noise phobia is usually quite straightforward. In most cases, the fear-eliciting sound is loud and quite distinct (e.g., gunshot, thunder). Also, the owner can usually identify exactly when the problem will occur and describe the fearful response of the animal (e.g., hide under couch, run away, attention-seeking).

Many noise phobias can be managed successfully with behavioral modification. The prognosis varies greatly depending on the individual, the duration of the phobia, the ability to control strong stimuli during treatment, and the success in finding an effective, controllable artificial stimulus to use during exposure exercises. Successful treatment of **thunderstorm**

Step	Comments
Identify stimuli	• All stimuli and situations that cause the pet to be fearful must be identified so that behavioral modification can be effective. For example, the pet may not be afraid of all dogs, just large ones, or the pet may be fine in its garden but anxious around dogs in the park. Specific types of behavior by other animals that trigger fear must also be identified, such as barking, quick movements or approaches
Identify the threshold for fear	• Identify the distance to other animals at which the pet shows signs of fear or the minimum size of an animal that elicits a fear response
Establish a gradient of stimuli	• The gradient should begin below the threshold for fear and should extend in small increments to the strongest presentation of the fear-eliciting stimuli • Exposure exercises should start between the distance at which the pet recognizes another animal and the distance at which it begins to show signs of fear. An alternative approach would be to start with an approaching animal that is smaller than that required to elicit fear and then use larger and larger animals in subsequent trials • The pet with a fear of large dogs might first be introduced to small dogs. Cats with a fear of dogs can be exposed to a tape recording of a barking dog played at a low volume
Desensitization and counterconditioning	• Choose a quiet, non-threatening location with few distractions where the pet feels comfortable to begin training, such as the pet's own home or garden • The pet should be under control so that it cannot harm itself or others • Begin with the pet under full control and at a distance from an animal where the pet recognizes it but at which the pet shows no signs of fear. Associate favored rewards with non-fearful responses. Food and/or clicker training generally works best for dogs while food, petting, or play can be used for cats • Very gradually decrease the distance between the animals in subsequent trials • Later, the pet should gradually be exposed to animals with slightly different characteristics in a variety of situations
Response substitution and differential reinforcement	• Develop a stimulus gradient as with desensitization above • Ensure that both pets are entirely under control and that the target pet is non-fearful and non-threatening. Using a previously trained command, e.g., sit, focus (a food lure can also be utilized), an acceptable response that is incompatible with the undesirable response must be achieved • Favored reinforcers are then given to mark and positively reinforce the correct response (i.e., sit/stay or heel in the presence of the other animal) • Use reinforcer assessment to determine the pet's favored rewards so that these can be saved and used for these counterconditioning sessions • A head halter allows for additional safety and control to achieve the desirable response in a more immediate manner. An immediate release when the appropriate response is achieved also provides a form of negative reinforcement • Disruptive devices such as air horns, squeaky toys, or citronella sprays may also be useful for interrupting the undesirable response so that the desirable response can be reinforced • Very slowly decrease the distance between the pet and the person • The pet is gradually exposed to animals with slightly different characteristics in a variety of situations
Flooding	• If the owner has good control of the pet and the fear is mild, controlled flooding can be used by exposing it to a level of the stimulus that is just above the fear threshold so that a mild fear response is elicited • Escape is prevented until the pet shows no sign of fear. Once the pet shows no sign of fear, rewards should be given • Confinement crates and head halters may be helpful accompaniments. Use of any of these devices is only appropriate if they do not result in increasing the pet's fear
Drugs and pheromones	• Feliway™ may be useful in reducing anxiety. Specifically Felifriend™ and a dog appeasing pheromone (D.A.P.™), which are presently available in Europe, may help to reduce interspecific and intraspecific fears and anxiety • Drugs are generally not effective when the fear is toward a specific stimulus as these dogs and cats will still be fearful of that stimulus even after drugs are administered. In addition anxiolytic drugs may disinhibit and lead to increased aggression. On the other hand, for mild fears and anxiety, buspirone might be effective, while for more generalized anxiety, states of panic, or responses that appear impulsive or excessive (e.g., long refractory period) tricyclic antidepressants such as clomipramine or amitriptyline or SSRIs such as paroxetine or fluoxetine might be useful

Figure 11.12 Steps in the management of pets with fear of other animals.

| Drugs and pheromones (*continued*) | • For pathological states that might be associated with anxiety and aggression, see the discussion of the European approach in Chapter 3
• Alternative therapy and dietary adjustments might occasionally be useful (see Ch. 5)
• Drug desensitization might be another option (see Ch. 4 for details). Benzodiazepines such as alprazolam might be utilized before an exposure session. If the desired response can be achieved for three or more consecutive sessions then the drug might be reduced by 25% and the program repeated until the pet can be retrained without medication. Alternately the benzodiazepine might be used on an ongoing basis (e.g., clorazepate tid and reduced by 25% weekly if the pet has improved) |

Figure 11.12   (*continued*)

phobias using only behavioral modification can be very difficult because of the presence of multiple stimuli, difficulty producing an effective artificial storm for desensitization, and inability to control naturally occurring stimuli during therapy.

Management

An important step in managing noise phobias is to have sufficient control over the pet and the environment (Figs 11.13 and 11.3, client handout #8 on the CD). Except during training sessions, the pet should not be exposed to the fear-evoking stimuli at all. Sometimes this is beyond the owner's control. For example, during a thunderstorm, it is usually not possible to insulate the pet completely from the noise. In this case, it may be necessary to tranquilize the pet initially, or to train during parts of the year when thunderstorms are not prevalent. Keeping the pet indoors, temporarily relocating the pet when problem situations are expected, or utilizing 'sound-proofing' are additional options.

First, identify all stimuli causing the phobic behavior and attempt to isolate the pet from exposure to these stimuli except during conditioning sessions. A pet that panics will often get worse with each exposure to a strong stimulus. The pet can be kept indoors, boarded, moved to a quieter neighborhood, or an area of the home can be sound-proofed.

Next, you'll need to find a method of controlling or modifying the stimuli for desensitization and counterconditioning sessions or training by differential reinforcement (response substi-

tution). A starter pistol can be muffled with a towel or enclosed in a box for dogs with gunshot phobia. Tape and video recordings of thunderstorms and camera flashes are often used with dogs that are afraid of storms. Controlling the distance from the stimulus to the subject can also be used to set up a gradient of stimuli.

Conditioning should take place in controlled environments with few distractions. Sit-stay and down-stay training should be practiced until the pet will respond dependably. Highly valued rewards, such as the pet's favorite toy or treat, should be given for proper responses. Favored treats and toys should be restricted except during these training periods. Once the pet responds to training commands, the owner should begin to train the pet in a variety of locations.

To begin desensitization and counterconditioning, select a suitable location for training where the pet feels comfortable and secure. Expose the pet to a low level of the fearful stimulus. The intensity of the stimulus should be just below the threshold that will evoke the fearful response. In an upbeat tone, give the pet a command to sit or lie down. Reward the pet if it responds without any sign of fear or anxiety. The key is to associate a positive experience and a relaxed state with the presence of the stimulus. Repeat, gradually increasing the strength of the stimulus until exposure to the full strength of the stimulus is achieved. Once the pet learns to tolerate full levels of the controlled stimulus, training should be done in a variety of environments. Some dogs may be easier to con-

Step	Comments
Identify stimuli and thresholds	• Make sure that all noises that evoke fear have been identified • Attempt to isolate the pet from exposure to these sounds during the periods between training sessions
Establish a gradient of stimuli	• For flooding and desensitization techniques, one must be able to control the intensity of the stimuli in order to establish a gradient • An audiotape or videotape of the stimulus can be used at varying volumes • A starter pistol in a sound-insulated chamber can provide control of the intensity of a gunshot. Nested cardboard boxes over the gun will reduce the volume
Retrain with rewards	• Teach the pet to respond to verbal commands or sound/visual cues with a 'sit-stay' or 'down-stay' response. Use highly motivating rewards • By repeatedly associating strong, primary reinforcers such as food with obedience commands and responses, secondary reinforcers are developed. Eventually, these can be used to elicit a state of happy anticipation when the pet is asked to sit in the presence of a likely fear-eliciting stimulus, even when no food is available
Desensitization and counterconditioning	• Select a calm location with few distractions for training. Make sure the pet is controlled and cannot harm itself or others. Give a training command in a very happy tone of voice and expose the pet to very low levels of fear-evoking sounds. Associate favored rewards with non-fearful behavior. Very gradually increase the intensity of the stimulus until it approximates actual levels • If actual fearful situations arise during retraining and trigger a fear response, the pet's behavior should be ignored. If the pet calms down or can be sufficiently distracted, it should be praised and rewarded. During the following training session, a lower intensity of stimulus should be used
Response substitution	• The technique is similar to desensitization above, but is an intervention that may be useful when the pet is exposed to stimuli that are somewhat above the fear threshold • The goal is to minimize exposure so that the pet is more amenable to therapy, and to train the pet to display a response incompatible with the fear and retreat response (such as sit or down or settle), which can then be reinforced with one of the dog's favored rewards • A head halter and leash or disruptive device may help to interrupt the undesirable behavior and direct the pet into the appropriate response • Success might be better achieved in a room where the stimuli are muted or where there are distractions, such as a music CD • As success is achieved at a particular level of the stimulus, the stimulus can then be gradually increased in intensity and the steps above repeated
Flooding	• If the owner has good control of the pet and the phobia is mild, the pet can be treated using flooding by being exposed to a level of the stimulus that is above the fear threshold while escape is impossible until it shows no sign of fear • Once the pet shows no sign of fear, rewards should be given • Confinement crates or head halters may be helpful. Use of any of these devices is only appropriate if they do not result in increasing the pet's fear
Punishment	• Under no circumstances should punishment be used
Drug therapy	• Medication may be helpful in managing fearful situations. Drugs prescribed for fears and phobias might include anti-anxiety drugs (e.g., alprazolam, clorazepate, buspirone) and antidepressants (e.g., clomipramine, amitriptyline, fluoxetine, paroxetine). Often, a combination of an antidepressant throughout the thunderstorm season and a benzodiazepine administered just prior to an event can be successful. D.A.P.™ or propranolol might also be used concurrently.

Figure 11.13 Steps in the management of pets with noise phobias.

trol, distract, and retrain using a head halter system for training. These dogs may then be easier to settle as soon as the head halter is applied.

Despite the best of intentions, actual fearful situations may arise during the training program. Should the pet show any fear or anxiety, the owner should try to ignore it. If the pet calms down or can be sufficiently distracted to the point that the fear ceases, rewards in the form of affection, play, or treats should be given. It may be possible to take the pet to an area where the stimuli are more muted or where there are sufficient distractions (CD, other pets, etc.) that the dog will settle and calm on command. A head halter may also be possible to achieve the desired response. As soon as the response is achieved the tension on the head halter can be released (negative reinforcement) and the acceptable response rewarded with a favored treat.

Severe thunderstorm phobias present quite a challenge and can be extremely difficult to treat solely using conventional behavior modification. Multiple stimuli are involved in this problem and it is difficult to find artificial stimuli for use in desensitization and counterconditioning to which most pets will respond. It is also difficult to protect the pet from storm exposure between training sessions. It is not uncommon for a storm to appear suddenly with little warning or when the owner is not home, so that medication cannot be given early enough to be optimally effective. For pets that are at a very high risk for severe injuries related to the phobia or who may cause extensive damage in the home, extended pharmacological treatment for days or weeks at a time during storm season may be necessary.

If a family member is home with the pet when a mild storm occurs, it may be helpful to distract the pet and then have a 'thunderstorm party.' When the pet begins to show mild anxiety, the person should ignore the pet and make an unusual noise (squeaker, whistle, tap table top, crinkle paper, clicker) so that the pet orients and stops acting anxious. After about 10 seconds or more, but before the pet begins acting anxious again, the owner should jump up, run to the kitchen, and grab a handful of meat or cheese treats. Next, the person should run through the home acting very animated, saying happy things loudly in an upbeat tone and tossing food about for the pet to eat. Unless the storm becomes strong enough to make the pet fearful and take its focus from the owner and the food, the 'party' will serve as a counterconditioning session.

Benzodiazepines (e.g., alprazolam, clorazepate, lorazepam) and tricyclic antidepressants (e.g., clomipramine, amitriptyline) may be helpful for difficult cases. The benzodiazepines are the best choice to use on an as-needed basis, and

alprazolam may prove to be the most potent for panic-type responses, although its duration of effect may only be a couple of hours. Tricyclic antidepressants may take several weeks or more to become effective and are probably best reserved for chronic problems. A dose of benzodiazepine may also be added to the therapy on an as-needed basis an hour or two before a storm is expected. Other options are the use of D.A.P.™, buspirone, alone or concurrent with other medications, or a phenothiazine given one to three hours prior to the event (which does not reduce anxiety but may be sufficiently sedating to avoid the problem entirely).

Prevention

The best way to prevent fears and phobias is to expose pets to as many different stimuli as possible while they are still young. As early as two weeks of age, puppies and kittens should be exposed to a wide variety of mild stimuli including different types of noises, lights, handling, and movement. Habituation during early, critical periods of development will help prevent many of the fears and phobias that might otherwise occur in adult cats and dogs.

Case example

The owners were concerned about Bernice, their three-year-old intact female Bernese Mountain Dog. Bernice became very fearful and distressed around the Fourth of July weekend each year when neighborhood children were setting off fireworks. She would pant, pace, hypersalivate, and whine endlessly.

The owner ensured that all exposure to fireworks was avoided until the dog was properly retrained. On one occasion, when prevention was not possible, Bernice was treated with alprazolam one hour before the fireworks were expected and was kept in the basement while a CD was played that had been used during Bernice's relaxation exercises. A recording of fireworks was made. To test whether the recording would sufficiently resemble the natural stimuli, it was played for the pet starting at a low amplitude, then gradually increased until the pet exhibited the very least sign of anxiety.

At least five times each week the owner would conduct exposure sessions for 15–20 minutes. The tape was played just below the volume that elicited anxiety while the pet was asked to respond to obedience commands for tasty food treats or was engaged in play with the owner. It was also played at a very low volume when the pet ate its regularly scheduled meals. Gradually, the volume was increased until the pet did not become anxious when hearing fireworks. The exercises were held in all rooms of the house and outdoors, with the sound coming from a variety of directions.

FEAR OF PLACES

Pets can become anxious about locations just as they can about people or other animals. Every veterinarian is familiar with the pet that is fearful of the veterinary clinic. Many owners testify that their pet loves to ride in the car but becomes anxious when they approach the clinic or even pass it on the street. Other animals are afraid to be kept in a kennel, or even a crate at home. Pets may also become fearful of a particular environment or a particular type of flooring. Some pets may be fearful of travel in moving vehicles and some may have a generalized fear of going outdoors or into the owners' backyard.

Diagnosis and prognosis

Predictable, recurrent signs of fear or anxiety (shivering, pupil dilation, submissive urination, escape behavior) when exposed to visual, auditory, and/or olfactory stimuli associated with a specific environment. The problem environment might be a room, building, yard, area of the neighborhood, or car.

The prognosis depends on the duration and intensity of the fearful behavior, as well as how often the pet has to visit the place where it is uncomfortable and endure strong fear-evoking stimuli before behavior modification is complete. If the pet is fearful of entering the veterinary clinic, repeatedly has to visit for uncomfortable treatments, and the owner is unable to work frequently with the pet to reduce fear, the prognosis is guarded to poor.

Management

Exposure techniques involving habituation, desensitization and counterconditioning, response substitution and flooding are used to treat this problem. The pet should repeatedly be taken near or to the place that causes fear to be given treats or to engage in play (Figs 11.14, 11.15). The goal is to provide numerous positive experiences in a controlled, calm manner at the site where fear is experienced and to reduce the occurrence of the fear responses. Identifying all possible fear-inducing stimuli and presenting them to the dog in a controlled manner for desensitization and counterconditioning or

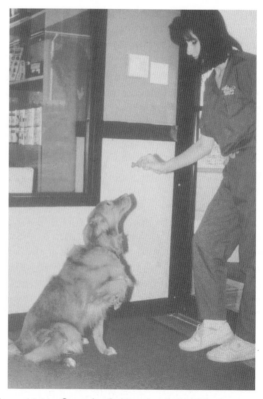

Figure 11.14 Grace is afraid on her first visit to the veterinary clinic. A technician uses a food lure to request a 'sit-stay' and then 'give a paw.'

Step	Comments
Identify aspects about the place that elicit fear Establish a gradient of stimuli Retrain with rewards	• Make sure that all stimuli (odors, sounds, visual elements) that evoke fear are identified • Attempt to avoid fear-eliciting stimuli or places between training sessions • If the pet is most fearful in a room in a specific building, the gradient would extend from the car parking lot or an adjacent property to the room • Teach the pet to respond to verbal commands or sound/visual cues with a 'sit-stay' or 'down-stay' response. Use highly motivating rewards • Secondary reinforcers can be developed by repeatedly associating strong primary reinforcers such as food with obedience commands and responses. Eventually, these can be used to elicit a state of happy anticipation when the pet is asked to sit near the place that elicits the fear
Desensitization and counterconditioning	• Approach as close as possible to the site that causes the fear response but stop before the pet becomes anxious. In a very happy tone of voice, request and reward an obedience response with a very tasty food reward. Subsequent exercises should take place at closer and closer distances from the problem area • If a fear-eliciting situation arises during retraining and triggers a fear response, the pet's behavior should be ignored. If the pet calms down or can be sufficiently distracted, it should be lavishly praised and rewarded. The following training session should occur at a greater distance from the site
Response substitution	• Identify all stimuli that might incite the fear and anxiety and develop a gradient for exposure – for example dogs fearful of car rides may be able to be exposed to the car when stationary in the driveway • Train the pet to exhibit an alternative, incompatible response to fear and escape (such as sit, down, or relax) and use the highest value reinforcers for success • If necessary use a head halter and leash or interruption device to help disrupt the inappropriate response and direct the pet into the appropriate response (which can be reinforced) • With each successful step, progress slowly through the gradient always ensuring the desirable response can be achieved and giving rewards before proceeding
Flooding	• If the phobia is very mild, flooding can be used to treat the pet by taking it to the site that causes anxiety on a leash and preventing it from escaping until it shows no sign of fear • Once the pet shows no sign of fear, rewards should be given • Confinement crates or halters may be helpful. Use of any of these devices is only appropriate if they do not result in increasing the pet's fear
Punishment	• Under no circumstances should punishment be used
Drug therapy	• Medication may be helpful in managing fearful situations • Drugs prescribed for fears and phobias include anti-anxiety drugs for short-term or as needed use, antidepressants to control the panic or anxiety state, and propranolol or buspirone. Combinations of antidepressants and benzodiazepines may be helpful. Phenothiazine tranquilizers do not reduce anxiety but may be useful as a sedative for some pets since they may be less aware of the stimuli in their environment

Figure 11.15 Steps in the management of pets with fear of places.

response substitution, ensuring a positive response, and progressing slowly to more intense stimuli that approximate the ultimate goal (i.e., problem situation) are the basic steps in a treatment program.

Feliway™ spray or room diffuser may be helpful in reducing the anxiety a cat experiences in its home, carrier, car, or new environment, and D.A.P.™, the dog appeasing pheromone, may reduce anxiety in similar environments in dogs. Drug therapy may also be useful as an adjunct to the behavior therapy program.

Prevention

Frequent exposure to all types of environments should be employed in a controlled, positive way during the early months of the pet's life so that the pet habituates to a variety of environments and situations.

Case example

Bijou, a young Toy Poodle, shook uncontrollably and crouched against the back of her cage during each visit to the grooming shop.

The owner was instructed to visit the grooming shop two to three times each week for food and play. They started the exercises in the side yard and car park, progressed into the waiting room, and finally moved into the grooming shop. At home the owner would frequently turn on an electric razor that was muffled with a towel for short durations while the pet was eating and during play sessions. The owner sent along very tasty treats with the pet when it had grooming appointments. The groomer would frequently give the treats throughout the visit. Within a few weeks, Bijou was allowing the groomer to play with her in the owner's absence, without signs of fear. Within six weeks, Bijou could be groomed entirely while showing no evidence of fear.

SEPARATION ANXIETY

Introduction

Separation anxiety is a distressing behavior problem with serious consequences for the owner as well as the pet. Dogs with this disorder exhibit exaggerated signs of anxiety when they do not have access to family members. This problem usually occurs when the owner is away from home, but may occur when the owner is home but the pet's access to the owner is blocked or the dog can't get the owner's attention. Approximately 14% of pet dogs seen in veterinary hospitals in the United States are suspected to suffer from separation anxiety. There are no notable differences between sexes or breeds of dogs in regard to risk of development of separation anxiety, but studies have indicated that there are significantly more mixed breeds, dogs adopted from humane societies, and dogs over 10 years of age that present for this problem.

Highly social species, such as dogs, exhibit attachment behaviors that serve to maintain social contact and bonds between adult individuals as well as between parents and offspring. In situations where an individual loses contact with the group, the resultant anxiety can trigger behaviors that will attract other members (vocalizations), behaviors that help remove barriers (digging, chewing), or ones that facilitate the restoration of contact (increased activity) with other members. It is this underlying drive to be with members of the established social group that provides the foundation for the development of hyperattachment problems.

The underlying issue involves hyperattachment to one or more family members. The onset of problems often coincides with changes in the amount of time that the owner spends with the pet. A new social relationship, working late, or returning to work after an extended stay at home are all examples of changes in the owner's life that can be anxiety-evoking for the pet. Environmental stress such as a move to a new home or a traumatic event might also contribute to a separation anxiety problem. In some older pets, the problem may gradually develop on its own without any major environmental changes. Although the exact etiology of these types of changes in senior and geriatric dogs is unknown, changes in the physiology of the aging canine brain may serve to facilitate the development of separation anxiety (Fig. 11.16).

Some owners are convinced that the destructive behaviors are purposefully directed toward them because the pet is 'retaliating' about being left alone or confined. Part of this reasoning is due to the fact that the objects that are commonly damaged include personal items belonging to the owner, such as books, clothing, shoes,

---

Initiators of separation anxiety include:
- Change in the owner's routine
- Owner returning to school or work
- Move to a new home
- Visit to a new environment
- Following a stay in a kennel
- Altered social relationships (new baby, new pet)
- Medical, cognitive

Figure 11.16 Initiators of separation anxiety.

and sofa cushions. What these objects have in common is that they are frequently handled by the owner and carry the owner's scent. Contact with these items may serve to remind the pet of the absent owner, which causes anxiety that triggers destructive displacement behaviors.

Treatment for separation anxiety involves developing independence for the dog by adjusting the relationship with the owner and promoting calmness when the owner is gone. This is done by managing the environment, teaching the owner alternate ways of interacting with the pet, using behavior modification and, for severe or refractory cases, prescribing medication.

Diagnosis

The diagnosis involves collecting historical information about the pet that reveals hyperattachment to the owner, anxiety at the time of the owner's departure, and owner-absent behavior problems for which other medical and behavioral causes have been ruled out (Fig. 11.17). A videotape can be an especially valuable means of assessing the problem (as well as monitoring response to therapy). It is also critical to evaluate the pet's behaviors as a whole, since there may also be other concurrent forms of fear or anxiety. These may be caused by medical problems, cognitive dysfunction syndrome, behavioral pathologies leading to anxiety (see Ch. 4), or other anxiety states such as thunderstorm phobias. As the anxiety increases the dog may seek out the owner for attention and reassurance (then receiving owner reinforcement).

Common features of separation anxiety:
- The pet is hyperattached to the owner
- The pet shows signs of anxiety as the owner leaves
- The problem behaviors usually only occur when the owners are absent or when the pets cannot gain access to the owners when they are at home
- The anxious behaviors begin very shortly after the owner leaves and may occur even during very short absences by the owner
- The pet shows exaggerated greeting behavior

Figure 11.17   Features of separation anxiety.

Anxiety is likely to increase when these dogs are separated from their owners, and for these dogs all causes of anxiety must be diagnosed and treated.

Medical workup

The initial step is the medical workup. Each pet should receive a thorough physical exam. Depending upon the specific behaviors the individual is exhibiting and the physical exam findings, a full neurologic exam, chemistry panel, CBC, thyroid evaluation, fecal exam, and/or urinalysis may need to be performed.

Hyperattachment

The typical home situation in which a separation anxiety problem develops is one in which the relationship between the pet and the owner is extremely close. When the owner is home, the pet may continuously keep the owner within eyesight or may constantly stay at the owner's side. A prime candidate for this type of problem is the dog with a slightly anxious temperament that successfully solicits attention from the owner whenever it wants, and is very sensitive to environmental changes. This is not a consistent finding, though, since there are some pets with separation anxiety that do not seek continuous physical contact when family members are at home.

Predeparture anxiety

As the owner prepares to leave, the pet usually shows salient signs of anxiety including increased activity (restlessness, pacing, whining), depression (withdraws, reluctant to move, 'downcast' look, refuses to take treats), or physiologic changes (panting, tachycardia, hypersalivation, vomiting). These occur in response to recognizable departure cues, such as picking up car keys, putting on a coat, picking up a brief case, etc.

Owner-absent problems

During the owner's absence, the dog may exhibit a wide range of behaviors including chewing, scratching, housesoiling, vocalizing, and hypersalivation. The targets of the destructive behavior are usually areas around windows or doorways where the owner leaves the home, or items that bear the owner's odor. The problems may occur every time the owner leaves or only after specific absences. For example, the pet may be fine when the owner leaves for work each day, but become distressed and destructive during absences by the owner in the evening.

Greeting behaviors

When the owner returns, the dog usually exhibits exaggerated greeting behaviors.

Ruling out other behavior problems

Destructive behavior

There are a variety of reasons why a dog might exhibit destructive behaviors. If the destructive behavior is usually directed toward doors and nearby windows where the owner exits, it is likely that the pet is suffering from separation anxiety. Other targets for destructive behavior include personal possessions of the owners or things they contact, such as hair brushes, books, clothes, and furniture. The dog will target those items because they carry the owner's scent, not because the dog is 'getting back at that person' for being left alone, as some owners might suspect. Much of the destructive behavior begins shortly after the owner's departure. This is a time when the pet's anxiety and arousal level is the highest.

Other causes of destructive behaviors in the owner's absence include teething, play, investigative behavior, hunger, nesting (during pseudocyesis), noise phobias, barrier frustration, and inadequate exercise or stimulation. Some pets will scratch and dig at walls and flooring when they hear mice scurrying about. Another explanation for intermittent destructive chewing around windows and doors is territorial behavior. Displaced chewing or destructive escape behaviors can be triggered when the pet sees another dog or a person outdoors.

Vocalizations

Vocalizations associated with separation anxiety may include crying, whining, yipes, howls, and barking. The tone is typically somewhat more high pitched than what is observed with other types of barking. These usually begin as the owner is leaving home. Excessive anxious vocalizing may also occur if the owner is home and the pet's access to the owner is blocked. Other causes of excessive vocalization that should be ruled out include physical discomfort, alarm barking, predatory response to prey animals seen through the window, compulsive disorder, territorial aggression, social response to hearing other dogs, cognitive dysfunction, and other anxiety-related disorders.

Housesoiling

Pets with separation anxiety will usually eliminate in the home every time the owner leaves. They will do this shortly after the owner leaves, even if they have just eliminated outdoors prior to the owner's departure, and in the absence of any medical problems. Some may even eliminate while the owner is in the act of departing. Unless the pet is also housesoiling due to a concurrent training problem, elimination in the home is unusual when the owner is present. An exception to this may occur when the owner is physically present, but mentally absent. This may happen when the owner is ignoring the pet and paying attention to a new baby or social partner.

Other causes of housesoiling when the owner is gone include training problems, schedule changes, diet changes, excessive confinement periods, gastrointestinal disease, lower urinary tract disorders, incontinence, medical problems that cause polyuria or diarrhea, medications that increase the volume or frequency of elimination, urine marking, and cognitive dysfunction. The most common cause of housesoiling is inadequate training. In most cases, these pets also housesoil when the owner is at home. Problems involving diet changes, disease processes, or medication should be discovered during the medical workup. Information about where the pet eliminates, as well as the pet's temperament, sexual status, and reactivity, may provide clues regarding marking problems.

Miscellaneous problems

In addition to excessive destructive behaviors, vocalizations, and inappropriate elimination, dogs with separation anxiety may also show signs of hypersalivation, emesis, diarrhea, self-mutilation, withdrawal, anorexia, depression, and lethargy. Many of these signs can be caused by a variety of diseases. Therefore, a good medical workup is important. But if the underlying problem is medical, you would expect to see the signs occurring when the owner is home as well.

Prognosis

The outlook is good if the duration of the time since the problem began is short, the pet doesn't exhibit significant signs of anxiety in a variety of other situations, the owners can be motivated to perform time-consuming exercises as well as change the way in which they interact with the pet and, in severe cases, the owners are willing to use psychoactive medication.

Management

The successful management of separation anxiety includes teaching the dog to tolerate owner absences and correcting the specific problems of chewing, scratching, digging, barking, or elimination. One study found that the fewer instructions the owners were given the more compliant and the more improvement. Therefore a simplified program that deals with proper homecoming and departures, teaching relaxed independence away from the owners, and decoupling departure cues from actual departures, in combination with drug therapy, may serve to improve most problems (Fig. 11.18).

Environmental considerations

(1) **Adding another pet**. In rare situations, providing another pet will provide a playmate or distraction for the dog. It does not necessarily have to be another canine. Turtles, ferrets, or cats might provide companionship or stimulation. But this will not always help since most dogs miss family member(s) in particular, and adding another pet is no substitute for the human companionship for which they yearn.

(2) **Temporary preventive and confinement techniques**. Confining the pet to a crate or small room in the home will immediately stop destructive behavior and housesoiling throughout the home, but is usually not well tolerated by pets that have little experience of confinement. Sudden confinement may actually add to the anxiety that the pet experiences during the owner's absence. Some pets become so determined to escape the confinement area that they cause major damage and even serious injuries to themselves. Ideally, the pet should be gradually introduced to the confinement area by using treats and toys when the owners are at home, and not left alone in the confinement area until it accepts confinement with the owners at home. Placing the crate near a patio window so the pet can see outdoors may help in some cases. In other cases, exercise pens or home-built indoor runs may be better tolerated. There may not be enough time for the frustrated owner to do confinement training properly. Day boarding, hiring a pet sitter, or using anxiolytic medication may initially be necessary when this is the case.

(3) **Distractions**. It may be helpful to provide certain types of chew toys and activities to keep the pet occupied during the high anxiety period immediately following the owner's departure. The best toys are those that are highly stimulating and keep the pet's attention. Although many dogs will not chew their regular toys or eat when anxious or stressed, new chew toys, or food-type chew toys (e.g., pigs' ears, rawhide dipped in bouillon, cow femurs stuffed with shrimp) may be attractive. Tasty food treats should be hidden inside toys, in packages that the dog must open, or hidden under bowls or

Step	Comments
Change the relationship	• Teach the pet independence • The pet should not be allowed to get attention on demand. When the pet gets what it wants every time it nudges or whines, it is more likely to be anxious when it is alone and cannot get social attention • The owners should know that they can give the pet the attention they desire, but it must always be on their terms, not the pet's
Departures and predeparture cues	• Departures should be kept as calm as possible • The presence of certain departure cues will typically create anxiety about an impending absence of the owner • The dog should be desensitized to those cues that cannot be avoided during departures. The owner should repeatedly pick up the car keys, open, shut, and handle the door, put on a coat or pick up a briefcase so that the pet habituates to these cues and they lose their strength in eliciting anxiety. Placing a dog in its cage, locking it in the kitchen, or opening and shutting the door are events that the dog should be constantly exposed to when the owner is at home, during sit-stay and reward training sessions • Until the pet has been desensitized to these cues, they should be avoided whenever possible during actual departures. Putting jacket and boots on in a different room, leaving a briefcase, handbag or keys in the garage, and leaving through a different door while the dog is otherwise occupied or distracted can greatly help reduce departure anxiety • Cues that are commonly associated with calmness, food, and the owner's presence can be provided during departures to reduce anxiety. During departures, a TV, radio, or videotape can be left on, or the dog can be provided with a favorite blanket to lie on. Some owners do not understand the principles of these techniques so that the dog is placed in a cage or a radio turned on only when the owner leaves, so that these cues become associated with anxiety and departure, not calmness
Greetings	• Homecomings should be kept very low-key and the pet should be ignored until it is calm
Obedience	• Teach 'sit,' 'down,' and 'stay' commands so the owner can begin teaching the pet to tolerate being alone
Teach the pet to be alone – phase I	• This phase should begin with the pet staying for a very short period before accompanying the owner to various rooms throughout the home • Gradually, the pet should be required to stay for longer periods of time, until it will remain in another room for 30–60 minutes or more
Teach the pet to be alone – phase II	• After the dog has been desensitized to the departure cues, the owner should practice short mock departures • The owner should initially leave for a very short period of only a few seconds to a few minutes. The duration should be shorter than the time in which it takes the pet to show signs of anxiety. Periods can be lengthened gradually as the pet responds without associated anxiety • The duration of departure should be lengthened on a variable schedule, so that the pet cannot predict exactly how long the owner will be gone
Exercise	• Lots of aerobic exercise should be provided
Distractions	• The pet may be less anxious when it has something to do while left alone • Highly stimulating toys should be provided • New chew toys, food chews (pigs' ears, rawhide), or strongly motivating food pieces hidden in the toys, such as meat or cheese, may get the pet's interest. These treats can be hidden inside toys so that they are difficult to remove, in packages that the dog must open, or hidden under bowls around the home • In rare situations, having another pet will provide a playmate (or distraction) for the dog
Confinement	• May result in increased anxiety unless the pet is already accustomed to confinement. Acclimating the pet to confinement should be done gradually. If this is not practical, anxiolytic medication (benzodiazepines, TCAs, SSRIs, buspirone) or D.A.P.™ may be useful
Punishment	• Punishment should be avoided, as should any other treatment modality that might cause anxiety

Figure 11.18   Management of separation anxiety.

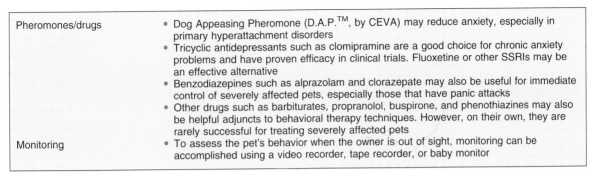

| Pheromones/drugs | • Dog Appeasing Pheromone (D.A.P.™, by CEVA) may reduce anxiety, especially in primary hyperattachment disorders
• Tricyclic antidepressants such as clomipramine are a good choice for chronic anxiety problems and have proven efficacy in clinical trials. Fluoxetine or other SSRIs may be an effective alternative
• Benzodiazepines such as alprazolam and clorazepate may also be useful for immediate control of severely affected pets, especially those that have panic attacks
• Other drugs such as barbiturates, propranolol, buspirone, and phenothiazines may also be helpful adjuncts to behavioral therapy techniques. However, on their own, they are rarely successful for treating severely affected pets |
| Monitoring | • To assess the pet's behavior when the owner is out of sight, monitoring can be accomplished using a video recorder, tape recorder, or baby monitor |

Figure 11.18 (*continued*)

boxes around the home in order to keep the pet busy. Reserving the dog's access to special treats to times when the owner is absent may actually teach the dog to look forward to the owner leaving. Leaving a radio or television on may help mask environmental noises that make the pet anxious and trigger barking or destructive behaviors.

(4) **Destructive behavior**. Environmental measures to stop destructive behaviors have varying degrees of success depending upon the individual dog's temperament. Applying aversive-tasting substances may help curb chewing. Removing or blocking access to chewed items may be protective. A low-volume motion alarm or area-avoidance device may help keep the pet away from an area. A basket muzzle (for safety, the pet must be able to open its mouth) may help immediately control destructive chewing, but should only be used if the pet can be taught to wear it without increasing its anxiety.

(5) **Housesoiling**. Clean up elimination odors and place food bowls, toys, or the pet's bed over previously soiled areas to discourage resoiling. Confining the pet to a relatively small area may decrease housesoiling. Large meals should be avoided prior to confinement. Providing a bowl of frozen water will prevent the pet from drinking large amounts at one time, and force it to sip throughout the day. For some cases, providing a doggie door may be helpful.

(6) **Vocalization**. Shock collars or any strongly aversive techniques should be avoided. Playing a radio at a volume that masks environmental noises or confining the pet to an area of the home where it cannot hear outside noises may be helpful. A citronella anti-bark spray collar may be beneficial and appropriate for some pets. It should be used for the first time when the owner is at home to ensure that it does not contribute to the pet's anxiety.

Behavior modification

Change the relationship with the owner – independence training

The owner should avoid giving the pet attention on demand. When the pet gets what it wants every time it nudges or whines, it is more likely to be anxious when it is alone and can't get social attention. The owners should know that they can give the pet the attention they desire, but it must always be on their terms, not the pet's. Strategies that involve having the owner completely ignore the pet at all times may be counterproductive and are not humane. Giving no rewards when the dog demands attention or follows the owner, while giving attention for long down stays and relaxing in its favored bed area (away from the owners) serves to remove reinforcement for following and overattachment and give reinforcement for independence. Not only would it be useful to train the pet to sleep or nap in a bedding area or crate (rather than constantly by the owner's side), it might also be useful to gradually adapt the dog to sleeping out of the owner's bedroom at night.

Departures and predeparture cues

Most dogs with separation anxiety have learned to associate specific cues with the owner's departure. The presence of these departure cues will typically create anxiety about an impending absence of the owner. Until the pet has been habituated to these cues, they should be avoided whenever possible during actual departures. Putting jacket and boots on in a room away from the pet, leaving a briefcase, purse, or keys in the garage and leaving through a different door while the dog is otherwise occupied or distracted can greatly help reduce departure anxiety. Departures should be kept as calm as possible.

To reduce the pet's anxiety at the owner's departure, the dog should be habituated to departure cues. This can be done by repeatedly picking up the car keys, opening the door, putting on a coat, or picking up a briefcase, etc., so that these cues lose their strength in eliciting anxiety.

Conversely, cues that have been associated with relaxation exercises, independence training, and the owner's presence (i.e., owner not departing), such as a favored mat, piece of owner's clothing, or a CD or television left on, can be used as conditioned inhibitors during the initial stages of departure training.

Greetings

Homecomings should be kept very low-key and the pet should be ignored until it is calm. When the greeting with the owner is the high point of the pet's day and the owner is late in arriving, the pet is likely to become distressed and engage in unacceptable separation behaviors.

Obedience

The pet must learn to respond to 'sit,' 'down,' and 'stay' commands so the owner can begin teaching it to tolerate being alone.

Teach the pet to be alone – phase I

The owner should introduce the pet to the idea that it cannot always be with family members by frequently requesting it to do down-stays and sit-stays. This phase should begin with the pet responding to a stay command for a very short period (one to two seconds) before accompanying the owner to various rooms throughout the home. Gradually, the pet should be required to stay for longer periods of time until it will remain in another room for 30 minutes or more. If the dog is confined to a particular room or area during normal departures, this is the area where a majority of the training should take place. Head halter training can sometimes be used to improve compliance.

Teach the pet to be alone – phase II

After the pet has been habituated to the departure cues, the owner should practice short mock departures. Prior to leaving, the pet should be ignored for 15 minutes. The owner should quietly leave for a very short period of only a few seconds to a few minutes. The duration should be shorter than the time in which it takes the pet to show signs of anxiety. Periods can be lengthened gradually when the dog repeatedly responds without anxiety. The duration of the departures should be lengthened on a variable schedule, so that the pet cannot predict exactly how long the owner will be absent.

Exercise

Frequent exercise sessions have a calming effect, decrease anxiety, and provide suitable social interaction. Providing vigorous, aerobic exercise two to three times daily can have a very positive effect in many cases.

Punishment

Punishment by the owner increases anxiety and plays no appropriate role in the successful management of separation anxiety. Unfortunately, it is the most commonly employed tool by the owner in an attempt to correct separation-related behavior problems. This approach is fraught with problems. First, since the behavior problem occurs when the owner is absent, punishment cannot be temporally associated with the behaviors and, therefore, the animal cannot learn from it. Second, punishment by the owner often causes conflict and more anxiety. Consider the dog that becomes very anxious and chews on the door because of the owner's absence. All this poor creature thinks about during the owner's absence is resuming contact. When this finally occurs, what happens? The owner scolds and possibly beats the dog. This causes conflict, even more stress, and the anxiety-related problems increase. At the worst, other problems can develop such as compulsive disorders, avoidance, and fear aggression.

Medication

Pharmacologic intervention can be a very important treatment adjunct for dogs with severe problems. For situations when a frustrated owner can no longer tolerate the pet's behavior, it may be life saving. Pretreatment physical exams and lab evaluations are important since most psychoactive medications require normal hepatic and renal function to assure proper metabolism. Dog appeasing pheromone (D.A.P.^{TM}) may also help to calm the dog and reduce anxiety.

Tricyclic antidepressants

Tricyclic antidepressants such as clomipramine and amitriptyline can be very helpful for treating pets with separation anxiety by providing relief from anxiety as behavior modification begins. Clomipramine (Clomicalm^{TM}, Novartis) is the only medication specifically labeled for treating canine separation anxiety and has been shown, in conjunction with behavior therapy, to improve the rate at which pets improve and the number of pets that have improved at the end of an eight-week trial. Although amitriptyline and perhaps imipramine might also be used for

separation anxiety, they have not been shown to be as effective as clomipramine, and their effects on serotonin may not be as 'potent.' Selective serotonin re-uptake inhibitors such as fluoxetine or paroxetine are another option with somewhat different side effect profiles and more selectivity for serotonin re-uptake blockade (which may or may not be advantageous).

Benzodiazepines

Benzodiazepines such as alprazolam and clorazepate may also be useful for immediate control of severely affected pets. For those that experience a major panic attack as the owner leaves, alprazolam or clorazepate can be given one to two hours prior to departures. They can be given concurrently with the daily tricyclic antidepressant or SSRI medication.

Selegiline hydrochloride

Selegiline hydrochloride is a monoamine oxidase B inhibitor and may help some cases. It should be considered for use in older pets that may also be showing signs of cognitive dysfunction (confusion, disorientation, changes in sleep–wake cycle, inappropriate vocalization, loss of learned behaviors, alterations in social interaction with the family).

Phenothiazines

These drugs may provide some sedation and decreased activity, but are generally not effective choices for anxiety. The dosage required to completely stop undesirable behaviors by severely affected dogs will usually cause excessive sedation.

Prevention of separation anxiety

Some time should always be spent discussing similar situations in the future that might trigger a recurrence and how to best avoid problems. When the owner anticipates a significant alteration in schedule or in the amount of time spent with the dog, the changeover should be made as slow as possible. Changes should be made very gradually in a way that can easily be tolerated by the pet. Medication might be considered as a preventative, but should be started at least four weeks prior to major changes. A little fore-thought will help prevent the anxiety that can develop in association with sudden, major changes in the pet's life.

Case example

Dolores was a four-year-old spayed female German Shepherd Dog that started exhibiting destructive behavior soon after her owner went back to work following an extended illness and stay at home. Dolores was constantly at the own-er's side whenever she was home and frequently nudged, pawed, or whined to get attention from the owner. When the owner was getting ready to leave, the pet would pace, whine, and tremble. While the owner was at work, she would scratch and chew at the front door and occasionally chew holes in pillows and stuffed furniture.

Upon the owner's arrival at the end of the work-ing day, the dog became extremely excited. Dragging Dolores back to the areas where she was destructive and spanking her had no effect on curtailing the problem.

Behavioral modification techniques were out-lined to the owner, but she didn't think they were practical, especially in the short term. Instead, the owner requested drug therapy, as euthanasia was her next consideration. The dog was started on clomipramine (2.0 mg/kg PO bid) for eight weeks and then gradually tapered off. The owner was instructed to review the pet's obedience training and to practice stays frequently, leaving the pet for gradually longer periods in a variety of areas throughout the house. During the owner's meals, the dog was given her favorite rubber toy, with a piece of liver and a few dog biscuits placed inside. The dog was taught to lie on its mat in the corner of the kitchen, while the owner turned on a favorite CD. Throughout a meal the dog was taught to stay in place while the owner ate, read a news-

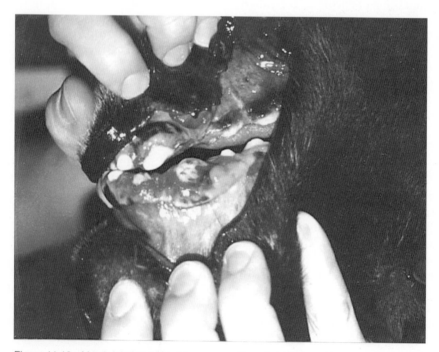

Figure 11.19 Mouth injuries caused by escape attempts in a dog with separation anxiety. Photo courtesy of Dr Kelly Moffat.

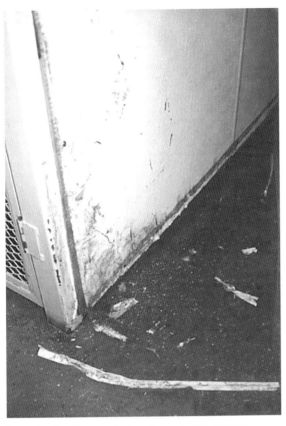

Figure 11.20 Damage to door frame during escape attempts in a dog with separation anxiety. Photo courtesy of Dr Kelly Moffat

paper, had coffee, and left the room on a number of occasions. During actual departures the owner was instructed to exercise the dog, return home, and have the dog lie on its mat. The owner then turned on the CD, gave the dog a new rawhide toy and its rubber toy with food and treats packed inside. The owner was to ignore the dog completely, and leave the room once or twice while the dog remained on the mat. While the dog was working on its toys, the owner was to leave and return to the room, and on the second or third occasion, depart quickly without giving the dog any attention or any indication of departure. This technique provided the dog with an enjoyable distraction, and a departure associated with minimal anxiety. Combined with drug therapy, the dog improved.

REFERENCES

Allpoints Research 1997 Pet owner survey, February

Baum M 1989 Veterinary use of exposure techniques in the treatment of phobic domestic animals. Behaviour Research and Therapy 27(3):307–308

Beaver BV 1983 Fear of loud noises. Veterinary Medicine, Small Animal Clinics March:333–334

Chapman BL, Voith VL 1990 Behavioural problems in old dogs: 26 cases (1984–1987). Journal of the American Veterinary Medical Association 196:944–946

Goddard AW, Charney DS 1997 Toward an integrated neurobiology of panic disorder. Journal of Clinical Psychiatry 58 (Suppl 2):4–11

Hart BL, Voith VL 1976 Fear induced aggressive behaviour. Canine Practice 3:14–20

Hothersall D, Tuber DS 1979 Fears in companion dogs: characteristics and treatment. In: Keehn JD (ed) Psychopathology in animals. Academic Press, New York, p 239–255

McCrave EA 1991 Diagnostic criteria for separation anxiety in the dog. Veterinary Clinics of North America, Small Animal Practice 21:247–255

McCrave EA, Lung N, Voith VL 1986 Correlates of separation anxiety in the dog. In: Abstracts of the Delta Society international conference, Boston

McEwen BS 1998 Protective and damaging effects of stress mediators. New England Journal of Medicine 338:171–179

McEwen BS, Magarinos AM 1997 Stress effects on morphology and function of the hippocampus. Annals of the New York Academy of Sciences 821:271–284

Novartis 1998 From Clomicalm™ clinical and technical review. Novartis Animal Health, Greensboro, NC

Rush AJ, Stewart RS, Garver DL et al 1998 Neurobiological bases for psychiatric disorders. In: Rosenberb RN, Pleasure DE (eds) Comprehensive neurology, 2nd edn. John Wiley, New York, p 555–603

Russell PA 1979 Fear-evoking stimuli. In: Sluckin W (ed) Fear in animals and man. Van Nostrand Reinhold, New York, p 86–124

Shull-Selcer EA, Stagg W 1991 Advances in the understanding and treatment of noise phobias. Veterinary Clinics of North America, Small Animal Practice 21:353–368

Tuber DS, Hothersall D, Peters MF 1982 Treatment of fears and phobias. Veterinary Clinics of North America, Small Animal Practice 12:607–623

Ursin H 1964 Flight and defense behaviour in cats. Journal of Comparative Physiology and Psychology 58:180–186

Voith VL 1979 Treatment of phobias. Modern Veterinary Practice 60:721–722

Voith VL, Borchelt PL 1985 Separation anxiety in dogs. Compendium of Continuing Education for Practicing Veterinarians 7(1):42–53

Voith VL, Borchelt PL 1996 Fears and phobias in companion animals. In: Voith VL, Borchelt PL (eds) Readings in companion animal behaviour. Veterinary Learning Systems, Trenton, NJ, p 140–152

12

The effects of aging on behavior in senior pets

DISTRIBUTION OF BEHAVIOR CASES

Studies of case distribution in senior pets with behavior problems can be misleading with respect to the type of problems that are most commonly seen. Most published studies refer only to those cases seen at behavior referral practices. While the cases seen by behavior consultants may be indicative of the more serious or complex problems that might be seen in some older pets, they only represent a small fraction of the many behavior problems and changes that can occur in senior pets and that might be observed by family members.

Data can be found for 70 cases in dogs and 83 cases in cats over nine years of age that were seen at behavior referral practices. In older dogs, 30% of referrals were for separation anxiety, 26% for aggression toward people, 23% for housesoiling, 19% each for excessive vocalization and phobias, 7% for waking at nights, 5% for compulsive disorders, and 4% for aggression toward other dogs. In a recent study of 103 dogs over seven years of age referred to a St Louis area behavior referral practice, separation anxiety (30%) was also the most common reason for referral, followed by aggression toward people (27%), with the new diagnostic category of cognitive dysfunction appearing in 7% of cases (see Fig. 12.1 for details). Reasons for behavior referrals of older cats were inappropriate elimination (73%), intraspecific aggression (10%),

Presenting sign	Under 9 years[a] (n = 431)	Over 9 years[b] (n = 70)	Over 7 years[c] (n = 103)
Aggression			
(a) humans	53%	26%	27%
(b) intraspecies	7%	4%	17%
Housesoiling	19%	23%	3%
Destructive	19%	29%	n/a
Excitable/unruly	14%	0	0
Phobias	7%	19%	5%
Separation anxiety	5%	30%	30%
Vocalization	5%	19%	1%
Excessive submission	5%	0	0
Compulsive – stereotypic	3%	5%	8%
Waking/restless at night	0	7%	0
Other anxiety	0	0	8%
Cognitive dysfunction	n/a	n/a	7%

[a]Landsberg (1991). [b]Landsberg (1995). Note the diagnostic category of cognitive dysfunction had not yet been established.
[c]Horwitz (2001). Note that the cases of destructiveness were not listed separately as they were all components of other anxiety disorders.

Figure 12.1   Canine behavior referral cases by age group.

vocalization and aggression to owners (6% each), and a few cases of fear, overgrooming and furniture scratching. It is important to note that the number of senior pet behavior cases seen at referral practices is relatively small. In dogs, only 62 of 1094 referred cases, or approximately 6% of all referred cases, were over the age of nine years. In cats, approximately 11% of 420 cases were over the age of nine years. The relatively small numbers of behavior cases in older dogs may reflect the decrease in aggressive cases (particularly dominance aggression). Inappropriate elimination represents the primary reason for referral in young, as well as geriatric, cats. Behavior problems are due to a combination of genetic influences, social and environmental experiences during development, and the effects of training and learning. It is not surprising that most behavior problems emerge within the first few years of life. By the time pets are behaviorally mature (two to three years of age), it is likely that most owners would have recognized and dealt with significant problems by correcting them, learning to live with them, or removing the pet from the home.

When presented with these problems the practitioner must evaluate each case to first determine whether there may be a medical cause for the problem. If the problem cannot be resolved with medical therapy alone, then the case will need to be managed as would any of the other behavior problems discussed in this text. However, there are some issues in the diagnosis and treatment of behavior problems that are specific to the senior pet and must be considered. Although problems in the older pet can be due to many of the same changes in the household that might affect younger pets (moving home, schedule changes, new members of the family through birth or marriage, family members leaving the home through death, divorce, or marriage), the older pet may be more resistant to change. In addition, medical conditions and cognitive decline could also have an impact on behavior, even if they do not directly cause the problem.

In general practice, there are a number of behavioral changes that might be noticed by owners that may not be severe enough to require referral or even a mention to the family veterinarian. Since the effects of aging on the brain can be subtle and slowly progressive, it is extremely important for owners to know about these signs and report them to their veterinarian as soon as they emerge. Behavioral changes may also be the first sign of any physical or health problem, so that early and timely reporting by the owners may lead to early diagnosis and earlier medical intervention, at a time when it might be more effective. Some studies have found that greater than 50% of dogs over the age of 11 have at least one sign of cognitive decline. This number may even be low, since deficits in learning ability and memory can be detected long before clinical signs develop using more sophisticated testing apparatus in a laboratory environment (Fig. 12.2). With over 7 million dogs aged 10 or older in the United States, there are millions of dogs that may have varying degrees of cognitive decline that are at present undiagnosed or untreated.

COGNITIVE DYSFUNCTION AND AGE

Aging pets often suffer a decline in cognitive function (memory, learning, perception, awareness). Traditionally an acronym of DISH (Disorientation, Interaction changes with owners or other pets, Sleep–wake cycle alterations, and Housesoiling) has been used to describe the signs of cognitive dysfunction. However, this is far from a complete list of the clinical signs that might be associated with brain aging. These might include a variety of signs related to confusion, social relationships, activity level changes, depression or apathy, increased anxiety, alterations in sleep–wake cycles, and effects on learning and memory (Fig. 12.3). For a more comprehensive client screening checklist see Figure 12.4.

Data from a study at UC Davis veterinary college involved interviews with owners of 180 dogs aged 11–16 years whose pets had no illnesses that would account for behavioral signs, including decreased social interaction with owners, sleep–wake cycle changes, activity level changes, housesoiling, and disorientation. In the 11- to 12-year-old dogs, 28% were positive for at least one category and this rose to 68% of 15- to 16-year-old dogs; 10% of owners of 11- to 12-year-old dogs and 36% of owners of 15- to 16-year-old dogs had signs in two or more categories (Nielson et al 2001). By contrast, a survey of 250 veterinarians found that only 7% of

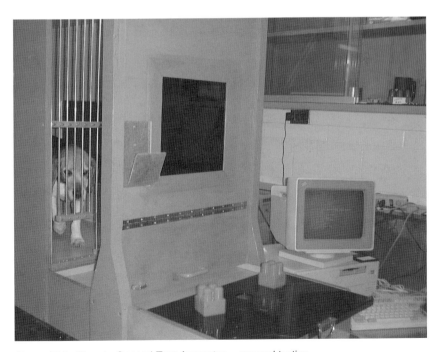

Figure 12.2 Toronto General Test Apparatus – reversal testing.

Signs of brain aging – cognitive dysfunction syndrome

A: Confusion, decreased awareness, deficits in spatial orientation
B: Altered social relationships with people or other pets
C: Activity increase – increased locomotor activity, restlessness, repetitive behaviors
D: Activity decrease – apathy, decreased responsiveness to stimuli
E: Anxiety
F: Altered sleep–wake cycles; reversed day/night schedule
G: Learning and memory problems – housesoiling, decreased ability to learn or remember work, tasks, commands
H: Appetite changes – increase or decrease
I: Increased irritability

Figure 12.3

owners of older dogs spontaneously report such problems to their veterinarian.

By tracking the above cases from the time of onset of one or more signs, it was found that they were likely to progress and more signs were likely to develop: 22% of dogs that did not have any signs of cognitive impairment at the first interview developed signs after 12 to 18 months, while 48% of dogs that had impairment in one category had impairment in two or more categories after 12 to 18 months.

Similarly in preliminary results from a study by Moffat (2001) of cats 11 years of age and older that were presented for routine care to a private veterinary hospital, 43% of 154 cats had at least one sign consistent with cognitive dysfunction (change in social relationships, disorientation, sleep–wake cycle alterations, anxiety, memory and learning problems). After removing 19 cats from consideration due to concurrent medical problems (which may or may not have been causing the cognitive signs), 35% had signs consistent with cognitive dysfunction and no other detectable health problem. In cats aged 15 years and older, more cats were affected (48%) and more signs were observed (2.5 per cat) compared to young cats aged 11 to 14 (30% affected, 1.8 signs per cat).

Neuropsychological tests that rely on quantitative measures rather than subjective owner assessments have been designed to evaluate the cognitive function of dogs (Fig. 12.2). In a number of tests, it has been possible to clearly identify age-related differences in cognitive ability. As with humans, the aging process in dogs does not affect all cognitive abilities equally. This may be due to the fact that age-related

pathology affects different parts of the cortex at different times. For example, visual discrimination learning (learning which of two objects covers a reward) is not usually affected by age in most animals including dogs. However, if the task is more difficult, such as in size discrimination (i.e., the dog must learn whether a small or large object covers the food – Fig. 12.5), aged animals have more difficulty in learning the task compared with younger animals. Tasks requiring the inhibition of a previously learned behavior, as in reversal learning (the dog must learn that the food is now under the opposite object), are also sensitive to age. This may be due to the fact that reversal learning but not discrimination learning in dogs requires the intact function of the prefrontal cortex. This is a brain region in dogs in which the earliest and most consistent neuropathology of the cortex tends to arise.

Memory decline in dogs is also age-dependent and provides more information about individual differences between young and old dogs. Researchers have used memory tasks that are age sensitive in dogs; such as an object recognition memory task, where the dog is required to recall which object covered the food 10 seconds earlier. Object recognition memory is impaired in aged dogs and some old animals cannot recall having seen an object presented 5–10 seconds previously. Memory testing reveals three groups of aged dogs: (a) unimpaired, (b) impaired, and (c) severely impaired (Fig. 12.6). This is consistent with the findings in the geriatric human population.

Age-related differences have also been demonstrated in exploration and locomotion.

COGNITIVE DYSFUNCTION SCREENING CHECKLIST

Owner's Name: **Species: Canine** _____ **Feline** ___

Pet's Name: **Breed:** **Age:** **Date:**

Key: 0 – none, 1 – mild, 2 – moderate, 3 – severe	Date:	Date:	Date:
A: Confusion – Awareness – Spatial orientation			
– gets lost in familiar locations			
– goes to wrong side of door (e.g., hinge side)			
– gets stuck, cannot navigate around or over obstacles			
– decreased responsiveness to stimuli			
B: Relationships – Social behavior			
– decreased interest in petting/contact			
– decreased greeting behavior			
– alterations/problems with social hierarchy			
– in need of constant contact, overdependent, 'clingy'			
C: Activity – Increased/repetitive			
– stares/fixation/snaps at objects			
– pacing/wanders aimlessly			
– licking owners, household objects			
– vocalization			
– increased appetite (eats quicker or more food)			
D: Activity – Decreased – Apathy			
– decreased exploration/activity/apathy			
– decreased responsiveness to stimuli			
– decreased self-care			
– decreased appetite			
E: Anxiety – Increased irritability			
– restless/agitation			
– anxiety about being separated from owners			
– increased irritability			
F: Sleep–wake cycles; Reversed day/night schedule			
– restless sleep/waking at nights			
– increased daytime sleep			
G1: Learning and Memory – Housesoiling			
– indoor elimination at random sites or in view of owners			
– decrease/loss of signaling			
– goes outdoors, then returns indoors and eliminates			
– elimination in crate or sleeping area			
– incontinence			
G2: Learning and Memory – Work, Tasks, Commands			
– impaired working ability			
– decreased recognition of familiar people/pets			
– decreased responsiveness to known commands and tricks			
– decreased ability to perform tasks			
– inability/slow to learn new tasks (retrain)			
Discuss any additional concerns or use this space to describe details of any of the above			

Figure 12.4 Cognitive dysfunction screening checklist (form #4 – printable from the CD).

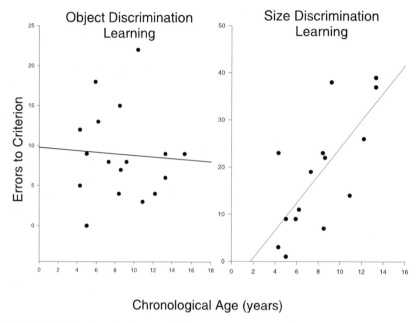

Chronological Age (years)

Figure 12.5 Object discrimination learning is not sensitive to age in dogs (correlation between age and error scores on object discrimination is $r = 0.05$). In contrast, size discrimination error scores increase significantly with age (correlation between age and error scores on size discrimination is $r = 0.728$). Reprinted from Head E, Callahan H, Muggenburg BA et al 1998 Discrimination learning ability and beta amyloid accumulation in the dog. Neurobiology of Aging 19:415–425 with permission from Elsevier Science.

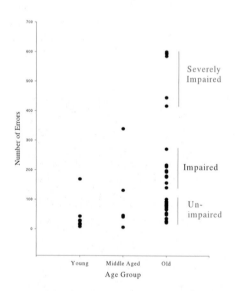

Figure 12.6 Spatial memory is unimpaired, impaired, or severely impaired in three different subsets of aged dogs. Reprinted from Head E, Milgram NW, Cotman CW 2001 Neurobiological models of aging in the dog and other vertebrate species. In: Hof AP, Mobbs C (eds) Functional neurobiology of aging. Academic Press, San Diego, p 457–468. Reprinted with permission from Academic Press.

The curiosity test allows the dogs to play with a variety of novel toys. In this test young dogs show more exploration and curiosity than old dogs, and the age-impaired dogs show almost no exploration (Fig. 12.7). Locomotor activity generally declines with age. Although this may be true for age-unimpaired dogs, age-impaired dogs exhibit increased levels of locomotion. This raises the possibility that the mechanisms underlying cognitive impairment might also affect locomotion. Similarly, in a human interaction test, where dogs are exposed to a familiar person, the young dogs spend significantly more time in contact with the person, the cognitively unimpaired dogs spend time close to the person but do not initiate as much contact, and the cognitively impaired dogs tend to ignore the person. By developing tests in which older dogs do not statistically perform as well as younger dogs, it then becomes possible to use objective criteria for assessing the response of animals to dietary or pharmacological intervention.

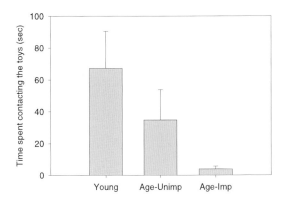

Figure 12.7   The amount of time spent playing or contacting the various toys in the room is plotted against cognitive group. Young dogs play with the toys more than age-impaired ($p < 0.027$) dogs who rarely touched the toys. Aged, unimpaired dogs explored the toys a little. (Courtesy of Christina T Siwak, Institute of Medical Science, University of Toronto, Scarborough, Ont.)

AGING AND ITS EFFECT ON THE BRAIN

There are a number of degenerative changes in the brains of older dogs that may be associated with behavioral signs of CDS, but a clear cause and effect relationship has not been established with the clinical syndrome. With increasing age in dogs, there can be cerebrocortical and basal ganglia atrophy, an increase in ventricular size, narrowing and retraction of the gyri, widening of the sulci, leptomeningeal thickening in the cerebral hemispheres (but not the cerebellum), occasional meningeal calcification, demyelination, an increase in the size and number of glial cells, and a reduction in neurons (Figs 12.8, 12.9). In one study an 18.5% reduction in neurons was found in dogs over 19 years of age, compared with younger dogs. The cortical regions overlying the hippocampus in particular can be affected. Other neuronal changes in older dogs include increasing amounts of lipofuscin, apoptotic bodies, and neuroaxonal degeneration. There is also an increased accumulation of ubiquitin granules and an accumulation of diffuse beta amyloid plaques and perivascular infiltrates (Fig. 12.10). Although the role of beta amyloid accumulation in the development of cognitive dysfunction is yet to be determined, it is neurotoxic, correlates with the severity of cognitive dysfunction in laboratory tests, and can lead to compromised neuronal function, degeneration of synapses, apoptosis-induced neuronal loss, and a depletion of neurotransmitters. Studies have shown that beta amyloid is undetectable in young dogs and is most extensive in the oldest canines, and that the greater

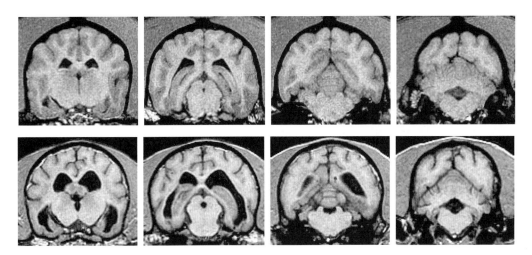

Figure 12.8   Selected MR images from a two-year-old (above) and a 15-year-old (below) dog. The old dog showed marked ventricular enlargement and cortical atrophy (deep gyri and widened sulci). (Photo courtesy of Lydia M-Y Su, Center for Functional Onco-Imaging, University of California, Irvine, CA.)

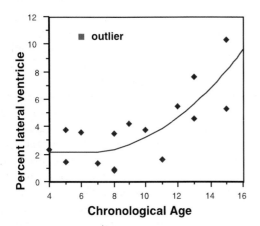

Figure 12.9 The plot of percent lateral ventricle volume (normalized by the total cerebral volume) with age. The relationship with age was not linear, rather it was stable before age 10 and progressed very rapidly thereafter. A six-year-old dog was obviously falling out of the age-dependence trend, and was marked as an outlier. Excluding the outlier, the age-correlation was significant. The solid curve is for visual guidance. Reprinted from Su M-Y, Head E, Brooks W et al 1998 Imaging of anatomic and vascular characteristics in a canine model of human aging. Neurobiology of Aging 19:479–485 with permission from Elsevier Science.

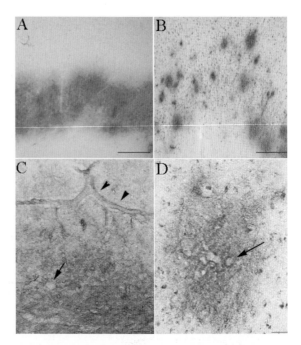

Figure 12.10 Diffuse Aβ deposition in the parietal cortex of (A) an aged cat with symptoms of CDS (tissue provided by Dr Kelly Moffat) vs (B) in the aged canine brain. Note that Aβ in the cat is present as a large diffuse cloud whereas in the dog, more discrete deposits form. Higher magnification of Aβ in (C) cats and (D) dogs. Note the Aβ deposition associated with blood vessels (arrowheads) in the cat and that in both animals, intact neurons (arrows) are present within diffuse clouds of Aβ. Bars in A and B: 500 μm; C and D: 50 μm. Slides printed with permission from the collection of Dr Elizabeth Head, Institute for Brain Aging, University of California, Irvine, CA.

the beta amyloid accumulation, the greater the cognitive impairment. In dogs, errors in learning tests including discrimination, reversal, and spatial learning were strongly associated with increased amounts of beta amyloid deposition.

Although atherosclerosis, cerebral ischemia, and cerebral hemorrhage are rare in dogs and cats, numerous vascular and perivascular changes have been identified in older dogs, including occasional cases of microhemorrhage or infarcts in periventricular vessels. Arteriosclerosis of the non-lipid variety may be commonly seen in the older dog (due to fibrosis of vessel walls, endothelial proliferation, hyalinization, mineralization, and beta amyloid deposition). The angiopathy present within some aged dogs may compromise blood flow and glucose utilization. In addition, the brain of the elderly pet may be subjected to hypoxia due to decreased cardiac output, anemia, blood hyperviscosity and platelet hypercoagulability, and conditions that lead to hypertension (diabetes, hyperthyroidism, renal disease, respiratory insufficiency). Cholinergic depletion and an increase in noradrenergic tone may also compromise cerebral blood flow by leading to a net vasoconstrictive effect. The first signs of these changes may be decreased physical activity and sensory acuity. Over time, limbic tremors, decreased sensory orientation, attitude and personality changes, soiling and incontinence, decreased responsiveness, and decreased ability to perform learned tasks may arise. Although there is a great deal of speculation as to the mechanisms that contribute to the onset of these signs, there seems to be sufficient data to indicate that alterations in neurotransmitter function (based on response to drug therapy) and increasing beta amyloid accumulation are at least in part responsible.

There are a number of parallels between canine cognitive dysfunction and human Alzheimer's disease. Dogs and humans both develop cognitive impairment with age, and a subset of each group develops severe impairment, although some dogs and people show no impairment whatsoever. There are also similarities in the neuropathology of dogs with cognitive dysfunction. Diffuse beta amyloid plaques within the cerebrum and hippocampus as well as vessel associated beta amyloid angiopathy have been identified in geriatric humans, dogs, and cats with signs consistent with cognitive dysfunction (see Fig. 12.10). In older dogs and cats, the plaques are diffuse and lack a central core. Beta amyloid negative neurons may be found trapped within plaques and beta amyloid positive neurons are also observed in areas with no plaque distribution. There are also numerous cerebrovascular beta amyloid deposits. Both dogs and humans develop senile plaques with the more severe cognitive impairments being associated with more extensive plaque formation. In another study of seven cats aged 12 to 20 years, beta amyloid angiopathy and senile plaques were identified in three cats aged 18 to 20 years. In addition, beta amyloid was found distributed around degenerated neurons and capillaries without forming plaques. In dogs and cats, neuritic plaques with associated nerve terminals containing hyperphosphorylated tau, and neuro-fibrillary tangles, which are found in human Alzheimer's patients, have not been observed. Beta amyloid load tends to accumulate earlier and in greater amounts in the prefrontal cortex, beginning at about age nine years in dogs, and then progresses to the temporal and pyriform regions, and is latest and slowest to accumulate in the occipital region. In addition, beta amyloid deposition spreads from the deeper cortical layers to the superficial layers with increasing age.

The appearance of cognitive deficits may reflect this progression in neuropathology with frontal-dependent tasks appearing to decline the earliest. Prefrontal tasks in the laboratory that

would be sensitive to beta amyloid pathology in this area of the brain might include reversal learning and memory tasks (object and spatial memory). It is possible that clinically affected pets might display stereotyped behavior such as pacing and circling, behavioral rigidity, perseveration (hard to break old tasks), and an inability to inhibit responses (e.g., elimination). If dysfunction were to involve the temporal cortex then auditory association might be affected, leading to increased vocalization. With parietal involvement, spatial disorientation, wandering, getting lost, and a decline in visual processing might arise. While beta amyloid extending into the entorhinal cortex is generally not observed until dogs reach 14 years, a subgroup of dogs may be affected by nine years of age. The thalamus and basal ganglia are rarely affected. Genetics may be a contributing factor in the extent of amyloid distribution, as some breeds develop beta amyloid at an earlier age and there is high concordance within litters in the extent of beta amyloid.

Functional changes that may occur in the aging brain include depletion of catecholamine neurotransmitters (norepinephrine, serotonin, dopamine), increased monoamine oxidase B activity, and increased free radical production. With age, mitochondrial function declines so that there is less efficient production of energy and an increased production of free radicals. Increased monoamine oxidase activity may result in liberation of oxygen free radicals, which in turn are damaging to cell membranes. The role of vascular insufficiency (decreased cardiac output, anemia, arteriosclerosis, blood viscosity changes, vasospasm) in enhancing the neurodegenerative process is unknown, but there may be a link between hypoxia and CDS.

REACTIVE OXYGEN SPECIES (TOXIC FREE RADICALS)

Although oxygen is required to survive, a small amount of oxygen that is used by the mitochondria for normal, aerobic, energy production is converted to reactive oxygen species (also known as free radicals) such as hydrogen peroxide, superoxide, and nitric oxide within the mitochondria. As mitochondria age, they become less efficient and produce relatively more free radicals and less energy, compared with younger mitochondria. In addition, neutrophils and macrophages respond to infection and inflammation by increasing amounts of free radicals. Finally, exogenous sources of free radical damage, such as ionizing radiation, carcinogens, or air pollutants, may result in production of free radicals within cells. Although these latter sources may be producers of free radicals, it is clear that the major source and production of free radicals is from endogenous metabolic processes.

Normally, the body's antioxidant defenses, including enzymes such as superoxide dismutase, catalase, and glutathione peroxidase, and free radical scavengers such as vitamins A, C, and E, eliminate free radicals as they are produced. If free radicals escape these physiologic mechanisms, they may react with DNA, lipids, and proteins, leading to cellular damage, dysfunction, mutation, neoplasia, and even cell death. It is this balance of detoxification and production that is in a controlled balance in the cell, and if tipped in favor of overproduction, a state of oxidative stress is manifest. The brain, of all tissues, is particularly susceptible to the effects of free radicals because it has a high lipid content, a high demand for oxygen, and limited ability for antioxidant defense and repair.

There is limited information available regarding oxidative damage in the aged canine or feline brain. The levels of endogenous antioxidant enzymes in the aged canine brain are reduced with age, suggesting a loss in the ability to scavenge free radicals. The extent of oxidative damage to proteins and lipids also rises with age in the canine brain. If oxidative damage plays a key role in neurodegenerative processes causing cognitive dysfunction, then we might expect that antioxidants would improve learning and memory in aged animals. Recent evidence in the laboratory supports this hypothesis and aged dogs provided with a diet rich in a broad spectrum of antioxidants show improved learning ability.

SENIOR CARE AND BEHAVIOR

Health care programs designed specifically for the needs of the senior pet should be an integral part of any veterinary practice. They are essential for the physical and behavioral well-being of the senior pet, since they provide the best opportunity for early diagnosis and intervention. Many disease processes in the older pet can be slowed, or the pet's quality of life improved with early diagnosis, as well as with intervention with drugs, diet, or supplements.

The optimal senior health care program includes three integral parts: (1) identification of clinical signs by asking the owners to report any changes in health or behavior as soon as they emerge; (2) regular physical examinations to detect changes that might not be noticeable to the owner; and (3) diagnostic or screening tests to detect abnormalities as early as possible.

(1) *Owner reporting.* Many of the signs of illness, disease, or failing health will be observed only by the owners in the home environment. Alterations in eating habits, waking the owners at night, housesoiling, and a decline in activity or social interactions with the family will not be detected on physical examination or laboratory testing. Yet many families fail to discuss geriatric-onset behavior or health changes with their veterinarian because they incorrectly assume that these problems are an unfortunate but untreatable aspect of aging. In addition, unless the veterinarian goes through a comprehensive list of questions, something of importance may be forgotten or overlooked. A questionnaire/checklist can be used to save time and to identify problems that owners might not otherwise mention and about which veterinarians might not otherwise ask (Fig. 12.11). Handouts can be used to demonstrate the practice's interest in geriatric care and educate the owners about the need for regular comprehensive geriatric evaluations. Owners that prefer to wait until their pet begins to exhibit problems before authorizing diagnostic testing may better accept the need for tests if problems are identified on the questionnaire. The questionnaire should then be kept in the medical record for future comparison.

SENIOR PET SCREENING CHECKLIST

Owner observations are an important aspect of health care of all pets, but are especially important in the senior pet. Please complete this questionnaire and return it to our receptionist before you see the doctor. It helps us to ensure that nothing is overlooked, and tells us about some of the signs that might not be evident on a physical examination.

Owner's Name
Pet's Name: Age:

Species: Canine _____ Feline _____
                                   Date:

Key: 0 – No problem, M1 – Mild, M2 – Moderate, M3 – Severe	0	M1	M2	M3	When problem began?
Weight gain _____ loss _____					
Appetite increase _____ decrease _____					
Vomiting _____					
Diarrhea _____ Colitis (stool with mucus or blood) _____					
Constipation/difficult defecation _____					
Increased drinking _____ Increased urine _____					
Coughing _____ Weakness after exercise _____ Panting _____					
Lumps/tumors _____ Skin problems _____ Describe:					
Bad breath/sore gums/difficulty chewing _____					
Muscle tremors/shaking _____					
Weakness/incoordination _____					
Difficulty climbing stairs/increased stiffness _____					
Diminished vision _____					
Diminished hearing _____					
Housesoiling: Urine _____ Horizontal surface _____ Vertical _____ Bowel movement _____ Urinary incontinence _____ Indoor elimination in view of family _____ Goes outdoors, eliminates indoors on return _____ Elimination in crate or sleeping area _____					
Impaired learning/memory: Decreased ability to work _____ Forgets name/commands/previously learned tasks _____ Decreased recognition of familiar people/animals _____					
Social: Decreased interest in petting/affection _____ Decreased tolerance of handling _____ More possessive _____ Increased need or demand for affection/attention _____ Problems with social relationships with other pets _____					
Disorientation: Gets lost _____ Goes to wrong side of door _____ Confused _____ Can't maneuver over or around obstacles _____					
Anxiety: Decreased tolerance of being left alone _____ Increased irritability _____ Restless/agitated _____ Anxiety _____ Fearful _____ Phobias _____ Aggression _____ Describe:					
Purposeless/repetitive activity: Vocal/whining _____ Pacing _____ Circling _____ Licking _____ Stares into space _____ Self-trauma _____ Sucking _____ Hallucinates _____ Describe:					
Sleep–wake cycles: Wakes at night/restless sleep _____ Decreased activity during the day/sleeps more _____					
Apathy/depression: Less reactive _____ Listless _____ Decreased interest in food _____ Decreased self-grooming _____					

Other problems/concerns (or use this space to describe any of the above in more detail)

List medications, diet or supplements your pet is taking:

Has your pet been previously diagnosed as having any medical problems? Y/N Describe:

Figure 12.11   Senior pet checklist (form #10 – printable from the CD).

(2) *Physical examination.* The physical examination may help to detect some problems before the presence of any obvious clinical signs. Examination of the sensory system, oral cavity, heart and lungs, and palpation of the joints, lymph nodes, prostate and abdomen is necessary at least once or twice a year to assess the health of systems and structures that cannot be properly evaluated by the pet owner.

(3) *Diagnostic and screening tests.* Based on the pet's age, breed, sex, and history, as well as the results of the physical examination, a series of screening or diagnostic tests is an invaluable part of every senior health care program. Blood pressure evaluation, tonometry, or a screening set of blood and urine tests are generally indicated, even if no abnormalities have been found. One study examined 90 dogs and 100 cats, eight years of age and older, that were in good general health according to their owners and had no previously diagnosed medical condition (Garcia JL, Bruyette DS 1998 Unpublished data, presented at ACVIM poster session). Of the dogs, 29% had low total T4, 17% had an elevated alkaline phosphatase, 16% had an elevated UCCR (three had both an elevated UCCR and alkaline phosphatase), and 12% had pyuria or bacteriuria. Of the cats, 6% had an elevated total T4 level, 9% were azotemic (five of these had urine specific gravity <1.035), one cat was diabetic, and one cat had a urinary tract infection (UTI). On a similar note, in a retrospective evaluation of 101 dogs with hyperadrenalcorticism or diabetes mellitus or both, 42 had UTI but less than 5% of the dogs with UTI showed clinical signs (e.g., stranguria, pollakiuria).

DIAGNOSING THE CAUSE OF BEHAVIORAL SIGNS/CHANGES IN OLDER PETS

As mentioned, the senior pet may be presented with a variety of behavior signs. These can be severe, such as destructiveness, anxiety and phobias, repetitive or compulsive disorders, night waking, housesoiling, increased vocalization and aggression, or more subtle, such as a decrease in responsiveness to the owner or decreased activity levels, which might be more indicative of cognitive decline. When presented with any newly emerging health or behavioral sign, the practitioner will need to diagnose the cause of those signs so that an appropriate treatment program can be implemented. Even though a pet with a behavior problem might be presented to the veterinarian at an older age, the age of onset of the problem may be much earlier. In some cases, the behavior problem may have begun at a relatively young age. This can be due to changes in intensity or frequency of the problem, or changes in the household that preclude living with the problem any longer. Therefore, a critical part of history taking is to determine the age at which the problem began to emerge and, if it is of long standing, why the owners have waited until this time to seek assistance.

Clinical history

By questioning the pet owner about any emerging health, physical, or behavior changes that might be exhibited by the pet, the practitioner should be aware of any and all signs that might be contributing to the problems at hand (see Fig. 12.11). Additional history will then be required to determine the cause of the behavioral changes. Of course, underlying physical and medical conditions may be identified, but there may also be elements of the history that reveal environmental factors and behavioral management techniques that have caused or aggravated the problem.

The behavioral and medical history from just before and at the time of onset is often the key to separating a primary behavior problem from one associated with medical conditions.

- Age of onset is an important factor in both diagnosis and the determination of a prognosis. Looking for a cause that is unrelated to aging will need to be considered if the clinical signs began to emerge at a younger age.
- Look for changes in the environment, the pet's schedule or routine, or the people and pets in the home, around the time of onset

of the problem that might indicate a behavioral cause.

- Look at the responses and actions on the part of the owner or other pets that might be aggravating, maintaining, or reinforcing the problem.
- Consider any possible genetic and medical conditions associated with the age of onset of the problem.
- Evaluate all signs in combination to determine if there is a pattern that would indicate a medical or physical cause or cognitive dysfunction.

Physical examination

Although a physical and dental examination is required for every behavior case, neurological examination, joint evaluation, sensory evaluation, and a prostate exam in male dogs may also be necessary in the older pet. The combined findings of the physical examination and the history will then be used to determine what additional tests will be needed to diagnose the cause of the signs.

Laboratory/radiographic assessment

Laboratory tests should be selected based on the signalment, history, and physical examination findings. Consider all possible medical differentials that might cause the presenting signs and run appropriate diagnostics. A minimum database might include a complete blood count, urinalysis, serum biochemistry, and endocrine screening tests (e.g., total T4 and perhaps a urine cortisol/creatinine ratio in dogs). Additional tests would be based on the presenting signs, the list of possible differential diagnoses, and the results of any preliminary testing. These might include fecal analysis, endocrine profiles, organ function tests, water intake measurement, additional blood testing, or more specialized tests such as endoscopy, ECG, ultrasonography, BAER, CSF evaluation, or even CT or MRI scans. See Figure 12.12 for a list of some of the age-related medical problems that might lead to behavioral signs.

CAUSES OF BEHAVIOR PROBLEMS IN THE AGING PET

Aging can have an effect on virtually every body system, which may in turn have a direct or indirect affect on the behavior of a pet (Fig. 12.12). Aging changes are generally progressive and irreversible. Disease, stress, nutrition, exercise, genetics, environment, and the effects of oxidative damage all play a role in the aging process. As pets age, each organ system can be affected, so that the practitioner must consider the pet as a whole rather than looking for a single cause of the pet's clinical signs.

In general, the presenting signs may arise as a result of a disease process, age-related effects on the body systems, age-related effects on the brain, primary behavior problems, or some combination of these factors. If the medical evaluation does not reveal an underlying physical or health problem that might be causing the behavioral signs, the practitioner will then need to determine whether the signs might be related to cognitive dysfunction (brain aging) or whether there might be a primary behavior problem. Of course the presence of a medical problem does not rule out the possibility of concurrent cognitive dysfunction or behavior problems. For example, it would not be unusual for an older pet with hearing and visual deficits and arthritis to also have some degree of cognitive decline. Therefore it might be difficult to determine which condition is most responsible for a specific behavioral change, such as decreased interaction with the owner. In some cases, a therapeutic trial (i.e., response to therapy) might be the most practical means of determining which signs are attributable to which problems.

Medical and physical health and its effects on behavior

The aging process is associated with progressive and irreversible changes in the body systems that could affect the pet's behavior. The most common causes of age-related death in dogs are cancer, cardiovascular disease, renal failure,

Age-related change	Possible behavioral implications
Dehydration – less responsive to thirst	Constipation, housesoiling, irritability
Degeneration of organ function – tissue hypoxia	Signs related to organ system affected
Weight loss due to organ dysfunction, metabolic, gastrointestinal or oral disease, decreased muscle, sensory decline, CDS, food aversion due to illness	Might lead to decreased activity, weakness, lethargy, housesoiling, increased irritability Some metabolic problems may induce weight loss but lead to compensatory polyphagia, garbage raiding, picas, or increased food possessiveness
Obesity due to decreased activity and metabolic rate	Less responsive, mobile, or active
Decreased immune competence, tumors	Signs related to infection, immune disease, or tumor
Hypothermia; decreased metabolism, decreased thermoregulation, and decreased vasoconstriction	Less interactive/hiding, trembling, reluctant to go outdoors, altered sleep–wake cycle
Decreased REM sleep, altered circadian rhythms	Night waking, increased sleep, daytime restless
INTEGUMENTARY	
Hyperkeratosis, pigment loss, follicular atrophy, decreased sebum, brittle nails	Increased discomfort, increased irritability, behavioral effects of endocrinopathies
GASTROINTESTINAL	
Increase in dental disease, oral tumors	Decreased appetite, increased irritability, aggression
Digestive – decreased absorption, decreased pancreatic and salivary secretion, and decreased colonic motility	Nutritional imbalances may have varying effects on behavior due to deficiencies – altered elimination habits, decreased appetite
RESPIRATORY/CIRCULATORY	
Decreased respiratory capacity, reduced efficiency, reduced oxygen to the CNS and other tissues	Altered mentation or personality, decreased exercise tolerance, decreased activity, CDS signs
Anemia, cardiac disease, hypertensive and hypotensive diseases, decreased CNS perfusion	Altered mentation or personality, decreased exercise tolerance, decreased activity, CDS signs
UROGENITAL	
Decline in renal function, incontinence, infection	Polyuria, decreased control, housesoiling
Prostatic hypertrophy	May affect frequency and control of urine or stools
ENDOCRINE	

Decreased gonadal production
Functional testicular tumors in 60% of older dogs:
    Ovarian tumors – granulosa cell
    Thecoma
	Sertoli cell tumor, effects of increased estrogens, male feminizing syndrome, e.g., mounting by males
	Thecoma/interstitial cell tumor – effects of testosterone increase; marking, increased aggression
	Granulosa – persistent estrus, anestrus, aggression

Hyperadrenocorticism	Panting, polyphagia, restlessness, waking, altered elimination habits, CDS signs
Diabetes mellitus, insulinoma, hyper/hypothyroid, parathyroid disorders, hypoadrenocorticism	Behavioral effect depends on hormone affected
MUSCULOSKELETAL	
Decreased muscle and bone mass, degenerative joint disease, neuromuscular deterioration	Weakness/decreased mobility, increased pain, irritability, and aggression, housesoiling
NERVOUS SYSTEM	
Altered neurotransmitter function affecting cholinergic, dopaminergic, serotonergic, noradrenergic transmission	Signs associated with CDS involving learning, memory, disorientation, sleep–wake cycles, social interactions, activity, altered mentation or personality
Neuromuscular dysfunction – tremors	Weakness, decreased mobility, housesoiling
Primary or secondary intracranial neoplasia	CDS signs – see Figure 12.4, seizure-related signs
Age-related pathology – brain hypoxia	CDS signs – see Figure 12.4
CNS effects secondary to hypoxia, electrolyte disturbances, tumors, toxic effects of organ failure	CDS signs – see Figure 12.4
SPECIAL SENSES	
Decreased sight/smell/hearing	Increased irritability/anxiety, decreased response to stimuli, increased vocalization, altered sleep–wake cycle, decreased ability to perform tasks, change in appetite

Figure 12.12   Effects of age on the behavior of geriatric pets.

epilepsy, and hepatic disease, while cats are most likely to die from cancer, renal failure, cardiovascular disease, or diabetes mellitus.

Any condition that is associated with pain or discomfort (e.g., arthritis, dental disease) can lead to increased irritability or fear of being handled. If mobility is affected, the pet may become increasingly aggressive rather than retreat. A decrease in mobility could also reduce the pet's ability to access its elimination area. Dogs with impaired sight or hearing might be either less responsive or more reactive to stimuli. The family's recognition of visual and hearing impairment in older dogs ranged from 41% of 11- to 12-year-old dogs to 68% of 15- to 16-year-old dogs for vision, and from 48% of 11- to 12-year-old dogs to 97% of 15- to 16-year-old dogs for hearing. Organ failure, tumors, degenerative conditions, immune diseases, neurological deterioration, and endocrinopathies are more common in the aging pet, and can have profound effects on behavior. For example, diseases of the urinary tract can cause or contribute to inappropriate urination. Any disease that affects the central nervous system or its circulation, whether directly (tumors) or indirectly (e.g., anemia), can affect behavior. Behavior changes ranging from lethargy to aggression have been reported in hypothyroid dogs, while Cushinoid dogs may exhibit altered sleep–wake cycles, lethargy, housesoiling, panting, and polyphagia. Hyperthyroid cats may be more active or irritable, and may have increased appetite. For a more detailed look at possible medical differentials see Figure 12.12.

Cognitive dysfunction syndrome

When the behavioral signs are due to the effects of aging on the brain, this is referred to as cognitive dysfunction syndrome. The diagnosis of cognitive dysfunction is made by exclusion. This is done by ruling out medical problems for a pet that is presented with signs consistent with impaired cognitive function. If there is the presence of one or more clinical signs in a cognitive screening checklist and no underlying

medical causes for the signs can be identified on physical examination and diagnostic tests, the owner can then be asked to fill out a more comprehensive checklist to determine all of the signs that might be consistent with cognitive dysfunction (Fig. 12.4). Primary behavioral conditions are also a possibility, so additional history may be required to rule out any changes in the pet's environment, household, or relationships that might account for the behavioral changes. The cognitive questionnaire can also be used to track response to therapy.

Medical contributing factors: surpassing the threshold

The threshold theory, as it applies to dermatology, is that each animal will tolerate a certain number of pruritic stimuli without itching. However, when stimulation exceeds the threshold, or when multiple stimuli (e.g., allergens) act together, clinical pruritus may be exhibited. Similarly it may take multiple stimuli to 'push' the pet beyond a threshold to where a behavior problem is exhibited. Medical conditions might also lower the threshold or level of tolerance. This is especially important in aging pets, where organ decline, sensory decline, painful conditions, age-related nervous system pathology, and an increasing number of medical problems can all affect behavior. For example, a pet that is fearful of children, but has never before displayed aggression, may begin to threaten or bite as it becomes more uncomfortable (as with dental disease) or less mobile (as with arthritis). Cats that are anxious but do not spray when other cats enter the property may begin to spray if they develop hyperthyroidism.

Primary behavior problems

Changes in the pet's environment may also contribute to the emergence of behavior problems. Schedule changes, a new member of the household (e.g., baby, spouse), a new pet, or moving can have a dramatic impact on a pet's behavior. Medical or degenerative changes associated with aging may cause the pet to be more sensitive or less adaptable to change. Many owners then inadvertently reward the undesirable behavior or become anxious or upset about the problem, which adds to the pet's anxiety. In addition, the owners may attempt to punish the pet for undesirable behavior, which might lead to further anxiety and conflict on the part of the pet. Some behavioral signs such as disorientation and decreased responsiveness to stimuli are not likely to be primary behavior problems. However repetitive, stereotypic, or compulsive behaviors, waking at night, housesoiling, and increased irritability, anxiety, and phobias could all be primary behavior problems. Of course, concurrent medical, physical, and cognitive changes would have a further impact on the expression (and prognosis and treatment) of these behavioral changes. Diagnosing a behavior problem requires intensive history taking, with particular emphasis on the onset and progression of the problem.

PRESENTING COMPLAINT – DIAGNOSTIC CONSIDERATIONS

Anxiety (including separation anxiety)

Increasing anxiety is a relatively common complaint of owners of older pets. Increasing sensitivity to stimuli, increasing fear (with or without aggression) of unfamiliar pets and unfamiliar people, increased irritability, and decreased tolerance of handling and restraint, increased following and desire for contact, and increasing anxiety during owner departures are some of the more common family concerns. Medical problems that affect CNS function including cognitive dysfunction, decreased sensory acuity, endocrine imbalances (hypothyroidism, hyperthyroidism, Cushing's disease), painful conditions such as arthritis and dental disease, and any condition that might have an impact on urine or stool control can contribute to the development of many of these signs. The owner's response to the pet then further molds the behavior. Owner anxiety, frustration, or distress over

the pet's behavior may further add to the pet's anxiety, while giving attention to the pet (perhaps in an attempt to calm it down) may reinforce the behavior. Noise sensitivity, perhaps related to hearing loss, may lead to increased anxiety and vocalization in some dogs.

Although the signs of separation anxiety in the older dog may be similar to those in younger dogs (i.e., hyperattachment when the owners are home, anxiety in the form of destructiveness, vocalization, housesoiling, salivation prior to and during owner departures), the cause is usually quite different. Of course it is possible that there has been a change in the owner's schedule or daily routine, and the older pet may have difficulty adapting to the new schedule or routine. However, due to medical problems or age-related cognitive changes, some older pets may be less tolerant of being left alone or may learn to increasingly seek out family members. The attention the pets receive reinforces the behavior. Over time, these pets then become increasingly anxious when the family leaves them alone. Crating or confinement of an older pet to deal with one behavior problem, such as housesoiling, may lead to anxiety and escape attempts, especially if it is an older pet that is not used to confinement, cannot get comfortable in the crate, or cannot control its urine or stools while in the crate. It is the confinement, not the owner absence, that may be leading to the anxiety in these cases. Therefore, the history, physical assessment, and findings of diagnostic testing as well as perhaps a videotape of the pet's behavior during departure are useful in making a diagnosis and developing a treatment plan. On review of a video, the owner might note that the anxiety is related to specific stimuli (noises, people coming onto the property) or that the clinical signs begin well after the owner's departure (which might indicate another cause for the signs). One of the most important factors in diagnosis is whether the pet exhibits any of these signs (anxiety, salivation, destructive behavior, vocalization, or housesoiling) while family members are at home and has access to them. If this is the case a cause other than separation anxiety should be considered.

Excessive vocalization

In both cats and dogs, vocalization may become a problem if it is increased, uncontrollable, or occurs at inappropriate times (e.g., at night). Sensory dysfunction (particularly auditory dysfunction), age-related cognitive dysfunction, CNS pathology, and age-related medical conditions may contribute to increased anxiety, noise sensitivity, and vocalization in older dogs and cats. Vocalization that is primarily a problem when the owners are absent might be related to separation anxiety (discussed above). Vocalization associated with anxiety is generally a plaintiff howl, or excessive whining. If the excessive vocalization occurs when the owners are at home, then the history will need to be evaluated to determine when and under what circumstances the dog or cat vocalizes. Cats or dogs with polyphagia might vocalize in an attempt to acquire food, which might then be reinforced if the owners acquiesce. Dogs might vocalize as a form of signaling if they have an increase in volume, frequency, or urge to eliminate. Painful conditions might lead to increased vocalization, which might be exacerbated by certain types of movement or handling. Dogs may begin to vocalize in response to specific stimuli (noises, visitors), as they become more fearful or anxious. In addition, both dogs and cats may begin to vocalize and wake the owners at night (see below). If the owner then attends to the vocalizing pet or tries to quiet the pet with food or toys, the behavior has been reinforced. Owner anxiety and punishment may increase the pet's anxiety and further aggravate the problem.

Restlessness/waking at nights

Dogs and cats that are restless or do not sleep through the night should be closely evaluated for medical problems that might lead to an increased frequency of elimination, restlessness, or discomfort. Sensory changes can affect the pet's depth of sleep. With age there may also be altered sleep–wake cycles and decreased REM sleep, which may be a component of cognitive dysfunction or other forms of CNS pathol-

ogy. Pets that sleep more during the day and evening hours may be more awake through the night. In dogs, an altered response to environmental stimuli, such as paper delivery or a garage door opening, may trigger nocturnal activity and vocalization. Keeping a diary may be helpful for identifying that type of problem.

Housesoiling

Housesoiling in dogs and cats may be indicative of a variety of medical problems in the older pet. Sensory decline, painful neurological or neuromuscular conditions that affect mobility, age-related cognitive dysfunction, other forms of CNS pathology, any medical condition that might affect behavior (e.g., endocrinopathies, hepatic encephalopathy), and medical conditions that increase the frequency of elimination or cause a decrease in control may all be contributing factors. In cats, litter avoidance may arise from medical problems that make accessing the litterbox difficult, uncomfortable, or more frightening (e.g., sensory decline, arthritis, obesity, conflict with other cats). Pets with disease conditions that affect the CNS (e.g., brain tumors, cognitive dysfunction) may begin to eliminate in the home, often in more random locations. This may be a more significant sign of cognitive dysfunction in dogs than in cats, since there may be numerous learned components including (a) voluntary control of elimination when the pet feels the urge, (b) signaling the family to be taken outdoors to eliminate, (c) seeking out the appropriate location, (d) responding to an elimination command (if trained in this manner), and (e) voluntarily voiding at the appropriate site. Housesoiling may also be a sign of cognitive dysfunction, but is more likely to be associated with advanced disease so that other signs are likely to be present. Housesoiling in dogs that occurs only when the dog has no access to the owner, such as when the owner departs, may also be a component of separation anxiety. However, just because a pet only eliminates when the owner is away from home is not diagnostic of separation anxiety. Many pets do not soil when the owners are at home because the owners are available to take the dog outdoors to eliminate or change the cat's litter and most pets will inhibit indoor elimination when the owner is present. In separation anxiety, there would generally be some other indication of anxiety as the owner prepares to leave or shortly after the owner departs. Crating the pet may lead to further anxiety, which could add to the elimination problem.

Although a change in schedule, environmental change, new sources of conflict or stress may contribute to housesoiling (including marking), aging may contribute to the problem as the pet becomes more rigid and less adaptable to change. Once a pet uses an indoor location when the owner is not around, a new indoor toilet area will have been established and, even with sufficient cleaning, the pet may continue to use this new site.

In addition to the medical assessment and diagnostics, the history is often critical in reaching a diagnosis, and in the older pet there may be multiple contributing factors. It will be necessary to determine whether there is a marking component, when the pet eliminates (owner present or absent), where the pet eliminates, and whether there is a random distribution, whether there is any evidence of incontinence, whether there are other concurrent changes in health or behavior, whether there were any obvious changes in the pet or the household when the problem began, and details on the family's attempts to alter the behavior to date (including what has worked, made no difference, or aggravated the problem).

Destructive behavior

Destructive behavior may have a variety of presentations, each with a different possible cause. For example, picas, licking, sucking or chewing of household objects (or family members or self-directed), scratching and digging may all have different causes. In addition, whether these problems are exhibited in the owner's presence, absence or both may indicate different etiologies. In dogs, destructiveness at doorways, win-

dows, and exit points (e.g., from a room or crate) might be indicative of separation anxiety, increased anxiety, and defensiveness in response to external stimuli or escape behavior (as might be associated with confinement or noise phobias). Combining the medical evaluation with the findings of the medical and behavioral history should help to determine the list of diagnoses that need to be considered. If other medical problems have been ruled out, cognitive dysfunction may be a consideration for pets with increased licking, chewing, or picas. Anxiety and conflict may also be a factor.

Fears and phobias

A number of medical and age-related conditions might cause or contribute to phobias. These might include sensory dysfunction (which might increase or decrease phobias), cognitive dysfunction, and other forms of age-related brain pathology. The locus ceruleus and its neurotransmitter noradrenaline are vital in the genesis of fear and panic, so that age-related changes that affect the limbic system, the locus ceruleus, and noradrenaline transmission can either aggravate or reduce fearful and phobic responses. Anxiety may also be influenced by other medical conditions that lead to pain or discomfort, endocrinopathies, and organ failure. Fearful responses may then be further reinforced or aggravated by the consequences of the pet's behavior. Owners may inadvertently reinforce the behavioral responses by trying to calm or comfort the pet, while owner anxiety or punishment in response to the pet's behavior might further aggravate the problem. Although excessive reactivity to noise and thunderstorms appears to be the most common phobias of older dogs, other less common presentations might include fear of going outdoors, entering certain rooms, or walking on certain types of surfaces. Excessively fearful and even aggressive responses may be seen in cats in response to certain stimuli (including noise) due to medical causes, anxiety, and conflict, or some combination of these.

Compulsive and stereotypic behaviors

Compulsive and stereotypic behaviors encompass a wide spectrum of behaviors with numerous causative factors. Conflict, stress, or anxiety-producing stimuli or situations may lead to displacement and redirected behavior, which over time might become compulsive. Owner responses may further reinforce or aggravate the problem. Medical conditions, cognitive dysfunction, and other related brain pathology and alterations in neurotransmitters may cause or contribute to the problem in the aging pet.

Aggression

Aggression may also arise in the older pet, although it is much more common earlier in life as the pet grows and matures. Aggression to family members may arise from changes in family makeup, such as the birth of a new baby or marriage, or other changes in the schedule or household that lead to increasing anxiety or conflict. Aggression to other family pets might arise from the introduction or maturation of a younger pet, or aging-related changes in the older pet that alter the way in which the pet responds to, or interacts with, the other family pets. Increased aggression toward unfamiliar animals and people may result from increasing anxiety and sensitivity to stimuli with age. In addition to the effects of any new sources of conflict, anxiety, or stress, the pet's health and cognitive status may cause or influence aggression. Medical conditions affecting appetite, mobility, cognition, sensory function, or hormonal status, and conditions leading to increased pain or irritability, might contribute to an increase in aggression.

TREATMENT OF COGNITIVE DYSFUNCTION

If medical problems have been ruled out and cognitive dysfunction is a presumptive diagnosis, then a therapeutic trial with selegiline and an antioxidant-fortified senior diet should be implemented in an attempt to improve the clinical signs and perhaps slow the progress of the disease. There is also good evidence that, as in people, continued stimulation in the form of games, play, training, and exercise can help to maintain cognitive function (i.e., use it or lose it). Pets diagnosed with medical problems and/or primary behavioral problems can also have concurrent cognitive dysfunction. Although it might be prudent to maintain an older pet on long-

---

Management of behavior problems in senior pets

1. Treat underlying medical problems (resolution or improvement will not be possible for many medical conditions). Therefore, the owner's expectations and the environment may need to be modified to meet the needs or limitations of some senior pets
2. Treat cognitive dysfunction if present or suspected. This may lead to an improvement in clinical signs. Retraining may not be possible if cognitive function is impaired
3. Assess response to therapy
    i) If behavioral signs have been resolved following medical treatment, then the medical problem or cognitive dysfunction has likely been the cause of the behavioral problem
    ii) If there has been some, but incomplete improvement then review the diagnosis to determine if there are additional contributing problems that might be improved with treatment
    iii) Consider the impact of any drug, dietary, or alternative therapy on behavior, and if this is a factor consider whether an alternative drug or dose might be appropriate and whether the benefits outweigh any side effects
    iv) Review the progress of the problem as there may be learned and conditioned factors that will also need to be addressed with behavior therapy and environmental modification
4. Treat primary or secondary behavior problems
5. Continue play, exercise and training through life (use it or lose it)

Figure 12.13

term therapy in an attempt to slow the progress of disease, many owners may not want to continue the treatment unless there is some evidence of improvement in the pet's condition. The cognitive dysfunction checklist can be used as an assessment baseline and then filled out after a specified course of treatment to determine if there is any improvement or deterioration (Fig. 12.4).

Selegiline

Selegiline is a selective and irreversible inhibitor of MAOB in the dog. It is the only drug presently licensed for the treatment of cognitive dysfunction in North America, and has been shown to be effective in placebo-controlled drug trials in 69–75% of patients. In a recent field trial, 641 dogs showed an overall improvement of 77% at day 60. In this latter study, activity and sleep–wake cycles were improved in 67% of dogs, while 78% of dogs with confusion or disorientation showed improvement (Campbell et al 2001).

Although the mechanisms by which selegiline produces clinical improvement in dogs with CDS are not clearly understood, enhancement of dopamine and perhaps other catecholamines in the cortex and hippocampus is presumed to be an important factor. Selegiline may help to restore dopamine balance through its actions as an MAOB inhibitor. In rodent studies, selegiline has also been shown to enhance dopamine synthesis, increase the release of dopamine into the synapse, and decrease the presynaptic re-uptake of dopamine. Recent human studies with a dopamine receptor agonist piribedil have shown significant short-term improvement in patients with mild cognitive impairment, suggesting that dopamine insufficiency plays some role in age-related cognitive impairment. Dopamine depletion has not, however, been identified in the elderly dog. Selegiline has also been shown to increase 2-phenylethylamine (PEA) in the dog brain. PEA is a neuromodulator that enhances dopamine and catecholamine function and may itself enhance cognitive func-

tion. Selegiline may also alleviate CDS through a number of other mechanisms. Release of noradrenaline may be enhanced, and re-uptake of noradrenaline may be inhibited. Catecholamine enhancement may lead to improved neuronal impulse transmission. Selegiline metabolites, l-amphetamine, and l-methamphetamine may also enhance cognitive function.

Selegiline may contribute to a decrease in free radical load in the brain. Free radicals are oxygen-containing molecules that may contribute to aging and the development of neurodegenerative disorders. Because MAOB is inhibited, fewer toxic free radicals may be produced. Selegiline may directly scavenge free radicals and enhance scavenging enzymes such as catalase and superoxide dismutase (SOD). SOD is increased in dogs on selegiline therapy. Selegiline also has neuroprotective effects on dopaminergic, noradrenergic, and cholinergic neurons. For example, it has been shown to protect against the toxic effects of the neurotoxin MPTP (l-methyl-4-phenyl-1,2,3,6 tetrahydropyridine).

Some dogs improve within the first two weeks, while a few do not show improvement until the second month. For CDS, selegiline is dosed at 0.5–1 mg/kg each morning and, if there is no significant improvement in 30 days, the dose can be adjusted up to the next tablet size for another month. Although not licensed for cats, selegiline has been reported to improve signs of cognitive dysfunction in cats, most of which were 14 years of age or older. Signs that have been improved include increased irritability, increased vocalization, disorientation, aimless pacing or wandering, stereotypic behavior such as circling and staring into space, decreased affection, housesoiling, decreased appetite, and overgrooming. There have been no reported adverse effects except occasional gastrointestinal upset, despite the presence of concurrent illnesses in some cats (seizures, chronic renal failure, and hyperthyroidism).

For more details on selegiline's other applications and drug contraindications and side effects, see Chapter 6.

Nutritional and dietary therapy

Two strategies have been utilized to try and prevent the production of damaging free radicals within animals. The first is caloric restriction, which is well known to extend lifespan in all species studied to date. The second is administration of supplemental antioxidants, with the idea of improving the endogenous antioxidant defenses and mitigating the effects of free radicals.

The use of antioxidants to decrease free radical damage may slow cognitive decline as well as improve the behavioral signs associated with cognitive dysfunction syndrome. Antioxidants act to scavenge and minimize production of reactive oxygen species, bind metal ions that may make poorly reactive species more toxic, and repair damage to target tissues. One study found that high doses of vitamin E (2000 IU per day) may slow the progression of Alzheimer's disease. Vitamin E acts to protect cell membranes from oxidative damage by scavenging radicals within membranes and interrupting lipid peroxidation. More recently, in a non-controlled study, the addition of the mitochondrial cofactor/antioxidant lipoic acid to the diet of patients with Alzheimer's slowed progression of behavioral signs. Finally, a variety of studies in other species have shown that high intakes of fruits and vegetables, or vitamin E and C, decrease the risk for developing age-related cognitive decline. Interpretation of the above data would indicate that antioxidants appear to work in a networking type of fashion, and thus complex mixtures may be of more benefit than single source additions.

A recent development in canine preventive health care is a senior diet supplemented with antioxidants, mitochondrial cofactors, and essential fatty acids (Hill's canine b/d®), which has been shown to improve the performance of a number of cognitive tasks when compared with older dogs on a non-supplemented diet (Figs 12.2, 12.14). In the study, 48 older dogs (seven to 11 years of age) were trained on a series of problem-solving tasks in which they had to make correct choices to get a food reward. The

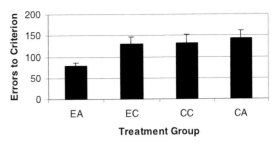

Figure 12.14 Long-term effects of food and cognitive enrichment on object reversal and size reversal learning. EA = cognitive enrichment and antioxidant food, EC = cognitive enrichment and control food, CC = no enrichment and control food, CA = no enrichment and antioxidant fortified food. (Courtesy of NW Milgram, Department of Psychology, University of Toronto, Scarorough, Ont.)

dogs were then divided into four groups: one with environmental enrichment (i.e., exercise, novel play toys, and continued testing); one with an antioxidant-enriched diet but no ongoing testing; one with the enriched diet and ongoing testing; and a control group. Over 30 months the dogs were tested on a number of tasks and in each case the dogs on the enriched diet outperformed the dogs on the control diet. In addition, at 12 and 24 months the dogs in the enriched behavior program were tested against the dogs that had received no enrichment and the dogs that had a combination of the enriched diet and environmental enrichment performed the best. In placebo-controlled home trials, the diet led to improvement in older dogs with disorientation, interaction with the owners or other pets, sleep patterns, housesoiling, and altered activity levels. In addition to vitamin E, the diet is supplemented with antioxidants including vitamin C (which helps to regenerate vitamin E), and a number of flavonoids and carotenoids from fruits and vegetables that help to inactivate free radicals such as spinach flakes, tomato pomace, grape pomace, carrot granules, and citrus pulp. The addition of lipoic acid and l-carnitine is intended to enhance mitochondrial function, and the addition of omega-3 fatty acids helps to promote cell membrane health. Human studies have also found that omega-3 fatty acids may be helpful in the treatment of dementia. In theory, similar dietary adjustments for cats may also have beneficial effects in preventing or reducing signs of cognitive decline, but this has not been studied to date.

Other medications for cognitive dysfunction

A number of other medications or supplements are either licensed in other countries or might be considered for the treatment of cognitive dysfunction in dogs based on findings in other species.

Nicergoline is an alpha 1 and alpha 2 adrenergic antagonist that is available in the UK for the treatment of aging-related behavior disorders in dogs. It may increase cerebral blood flow, enhance neuronal transmission, and have a neuroprotective effect on neural cells. It may also increase dopamine and noradrenaline turnover and inhibit platelet aggregation (Fitergol®, Rhone Merieux health registration document, UK). The drug is recommended for elderly dogs with decreased activity, sleep disorders, decreased exercise tolerance, housesoiling (including incontinence), reduced appetite, and decreased awareness. In one open label trial there was an overall improvement of 75% over 30 days, but this was not compared with placebo. The suggested dose is 0.25–0.5 mg/kg/day each morning for 30 days and then maintained if effective. Although cerebral vasodilators in general have not been effective in Alzheimer's patients, some clinical improvement has recently been demonstrated with nicergoline in human cases of vascular and degenerative dementia.

Nylidrin hydrochloride (Arlidin®, Rhone-Poulenc Rohrer), a beta-adrenergic agonist, is a vasodilator that may also be useful in improving cerebral blood flow. It has been effective in improving mental alertness in human patients with mild to moderate symptoms of cognitive impairment, and may therefore be a consideration in some dogs with cognitive dysfunction. A dose of 3–6 mg three times per day per dog has

been suggested, although there are no published safety or efficacy studies in dogs and cats.

Propentofylline is licensed for the treatment of dullness and lethargy in old dogs in a number of European countries including the UK, Germany, and Spain. It has been advocated to increase oxygen supply to the CNS without increasing glucose demand, and there is weak evidence that it may also slow the progression of Alzheimer's in people. It is purported to inhibit platelet aggregation and thrombus formation, make the red cell more pliable, and increase blood flow. It is dosed at 3 mg/kg bid in dogs (Karvisan®, Germany; Vivitonin®, UK – Hoechst Rousell Product Monograph). In North America, where propentofylline is not available, there have been anecdotal reports of improvement with pentoxifylline, which may also have effects on blood flow and inflammation.

Drugs that may enhance the noradrenergic system, such as adrafanil and modafinil, might be useful in older dogs to improve alertness and help maintain normal sleep–wake cycles (by increasing daytime exploration and activity). The noradrenergic systems help to maintain alertness, wakefulness, attention, memory and learning, and neuroprotection. With age, alterations in the noradrenergic system may contribute to declining cognitive function, decreased alertness, mood alterations, as well as neurodegenerative diseases. Adrafanil is licensed for humans in Europe to improve alertness in the elderly. In laboratory studies in dogs adrafanil has been shown to have cognitive enhancing potential. In open field testing in dogs adrafanil caused increased locomotion without producing stereotypical activity at a dose of 20 mg/kg and higher at both two and 10 hours postdosing.

In a recent comparative study by Siwak et al (2000b) at the University of Toronto, dogs aged nine to 16 years were given either adrafanil at 20 mg/kg daily, propentofylline at 5 mg/kg bid or nicergoline at 0.5 mg/kg daily for 33 days. Treatment with adrafanil led to a significant increase in locomotion, which was unaffected by nicergoline or propentofylline.

Tacrine is a cholinergic agent that is being used in humans in an attempt to slow cognitive decline, but improvements have been modest and the drug can cause gastrointestinal upset, hepatic dysfunction, and headaches. Donepezil HCl is an acetylcholinesterase inhibitor that has led to modest improvement in some humans with dementia of the Alzheimer type, although there is no evidence that it alters the underlying pathophysiologic process. Common side effects included nausea, vomiting, diarrhea, sleep–wake disturbances, headache, and other non-specific pains. The authors are unaware of any reports of safety or efficacy in dogs and there is no data to support their use.

Ginkgo biloba and phosphatidylserine are natural supplements that might be considered for cognitive dysfunction in pets. There is some evidence in humans that Ginkgo biloba may improve some cases of Alzheimer's disease or delay its progression. Ginkgo biloba is licensed in Germany for the treatment of humans with cerebral dysfunction related to vascular insufficiency or depression and the early stages of Alzheimer's disease. The mechanisms of action may include reversible MAO inhibition, and free radical scavenging. Phosphatidylserine is a membrane phospholipid that is purported to facilitate neuronal activities such as signal transduction, and it might help to maintain normal neurotransmitter levels (acetylcholine and dopamine). Also, see Chapter 7.

In humans, women develop Alzheimer's three times more frequently than males, but by the age of 84, men and women are affected equally. In recent studies, evidence to support the use of estrogen therapy in postmenopausal women with Alzheimer's disease could not be validated, although there may be a protective effect prior to the onset of memory decline. Estrogen may have an anti-inflammatory effect as well as antioxidative effects, and may lead to an increase in cerebral blood flow. In dogs, estrogen-treated females made significantly fewer errors in a size-reversal learning task than estrogen-treated males or placebo-treated males and females. However, estrogen-treated aged females made more errors in spatial memory tasks than estrogen-treated males and controls. In a recent study of a small group of

dogs, intact aging male dogs showed less evidence of cognitive impairment than neutered dogs. Recent studies in humans may support testosterone as being neuroprotective against Alzheimer's. If supplementation is considered with testosterone or estrogen, they should only be given at physiologic levels since high levels can be toxic.

Other homeopathic and natural supplements that have been suggested for calming, reducing anxiety, or inducing sleep include melatonin, valerian, D.A.P.™, Feliway™, and Bach's flower remedies. Anti-inflammatory drugs may also be effective in improving cognitive dysfunction.

Alterations in neurotransmitters or their receptor sites may lead to behavior changes such as increased irritability, decreased responsiveness to stimuli, fear, agitation, and altered sleep–wake cycles. Although pets with these problems may improve with selegiline therapy, antidepressants and anxiolytics might also be a consideration. Since the elderly are particularly susceptible to the effects of anticholinergic drugs, it would be prudent when selecting this class of drugs for older pets to consider those with less anticholinergic effects and less sedation when there is an option. Therefore, serotonin re-uptake inhibitors such as fluoxetine, fluvoxamine, or paroxetine and the non-sedating anxiolytic buspirone might have the least potential for side effects. In addition, a lower initial dose should be utilized and the drug slowly increased if necessary. Elderly patients may have decreased hepatic function, which can result in decreased clearance of drugs such as diazepam and clorazepate. These are drugs that are metabolized by oxidative pathways to active intermediate metabolites in the liver. Therefore, when benzodiazepines are considered in the senior pet for anxiety or inducing sleep, oxazepam and lorazepam, which have no active intermediate metabolites, might be safest. In humans, clonazepam, gabapentin, or carbamazepine might be considered to stabilize mood and treat aggression in the elderly and may therefore be a consideration in elderly dogs with dementia or anxiety disorders.

TREATMENT OF SPECIFIC BEHAVIOR PROBLEMS OF GERIATRIC DOGS AND CATS

Treatment will vary based on diagnosis. Treating or controlling underlying medical problems including cognitive dysfunction and treating primary behavioral problems are relatively straightforward. However, as mentioned, the senior pet may have a combination of many medical and behavioral factors that will need to be assessed and treated both individually and in combination.

For most behavior problems in senior pets, the behavioral program (behavior modification, environmental modification, surgery, and drugs) will be similar regardless of age. However, in the older pet, it will be increasingly more likely that some form of medical therapy will need to be implemented to control underlying health problems. If these medical problems cannot be entirely controlled, then this must be taken into account with respect to behavioral management. For example, in cats and dogs with renal failure, litterbox management and access to elimination areas will need to be modified to adjust for this increased volume and frequency, there will likely be a need for more frequent cleaning, additional litterboxes, a larger litterbox, and perhaps a relocation of the litterboxes to accommodate the larger volume of urine and more frequent need to eliminate. In dogs with renal failure, more frequent access to elimination areas or a new indoor toilet area may need to be provided. Not only will the pet's health have an impact on the behavioral program, it will also have an impact on what might be achieved. In addition, any drugs needed to control underlying medical problems may have an impact on behavior or the techniques that will need to be utilized. Another important consideration is the selection of drugs for behavioral modification, as some medications may have greater potential for adverse effects (e.g., anticholinergic drugs) or may be entirely contraindicated with certain medical conditions or with other drugs that are being utilized.

Anxiety (including separation anxiety)

Treatment for both dogs and cats involves controlling underlying medical problems and identifying and correcting any owner responses that might be reinforcing or aggravating the behavior. Behavior modification and environmental modifications for various forms of anxiety are discussed in appropriate sections throughout this text. For example, dogs with signs of separation anxiety will need to be taught to settle and relax for progressively longer periods of time away from the owner. It may not be possible to leave the older pet alone as long because of the need for additional opportunities to eliminate, so that a midday visit, doggie door, or a papered indoor elimination area may be necessary. For cats attention on demand must be avoided and the owner should initiate regular and structured play and interaction throughout the day, along with some simple reward-based training for commands. Pheromones and drugs to reduce anxiety and improve the pet's cognitive function may also be needed to improve outcome (see Ch. 11 for more details on separation anxiety).

Excessive vocalization

In addition to treating underlying medical problems and cognitive dysfunction, treatment generally requires identifying and correcting any owner responses that might be reinforcing or aggravating the behavior. For dogs, bark control collars (non-shock) and bark control training as discussed in the section on vocalization may be useful, while cats can be disrupted in the act with a water sprayer or compressed air. Non-vocal behavior should then be reinforced. Concurrent drug therapy may also be required if there is an anxiety or cognitive component to the problem. Pets that vocalize when they should otherwise be sleeping through the night are discussed below (see Chs 13, 14 for more information on the diagnosis and treatment of excessive vocalization in dogs and cats).

Housesoiling

Because there may be numerous factors that cause or influence housesoiling, the treatment program will vary by diagnosis. Cognitive dysfunction and medical problems should be treated with appropriate drugs or diet. However, once the inappropriate elimination or litter avoidance has been established, additional behavioral and environmental management will likely also be needed. Addressing any initiating or maintaining factors that still remain should be the first issue. For example, housesoiling due to anxiety requires treatment of the underlying issues that are leading to anxiety. Pets with polyuria will have a need to void more frequently. The frequency of defecation may also increase due to medical problems or a change to higher fiber diet. In cats, more frequent litterbox cleaning, additional litterboxes, a larger litterbox, and perhaps a relocation of the litterboxes to areas of easy access may be necessary. In dogs that have been trained to eliminate outdoors, the owners may need to change their schedule to accommodate the dog's need for more frequent elimination. Alternately they may need to provide a dog door or an indoor toileting (e.g., paper training) area. Musculoskeletal problems, such as weakness, muscular atrophy, and arthritis, can make it difficult for the dog to get outdoors to eliminate or for the cat to navigate stairs to get to its litterbox. Medication to control pain, carpet runners on stairs for traction, and control of obesity might help. Adjusting the height, size, or location of the litterbox may increase a cat's ability or desire to use its litterbox.

Once the pet's medical needs have been met, it will also be necessary to re-establish proper training by increasing indoor supervision and immediately taking the dog outdoors if there are any signs that elimination is needed, re-establishing a routine and schedule by taking the dog outdoors as often as necessary and rewarding outdoor use, and confinement (with or without paper for elimination) of the dog away from previously soiled sites. Similarly cats may need to be supervised to prevent inappropriate elimination and may have to be confined away from previously soiled sites when the owner cannot supervise. If there is evidence of cognitive decline then drug and/or dietary therapy may be useful to improve the success of retraining (see Chs 17, 18 for more information on the diagnosis and treatment of elimination problems in dogs and cats).

Destructive behavior

Treatment will need to first address the underlying cause of the destructiveness. Treatment of underlying medical problems and cognitive dysfunction may resolve some problems, but will not be successful for all cases. Treatments of destructive behavior caused by separation anxiety, phobias, or fear-evoking stimuli are discussed elsewhere in this text. Medical problems such as cognitive dysfunction should be addressed. Preventing access to sites or objects where inappropriate destruction might occur, using deterrents or booby traps to keep pets away from problem areas, utilizing preventive techniques such as confinement, and providing novel and appealing alternatives for chewing may need to be considered (see Ch. 5 for more information).

Restlessness/waking at nights

If medical problems or cognitive dysfunction are a factor, they will first need to be treated. However, many medical problems of the elderly pet cannot be entirely resolved and once the altered cycle has been established the owner will need to try and re-establish a normal sleep–wake cycle.

Increasing daytime and evening activity and limiting daytime sleep may help to re-establish sleep through the night. Drugs to induce sleep or alternatively to keep the pet more alert and active during the daytime may be needed to complement this therapy. Attention-seeking behavior must be ignored and not reinforced (e.g., locking it out of the room) or disrupted using a device such as a water gun, compressed air canister, an audible alarm or an ultrasonic alarm. SSRIs such as fluoxetine might help re-establish normal sleep–wake cycles. Sedating hypnotic benzodiazepines or even an antihistamine such as diphenhydramine might be useful to help induce sleep for a few nights until night-time sleep can be re-established. Increased day-time activity and a normalization of circadian rhythms might be re-established with drugs, diets, or supplements that enhance cognitive function or that increase daytime activity (such as adrafanil).

Fears and phobias

Treatment requires that underlying medical problems and cognitive dysfunction first be controlled. Noise phobias in dogs may begin as sensory dysfunction declines, although with further loss of hearing the problem might ultimately be resolved. Housing the pet away from stimuli, masking the stimuli with background music, training the pet to calm and settle in the rest area, using cues to condition a pleasant response, and drug therapy or pheromone therapy for panic and anxiety might be utilized. Owners must ensure that their responses do not further aggravate or reinforce the behavior. Also see Chapter 11 for treatment of specific fears and phobias.

Compulsive and stereotypic behaviors

Treatment would require controlling or resolving underlying medical problems including cognitive dysfunction, identifying and correcting any source of conflict or anxiety, correcting any owner responses that might be aggravating or reinforcing the problem, finding alternative forms of stimulation to occupy and calm the pet, and drugs that would treat the underlying neuropathology. A more comprehensive review of the treatment of compulsive disorders is discussed in Chapter 10.

Aggression

The contribution of medical problems (including pain) and cognitive dysfunction to the development and perpetuation of aggression may be difficult to assess until treatment has been implemented and any improvement can be evaluated. Of course, medical problems that cannot be entirely resolved, such as a decline in sensory function, may contribute to a more guarded prognosis or limitations in what can be achieved. Prevention by avoiding situations that trigger aggression may be the best option for some of these pets. Aggression in the older pet is often associated with anxiety, so drugs that reduce anxiety or improve serotonergic transmission may prove to be helpful.

Aggression cannot be effectively treated until a proper diagnosis is made and the cause of the aggression has been determined. Drug selection, behavior therapy, and environmental modification for specific types of aggression are discussed in detail in the sections on aggression. For example, the treatment program for fear-related aggression involves desensitization and counterconditioning, as well as training the pet to be more responsive to the owner's commands so that appropriate behavior can be achieved in the presence of the stimulus. Head halters can provide control, safety, and enhance the owner's ability to immediately and effectively communicate with the pet.

Whether medical problems are a factor or not, learning and conditioning are likely to have an impact on the development and perpetuation of the problem. Therefore, the family's response to the pet's behavior should be assessed to see whether it may be aggravating the problems or reinforcing undesirable behavior.

As the family dog or cat gets older, two types of social problems with other pets may occur. These include problems associated with the addition of a new pet to the home and alterations in the relationship between existing pets. The introduction of a new pet may lead to increasing anxiety in the existing pet because of the alterations in the attention, play, or exercise the pet receives, or competition over resources. Generally, if the existing pet is sufficiently healthy and has had adequate socialization, there are likely to be few problems. However, if the elderly pet has any medical problems, has been inadequately socialized to other pets, or is fearful or anxious about the introduction of the new pet, aggression (or other behavior problems such as fear and inappetance) may arise.

If an older dog becomes overly fearful or aggressive when a new puppy is introduced, the dogs should be separated whenever someone is not around to supervise. Before the puppy and the older dog are allowed to interact, the owner should provide enough exercise or play to fatigue the puppy. This will help ensure desirable interactions. The owner should reward all gentle play. The noise of a squeak toy may help distract the puppy from engaging in play attacks. A long lead on the puppy can be used for control and to apply a light correction. A head halter and lead can be very helpful for control. Occasionally, a timely squirt from a water gun or a toy tossed near the puppy will provide the distraction necessary to prevent or stop rough play. As the puppy learns to settle on command, and communication skills are further defined, a healthy social relationship should begin to emerge.

Sometimes, aggression between two adult dogs that have lived together for years develops when the older, dominant dog becomes unhealthy, weaker, or less assertive. Medical problems, including pain and sensory decline, cognitive dysfunction and increasing anxiety, may alter the relationship between young and older dogs. As the older dog ages, or as the younger dog matures, the younger dog may begin to challenge the older dog in competitive or social situations. These may include soliciting attention from the owner, greeting visitors, exhibiting territorial displays, and guarding food or toys. The owners may make the situation worse by trying to protect one dog from the challenges of the other, rather than allowing the dogs to work out their relationship on their own. In some cases, muzzles or head halters may be necessary for control and safety. Treatment

involves improving safety with more supervision or separation, controlling the pets' environment and resources, rebuilding the bond between the pets with shared physical activities, obedience training and leadership exercises with both pets.

The main social problem between cats occurs when another cat is introduced into the home. The older cat, especially if it has lived alone for a long period, may be particularly resistant to accepting another member of the same species into the home. An initial separation period, gradual exposure, and counterconditioning exercises may help. A quiet kitten (seven to nine weeks old) of the opposite sex is most likely to be accepted, although some older cats will not accept another cat into the home, no matter what choice is made or what the owner does to try to facilitate the introduction. As the older cat ages and medical problems arise, there may be increasing anxiety or defensiveness toward other cats in the home. As the relationship deteriorates, the younger cat (or cats) may react to the changes in the health or behavior of the older cat with increasing aggression, further aggravating the problem. Although treatment of underlying medical problems, desensitization, counterconditioning, drug therapy, and Feliway® may be effective, it can be difficult to re-establish a healthy social relationship between an aging cat and younger cats once they have been disturbed. See Chapters 19 and 20 for more information on canine and feline aggression.

Case examples

Case 1 Tony, an 11-year-old orange male tabby cat, began to spray on the patio doors. Neighborhood cats often frequented the patio but until recently Tony had exhibited no indoor spraying. A complete behavioral assessment revealed no obvious changes to Tony's household or environment, and there were no obvious changes on physical examination. Before behavior therapy was instituted, a complete laboratory workup was performed, including complete blood counts, serum biochemistry, a thyroid profile, and urinalysis. Tony's thyroxine

(T4) level was markedly elevated and a diagnosis of hyperthyroidism was confirmed with further imaging studies. Thyroidectomy was performed and Tony's spraying immediately ceased.

Approximately six months later Tony began to spray again near the patio door. A cause could not be found. Tony was on thyroxine supplementation and laboratory testing revealed that levels were in the normal range. The owners were able to prevent further spraying by confining Tony away from the patio doors when they were out and installing vertical blinds and supervising him when they were at home.

Case 2 Jody was a 13-year-old, 6 kg, spayed female Beagle cross who had begun to wake the owners every night by pacing and vocalizing. Jody traditionally slept on the bedroom floor and when the problem first began the owners attempted to leave Jody outside the bedroom with the door closed. This only led to louder vocalization as well as digging and scratching at the door. The owners would attempt to put Jody outdoors to eliminate but she merely waited outside the door to be allowed back in.

Medical evaluation, routine laboratory testing, and physical examination revealed no significant abnormalities, except for a moderate increase in serum alkaline phosphatase. Further studies were conducted in consideration of a possible diagnosis of hyperadrenocorticism. Results of a low-dose dexamethasone suppression test were equivocal but there was no measurable increase in water intake. A diagnosis of hyperadrenocorticism could not be confirmed at this time. During the daytime there was no apparent increased frequency of elimination and the owners noted no other apparent changes except a decreased responsiveness to previously trained commands and occasional restless pacing. The owners also felt there was a decrease in hearing ability, although the dog could be successfully distracted with an ultrasonic device.

Although specific causes for the night waking and increased restlessness could not be identified, the decrease in hearing ability and age-related cognitive decline were presumed to play a role in the problem. The owners were instructed to provide additional play, attention, and exercise during the late afternoon and evening, and to attempt to keep Jody awake by denying her access to her bedding area and using play and chew toys to keep her awake and active for a few hours prior to bedtime. They were also instructed to review obedience training including extended 'down-stays.' When this was unsuccessful, the owners attempted to change the feeding schedule from once daily in the morning to half at 8 a.m. and half at 8 p.m. If Jody did wake at night, the owners were instructed to ignore her or to utilize a 'down-stay' command. If she did not respond, she was to be locked into the basement until she quietened down. Jodie was placed on a senior antioxidant-supplemented diet and selegiline and overall she made good improvement. She appeared to be more responsive to commands, more enthusiastic about greeting and playing with the owners, and exhibited less daytime pacing. However, the night waking continued and the owner requested drug therapy, as a last resort.

Oxazepam was dispensed at 2 mg prior to bedtime and the owners purchased a can of compressed air to spray at Jody if she approached the bed at night. The first few nights Jody slept through the night and on the third night when Jody awoke and approached the bed, the owner used a spray of compressed air to deter the behavior. Jody backed away and after another attempt was interrupted with a spray, she lay down and returned to sleep. After another week the medication was reduced by 50% and after the second week it was withdrawn completely.

AGE-RELATED COGNITIVE AND AFFECTIVE DISORDERS (ARCAD)

In addition to an evaluation of the clinical signs through a careful and comprehensive assessment of the history, French behaviorists have developed some scales to give practitioners more objective tools for diagnosis and treatment. One scale has been designed to assess aggressiveness and a second to help identify emotional and cognitive disorders (EDED scale). Details of these two scales can be found in Chapter 21. In addition a scale has been developed specifically for the older pet to evaluate for cognitive decline and affective disorders (the ARCAD scale). According to Dr Patrick Pageat, 'the calculation grid of the ARCAD score was constructed according to the same rules as the emotional and cognitive disorder (EDED) scale. While the parameters that make up both scales are very similar, they can have different diagnostic meanings. Therefore, while the EDED scale helps evaluate dogs of all ages, the ARCAD measurement provides a better means of assessing problems that might be specific to the older dog. For example, old dogs can obtain an EDED score of the anxious type, while their ARCAD score suggests a temperament disorder. The EDED scale would seem too sensitive to assess thymic disorders that have a more discreet symptomatology in old dogs. Moreover, the ARCAD scale helps discriminate affective disorders (emotional score) from cognitive disorders to determine if drugs such as selegiline might be indicated.'

The information in Figure 12.15 on the ARCAD scale and some specific behavior disorders of older dogs has been provided by Dr Pageat. It is interesting to note that, although the methods of evaluating cognitive disorders may differ, there is a significant correlation between the ARCAD score and the occurrence of beta amyloid deposits in the brain (just as there appears to be a correlation between beta amyloid deposition and the clinical signs of cognitive dysfunction based on the more subjective North American scoring system). Dogs with high ARCAD scores were shown to have deposits of beta-amyloid substance in the temporal cortex and the hypothalamus. The correlation is stronger between the affective sub-score and the occurrence of these deposits.

BEHAVIOR DISORDERS IN AGING DOGS

This section only comprises one nosological entity: hyperaggressiveness in old dogs.

Hyperaggressiveness in old dogs

Description

These are dogs aged seven years and over that display a permanent increase in the tendency to produce aggression in all sectors of their social life. The aggression is de-structured in that the bite precedes the threat, and there is no appeasement phase. Aggression may no longer be inhibited in response to submissive postures or when the opponent is immature (pups and children). Most of these dogs are also bulimic.

Etiology and pathogenesis

Based on response to therapy, there appears to be a dysfunction in the serotoninergic structures. Although piracetam helps to re-establish the normal sequence of the aggressive episodes, it does not decrease their frequency. A decrease in the frequency of aggression is only observed when drugs that increase serotoninergic transmission are administered. Dogs that are administered fluoxetine, clomipramine, or fenfluramine improve, whereas substituted benzamides, anti-productive neuroleptics, or risperidone worsen the disorder. Tumors of the cerebral cortex may be the source of this clinical picture.

Epidemiology

There appears to be no breed, gender, or family predisposition.

Diagnosis

- Increase in the frequency of the whole set of aggressive behaviors.
- Inversion of the first two phases of aggression, bite then threat.
- Disappearance of aggression inhibition in response to submission of the opponent or if it is immature.
- Bulimia.
- Onset after the age of seven years.

THE ARCAD SCALE – AGE-RELATED COGNITIVE AND AFFECTIVE DISORDERS

AFFECTIVE OR EMOTIONAL PARAMETERS

Behavior	Item	Score
Eating	Hyperphagia/tachyphagia	5
	Anorexia or hyporexia	3
	Dysorexia	3
	Regurgitation and reingestion	2
	Normal appetite	1
Drinking	Polydipsia	4
	Champing at water without swallowing	3
	Normal	1
Auto-stimulatory behavior	Repeated movements of licking, nibbling	5
	Stereotyped nibbling, tail-chasing	3
	Attention-seeking licking and nibbling	2
	Normal body care	1
Elimination behavior	Defecates and urinates where he stands (including sleeping area)	5
	Defecates and urinates where he stands (sparing sleeping area)	4
	Defecates and urinates in small scattered amount	3
	No change	1
Sleep	Restless at bedtime	5
	Switches between insomnia and hypersomnia	3
	Sleeps over 15 hours a day	2
	Unchanged	1
Total emotional score =		

COGNITIVE PARAMETERS

Behavior	Item	Score
Learned specific behaviors	Virtually no response	5
	Random responses	3
	Unchanged	1
Self-control	Tends to generalize aversive experiences	5
	Difficult to calm down after a stressful event	3
	No apparent changes	2
Learned social behavior	Steals and retains the stolen objects	5
	Bites without warning	2
	Does not submit itself when rebuked	3
	Unchanged	1
Adaptive capabilities	Looks indifferent to changes	5
	Unable to stand changes in routine	3
	Retreats from novel situations	2
	Changes induce normal interest	1
Total cognitive score =		
Total ARCAD score = total emotional score + total cognitive score =		

INTERPRETATION OF ARCAD SCORING

Interpretation	Score
Normal aging	9 to 15
Re-evaluate in 6 months	16 to 21
Dysthymia (depression)	22 to 30
Old dog hyperaggression	18 to 30*
Involutive depression	31 to 44

*With a score of 3 or 4 for social learning and a score of 3 for self-regulation; in association with a measurement from the aggressiveness index (see Chapter 21 for details).

Figure 12.15   ARCAD scale (form #16 – printable from the CD).

Differential diagnosis

One must consider sociopathy at the 'secondary hyperaggressivity' stage and dysthymia of old dogs. In the first case, the dog would have been behaving aggressively for several years and the aggression sequences observed at the time of the diagnosis are characterized by the disappearance of the intimidation and appeasement phases. In dysthymia of old dogs, the aggressions observed are irritable aggressions with a normal sequence. Moreover, these only appear during the productive phases, whereas the dog is 'normal' or depressed during the rest of the time.

Prognosis

This is guarded. If young children are at risk it may be preferable to consider euthanasia of the dog. It is difficult to get a complete and definitive cure. Relapses are frequent (44%) and so require continuous vigilance of the dog.

Treatment

Therapy relies on serotonin re-uptake inhibitors such as fluoxetine (2 mg/kg), clomipramine (1–4 mg/kg), or perhaps fenfluramine, which helps control the disorder very rapidly. This is used at a dosage of 0.5 to 1 mg/kg spread over one to two daily doses. During the use of serotonin re-uptake inhibitors, piracetam (20–40 mg/kg) can be added to the treatment.

Author's note: fenfluramine is an amphetamine that selectively stimulates the release of 5HT and blocks its re-uptake. Chronic use leads to serotonin depletion. It was primarily used as a weight loss agent for humans and has been removed from the market in North America due to the potential for pulmonary hypertension and valvular heart disease. Serotonin is a potent vasoconstrictor. Piracetam is used for cognitive enhancement in Europe for humans with Alzheimer or vascular dementia. It is not licensed in North America. It may act to increase oxygenation and improve blood flow in the brain and increase glucose utilization.

Confusional syndrome of old dogs

This category encompasses disorders characterized by a profound alteration in the cognitive capacities of the animal and thus an alteration in all forms of learning. A clinical entity can be defined in this category: 'the confusional syndrome of old dogs.'

Description

The clinical picture resembles what has been described by American authors as 'cognitive dysfunction.' The animal shows a general alteration in learned behaviors, which manifests itself in a discordance of its habits (it doesn't come for its usual walk, it doesn't 'greet,' it doesn't recognize familiar people, etc.), housesoiling, and disorganized activity. The owners may describe episodes of spatial disorientation (e.g., lost in a familiar room, cannot find exit). We also notice a temporal disorientation, with the dog becoming active in the middle of the night. This state may alternate, especially at the start of the development, with almost normal periods.

Etiology and pathogenesis

Cerebral aging is its cause and may be related to lesions of the Alzheimer type observed in some subjects.

Diagnosis

- Episodes of spatial disorientation.
- Episodes of temporal disorientation with no disorder in the structure of sleep, nor the total length of sleep.
- An alteration in learned responses (rituals, specific forms of learning, and cleanliness).
- Disorders appear intermittently at the start of the development.

Differential diagnosis

In relation to thymic disorders (depression), the absence of an alteration in the structure of sleep is a major factor in differential diagnosis. The cognitive disorders of old dogs can be distinguished from a confusional state due to phenothiazines by the absence of fright or irritable aggressions as well as the absence of any recent therapy.

Prognosis

This is guarded since no treatment provides a definitive resolution.

Treatment

Only selegiline provides lasting improvement. Behavior therapy can only be instituted if sufficient cognitive function can be re-established. (*Author's note*: at the time of writing Hill's Canine b/d® had not yet been assessed by Dr Pageat.)

Thymic disorders of old dogs: 1) Involutive depression

Description

This depression is of a chronic type. Affected dogs display very deep cognitive and affective disorganization. We observe an increasingly marked loss in acquired behavioral knowledge, which comes from socialization and living with humans. As a result, the dogs may housesoil, they may resume oral exploration of the environment, they no longer respond to known commands, and are unable to organize social interactions. Housesoiling is characterized by enuresis and encopresia, as well as a loss in capacity to choose a specific location for elimination. As with pups below the age of four months, the old depressive dog may relieve itself wherever it is at the time it feels prompted. Oral exploration often leads to the ingestion of foreign bodies. As a result, the vet must suspect involutive depression in any old dog presented for consultation because of this. Exploratory

behavior is then completely disorganized. Social interactions are considerably modified. Dogs are no longer capable of maintaining their hierarchical position, they tend to hide away. Sleeping disorders are particularly severe. Their nature is identical to the one seen in humans with chronic depression, but awakenings are much more sudden and usually accompanied by autonomic disorders (micturition, defecation, ptyalism, and vomiting), as well as howling or sharp cries.

Etiology and pathogenesis

Endogenous and exogenous factors can be identified. In addition to cerebral aging, cerebral lesions and endocrinopathies can be involved in the genesis of the disorders. The most frequently associated cerebral lesions are tumors of the diencephalon and intracranial hypertension. Hypothyroidism and hyperadrenocorticism may also play an important role. Hypothyroidism seems less tolerable to old subjects because the bioavailability of thyroxin is decreased with age. Hyperadrenocorticism may be associated with an involutive depression, but is usually encountered in dysthymias. The most important exogenous factor is the existence of an untreated anxious state in the adult. This predisposition factor is usually aggravated by the attitude of the owners to the signs, particularly housesoiling. Owners frequently tend to keep the dog confined in order to limit soiling, which increases stress of the animal and thus worsens its depression. Therapy techniques, such as systematic desensitization, which aim to decrease the occurrence of certain emotional responses when exposed to well-identified stimuli, may worsen the state of distress in these dogs.

Epidemiology

This condition affects mainly dogs aged seven years and above. There is no breed predisposition. Females represent 65% of the animals affected. The most useful epidemiological factors to highlight concern the impact of a halt to a specific activity and socioaffective disturbances (arrival of a pup).

Diagnosis

Compulsory conditions:
- A chronic depressive state (with sleeping disorders).
- At least two involutive manifestations: oral exploration, housesoiling, the disappearance of learning, social contact via a sucking or nibbling of the skin of the partner (human or dog).

Complementary signs (at least two):
- Continuous moaning.
- An acral lick dermatitis (often discreet lesions limited to the skin thickening without alopecia).
- Hyperattachment.
- Destruction of furniture during separation.
- Wandering, 'dragging its feet,' and the use of stereotyped routes.

Differential diagnosis

Possible diagnoses are a chronic depression of adults or dysthymia of old dogs. The difference with a chronic depression in adults relies on the absence of an involutive process in this condition. In the case of dysthymia of old dogs, hyposomniac episodes of the productive phase must be sought, as well as aggression.

Prognosis

This is generally good; the only limiting factor may be the lack of patience of the owners.

Treatment

For chemotherapy, two approaches can be considered. The one which gives the most consistent results is clomipramine (1–4 mg/kg) in association with piracetam (20–40 mg/kg). When anxiety manifestations complicate the clinical picture, it may be useful to associate an anxiolytic drug. Trioxazine (0.14–0.28 per day) provides a good complement to this treatment. The other

solution, in subjects whose cognitive processes are severely altered, consists of prescribing selegiline (0.5 mg/kg). However, this treatment does not provide a decrease in the soiling rapidly enough and may not be acceptable to owners who demand immediate modifications. Behavior therapy is to reinstate contact with the dog by the owners who had kept it away because of the soiling.

Thymic disorders of old dogs: 2) Dysthymia

Description

Dysthymia evolves in two stages, with the first one corresponding to a unipolar disorder, then a second one characterized by a move to bipolar disorder. The most typical characteristic of this condition is the loss of capacity to evaluate the passage and length of one's body. Old dysthymic dogs tend to force their way through and may remain stuck for hours growling and whining. Any external attempt to help might trigger an aggressive response.

Etiology and pathogenesis

This is similar to involutive depression and may follow the same process as the disorganization of mood. Hypothyroidism does not seem to be associated with dysthymias, whereas hyperadrenocorticism must always be considered. In fact, dysthymias can be observed both in animals suffering from hyperadrenocorticism and with animals that have received injections of long-acting corticosteroids.

Epidemiology

There appears to be no breed, gender, or familial group predisposition.

Diagnosis

This is based on the appearance after the age of seven years of a unipolar then a bipolar dysthymia and the incapacity to evaluate a passage with obsessive attempts to force its way through.

Differential diagnosis

Rule outs are either bipolar dysthymia of adults or involutive depression. In bipolar dysthymia of adults, the move from a unipolar initial form as well as the tendency to move into impossible passages is absent. In involutive depression, there is the presence of involutive

manifestations and an absence of the productive signs of dysthymia.

Prognosis and treatment

Prognosis is guarded. Treatment must be maintained during the whole life of the dog. This is only biological. The only molecule that currently provides consistent results is selegiline (0.5 mg/kg).

FURTHER READING

Arnstein AFT 1993 Catecholeamine mechanisms in age-related cognitive decline. Neurobiology of Aging 14:639–641

Aronson L 1998 Systemic causes of aggression and their treatment. In: Dodman NH, Shuster L (eds) Psychopharmacology of animal behavior disorders. Blackwell Scientific, Malden, MA, p 64–102

Bain MJ, Hart BL, Cliff KD et al 2001 Predicting behavioral changes associated with age-related cognitive impairment in dogs. Journal of the American Veterinary Medical Association 218(11):1792–1795

Beaver B 1994 Owner complaints about canine behavior. Journal of the American Veterinary Medical Association 204:1953–1955

Bobik M, Thompson T, Russel MJ 1994 Amyloid deposition in various breeds of dogs. Society of Neuroscience Abstracts 20:172

Borchelt PL, Voith VL 1986 Elimination behaviour problems in cats. Compendium of Continuing Education 8:197–205

Borras D, Ferrer I, Pumarola M 1999 Age related changes in the brain of the dog. Veterinary Pathology 36:202–211

Campbell S, Trettien A, Kozan B 2001 A non-comparative open label study evaluating the effect of selegiline hydrochloride in a clinical setting. Veterinary Therapeutics 2(1):24–39

Cantuti-Castelvetri I, Shukkitt-Hale B, Joseph JA 2000 Neurobehavioral aspects of antioxidants in aging. International Journal of Developments in Neuroscience 18:367–381

Carillo MC, Ivy GO, Milgram NW et al 1994 Deprenyl increases activity of superoxide dismutase. Life Sciences 54(20):1483–1489

Chapman BL 1993 Geriatric behaviour. In: Animal behaviour. Proceedings of the TG Hungerford refresher course, Sydney. Postgraduate Committee in Veterinary Science, University of Sydney, Sydney, p 133–143

Chapman BL 1995 Behavioural disorders. In: Goldston RT, Hoskins JD (eds) Geriatrics and gerontology of the dog and cat. WB Saunders, Philadelphia, PA, p 51–62

Chapman BL, Voith VL 1990a Cat aggression redirected to people: 14 cases (1981–1987). Journal of the American Veterinary Medical Association 196(6):947–950

Chapman BL, Voith VL 1990b Behavioral problems in old dogs: 26 cases (1984–1987). Journal of the American Veterinary Medical Association 196(6):944–946

Colle M-A, Hauw J-J, Crespau F et al 2000 Vascular and parenchymal beta-amyloid deposition in the aging dog: correlation with behavior. Neurobiology of Aging 21:695–704

Cummings BJ, Su JH, Cotman CW et al 1993 B-amyloid accumulation in aged canine brain: a model of early plaque formation in Alzheimer's disease. Neurobiology of Aging 14:547–560

Cummings BJ, Head E, Ruehl WW et al 1996 Beta-amyloid accumulation correlates with cognitive dysfunction in the aged canine. Neurobiology of Learning & Memory 66:11–23

Davies M 1996 The nervous system. In: Canine and feline geriatrics. Blackwell Science, Oxford, p 48–68

Forrester SD, Troy GC, Dalton MN et al 1999 Retrospective evaluation of urinary tract infection in 42 dogs with hyperadrenocorticism or diabetes mellitus or both. Journal of Veterinary International Medicine 12(6):557–560

Gelfand M et al 2001 Testosterone medicated neuroprotection through the androgen receptor in human primary neurons. Journal of Neurochemistry 2:527–535

Gerlach M, Riederer P, Youdim MBH 1994 Effects of disease and aging on monoamine oxidases A and B. In: Lieberman A, Olanow CW, Youdim MBH et al (eds) Monoamine oxidase inhibitors in neurological diseases, p 21–30

Gerlach M, Reiderer P, Youdim MB 1996 Pharmacology of selegiline. Neurology 47(6 Suppl 3):137–145

Goldston RT 1995 Introduction and overview of geriatrics. In: Goldston RT, Hoskins JD (eds) Geriatrics and gerontology of the dog and cat. WB Saunders, Philadelphia, PA, p 1–9

Hart BL 2001 Effect of gonadectomy on subsequent development of age-related cognitive impairment in dogs. Journal of the American Veterinary Medical Association 219(1):51–56

Head E, Mehta R, Hartley J et al 1995 Spatial learning and memory as a function of age in the dog. Behavioral Neuroscience 109:851–858

Head E, Hartley J, Mehta R et al 1996 The effects of l-deprenyl on spatial short term memory in young and aged dogs. Progress in Neuropsychopharmacology, Biology and Psychiatry 20:515

Head E, Callahan H, Cummings BJ et al 1997 Open field activity and human interaction as a function of age and breed in dogs. Physiology & Behavior 62(5):963–971

Head E, McCleary R, Hahn FF et al 2000 Region-specific age at onset of beta-amyloid in dogs. Neurobiology of Aging 21:89–96

Head E, Milgram NW, Cotman CW 2001 Neurobiological models of aging in the dog and other vertebrate species. In: Hof P, Mobbs C (eds) Functional neurobiology of aging. Academic Press, San Diego, p 457–468

Heinonen EH, Lammintausta R 1991 A review of the pharmacology of selegiline. Acta Neurologica Scandinavica 84(Suppl 136):44–59

Horwitz D 2001 Dealing with common behavior problems in senior dogs. Veterinary Medicine 96(11):869–878

Hunthausen W 1994 Identifying and treating behaviour problems in geriatric dogs. Veterinary Medicine 89(9):688–700

Hunthausen W 1995 Housesoiling and the geriatric dog. Geriatric Medicine. Supplement to Vetinary Medicine August:4–15

Jurio AV, Li XM, Paterson A et al 1994 Effects of monoamine oxidase B inhibitors on dopaminergic function: role of 2 phenylethylamine and aromatic l-amino acid decarboxylase. In: Lieberman A, Olanow CW, Youdim MPH et al (eds) Monoamine oxidase inhibitors in neurologic diseases. Marcel Dekker, New York, p 181–200

Kalmijn S, Launer LJ, Ott A et al 1997 Dietary fat and the risk of incident of dementia in the Rotterdam study. Annals of Neurology 42:776–782

Kittner B, Rossner M, Rother M 1997 Clinical trials in dementia with propentofylline. Annals of the New York Academy of Science 26(826):307–316

Knoll J 1998 L-deprenyl (selegiline) a catecholaminergic activity enhancer (CAE) substance acting in the brain. Pharmacology and Toxicology 82:57–66

Landsberg GM 1991 The distribution of canine behavior cases at three referral practices. Veterinary Medicine 86(11):10–11

Landsberg GM 1995 The most common behavior problems of older dogs. Veterinary Medicine August(Suppl):18–24

Lebars PL, Katz MM, Berman N et al 1997 A placebo-controlled, double blinded, randomized trial of an extract of Ginkgo biloba for dementia. JAMA 278:1327–1332

Luttgen PJ 1990 Diseases of the nervous system in older dogs. Part 1. Central nervous system. Compendium of Continuing Education 12(7):933–945

Maitra I, Marcooci L, Droy-Lefoix MT et al 1995 Peroxyl radical scavenging activity of Gingko biloba extract Egb761. Biochemical Pharmacology 11:1649–1655

Mecocci P, MacGarvey U, Kaufman AE et al 1993 Oxidative damage to mitochondrial DNA shows marked age-dependent increases in human brain. Annals of Neurology 34:609–616

Milgram NW, Ivy GO, Head E et al 1993 The effect of l-deprenyl on behavior, cognitive function and biogenic amines in the dog. Neurochemical Research 18(12):1211–1219

Milgram NW, Head E, Weiner E et al 1994 Cognitive functions and aging in the dog: acquisition of nonspatial visual tasks. Behavioral Neuroscience 108:57–68

Milgram NW, Ivy GO, Murphy MP et al 1995 Effects of chronic oral administration of l-deprenyl in the dog. Pharmacology and Biochemistry of Behavior 51(2&3):421–428

Milgram NW, Adams B, Callahan H et al 1999 Landmark discrimination learning in the dog. Learning & Memory 6(1):54–61

Milgram NW, Estrada J, Ikeda-Douglas C et al 2000a Landmark discrimination learning in aged dogs is improved by treatment with an antioxidant diet. Society of Neuroscience Abstracts 26(1):531

Milgram NW, Siwak CT, Gruet P et al 2000b Oral administration of adrafanil improves discrimination learning in dogs. Pharmacology and Biochemistry of Behavior 66(2):301–305

Milgram NW, Head E, Cotman CW et al 2001 Age dependent cognitive dysfunction in canines: dietary intervention. In: Overall KL, Mills DS, Heath SE et al (eds) Proceedings of the third international congress on veterinary behavioral medicine. Universities Federation for Animal Welfare, Wheathampstead, UK, p 53–57

Milgram NW, Head E, Cottman CW 2002 The effects of antioxidant fortified food and cognitive enrichment in dogs. In: Symposium on brain aging and related behavioral changes in dogs, Orlando, FL. Veterinary Health Care Communications, Lenexa, KS, p 31–33

Moffat K 2001 Mesa Veterinary Hospital – Proceedings of the American Veterinary Society of Animal Behavior at the American Veterinary Association Conference, Boston

Mosier JE 1989 Effect of aging on body systems of the dog. Veterinary Clinics of North America, Small Animal Practice 19:1–12

Nagaraja D, Jayashree S 2001 Randomized study of the dopamine receptor agonist piribedil in the treatment of mild cognitive impairment. American Journal of Psychiatry 158(9):1517–1519

Nakamura S, Nakayama H, Kintipattanssakui W et al 1996 Senile plaques in aged cats. Acta Neuropathologica 91:437–439

Neer TM 1995 The nervous system. In: Goldston RT, Hoskins JD (eds) Geriatrics and gerontology of the dog and cat. WB Saunders, Philadelphia, PA, p 325–346

Nielson JC, Hart BL, Cliff KD et al 2001 Prevalence of behavioral changes associated with age-related cognitive impairment in dogs. Journal of the American Veterinary Medical Association 218(11):1787–1791

Peers RJ 1990 Alzheimer disease and omega-3 fatty acids: hypothesis. Medical Journal of Australia 153:563–564

Penaliggon J 1997 The use of nicergoline in the reversal of behavioural changes due to ageing in dogs: a multicentre clinical field trial. In: Mills DS et al (eds) Proceedings of the first international conference on veterinary behavioural medicine. Universities Federation for Animal Welfare, Potter's Bar, UK, p 37–41

Postal JM Effectiveness of nicergoline in improving behavioural modification associated with senility in dogs. In: Use of alpha-blocking agent Fitergol in the treatment of behavioural disorders in old dogs. Rhone-Merieux Publication, Pairault, France, p 15–18

Reedy LM, Miller WH 1997 Allergic skin diseases of dogs and cats, 2nd edn. WB Saunders, Philadelphia, p 34

Ruehl WW, Hart BL 1997 Canine cognitive dysfunction. In: Dodman NH, Shuster L (eds) Psychopharmacology of animal behavior disorders. Blackwell Scientific, Malden, MA, p 283–304

Saletu B, Paulus E, Linzmayer L 1995 Nicergoline in senile dementia of Alzheimer type and multi-infarct dementia; a double-blind placebo-controlled, clinical and EEG/ERP mapping study. Psychopharmacology 117:385–395

Salo PT, Tatton WG 1992 Deprenyl reduces the death of motoneurons caused by axotomy. Journal of Neuroscience Research 31:394–400

Sano M, Ernesto C, Thomas R et al 1997 A controlled trial of selegiline, alpha tocopherol, or both for the treatment for Alzheimer's disease. New England Journal of Medicine 336(17):1216–1222

Satou T, Cummings BJ, Head E et al 1997 The progression of beta-amyloid deposition in the frontal cortex of the aged canine. Brain Research 774(1&2) 35–43

Siwak CT, Gruet P, Woehrle F et al 2000a Behavioral activating effects of adrafinil in aged canines. Pharmacology and Biochemistry of Behavior 66(2):293–300

Siwak CT, Gruet P, Woehrle F et al 2000b Comparison of the effects of adrafinil, propentofylline, and nicergoline on behavior in aged dogs. American Journal of Veterinary Research 61(11):1410–1414

Siwak CT, Tapp NW, Milgram NW 2001 Age associated changes in non-cognitive behaviours in a canine model of aging. In: Overall KL, Mills DS, Heath SE et al (eds) Proceedings of the third international congress on veterinary behavioral medicine. Universities Federation for Animal Welfare. Wheathampstead, UK, p 133–135

Su M-Y, Head E, Brooks WM et al 1998 MR imaging of anatomic and vascular characteristics in a canine model of human aging. Neurobiology of Aging 19(5):479–485

Tapp PD, Siwak CT, Head E et al 2001 Sex differences in the effect of oestrogen on size discrimination learning and spatial memory. In: Overall KL, Mills DS, Heath SE et al (eds) Proceedings of the third international congress on veterinary behavioral medicine. Universities Federation for Animal Welfare, Wheathampstead, UK, p 136–138

Tighilet B, Lacour M 1995 Pharmacological activity of the Gingko biloba extract on equilibrium function in the unilateral vestibular neurectomized cat. Journal of Vestibular Research 5(3):187–200

Whilte HL, Scates PW, Cooper BR 1996 Extracts of Gingko biloba leaves inhibit monamine oxidase. Life Science 58(16):1315–1321

Yasar S, Goldberg JP, Goldberg SR 1996 Are metabolites of l-deprenyl (selegiline) useful or harmful? Indications from preclinical research. Journal of Neural Transmission 48(Suppl):61–73

13

Unruly behaviors, training, and management – dogs

JUMPING UP ON PEOPLE

This is a very common problem, especially for owners of young, friendly dogs. Pets that jump up on people can be a real nuisance at the very least, but can also be quite dangerous. Dogs will jump up on people as a greeting when they first meet someone, when they want to play, when they want food, and occasionally as a socially assertive gesture. Owners usually find this to be a very difficult behavior to stop. There are several reasons for this: (1) the family has no effective, humane way to interrupt the behavior; (2) little time is spent teaching a desirable way for the pet to interact in social situations; (3) the family is inconsistent in responding to the behavior; and (4) the pet may be getting insufficient exercise and is easily excited.

Diagnosis and prognosis

The diagnosis is evident from observing the dog jumping up on the family members or visitors. If the family and visitors are consistent, there is an excellent prognosis for complete correction of the problem.

Management

In order to manage this annoying behavior, it is very important that everyone follow the same basic rules in training (Fig. 13.1). The successful management of dogs that jump up on people

Method	Comments
Obedience training	• An owner with good control and a well-trained dog may be able to correct the behavior with a command to sit followed by a reward at each greeting
Exercise and play	• Regularly scheduled exercise and play, initiated by the owners, is needed to help reduce excessive arousal and calm the pet
Avoid eliciting the behavior	• Keep greetings very low-key. Don't encourage the behavior during play and don't allow jumping up during some situations, or on some people, if it is not allowed at others
Ignore the behavior	• Behaviors that are not rewarded will become extinct with time, but only if the owner has enough patience. One of the problems with this approach is that the behavior often gets worse before it decreases as the pet tries harder to elicit a response from the owner
Rewards	• The dog should be lightly and calmly praised when it approaches and does not jump up. Praise must immediately cease if the dog attempts to jump up
Interruption	• Stern verbal reprimands such as 'no!' accompanied by an unexpected stimulus (e.g., shake can, air horn, water gun), should be sufficient. The interruption should be sufficiently intense to deter the behavior without eliciting any sign of fear. A device should be chosen that is appropriate for the pet's temperament. The dog can then be commanded to perform an appropriate, acceptable, non-jumping behavior (see handout #24 on the CD)
Negative reinforcement	• An aversive device (horn, ultrasonic) is applied until the pet jumps down, at which time the aversive stimulus is immediately withdrawn
Response substitution (differential reinforcement)	• A behavior is taught that is incompatible with jumping up. For example, the dog can be taught to sit upon meeting someone, in exchange for food, a toy, or social reward. Make it maintain that position for a few seconds at first, and gradually shape the behavior so that the dog sits for 10 seconds or longer before giving the reward. Timing is important because you do not want to reinforce a chain of behaviors in which the dog first jumps up and then sits so it can be rewarded
Control devices	• For owners that have difficulty gaining verbal control, a head halter and long leash can be left attached to the dog and the leash used to enforce the 'sit' command as well as deter the jumping behavior
Punishment	• If punishment is the only treatment used, it is not uncommon for the dog to habituate to the aversive stimulus. Corrections that cause pain or elicit a fear response should never be used. Physical corrections, such as kneeing the pet, may result in excited, rough play as a response
Surgery	• Neutering has little or no effect on this behavior unless it is associated with male mounting behavior
Drugs	• There are no indications for using drugs with this behavior problem

Figure 13.1   Management for the dog that jumps up.

involves a balance of rewards and consistent, timely interruptions. A daily regime that includes play, exercise, and training is an important part of reducing arousal and improving control. Since the goal of treatment for jumping up is to train the dog to greet in an acceptable alternative manner, training the sit, down, and settle commands should be practiced regularly until they are immediately successful in non-greeting situations.

During greetings, family members and visitors should remain very low-key to prevent the pet from becoming highly aroused and excited. This will make it less likely to jump up on them. The dog should be lightly and calmly praised when it approaches and keeps its paws on the ground. By holding a biscuit in front of the pet at nose level as it approaches, the owner may be able to get the dog's attention, keep its feet on the ground, encourage it to sit, and give the food as a reinforcement. A leash can be used to ensure that the desired behavior (staying on the floor) can be achieved. Under no circumstances should the pet be praised for jumping up, and family members should not indulge the dog in games that involve jumping up (Fig. 13.2).

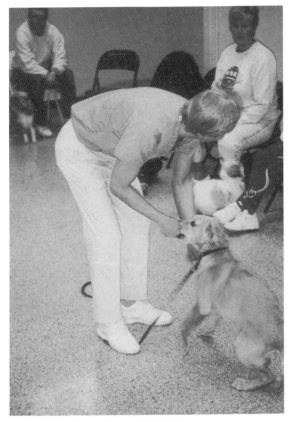 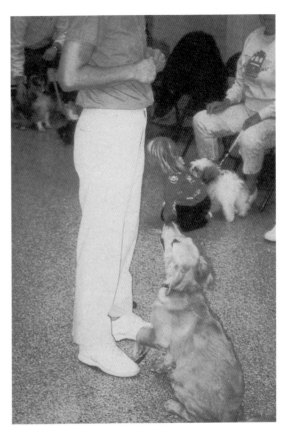

Figure 13.2 A leash can be used to ensure that the dog stays on the floor in a sit position rather than jumping up to greet (left). A desirable sit response can then be reinforced.

When the dog begins to jump up, it can be interrupted with a sharp reprimand. A verbal correction may be enough for some dogs, but for others the reprimand may need to be accompanied by a sharp noise, like the shake from a can containing several coins. A rare, exuberant dog may require the sound from a compressed airhorn or citronella spray to interrupt the behavior. The audible stimulus (verbal or noisemaker) must be strong enough, relative to the pet's temperament, to stop the behavior immediately without eliciting any sign of fear. A good interruptive stimulus should immediately stop the behavior without causing anxiety or avoidance. An interruption that is not sufficiently aversive could actually worsen the behavior by providing attention or by getting

the dog more excited. A timely interruption provides a window of opportunity in which the owner can calmly ask the dog to sit and give it praise and/or a food reinforcement. Another way of controlling the pet while teaching it how to greet people is to use a head halter. When the pet is controlled with the halter, jumping up can be turned into a calm sit, which can then be rewarded (see Figs 3.33–3.36). In order to successfully implement head halter training for jumping up, the owners can set up greetings by inviting friends to the home, or by having family members leave and return. With the head halter and a leash attached, the dog can first be commanded to sit and if the dog does not immediately comply, the sit can be accomplished with a pull up on the leash. Once the pet has learned that it can never attempt to jump up on someone without being interrupted, and that sitting quietly is always pleasantly reinforced, the behavior should stop. Punitive or painful corrections should be avoided. These include stepping on the dog's paws, throwing it on its back, pinching the ears, kicking the dog, thumping it with the knee, using a pinch collar, etc.

This type of approach works very nicely with most dogs. By spending a little extra time at greetings, though, the owner can increase the speed of resolution of the problem. After the pet has been corrected or rewarded for the initial greeting, the person should leave and re-enter multiple times in order to reward a number of correct responses in succession. This will result in more rapid learning. See client handouts #24 on unruly behavior (Fig. 13.3), #2 on basic training (Fig. C.4), #13 on head halters (Fig. 3.37), and #23 on settle (Fig. 5.13). The handouts can be printed from the CD.

Prevention

Jumping up can be effectively prevented by encouraging owners to use basic obedience training to begin taking control of the pet when it is a young puppy, by avoiding over-enthusiastic greetings, by not encouraging or reinforcing the behavior, and by teaching the pet appropriate greetings before it learns undesirable ones.

Owners should follow these basic rules:

- Attend early obedience classes with the puppy.
- From the beginning, ask the young dog to sit every time it approaches someone.
- Never reward the pet when it jumps up by picking it up, giving food, play, or attention.
- Reward the pet each time it approaches and does not jump up.
- Immediately interrupt the pet every time it begins to jump up.
- Make sure all family members and visitors abide by the same rules.

Case example

Lucy, an eight-month-old spayed female Irish Setter, would jump on the owners and most visitors when they came into the home. The owners had attempted to reprimand Lucy verbally and when that was unsuccessful, they attempted to knee Lucy in the chest. Despite these and even more physical techniques, such as toe pinching, the problem only seemed to escalate.

Lucy enjoyed greeting people and, as a young puppy, had been intermittently rewarded by the owners and some visitors with patting or attention during greetings. As Lucy grew, the owners attempted to punish the pet verbally and then physically but as the 'punishment' gradually escalated, Lucy habituated to the reprimands and physical contact. In fact, through 'punishment' the owners were inadvertently rewarding the behavior because Lucy enjoyed rough handling (play) and attention.

The owners were instructed to work on reward-motivated training techniques during non-greeting times. They were taught how to train Lucy to sit instantaneously on command and remain sitting for 10 seconds or longer. Since Lucy enjoyed playing with her ball, it was used as a reward for training. The owners then attempted to use techniques that would teach Lucy a desirable method of greeting (having Lucy sit and then receive ball playing as a reward) whenever anyone entered the home. When the owners entered the home, if Lucy did not immediately respond to a 'sit' or 'down' command, they were to ignore Lucy completely (no eye contact and as little physical contact as was practical when she greeted them. The owner then left a 10-ft leash and head halter attached to the dog so that when visitors arrived, a 'no' command followed by a quick pull on the leash could be used to interrupt the behavior. As soon as the jumping ceased the owners were instructed to call the dog to play ball. Numerous trial departures and arrivals were repeated with the leash and halter attached until Lucy began to approach the owners to play ball when visitors arrived at the door.

DEALING WITH PROBLEM BEHAVIORS – JUMPING UP, GETTING ON COUNTERS AND FURNITURE

Jumping up

1. From the beginning, every time the young pet walks up to a family member or visitor, it should be asked to sit, especially when children are present.
2. The key to changing this behavior is consistency. Jumping up should not be allowed by any pet at any time. Appropriate behavior should always be calmly rewarded.
3. Avoid accidentally encouraging or rewarding the behavior. Even verbal or physical discipline can actually reinforce the behavior if it is not strong enough to interrupt it.
4. Train your dog to exhibit an acceptable response at greetings. You can use a sit and settle command, or perhaps train it to expect a tummy rub when people enter the home. Encourage and reward the desired response.
5. Use a sharp noise, such as a shake can, as needed to interrupt the problem behavior. Don't use any method that involves a physical correction or discomfort, such as stepping on toes, kneeing the chest, pinching paws, alpha rolls, etc.
6. If your pet is incorrigible about jumping up on visitors, you may need to set up a training session that involves a series of repeated greetings.
   (a) Ask a friend to knock or ring the bell. Open the door for the person to enter
   (b) When the pet jumps up, immediately say 'no' and provide a sharp noise that will quickly interrupt the behavior without eliciting any fear or anxiety from the pet (e.g., shake can, water gun). This can also be done by using a head halter and leash.
   (c) Ask the friend to leave and repeat the entrance and greeting.
   (d) Anytime the pet jumps up, interrupt it. Anytime the pet doesn't jump up, ask it to sit and reward it with a very tasty treat.
   (e) Repeat the exercise until the ratio of rewards to interruptions is at least 2:1.
   (f) It is also helpful for family members to do repeated greetings involving interruptions and reinforcements as outlined above when they greet the pet.

Getting on the furniture or into rooms where the dog is not allowed

1. Once rules are established regarding what the pet is allowed to do, all family members must consistently follow the same rules.
2. Desirable behavior, such as lying on the floor or a dog bed, and staying away from rooms that are out of bounds, should be encouraged and reinforced. Whenever you are sitting on furniture and the pet approaches, ask it to sit and give it a toy or attention before it tries to jump up.
3. Provide acceptable alternatives for sleeping and play so that your dog can be encouraged and rewarded for sleeping on its own bed on the floor and staying in rooms that are acceptable.
4. Whenever you cannot supervise your dog, it must be consistently prevented from getting on the furniture or into rooms that are out of bounds. If your pet attempts to get onto the furniture or into the room, it must immediately be deterred as the behavior begins and not when the dog is already in the room or on the furniture
5. Physical punishment should be avoided. Rather, an immediate unpleasant disruption should be used to stop the undesirable behavior as it begins. A pull on a leash (if one has been left attached), a sharp noise (such as a shake can or audible alarm), a spray of water, or a remote control citronella collar can be used to deter the dog.
6. When you are away from home or not available to supervise, access to the area must either be prevented or deterred. This can be done by blocking access to the area, or using indoor avoidance units (e.g., citronella spray barriers, motion-activated alarms, upside down mousetraps, Snappy Trainer™, or alarm mats).

Raiding garbage or stealing food

1. Training the dog to stay away from garbage cans and food that has been left on a table or counter may be extremely difficult if the dog is highly food-motivated and exploratory.
2. If you are available to supervise your dog, you can prevent or deter access to the food or garbage with commands, a long leash left attached to the dog's collar so that it can be immediately interrupted with a gentle pull, a noise device such as a shake can, or a device such as a remote citronella collar or a water rifle.

Figure 13.3   Unruly behaviors in dogs (client handout #24 – printable from the CD).

Raiding garbage or stealing food (*continued*)

3. When you cannot supervise, the best advice is to always keep the food or garbage out of the pet's reach in inaccessible areas or containers with area avoidance devices (e.g., citronella spray barriers, motion-activated alarms, upside down mousetraps, Snappy Trainer™, or alarm mats), or by confining your dog away from the area.

4. Some dogs may learn to avoid areas booby trapped with bitter tasting repellents.

Figure 13.3 (*continued*)

STEALING, GETTING INTO TRASH CONTAINERS, AND JUMPING ON FURNITURE

Pets engage in these behaviors because of their inquisitive and investigative natures and because they are self-gratifying (the pet may obtain food, a desired object to chew, or a resting station). Attempts to use punishment usually fail because corrections are applied long after the behavior is finished. Owners are often certain that their pets know they have done wrong when they discover the problem but, in most cases, this logic is seriously flawed. They think the pet knows what it has done wrong because it looks guilty or runs away when the owner approaches. In these cases, the pet has learned that there are unpleasant consequences for being on the furniture or worktop, or in the rubbish when the owner approaches. It has also learned that there are no unpleasant (only pleasant) consequences when going onto the furniture or into the trash in the owner's absence. For a client review of correction techniques, see handout #24 on the CD (Fig. 13.3).

Diagnosis and prognosis

The diagnosis is made based on the owner's observation that the dog or cat performs the activities. For most situations, the prognosis for correction is good. These behaviors are typically young pet behaviors and may decrease or stop on their own as the pet grows older.

Management

Stealing

Teaching the pet what it is allowed to have in its mouth is the first course of action. The pet should have a variety of interesting toys available, and should frequently receive a food treat or lavish social reward for chewing on them. It should not be given discarded objects (e.g., old shoes) as playthings, as this only makes it more difficult for the pet to distinguish between household possessions and chew toys. The family should provide adequate play, exercise, and social attention to meet the pet's requirements.

If a pet is found chewing on a household item, it should be interrupted with a quick, sharp reprimand or sharp noise, and the possession retrieved. The pet can then be asked to sit, and a more suitable chew toy provided. Harsh correction, prolonged scolding, delayed punishment, and physical punishment should all be avoided. Preventing access to problem areas and safeguarding valuables by keeping them in pet-proof (or child-proof) containers or cupboards may be useful for some households. Booby traps such as a motion-activated alarm can also be a very successful tool to teach a pet to stay away from the owner's possessions (Fig 5.4, handout #21 on the CD).

Aversive-tasting substances can also be very helpful for curtailing this behavior. For example, if the pet steals shoes, three or four of the owner's old shoes can be coated with something that is bitter or hot to the taste (Fig 5.4, handout #21 on the CD). The shoes should be placed in a variety of areas around the home. Periodically, they can be moved to other locations. Every seven to 10 days, they should be replaced with other shoes that have a somewhat different appearance. Eventually, the pet will learn that any shoe found around the home, no matter what it looks like or where it is located, will taste bad. Concurrently, the owner should coat the dog's toys with something that tastes good that will help accentuate the difference between what it is supposed to chew and what it is not.

Getting into trash

Dogs may raid the trash bins and any food cupboards that might be accessible for both food items and play toys (e.g., pieces of tissue). Some of these items can be particularly dangerous if they are swallowed since they may be hard to digest (chicken bones, peach pits) or may have bacterial contamination (left-over pieces of meat). Although these problems are generally related to exploration and scavenging, the dog should first be assessed to ensure that it is not underweight and that there are no underlying medical problems that might lead to increased appetite (e.g., Cushing's disease). Dogs that have been placed on a calorie-restricted diet for weight control may begin to scavenge more intensely. Higher bulk diets may help to satisfy some of this need, while dental chew toys, dental diets, and food toys that are coated or stuffed with food (that require manipulation to release the food) may help to direct chewing to more appropriate outlets. Exercise, training, and play periods before departure should also help calm the pet and reduce exploratory behavior while the owners are out. The best solution is to prevent access to problem areas by using a more secure container or by placing the trash in a location where the pet does not have access unless the owner is present to supervise and deter access to the garbage. Another option is to place one of the taste aversives or booby trap devices such as a motion-activated alarm on the trash container.

Getting on furniture

This is another situation where consistency is very important. If the family decides that the pet should not be allowed on furniture, then no exceptions can be made. The dog should have a comfortable resting location (dog bed, crate, at the foot of a chair), where it is encouraged to rest and chew on its play toys. If a family member would like to have the pet in the lap, but not on the furniture, the person should get on the floor and then allow the pet to get in the lap. Whenever the pet approaches a family member sitting on a piece of furniture, the pet should be asked to sit and praised before it has a chance to jump up on the furniture. Another solution is to give the pet a toy stuffed with food as it approaches, to give it something to do other than jump up on the furniture.

Keeping the pet off furniture when the owner is not around requires a different strategy. Preventing access to the furniture is generally the most practical option until the dog can be 'trusted' to stay off the furniture. If the dog has access to the furniture, it should be supervised by the family so that jumping up can be deterred immediately and resting in the desired location reinforced. When the owner is not around, a less appealing covering or booby traps such as double-sided tape, motion detectors, avoidance mats or Snappy Trainer™ should keep most pets off the furniture (Fig. 5.4, handout #21 on the CD).

Prevention

These problems are most common in young pets. Large amounts of physical and mental stimulation, as well as a sufficient amount of supervision, are very important for keeping young pets out of trouble. Owners should constantly look for acceptable behaviors to reinforce and not focus on punishment to shape behaviors. When the untrained pet cannot be closely supervised, it should be confined to a safe area. Unacceptable behaviors should consistently be quickly interrupted, and the pet should then be directed to engage in appropriate behaviors.

Closing off doors to problem areas, using child locks, baby gates, long leashes, and tie-downs next to the owner may all be helpful for controlling the young pet while appropriate behaviors are being taught. As an adjunct to other forms of behavior therapy, short-term use of basket-type muzzles may be useful for dogs that might need to be placed in environments where problems (e.g., destruction) might occur (Fig. 13.4).

Case example

Gilligan, a two-year-old male Standard Poodle, could not be 'trusted' by the owners whenever he was out of their sight. His exploratory, playful, and destructive nature had persisted into adulthood, and whenever he was left alone or unsupervised he would go into rooms where he was not allowed, steal food off tables or out of cupboards, raid rubbish bins for items that could be eaten or chewed, and climb onto furniture where he would often chew on the upholstery. Gilligan enjoyed playing with the owners and other dogs outdoors and was kept confined to his owners' half-acre property with a citronella spray 'fencing' unit. The owners had attempted to confine Gilligan to a cage but this resulted in extreme anxiety on Gilligan's part (howling, salivating, chewing at the bars), and he was capable of escaping from or damaging most cages.

Because of Gilligan's size and the anxiety associated with being caged, confinement techniques were not practical in this case. Many of the potential problem areas could be closed off, but a few of the rooms had no doors and no physical means of denying entry.

Gilligan's highly energetic and exploratory nature was dealt with by increasing play periods and adding training sessions each day. The owners played chase and fetch games and took longer walks before each departure. Gilligan enjoyed playing with other dogs, so he was also given the opportunity to play with two of the neighbors' dogs every morning before the owners departed for their daily activities. Although obtaining a second compatible, playful dog for the household may have helped in this situation, the owners had no interest in pos-

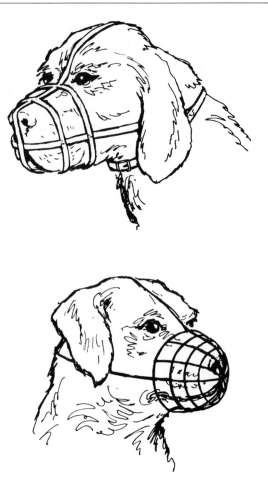

Figure 13.4 Basket-type muzzles might be used to prevent behavior problems such as stealing and destructiveness, as well as to prevent injury in situations of potential aggression.

sibly adding to their problems with another dog. When the owners departed, all bedrooms, the study, and the basement were closed off and the only remaining rooms that Gilligan had access to were the dining room and kitchen. Child locks were placed on the kitchen cupboards so that these could not be opened and all rubbish was placed in the garage before the owners departed. Three or four toys with treats (meat, peanut butter) hidden inside and a few small bowls of food (with a hidden treat of meat or cheese inside) were provided each time the owner had to leave home. Gilligan's problems were dramatically decreased, but his explorations into the dining room occasionally led to damage or destruction. Since motion detectors and other forms of booby trap had not been successful, the owner placed a child gate in front of the dining room, with an indoor transmitter dish for the citronella spray collar sitting directly behind the gate. Gilligan quickly learned to stay away from these rooms when wearing the receiver collar.

PULLING/FORGING AHEAD AND LUNGING ON LEAD

Many dogs have habits of lunging ahead on their leash and pulling their owners along during a walk. These behaviors are unsafe and not a pleasurable experience for the owner. Both will enjoy the walk more if the dog correctly maintains its position next to the owner during the walk.

Diagnosis and prognosis

The diagnosis is made based on history. The dog controls the owner during the walk, not the other way around. In some cases, the dog persists even if the owner uses a choke collar, but without correct technique. Fortunately, there is a good prognosis for correction of the problem.

Management

Lunging and pulling on the leash are much easier to prevent than to treat, but can be managed effectively with some behavioral modification and the use of proper equipment. Obedience classes are very useful for learning the heel command. A slip training collar or head halter and the guidance of a good trainer will usually put the pet under control quickly so that it can be taught how to walk on the lead without constantly pulling. Training typically involves a light correction with the leash, pulling the dog into position with the head halter, or abruptly changing direction to take charge of the pet and stop the pulling. The owner must then immediately release and reward the pet when it is in position with praise, affection,

food, or clicker. See handouts #2 (Fig. C.4), #13 (Fig. 3.37), and #21 (Fig. 5.4) on the CD.

Other harness-like devices deter or prevent pulling and lunging by means of straps that apply pressure to the axillary areas when the pet forges forward. These do not improve the owner's overall control of the dog, but may be more readily accepted by some owners who dislike having the pet wear a head halter that looks similar to a muzzle. Care should be taken to fit the harness properly so the axillary areas are not abraded. Because of potential abrasions, these halters are usually not acceptable for jogging with the pet. Distraction devices (e.g., ultrasonic and audible trainers) and conditioned reinforcers (clickers) may also be helpful for getting the dog's attention during a retraining program.

Prevention

Lunging and pulling on the lead are effectively prevented by teaching the 'heel' command to dogs when they are young or when they first learn to walk on a lead. Training collars and head halters are very useful for this purpose.

Case example

Fester, a four-year-old, 50 kg male entire Rottweiler, could not be physically restrained by his 50 kg female owner in the presence of male dogs. Fester threatened and lunged at other male dogs and would probably have attacked if not physically restrained. The husband, who weighed 85 kg and had taken Fester to obedience classes as a puppy, could physically restrain Fester on walks and could usually get him to respond to a 'heel' command with a strong tug on the choke collar and harsh verbal corrections. Fester had been fitted with a prong collar, which was of no benefit for the female owner. The prong collar helped the male owner gain better control over Fester, but Fester's aggression toward other male dogs had further escalated. Although the prong collar provided the male owner with a more intense means of suppressing Fester's aggression, it only served to fuel his aggression toward other dogs since Fester would now associate pain and increased fear and anxiety with the approach of other dogs. The only real control the male owner had was through physical suppression, and this was impractical and unsuccessful for the smaller female owner.

Fester was first retrained to the 'heel' command using a head halter and reward training by the female owner. The owners were advised to have Fester neutered as this might help reduce his aggression to other male dogs, but the owners preferred to defer this until all other aspects of training had been put into place. Once Fester could successfully 'heel' for both owners in dog-free environments, he was gradually reintroduced to other dogs, beginning first with female dogs, then neutered males and the occasional male dog that was housed or tied up on his own property. The halter provided exceptional control and Fester could be kept at the heel except when an unexpected male dog approached. Neutering and continued use of the head halter led to much greater improvement, so that within six months, the female owner reported that virtually all walks were enjoyable and problem-free.

EXCESSIVE BARKING

Barking is a normal and natural means of canine communication. This type of vocalization may be seen in conjunction with hunting, herding, territorial defense, threat displays, fear, distress, attention seeking, care seeking behaviors, and play. Aimless, repetitive barking may also be a part of canine cognitive dysfunction syndrome. Barking may increase in frequency when any type of reinforcement is associated with it. This is often the case when owners accede to their dogs' desires by providing food, play, or some other form of attention. Reinforcement may be inadvertent, such as when the owner attempts to stop the barking or calm the pet down by providing treats or by any verbal or physical attention. Attempts at punishment, especially light scolding, may also serve to reward the behavior if they are not sufficiently aversive. Barking is also reinforced when the threat (e.g., a stranger

approaching) is successfully removed (stranger retreats) by the barking.

Diagnosis and prognosis

The diagnosis for any barking case is based upon the history of the problem. Attention should be given to those situations in which the problem occurs. The owner's response to the barking and the dog's response to the owner's attempts at 'correction' are also critical issues in both the diagnosis and the prognosis. By the time the case is presented to the practitioner, the barking may have multiple contributing factors, and there may be more than one type of barking occurring. Barking can be quite difficult to correct since it is a highly innate behavior in some dogs, and often occurs in the owner's absence. Barking that occurs in the owner's presence and problems in which the stimuli can be controlled usually have a much better prognosis.

Barking categories

- Attention-getting, care-seeking, food-soliciting
- Conditioned
- Territorial defense, protective aggression
- Conflict, fear, anxiety-induced
- Separation – lone call
- Hunting
- Herding
- Play, social situations
- Group-facilitated behavior
- Cognitive dysfunction

Management

Behavioral modification is based on the following (see Fig. 13.5):

- Identify and eliminate the cause by controlling or avoiding stimuli that elicit barking.
- Remove reinforcing factors.
- Reward quiet behavior.
- Desensitization and counterconditioning to change the response to stimuli.

Step	Comments
Treatment based on diagnosis	• After determining why the dog is barking, a specific treatment program can be implemented for the problem (e.g., separation anxiety, territorial aggression, compulsive – see appropriate sections throughout the text)
Identify stimuli	• Determine all stimuli that lead to barking so that exposure can be prevented or the pet's response to the stimulus altered
Avoid access to stimuli	• Prevent access to the stimuli (e.g., prevent access to doors and windows) or modify the stimulus so that it does not lead to the response (e.g., change the doorbell). The stimulus itself might also be muted or controlled in order for desensitization and counterconditioning to be implemented
Alter owner response	• The owners must avoid responses that reinforce the vocalization including any punishment, anxiety-evoking, or verbal techniques that might increase the barking
Train quiet command	• Teach the dog to settle and quiet down on command (see below)
Desensitize and countercondition	• Identify all stimuli that lead to vocalization and develop a gradient for presentation. Use favored rewards to ensure a calm, positive response during exposure to the stimulus (counterconditioning)
Reward quiet behavior	• The owner should constantly look for quiet behavior, especially in response to provoking stimuli; and reward the pet
Response substitution – differential reinforcement	• The pet is taught to exhibit a quiet response when exposed to the stimulus. Muting or controlling exposure to the stimulus, and a well-trained quiet command (so that the dog responds immediately) should be used to ensure an immediate quiet response. A head halter, disruption device could be used to help ensure success
Head halter training	• A head halter can be used to reorient the head away from the stimulus, focus on the owner, and prompt the dog into a sit with its mouth closed. As soon as the pet is quiet, the leash is relaxed. It can be used as a form of negative reinforcement for teaching quiet behavior
Bark control devices	• Handheld devices (Barker Breaker™, Spray Commander™, or a shake can) used by the owners, or bark-activated devices requiring no owner interaction can be used to stop barking. These devices can be used to disrupt barking as part of a training program or may be successful at stopping barking (punishment) if they are sufficiently deterring and repeated consistently until the barking ceases (see Fig. 13.6)
Surgery	• Debarking surgery may reduce the volume of the bark but may fail due to regrowth and recurrence of some barking. It is considered inhumane in a number of countries and does not address the underlying cause
Drugs	• Drugs may be indicated for specific forms of barking such as compulsive disorders and separation anxiety. Sedatives may be helpful at low doses in some situations, but are usually not recommended for long-term use

Figure 13.5 Managing the dog that barks.

• Timely interruptions or punishment to achieve the quiet response.

While barking can be controlled by training the dog to be quiet on command, this approach is primarily effective when the dog barks in the owner's presence. With punishment-based techniques, the dog may learn to inhibit the barking in the presence of the owner, but is likely to continue in the owner's absence. However, with techniques that interrupt the undesirable response and consistently and repetitively achieve a desirable response, the problem may also diminish even when the owner is absent. In a study by Dr Patrick Pageat, the use of a punishment device such as a water hose was quickly able to reduce fence barking, but over a three-month period there was a recurrence in 86% of cases. There was only a 4% recurrence in barking at the fence over 90 days when a bark-activated citronella collar was used to disrupt barking and this was immediately followed by a play session when the dog was quieted.

Depending on the dog's level of motivation and the intensity of the stimulus, many of these owner-absent problems can be reduced by the use of bark-activated products. Devices that are intended to interrupt barking may act as a deterrent (punish inappropriate behavior) if they are aversive to the pet, may act to temporarily interrupt the behavior (allowing for a window of opportunity for retraining), or may be insufficiently novel or noxious to have any effect on some dogs, especially those that are highly motivated to bark. Some products are designed to sit on counters or attach to walls or cages and may be effective for dogs that bark in specific areas such as by the front door on in their cages. Bark-activated products that attach to the dog's collar are particularly useful for the pet that is not restricted to specific areas (see Fig. 13.6). In one study by Drs Juarbe Diaz and Houpt, barking was decreased in 88.9% of cases with the citronella spray collar, but in only 50% of cases with a bark-activated shock collar. In a study of 41 barking dogs at two veterinary hospitals, Drs Kelly Moffat and Gary Landsberg found that about 77% of dogs wearing a citronella spray collar and about 59% of dogs wearing a scentless spray collar had a significant reduction in barking in a veterinary hospital setting. The management of barking related to

separation anxiety is discussed in Chapter 11. Further discussion of behavior products can be found in handout #21 on the CD (Fig. 5.4).

Prevention

- The owner must never reward barking (e.g., by giving attention, food, play) and must not go to a barking or crying puppy or release it from a cage (unless the puppy is in distress) as this only serves to reinforce the behavior.
- The young dog should be socialized and habituated so that it is accustomed to sounds, situations, and people that might initiate barking.
- Teach basic obedience training for control.
- Immediately and consistently interrupt any undesirable barking at its commencement.

TRAINING THE 'QUIET' COMMAND

The goal is for the dog to respond to a 'quiet' command when it is barking. This can be accomplished by watching for every time that the dog

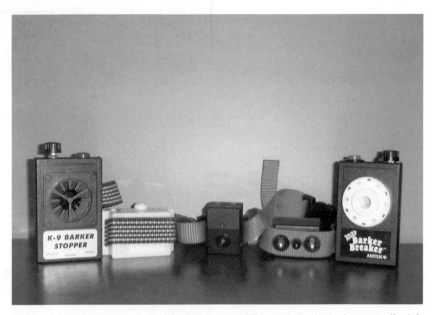

Figure 13.6 Bark-activated products that act as audible and ultrasonic deterrents (far left, far right) must be set up within a meter of where the dog barks. Bark-activated products that attach to a collar deter barking with a spray of citronella (Aboistop™, second from left; Gentle Spray™, center) or with electronic stimulation or shock (second from right).

barks and saying 'quiet!' immediately after the first vocalization (even if it is just a faint woof), calling the dog, and requesting a sit-stay. The dog should be given a food, social, or toy reward. The pet can then be released. The 'quiet' command and reward process should then be repeated for subsequent barks, but the dog should remain quiet for a few seconds longer each time before the reward is given. Timing is critical in this training, as the dog must learn that being quiet (not barking) is the reason for the reward.

If the pet ignores the 'quiet' command, the owner should immediately provide a disruptive stimulus (shake can, air horn, water spray, compressed air, Barker Breaker™) that is startling enough to stop the barking but not strong enough to elicit a fear response or make the pet reluctant to approach the owner when called.

This technique will not completely eliminate barking. This is important for many owners who want to decrease excessive barking and have some verbal control over the pet's vocalizations but not prevent it from alerting them when it hears something unusual.

A grasp of the muzzle accompanied by a verbal correction is an approach used by some owners for interrupting barking of a young and submissive pet. The grasp is released as soon as the dog is quiet (negative reinforcement) and the grasp (and release) is repeated if the barking resumes. This technique is generally impractical for most owners, as it is difficult to time and implement and may lead to hand-shyness or trigger biting (defensive, play). Therefore, a similar but more effective technique is to use a head halter and leash to train the quiet command. Unlike the use of a muzzle grasp, the dog does not become handshy and the upward pull of the leash can immediately and consistently stop barking. The owner gives the command to be quiet, pulls upward on the leash (which closes the mouth), then releases and rewards as soon as the dog stops vocalizing. However, if the barking resumes the pull and release can be repeated until the dog remains quiet. Owners should be advised that the proper timing of the release for quiet behavior (negative reinforcement) is as important as the immediate pull that is required to stop the barking (Fig. 13.7). Client handout #1 (reviewing bark control training) is reproduced in Figure 13.8.

Case example

Mr Ed was a two-year-old neutered male Shetland Sheepdog that barked at virtually any person or pet that approached the property. The owners lived in a townhouse development and the neighbors had recently lodged a complaint. The barking would continue until the person or pet was out of sight or until they came inside and Mr Ed had a chance to greet them. The only way that the owners could stop the barking was to get Mr Ed's tug toy and initiate play. Although the barking was primarily a form of territorial alert, Mr Ed was not exhibiting any aggression and seemed more interested in meet-

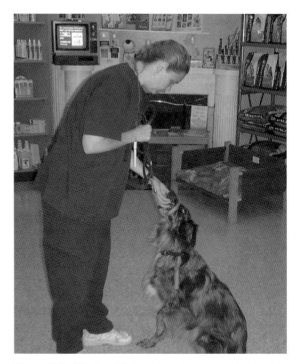

Figure 13.7 The head halter is used to prompt the dog into a quiet sitting position, using the second hand for additional support.

BARKING – TRAINING QUIET

1. Training the 'quiet' command

(a) Training a dog to be quiet on command requires that the dog first be barking. Training will therefore be most successful if you can anticipate a situation when the dog will bark (e.g., children playing, knocking at the door, etc.) so that you can be prepared to quiet the dog on command.

(b) As soon as you hear even the smallest first woof, say 'quiet,' call the dog to you, ask it to 'sit,' and praise a quiet response.

(c) If the puppy doesn't listen and barks after you ask it to be quiet, immediately shake a shake can or sound an air horn as you repeat the 'quiet' command. If the volume is correct for the temperament of the pet, it should immediately stop barking and show a slight startle response without acting afraid.

(d) Another alternative is to leave a head halter and leash attached to the dog. If the dog does not immediately become quiet on command, then a quick pull on the leash and head halter can guide the dog into a quiet sitting position. This is followed by a release of tension on the lead to indicate the correct response has been achieved.

2. Encouraging quiet behavior

(a) You should observe the dog for a calm, quiet response and provide attention, affection, play, or food to encourage this behavior.

(b) Barking must not be reinforced with any form of attention, affection, food, or play. Any attention that does not stop the barking may actually serve to reinforce the behavior. If barking cannot be stopped, it should be ignored until the dog is quiet, and then reinforcement can be given.

(c) Verbal corrections, yelling, punishment, or your own anxious behavior may further aggravate your dog's barking and anxiety.

(d) Use of a bark-activated device (audible alarm, citronella spray, bark-activated collar) may inhibit barking in some dogs. Once the barking stops, you should then immediately distract the dog with affection or a favored treat or toy so that the quiet behavior can be reinforced and barking is less likely to recur.

(e) Avoid leaving the puppy outdoors unsupervised for long periods. It may be stimulated to bark by passing stimuli (other dogs, strangers) or may bark to attract your attention. Opening the door or going out to the dog, even to settle the dog down, will only serve to reinforce the barking behavior.

3. Anxiety-induced barking

When barking arises out of anxiety, the treatment program will need to be designed to address the underlying cause of anxiety as well as any factors that might be reinforcing or aggravating the problem.

Figure 13.8   Training quiet (handout #1 – printable from the CD).

ing the visitor than in chasing him or her away. Barking only ceased when Mr Ed was rewarded (by the owner's greeting or the arrival of the visitor) or when the stimulus was removed (the visitor or animal was out of sight).

The owner began some basic obedience reward training, but although Mr Ed became much more responsive to commands, the owner was unable to interrupt the barking on command or train Mr Ed to the 'quiet' command. Mr Ed was then halter trained, and whenever the owners were available to supervise, Mr Ed was left with a head halter and 10-ft leash attached. At the instant barking began, the owner would command 'quiet!' and pull on the leash, releasing it after Mr Ed became

quiet. If Mr Ed remained quiet (training began with five seconds of quiet and was eventually extended to 30 seconds), he was rewarded. Within days, Mr Ed would stop barking on command. However, whenever the owners were away from home, the neighbors would still complain about barking. Since there was no way to successfully remove or reduce the sights and sounds that stimulated Mr Ed to bark, debarking surgery and bark-activated devices were discussed. Since the owners would be unable to keep Mr Ed if the barking persisted, surgical debarking was considered, but the owners first decided to test the effectiveness of the antibark devices. A collar-mounted product was chosen, since the dog would bark throughout the house and Mr Ed would exhibit anxiety-induced barking if confined. An audible bark collar and an ultrasonic bark collar were both unsuccessful as they were inconsistent and not sufficiently aversive, but Mr Ed responded immediately to the use of a citronella spray collar. Whenever Mr Ed wore the collar, barking was suppressed.

CANINE HYPERACTIVITY AND UNRULINESS

Although true hyperactivity disorders are very rare in dogs, hyperkinesis with or without hyperactivity can usually be diagnosed because of the paradoxical response to amphetamines. Most overactive dogs are either genetically predisposed to high levels of energy and activity, like working breed dogs, or their unruly behaviors have been inadvertently rewarded (or both). Problem situations are likely to occur when the need for exercise, proper social interaction, and control are neglected. Unruliness tends to be a catch-all phrase for dogs that the family cannot get under control, respond poorly to commands, and engage in behaviors the family finds obnoxious. In addition to the overactive dog, many of the behaviors discussed elsewhere in this text (jumping up, nipping and biting, destructiveness, digging, and some forms of barking) are examples of unruly behaviors that are bothersome for owners. Running away, chasing cars, refusal to come when called, and stealing items are also common owner complaints. Some dogs with compulsive disorders (spinning, shadow chasing, tail chasing) may present for being overly active and out of control. Some additional diagnostic considerations and treatment for stereotypic behaviors are discussed in Chapter 10.

Obedience training, leash control, head halter training, and other techniques designed to give owners more control over their dogs are required to correct these problems. However, there are great genetic differences between individuals so that training techniques may need to be adjusted to suit the individual.

Diagnosis and prognosis

Dogs with hyperkinesis or attention deficit disorders with hyperactivity (ADHD) may exhibit a paradoxical response to treatment with amphetamines. Unlike the CNS stimulation that these drugs produce in normal animals, dogs with ADHD become less active and more attentive when treated with these drugs. Dogs with ADHD may exhibit overactivity, poor attention span, lack of trainability, aggressive displays, and failure to calm down in neutral environments. In suspected cases of ADHD, dogs should be admitted to the veterinary hospital and baseline heart rate, respiratory rate, and activity level should be recorded.

The diagnosis can be confirmed by administering 0.2–0.5 mg/kg of dextroamphetamine orally and then observing every 30 minutes for one to two hours. Dogs with hyperkinesis become calmer and have lowered heart and respiratory rates. Alternatively the owner can be advised to monitor the dog's repetitive and overexuberant displays (to get a baseline) and then use methylphenidate as a therapeutic response trial. Low doses are initially used (e.g., 0.5 mg/kg in the morning and afternoon). If there is no improvement and there have been no adverse effects after three days, the dose can be adjusted upward in 0.25 mg/kg increments every three days until a response is achieved. At each dose level, if there has been no improvement or adverse effects, the dose can again be raised to a maximum of 2 mg/kg bid. If an improvement is noted, then long-term therapy might be considered with gradual adjustment of the dose every few days to achieve optimum response.

Caution should be taken if home monitoring is used because amphetamines can increase excitability, unruliness, activity, restlessness, and aggression. Therefore, if there are any of these or other adverse effects at any point during the trial, the drug should be immediately discontinued.

For those cases where a hyperactivity disorder is not the cause, the prognosis will be based on the ultimate cause of the overactivity. Those cases that have been inadvertently rewarded by the owners can usually be improved with behavioral modification techniques, while those with an innately high energy level and little opportunity to exercise may be much more difficult to resolve. Young dogs are generally more playful and active than adults, so that some hyperactivity problems may improve as the pets grow older.

Management

Treatment of unruliness and hyperactivity must be tailored to the individual pet. Important considerations include the breed of the pet, the owner's response to the dog's behavior, the environment, family social dynamics, and the amount of successful, previous training.

The most critical aspect of controlling and eliminating these types of problems is to identify and address the motivation or underlying cause for the behavior. Thought must be given to why the dog is acting in an undesirable manner. If the pet is not receiving enough exercise, increasing the amount of daily exercise and play should be helpful. Situations that cause the pet to become exceptionally excited, like greetings or reaching for a leash, should be kept low-key. If the pet won't listen to commands, obedience training will be very important. Once the pet learns basic command responses, sits and downs should be requested before the pet gets anything it wants or needs, and stays should frequently be practiced to constantly remind the pet that the owner is in control. Attention-seeking behavior must be ignored. The owner's role in the development of the problems should be examined and addressed. Inadvertent reinforcement of undesired behavior and inconsistencies in responding to the behaviors are common mistakes family members make. (See Fig. 13.9.)

Prevention

Dogs, especially puppies and adolescent dogs, should be provided with appropriate and sufficient amounts of play, exercise, mental stimulation, and social interaction to meet their individual needs (Fig. 13.9). Owners must give no attention and completely ignore their dogs when the pets are exhibiting undesirable behaviors. Ignoring, walking away, and shutting the door or 'time out' would be preferable to providing attention. All rewards (play, food, attention) should only be given for calmness and obedience. Since immediately providing a play period or exercise when the pet is acting in an unruly or overactive fashion may reward the behavior, it is best to apply some distraction that will quiet it for at least 10 seconds prior to engaging it in some form of play or exercise. Head halter training should be considered for dogs that are difficult to manage.

Case example

Dennis was an 11-month-old, 4 kg Toy Poodle, that the owner could never calm down and which would jump from the ground into his owner's arms when he wanted attention. The owner complied by patting Dennis, carrying him around for a few minutes, and sometimes playing ball or giving Dennis a few treats when he was put back down. During the behavior consultation, Dennis was placed on the office floor but barked excessively, ran back and forth to the door, or jumped on to the owner's lap. He was a very active and energetic young dog. During the course of the consultation the owner was advised to ignore Dennis and a long 10-ft leash was left attached to his body harness. Each time Dennis jumped on the owner's lap or began to bark, an ultrasonic training device, a water rifle, or a tug on the leash was used to deter the behavior. Remote corrective techniques were utilized so that the aversive stimulus was used to interrupt the behavior (which it did). After several interceptive distractions and 30 minutes of the owner's ignoring Dennis by avoiding eye contact and pulling or stepping on the leash when he tried to jump on the owner's lap, Dennis lay down by the owner's feet and relaxed or slept for the next 30 minutes.

Withdrawing all attention and rewards for demanding and excitable behavior, as well as

Method	Comments
Exercise, play and programming	• Provide a regular routine of play, and vigorous exercise that is designed to suit the dog's individual needs (e.g., retrieve, sled pulling, flyball, agility). Train the dog to settle and provide self-play toys after each session
Rewards	• Train a settle, or focus command. Make rewards contingent on calm behavior. Clicker training can be highly effective
Extinction	• The family must stop providing any reinforcement for undesirable behaviors. They must ensure that attention, rewards, and play are never given as a response to a pet's demand. This only serves to reward excitable and pushy behavior. Stopping play and ignoring, walking away, or 'time out' when the dog gets overly excited (negative punishment) may be successful in some cases
Obedience training	• Use sit, stay, and settle commands to train calm, quiet responses. Slowly extend quiet time during training. Excitable pets may do better in low-distraction, quiet environments or even with private lessons during initial training, then moving to group situations. Consider providing an exercise period before training sessions
Punishment/distraction	• For dogs that are overactive or excitable, punishment is seldom successful. It may be possible, in some cases, to identify a device or product that can be used to distract the dog or interrupt the behavior, so that calmness can be trained. Ultrasonic trainers, audible alarms, or water guns might be helpful. If the behavior is preceded by barking, antibark spray collars may provide interruption and distraction at the onset of the behavior
Training devices	• No-pull halters, head halters, and long leashes are particularly useful in gaining control over exuberant or hard-to-control dogs
Drug therapy	• ADHD or hyperkinesis may respond to amphetamines. Anti-anxiety drugs and sedatives may occasionally be helpful to gain control during initial training but may interfere with learning. Antidepressants such as imipramine, amitriptyline, or fluoxetine may be useful in some cases, and selegiline may also be a consideration as the effects of 2PE and enhanced catecholamine transmission may lead to a paradoxical inhibitory effect

Figure 13.9 Management of the overactive dog.

using timely interruptions, were successful in controlling Dennis's unruly behavior. At home, the owner left a long leash attached, continued to ignore all demanding behaviors, and used interruption devices to deter Dennis. Additional play and exercise periods were provided, but only when Dennis was calm and non-demanding. The owner took Dennis to obedience classes where he was too distracted and excitable to respond. The trainer suggested a few private lessons in a quiet environment and Dennis improved considerably, but continued to remain a high-energy, demanding, excitable dog.

NOCTURNAL ACTIVITY

Provided there are no underlying medical causes, it will be necessary to determine why the dog might be waking at night (fear, anxiety, schedule change, outdoor stimuli) so that the cause can be resolved. Increasing daytime and evening play and activity, developing a secure and comfortable night-time sleep area and ensuring the owner does not reinforce the behavior (ignore or use disruptive device) are the basics of treatment. Hypnotic benzodiazepines (see Ch. 6) to help induce sleep, D.A.P.™ to reduce anxiety, and antidepressants to help better regulate sleep–wake cycles might be considered as drug options. Night waking is discussed in further detail in Chapter 12.

UNDESIRABLE SEXUAL BEHAVIOR

Sexual and mating behavior is beyond the scope of this text. However, there are a number of undesirable behaviors that may have a sexual basis, with which owners may have problems. In North America, the relatively common practice of neutering can reduce or eliminate most sexual problems (Fig. 5.3). However, problems such as masturbation and mounting may persist even after castration. In fact, some female dogs may mount as part of their social repertoire with people or other dogs. Roaming, marking, inter-male aggression, and behavior changes associated with female sexual cycles might be other signs.

Diagnosis

Before behavioral issues can be addressed, the diagnosis first involves ruling out underlying medical problems and determining whether neutering is an option. If it is uncertain whether a pet has been entirely neutered (e.g., retained testicles), testosterone levels can be measured one and two hours following an injection of HCG (250 IU SC) or GnRH (2.2 μg/kg IM). For dogs mounting other dogs, be certain to assess the medical health of both dogs as odor and pheromonal changes associated with endocrine diseases, ear infections, anal sacculitis, cystitis, etc., may be factors. Also see Chapter 21 for Dr Pageat's diagnostic rule-outs.

Treatment

The sequence of events prior to the behavior, and the owner's response to the problem, should be assessed. Inciting factors might be avoided or immediately redirected to an appropriate response and any owner reinforcement is removed. For mounting, the treatment program would be similar to jumping up (described earlier in this chapter). For masturbation and mounting of other pets, the problem might be allowed to continue if it is doing no harm or directed to an alternative acceptable outlet or location. Other options are prevention, the use of remote punishment, or supervision and retraining with a leash and head halter. For anxiety-related disorders, drug therapy or D.A.P.™ spray might be useful. For intact males, drugs that reduce testosterone (Ch. 6) might be useful, while for neutered males, progestins might be effective, but the side effects are a major concern with these drugs.

FURTHER READING

Adams GJ, Johnson KG 1994 Behavioral responses to barking and other auditory stimuli during nighttime sleeping and waking in the domestic dog (*Canis familiaris*). Applied Animal Behavioral Science 39:151–162

Aubry X 1997 A comparison of different antibarking devices. Aversive and disruptive stimuli. In: Mills DS, Heath SE, Harrington LJ (eds) Proceedings of the first international conference on veterinary behavioural medicine. UFAW, Potter's Bar, UK, p 156–163

Beaver BV 1999 Canine behaviour: a guide for veterinarians. WB Saunders, Philadelphia, PA

Coppinger R, Feinstein M 1991 'Hark! Hark! The dogs do bark ...' and bark and bark. Smithsonian 21(10):119–129

Hart BL, Hart LA 1984 Selecting the best companion animal: breed and gender specific profiles. In: Anderson RK, Hart BL, Hart LA (eds) The pet connection: its influence on our health and quality of life. University of Minnesota Press, Minneapolis, MN, p 180–193

Houpt KA 1979 Sexual behavior problems in dogs and cats. Veterinary Clinics of North America, Small Animal Practice 27(3):601–615

Juarbe-Diaz SV, Houpt KA 1996 Comparison of two antibarking collars for treatment of nuisance barking. Journal of the American Animal Hospital Association 5(32):231–235

Luescher AU 1993 Hyperkinesis in dogs: six case reports. Canadian Veterinary Journal 34:368–370

Mathews SL 1984 Eliminating barking as an attention-getting device. Canine Practice 11(1):6–9

Moffat KM, Landsberg GM, Beaudet R 2003 Effectiveness and comparison of both a citronella and scentless spray bark collar for the control of barking in a veterinary hospital setting. Journal of the American Animal Hospital Association 39(in press)

Pageat P, Tessier Y 1997 Disruptive stimulus: definition and application in behavior therapy. In: Proceedings of the first international conference of veterinary behavioral medicine. Universities Federation for Animal Welfare, Potter's Bar, UK, p 187

Serpell J 1995 The domestic dog: its evolution, behavior, and interactions with people. Cambridge University Press, New York

Voith VL, Borchelt PL 1987 Advice for clients with overactive dogs. Veterinary Technician September:25–28

Wells D 2001 The effectiveness of a citronella spray collar in reducing certain forms of barking in dogs. Applied Animal Behavior Science 73:299–309

14

Unruly behaviors, training, and management – cats

FELINE NOCTURNAL ACTIVITY

The cat as a species can be fairly sedentary throughout the day, with the highest activity exhibited at dusk and dawn. This can cause problems in a household. Bothersome nocturnal behaviors are more common in kittens and usually decrease when the pet reaches 12–18 months of age. However, some cats are eternally 'young at heart' and the behavior can continue through adulthood. Not only can they provide unwanted attention to their owners during sleep, but they can also run through the house at night, during exuberant play sessions. Owners might complain of lack of sleep, or damage done to the house at night while they were sleeping. They may even report that the cat or kitten contacts them physically during the night, perhaps by trying to sleep on their face or nibbling their toes. Although many of these problems are more frequent at night, exuberant play and jumping on or pouncing at owners can also occur at any time during the day (see also feline excessive vocalization, below).

Diagnosis and prognosis

The diagnosis is made based on the history provided by the owner. The complaint is one of feline activity during the night that is not well tolerated by the owner. Pouncing, play bites, swatting, and noisy running over the bed or through the home may be bothersome for the

323

family. The cat is usually young, active, and may not be receiving enough physical and social activity during the day. Cats that previously slept through the night and have now become increasingly vocal or active should be assessed for underlying medical problems including cognitive dysfunction (see Ch. 12), as well as any recent change in the household or schedule that may have led to decreased daytime activity and increased night-time activity.

The prognosis for successfully stopping the behavior is fair to good for most situations. Exuberant play and pouncing behaviors have a much better prognosis in a young playful kitten and are more of a concern if they persist into adulthood. The prognosis for improving an adult cat with increasing nocturnal activity will vary based on the cause of the problem and whether it is amenable to drug therapy.

Management

The owner should avoid giving the cat attention or reinforcing it when it is performing an undesirable behavior. Scolding should also be avoided. Light scolding might reinforce the behavior, while harsh scolding may weaken the bond with the pet and cause avoidance behaviors. The cat may be more likely to sleep through the night if it is given more attention, activity, and play in the early evening before the family retires for the night. Play with the cat is best directed at moving objects so that toys thrown or dragged along by the owners, and those that can be batted along the ground or dangled from cat perches or door handles, work best. A second cat of the same age and temperament might provide an outlet for play behavior. Preventing access to the cat's favored sleeping areas during the daytime may also be helpful.

Restricting the areas accessible to the cat can also be helpful. This might involve closing the bedroom door, or confining the cat to another room or a crate during the night. Booby traps, such as upside down mousetraps or motion-activated sprayers, can be used to keep the pet away from particular areas where it scampers and makes noise. The cat that cannot be kept out of the bedroom during the night can be discouraged with a water gun, ultrasonic device, or the hissing sound from a can of compressed air.

For night-time vocalization related to medical problems, cognitive dysfunction, or excessive anxiety, drug therapy may be useful depending on the cause. Selegiline may be effective for cognitive dysfunction (see Ch. 12 for more details), while a pre-bedtime dose of a benzodiazepine, an antihistamine such as diphenhydramine, or a phenothiazine might help to induce night-time sleep in the short term.

Prevention

Providing interactive games and appealing play toys is very important for meeting the young cat's social and play requirements. Interaction with the pet that allows it to play with or attack body parts should be discouraged.

Case example

Ralphy Boy, a nine-month-old neutered male domestic shorthair cat, lived in an apartment with a couple in their late 60s. Ralphy was a gregarious kitten who liked to initiate play by jumping onto the owners' laps or shoulders. However, the major problem was that Ralphy loved to chase across the bedroom furniture and bedcovers at about 2 o'clock every morning. The owners had recently had Ralphy neutered, with no effect on this behavior, and had taken to locking Ralphy out of the bedroom at night where he would howl and run around knocking items off the table tops and work surfaces.

The owners were providing little if any interactive play, so that Ralphy Boy slept throughout the evening and was up and raring to go at night. The owners had no control over Ralphy Boy so that he was allowed to play, eat, and be patted whenever he desired. The owners began gaining more control by providing no further rewards of any kind (food, play, or affection) except on their own initiation. The cat quickly learned the 'come!' command, which the cat always had to respond to before rewards were given. Ralphy was also taught to sit on his owner's lap and be stroked for several minutes before each feeding or play session. Interactive cat wands for chasing and a cat play center with dangling toys were placed in the den, and play sessions were planned each evening. From 7 to 11 p.m. Ralphy was provided with numerous play sessions and a catnip treat so that he had less chance to sleep during the day. A feeding session was added at 11 p.m. and Ralphy was confined to the den each night. The situation improved dramatically but Ralphy continued to wake and vocalize on some nights. A playful six-month-old neutered male kitten was obtained from a local shelter. Although Ralphy Boy and his new friend 'Norton' occasionally woke and played at nights there was no further vocalization and the cats caused no problems for their owners as they were housed in the den at nights.

FELINE EXCESSIVE VOCALIZATION

Excessive vocalization is more common in the oriental breeds but can occur in virtually any cat. Since cats are quite active at dawn, it is not uncommon to have complaints of vocalization very early in the morning. There are many causes of nocturnal vocalizing very early in the morning, including territorial arousal, attention-seeking behavior, hunger, pain, and disorientation (e.g., geriatric cats with cognitive dysfunction). Cats placed on weight-loss diets may occasionally vocalize as a demand for food.

Diagnosis and prognosis

For successful diagnosis and treatment, the cause of the cat's vocalization must be determined. Medical problems could contribute to increased vocalization, restlessness, altered sleep–wake cycles, and increased nocturnal activity, so that an appropriate medical workup should first be performed based on the signalment and clinical signs. Knowing the time (nocturnal vs daytime) and situations in which the problem occurs can be helpful in making the diagnosis. It is usually beneficial for the family to keep a diary that includes time of night, day of week, month, when and where the behavior occurs, and comments on what else might be occurring in the environment at the same time. The goal is to identify the triggers for the behaviors so they can be addressed.

Except in oriental breeds, where the behavior can be highly innate and unrelated to specific stimuli, the prognosis is moderately good for successful correction, provided the owner is able to identify and remove those factors that are initiating or reinforcing the problem.

Management

The guidelines are as follows:

- Identify the owner's response to the cat's vocalization and remove any reinforcement (e.g., attention, food, affection, allowing outdoors). Attention should never be given for demanding or vocal behavior.
- Quiet, non-demanding behavior should be reinforced.
- Use an interruptive stimulus during vocalization (water gun, compressed air canister, audible or ultrasonic alarm). It is best to avoid eye contact and say nothing while interrupting the behavior. When quiet, the cat can be reinforced.
- Identify the stimulus for the cat's vocalization and reduce exposure. Closing windows so the cat cannot hear or see roaming cats may help. Anything that attracts roaming cats to visit during the night should be discouraged, such as feeding outdoors by the door or on the porch.
- Provide for all the cat's needs. For nocturnal vocalization, provide play, activity, and exercise throughout the evening. Sometimes, obtaining a second playful cat can provide an additional outlet for play. Providing food so that it is available just before bedtime and through the night may also be useful for some cats.

- Cats on weight-reduction diets that constantly demand and howl for food should be fed high-bulk diets.
- A benzodiazepine or sedating antihistamine prior to bedtime may be helpful for a few nights to help re-establish night time sleep.
- Cats with old age onset vocalization should be closely evaluated for any potential medical causes including painful conditions, sensory decline, and cognitive dysfunction. Although not approved for use in cats, selegiline may be effective in cases of cognitive dysfunction (see Ch. 12 for details).

Prevention

Avoid rewarding vocalization by allowing the cat outdoors or providing food, attention, or play on demand. Providing sufficient play and exercise during the daytime and evening will help provide the cat with sufficient attention and may help get it on to a schedule so that it sleeps through the night. A mentally stimulating environment with interactive toys may also help.

Case example

Jethro was a three-year-old neutered male Siamese cat that had always been excessively vocal. Whenever Jethro cried out, the owners tried to determine what Jethro might want so that they could give it to him. Since providing food was the only technique that consistently stopped vocalization, the owners assumed that the cat was constantly hungry.

At the time of consultation, Jethro was 7 kg. He had recently been placed on a diet by the referring veterinarian and the vocalization problem had further escalated. Rather than buy an expensive, low-calorie prescription food, the owners had merely cut back dramatically on the amount being fed. Because of the diet, Jethro was indeed howling for food. It is likely that the initial howling was merely the typical overvocalization of some Siamese cats. It became a conditioned behavior because the owners had consistently rewarded the behavior.

The first step in correction was to satisfy the cat's needs by changing to a high-bulk diet. Jethro was provided with multiple small meals of this diet whenever the owner was home but never on demand. When the owner was out, food was not provided. Whenever Jethro approached the owners and began to vocalize, he was sprayed with a can of compressed air. Whenever Jethro approached the owners and did not vocalize, a catnip treat, affection, interactive play, or a play toy was provided. Although Jethro continued to vocalize excessively, this was dramatically reduced after only a few days and could be easily interrupted with the compressed air.

STEALING, GETTING INTO TRASH, CLIMBING ON COUNTERS AND FURNITURE

Cats might engage in these behaviors because of their inquisitive and investigative natures and because they are self-gratifying (the pet may obtain food, a desired object to chew, or a resting station). Attempts to use punishment usually fail because corrections are applied long after the behavior is finished. Owners are often certain that their pets know they have done wrong when they discover the problem but, in most cases, this logic is seriously flawed. They think that the pet knows what it has done wrong because it looks guilty or runs away when the owner approaches. In these cases, the pet has learned that there are unpleasant consequences for being on the furniture or worktop, or in the rubbish when the owner approaches. Even if the owner punishes the pet while it is on the counter, this only teaches the cat to avoid the counter when the owners are present. This is because when the owners are not around, the cat has already learned that there are no unpleasant (only pleasant) consequences when going into these areas.

Diagnosis and prognosis

The diagnosis is made based on the owner's observation that the cat performs the activities. For most situations, the prognosis for correction is good. These behaviors are typically young pet behaviors and may decrease or stop on their own as the pet grows older.

Management

Stealing

This is not as common a problem as in dogs, but some cats will steal and sometimes cache (hide and store) rubber bands, knitting material, clothing, or child toys. Providing the cat with its own acceptable toys for chewing and carrying is therefore the first course of action. The pet should have a variety of interesting toys available, and be given a food or social reward for playing with them. With cats, moving the toy as if it were prey may further encourage the cat to play with this toy. Do not give the cat discarded items of clothing, as this only makes it more difficult for the pet to distinguish between household possessions and chew toys. The family should provide adequate play, exercise, and social attention to meet the pet's requirements.

If a pet is found chewing, stealing, or carrying a household item it should be interrupted with a quick, sharp noise, and the possession retrieved. The pet should then be directed to chewing and playing with acceptable toys. It may be prudent to identify the types of objects the cat prefers to chew so that all potential household targets can be kept out of reach and appropriate (similar texture, size, or shape) toys provided. For example, Kitty Kong™ has rubber whiskers that resemble rubber bands and cats that chew on wool may prefer a toy made of wool or similar material (as long as the objects are not ingested). Harsh corrections, prolonged scoldings, delayed punishment, and physical punishment should all be avoided in cats as they are likely to cause fear of the owner and may at best only deter the behavior in the owner's presence. Preventing access to problem areas and safe-guarding valuables by keeping them in pet-proof (or child-proof) containers or cupboards may be useful for some households. Booby traps such as a motion-activated alarm (see Fig. 5.4, handout #21 on the CD) can also be a very successful tool to teach a pet to stay away from the owner's possessions.

Aversive tasting substances can also be very helpful for curtailing this behavior. For example, if the pet chews on rubber, cords from blinds, computer cables, or plants, a cat repellent, or even a little cayenne pepper mixed with water, can be applied to the surface (see handout #21 on the CD). Concurrently, the owner should coat the cat's toys with an appealing taste or a little catnip to accentuate the difference between what it is supposed to chew and what it is not.

Getting into trash and food containers

Again, this is less of a problem in cats in comparison with dogs, but sometimes cats raid trash cans for food or items for play. If cats can gain access to packaged foods some cats may chew through the packages. Cats that have not raided food cupboards or trash bins in the past may begin to do so when they are put on a calorie-restricted diet for weight reduction or with medical problems that are associated with hyperphagia (e.g., thyroid disease, renal dysfunction). Providing more bulk or roughage in the diet, offering food-stuffed toys, dental diets to increase oral stimulation, and increasing play and exercise may help to reduce the problem. A simple solution is to use a more secure container or place the trash and any potential food targets in a location where the pet does not have access unless the owner is present to supervise and deter access to the garbage. Another option is to place one of the booby trap devices such as a motion-activated alarm on the trash container.

Getting on counters and furniture

One of the more common owner complaints is about the cat that explores table tops and counters. Not only might these be interesting areas to explore, they may have odors and tastes that attract the cat to the area. Therefore the first step is to ensure that nothing is left on the counters or table top that might be appealing to the cat. If the family decides that the pet should not be allowed on furniture or counters then all family members must consistently enforce the rules and no exceptions can be made. The cat should have a comfortable resting location (bed, crate, chair, cat condo), where it is encouraged to rest and play with its toys. If a family member would like to have the pet in the lap, but not on the furniture, the person should get on the floor and then allow the pet to get in the lap. Another solution is to give the pet a toy stuffed with food as it approaches to give it something to do other than jump up on the furniture.

Keeping the pet off counters and furniture when the owner is not around requires a different strategy. Preventing access to the furniture is generally the most practical option until the cat can be 'trusted' to stay away. If the cat has access to the furniture or counter, it can be supervised by the owner so that jumping up can be deterred immediately and resting in the desired location reinforced. However, when the owner is not around, the appeal of the surfaces can be greatly reduced by using surface coverings that the cat finds unpleasant (e.g., upside down carpet runners). Alternately aversive repellent or booby trap devices such as double-sided tape, motion detectors, avoidance mats, or Snappy Trainer™ should keep most pets off the furniture (see Fig. 5.4, handout #21 on the CD, and Fig. 14.1 for details).

Prevention

These problems are most common in young pets. Large amounts of physical and mental stimulation, as well as a sufficient amount of supervision, are very important for keeping young pets out of trouble. Owners should constantly look for acceptable behaviors to reinforce and not focus on punishment to shape behaviors. When the untrained pet cannot be closely supervised, it should be confined to a safe area. Unacceptable behaviors should consistently be quickly interrupted, and the pet should then be directed to engage in appropriate behaviors. Closing off doors to problem areas, using child locks, baby gates, long leashes attached to a body harness (used as a tie-down next to the owner) may all be helpful for controlling the young pet while appropriate behaviors are being taught.

Case example

Samantha, a four-year-old spayed female cat, lived in a one-bedroom apartment with her 23-year-old owner. Because of her owner's concerns about cleanliness and health, Samantha was not allowed on the kitchen worktops or tables. When the owner was present, the cat had been taught to stay away from the tables and counters with a water rifle, but whenever the owner went out of the room or out of the apartment, Samantha continued to climb on the worktops and table. The owner had tested this by leaving some food on the counter, which Samantha quickly ate when the owner left the room. Remote punishment techniques with the water sprayer had not been successful (presumably because the owner did a poor job of hiding out of sight and Samantha was able to determine when the owner was watching). The owner was not willing to confine Samantha to the bathroom, bedroom, or a crate.

Samantha continued to climb onto the tables and worktops as part of her daily exploratory and play behaviors and because food, leftovers, or tasty spills could occasionally be found in these areas (not to mention the test foods that the owner had purposely provided), that would intermittently reward her 'travels.' The first step was to provide Samantha with a play center that consisted of scratching surfaces, a few cubby holes for hiding, and a number of ledges and platforms for climbing and perching. On these platforms and dangling from the ledges were toys and small morsels of food and treats. Samantha soon began to explore and investigate the play center regularly, but continued occasionally to wander across the table and worktops. The owner purchased a

1. Once rules are established regarding where the pet is allowed to go, and what areas are to be off limits, all family members must consistently follow the same rules. Whenever a family member can supervise the cat it must be prevented from getting into these locations or onto the furniture or counters.
2. If the pet attempts to climb onto furniture or counter or enter an 'out of bounds' room, it should be immediately deterred as the behavior begins. Physical punishment should be avoided. Rather, an immediate unpleasant disruption should be used to stop the undesirable behavior as it begins. A sharp noise (such as a shake can or audible alarm), a spray of water, or a remote control citronella collar can be used to deter the cat. Cats can also be trained to wear a leash and body harness and the leash can be used to train the cat what areas to avoid.
3. It can be helpful to have a specific area or perch with bedding, treats, and toys where the cat sleeps or rests, so that it is attracted to that area rather than rooms or furniture that are considered out of bounds.
4. Make certain that there is nothing in the area that might attract the cat such as food, toys, or treats.
5. Whenever you cannot supervise your cat, it must be consistently prevented from getting on the counter or into rooms that are out of bounds. This might be accomplished by blocking access to the area, confining the cat to a particular room or area of the house where exploration is allowed, or even through crate training.
6. Deterrent devices are another option to keep cats away from specific areas when the owner is not available to supervise. A less appealing surface (e.g., upside-down vinyl carpet runner), unpleasant odors such as cat repellents, aversive tastes (if the cat chews items in the area), or booby traps such as motion-activated spray cans and alarms, upside-down mousetraps, Snappy Trainer™, or alarm mats (Fig. 5.4).

Figure 14.1 Getting on the furniture, counters, or into rooms where the cat is not allowed.

motion-detector spray that was used to keep the cat away from the worktop when she was out, and a piece of plastic carpet runner (nubs up) was draped across the table except at meal times. The cat was never seen on the work surfaces or table top again.

UNDESIRABLE SEXUAL BEHAVIOR

Sexual and mating behavior is beyond the scope of this text. However, there are a number of undesirable behaviors that may have a sexual basis, with which owners may have problems. In North America, the relatively common practice of neutering can reduce or eliminate most sexual problems (Fig. 5.3). However, problems such as masturbation, mounting, roaming, and urine marking may persist after neutering and female cats may exhibit display marking and excessive vocalization that might mimic sexual cycling.

Diagnosis

The diagnosis involves ruling out underlying medical problems, behavioral causes, and determining whether neutering is an option. If it is uncertain whether a pet has been entirely neutered (e.g., retained testicles), testosterone levels can be measured one and two hours following an injection of HCG (250 IU SC) or GnRH (25 µg/cat IM). To determine whether there might be ovarian remnants, the same dose is utilized and 10 days later blood is drawn for a progesterone level.

Treatment

Urine marking is discussed in Chapter 18. The sequence of events prior to the behavior, and the owner's response to the problem, should be assessed. Inciting factors might be avoided or immediately redirected to an appropriate response as soon as the sequence is likely to begin. For mounting of other cats, the relationship between the cats must be reviewed to determine the underlying cause and whether, in fact, the problem needs to be resolved. The problem may need to be prevented in the owner's absence and might be inhibited using a leash and harness or disruptive devices when the owner is supervising. Alternative acceptable forms of play and social interaction should of course be reinforced. For mounting of household possessions and masturbation, the cat might best be allowed to continue if it is doing no harm, or it could be provided with an alternative acceptable behavior in which to engage. Treatment options include ensuring that the owner is not inadvertently stimulating, reinforcing, or aggravating the problem; preventive techniques; increasing environmental stimulation; reducing sources of anxiety with behavior modification; Feliway™; and drugs. For neutered males, progestins might be effective but the side effects are a major concern with these drugs.

FURTHER READING

Beaver BV 1981 Modifying a cat's behavior. Veterinary Medicine Small Animal Clinics 76:1281–1283
Beaver BV 1992 Feline behavior: a guide for veterinarians. In: Canine communicative behavior. WB Saunders, Philadelphia, PA, p 106–136

Houpt KA 1979 Sexual behavior problems in dogs and cats. Veterinary Clinics of North America, Small Animal Practice 27(3):601–615
Milani MM 2000 Crate training as a feline stress reliever. Feline Practice 28(3):8–9

15

Canine destructive behaviors

A very common complaint of dog owners is destructive behavior that can result in damage to the home, injury to the pet, and a weakened family–pet bond. Chewing, scratching, and dig4-ging are clinical signs that can occur for a variety of reasons. In many cases it is simply a matter of normal behavior being directed toward an unacceptable object or area. Preventive counseling, including a thorough discussion of normal puppy behavior as well as the appropriate use of confinement and supervision, can help the family avoid these types of problems in young pets.

Some problems involving destructive behavior can have more serious and complex underlying etiologies. Separation anxiety, escape behavior resulting from an overwhelming phobia, or compulsive sucking and chewing of household objects may require more complete history taking and well thought out therapy plans. Other problems have causes that are basically simple but may not be obvious, such as chewing, scratching, or digging to get at rodents, chewing furniture to get to a toy, chewing or scratching of walls, windows and furniture due to territorial arousal, and chewing clothing or carpeting with an interesting odor or taste.

DESTRUCTIVE CHEWING BY DOGS

In some cases, family members contribute to the problem by providing inappropriate objects (e.g., old shoes, socks, blankets) for the dog to

331

chew and not providing enough appropriate ones. Chewing is a normal behavior for puppies and adolescent dogs that are investigative, have lots of energy, and are more playful than adults. Inappropriate chewing and destructiveness by young dogs can be a result of exploration, play, scavenging, hunger, and attempts at escape from confinement. It can also result from insufficient exercise and stimulation.

Diagnosis and prognosis

Destructive behavior by young dogs is usually a 'management' issue. A good portion of a young dog's non-sleeping day involves playing, exploration, eating, and chewing. Destructive chewing is therefore not unusual and should be expected by owners. Persistent damage reflects a lack of training and control by the owner rather than a pathological state in the dog. Some dogs learn to grab and chew on items to get the owner's attention, and engage in chase games. Owners of young dogs should be questioned about the dog's daily schedule including the amount of exercise and training the pet receives, the type of confinement and supervision provided, what steps have been taken to 'dog proof' the home, as well as the type of toys that are available.

The cause of destructive chewing in adult dogs can be more difficult to diagnose and manage successfully. Some underlying causes include hunger, predation, separation anxiety, noise phobias, confinement problems, compulsive disorders, and territorial behavior. Underlying medical problems might not be a major consideration, but certain types of destructiveness such as picas, destructiveness associated with increased anxiety and phobias, and destructiveness that increases with age may all be related to medical components. Concurrent signs such as weight loss, polyuria and polydypsia, gastrointestinal upset, sleep disorders, or changes in behavior may be indicative of a medical cause. Dogs placed on a calorie-restricted diet for weight loss may begin to explore and destroy in their 'quest' for more food. Any condition that leads to an increased appetite can contribute to picas, garbage raiding, and food stealing. At the very least, a set of baseline screening tests (hemogram, biochemical profile) and in some cases screening for endocrine dysfunction (thyroid, adrenal) might be warranted.

Clues to pursue include:

- What is chewed.
- When and where the behavior occurs.
- Situations in which the behavior occurs.
- Whether the pet seems hungry most of the time.
- How it responds to prey animals.
- Whether the chewing is associated with family member absences.
- Response to loud noises.
- How and where the pet is confined.
- The response of the pet to territorial stimuli.
- What the owner has done to try to stop the behavior.
- Other recent changes in health or behavior.

See Figure 15.1. The prognosis varies with the temperament of the pet, the pet's environment, family dynamics, and the underlying cause of the chewing. With proper diagnosis, training, and adequate supervision, the prognosis for complete control of most chewing problems is good to excellent.

Management

For puppies and adolescent dogs, treatment is relatively straightforward. Once chewing problems emerge, the owner should ensure that the pet has appropriate opportunities and objects for chewing, adequate mental and physical stimulation, an adequate amount of supervision and appropriate confinement as needed. Dog chew toys will only be successful in reducing the problem if the dog actually chews them. The family should begin by offering a variety of toys and determine the toys that the pet prefers. They should encourage the pet to interact with the toys and reward it each time it chews on them. Toys made of heavy rawhide, nylon, and durable rubber are most practical. Cheese or meat spreads can be lightly coated on the toys to stimulate interest, or small pieces of food can be

Causes of destructive chewing	Considerations
Play, toy retrieval	• Puppy, young adult dog • Edges of furniture chewed, toy found underneath
Investigative behavior	• Adolescent dog • Random objects, areas – may be increased interest if novel • Certain textures and materials may be preferable • May occur when the owner is home, but not supervising the pet
Improper toys or play	• Clothing, towels, etc., provided as play toys • Tug of war with objects similar to those the owner doesn't want chewed
Inadequate exercise or stimulation	• Adolescent dog • May occur when the owner is home, but not supervising the pet • May also show signs of hyperactivity, unruliness
Hunger	• Associated with a reduction in the amount of food fed • Associated with a delay in the normal feeding time • Directed toward object containing food odor
Predatory behavior	• Predatory responses observed that occur with high arousal • Evidence of prey animals in areas where the pet chews
Territorial behavior	• Escape or redirected behavior • Signs of high territorial arousal observed by the family • Curtains, furniture, woodwork near windows and doors are scratched and chewed • May be accompanied by urine marking in the above areas • Owner may be home or absent
Separation anxiety	• Occurs only or predominantly when the pet can't make contact with a family member • May occur when the family member is away from home in an area of the home that is inaccessible to the pet or when the pet can't gain the attention of the owner • Destructive chewing occurs at exit areas (doors, windows) or directed toward objects with the owner's scent • May initially occur in association with a change in a family member's schedule that results in less time spent with pet
Noise phobias (storms, fireworks)	• Evidence of high levels of anxiety associated with specific, strong stimuli • Targets for chewing are exit or escape areas (doors, windows) • Owner may be home or absent and behavior may be observable when owners home
Barrier frustration/escape behavior	• Associated with a change in the areas where the pet has access in the home or with the introduction of confinement • Owner may be home or absent
Compulsive disorder	• Destructive behavior occurs when chasing shadows or moving lights • Oral behavior may be directed toward household objects that are licked, chewed, or swallowed
Medical	• Based on the presenting signs rule out any potential medical problems

Figure 15.1   Causes of destructive chewing.

wedged into some toys. Toys that require manipulation for the food to be released are also good for keeping the pet's attention. The pet should have about eight to 10 toys, but not have all available at any one time. Periodically, a few of the pet's available toys can be replaced with other toys. Rotating toys will help ensure that the pet always has toys that are novel and interesting. When the pet initiates chewing on a toy, the owner should lightly praise it and covertly toss a small piece of kibble to land next to the pet as reinforcement. This should make the pet think that chewing toys makes food fall out

of the sky. The pet should receive lots of aerobic exercise each day. The more energy the pet uses in acceptable activities, the less is available to get into trouble.

Until the owner can trust the dog, it should be under constant supervision or confined to a safe area. Crate confinement during the day should be limited to about four to five hours if used on a daily basis. Larger confinement areas, such as exercise pens or small rooms, are preferable for situations where the family is away all day. When the pet can be trusted and is allowed to have more freedom, it can be taught to avoid previously chewed objects by making them taste bad by applying a small amount of cayenne pepper, oil of citronella, or a commercial antichew spray. Booby traps, such as motion detector alarms, may also be successful in keeping the pet away from objects it might chew. They provide an immediate, consistent interruption and don't require the owner's presence. A head halter with a 10-ft long leash can also be used for control and to interrupt undesirable chewing.

If hunger is a problem, management might include increasing the amount of the daily ration, switching to a higher bulk diet, or changing the feeding schedule. Trapping and removing rodents and other small animals around the home might stop digging into doors and walls in pursuit of prey. For pets with anxiety disorders, behavior modification and possibly medication may be necessary (see Ch. 11). Dogs that chew because of poor tolerance for confinement may be helped by providing food-laced toys, changing the confinement area, increased exercise, using D.A.P.™, and in some cases a benzodiazepine or sedative given prior to the owner's departure. Chewing on windowsills and drapes during territorial displays can be stopped by keeping windows closed, moving furniture to block access, wearing a citronella antibark collar, desensitizing the pet to the stimuli, or by using motion-activated alarms.

The consultant should counsel the owners against using any type of punishment that involves hitting or threatening the pet with a hand or something in the hand, delayed punishment, or anything that elicits a fear response from the pet. A treatment plan that concentrates on positive training, appropriate control of the pet, and uses minimal or no punishment is the most satisfactory. See Figure 15.2 and client handout #6 on the CD, on chewing and digging (Fig. 15.3).

Prevention

The best way to prevent destructive chewing is to provide puppies with appropriate chew toys and teach them early which items are theirs to chew, and which are not. Until the owner can trust the pet, it must be under constant supervision or confined to a safe 'puppy-proofed' area. Young dogs also need ample exercise time for them to dispel some of their boundless energy. Since anxiety can also prompt dogs to be destructive, emerging anxiety problems should be promptly addressed.

Dogs cannot easily discern which objects are acceptable for them to chew and which are not. This can be particularly challenging if owners play games like 'tug of war' with towels or socks, or give dogs household items like old shoes for chew toys. Owners should be instructed not to give the dog any household items for its chewing enjoyment. Proper guidance of the chewing behavior toward acceptable items should be considered a basic component of any dog-rearing program (see Ch. 3 for details on prevention).

Case example

Barney was a nine-month-old Labrador Retriever presented for his incredible propensity to destroy items around the house. The owners were busy and rarely had time to exercise the pet. During the day, while the owners were at work, Barney was left unconfined in the home. Since his adoption at two months of age, he had eaten holes in the carpet, chewed large holes in two expensive pieces of furniture, destroyed books, chewed spectacles, and dug up or chewed every plant in the home.

A dog run was set up in the basement to provide safe confinement when the owners could not supervise the pet. The dog was only allowed out of his run if and when he could be kept within sight. The owners were instructed to provide much more exercise, with the goal of fatiguing the pet. It was suggested that exercise should take place at least three times daily. A professional dog walker was recommended to help out. Several new toys were introduced. They were laced with a small amount of food to make them more attractive than the owner's possessions, and the owners spent time every day playing with Barney and the toys. Barney was taught to play fetch. Whenever the pet

Step	Comments
Provide acceptable and stimulating chew toys	• Owners must provide the dog with every opportunity to chew appropriately. The pet should be offered a wide selection until the owner can determine preferred chewing objects • Provide toys that are durable (nylon, plastic, rubber) that can be filled with biscuits, dog food, rawhide, or pieces of meat or cheese. Spread cheese or peanut butter on toys. Freeze food-filled toys to lengthen their desirability • A variety of chew toys should be available but replace and rotate toys regularly to keep them novel • Playing fetch with the chew toys may help stimulate interest in the items • Owners must not engage the dog in play with household objects and must not give the dog old household items for chew toys
Reward desirable behavior	• When the pet chews on one of its chew toys, it should receive a social or food reward to reinforce the behavior
Exercise	• A regular schedule of vigorous exercise such as long walks, retrieving games, or jogging will help the dog burn off excess energy • Activities such as catching a ball or frisbee, obedience trials, agility, or flyball will provide exercise as well as providing mental stimulation
Provide mental stimulation	• Additional outlets to help calm the pet might include interactive play toys, additional pets, and regular obedience training to teach the dog to calm and settle (Fig. 5.13, handout #23 on the CD) • Hiding stimulating toys and treats throughout the dog's play area can offer an enjoyable and time-consuming activity for the dog
Punishment	• The use of harsh, delayed, or physical punishment risks breaking the bond with the pet and should not be used • To be effective, punishment must be administered during or immediately following the act. A delay of even a few seconds is a contraindication for using punishment • Any aversive stimulus that is used for punishment must be appropriate for the pet's temperament. If a fear response is elicited, the stimulus is inappropriate • Environmental punishment, such as a motion-activated alarm, teaches the pet that chewing leads to something it dislikes whether the owner is present or not
Aversion	• Sprays or ointments which taste hot or bitter can be applied to household objects to make them less desirable for the pet to chew. Household items such as cayenne pepper or underarm deodorant may be successful deterrents
Provide supervision/confinement	• Whenever the owner cannot supervise the pet, it should be confined to a crate, exercise pen, or dog-proofed room so that it does not have the opportunity to engage in unacceptable chewing behavior. This may be necessary until the pet is nine to 24 months old
Treat territorial and anxiety disorders	• Change window or confinement areas so the pet is not aware of territorial stimuli • Use a motion-activated alarm to keep the pet away from windows • Use a citronella antibark collar • Desensitize the pet to territorial stimuli • See Chapter 11 for treatment of various phobic and anxiety disorders, and Chapter 19 for treatment of territorial aggression

Figure 15.2 Management of destructive chewing in dogs.

initiated chewing on any of its toys, the owners praised him and occasionally gave a small biscuit. Household items in which Barney had shown a special interest were painted with a hot-tasting substance. Small plants were placed out of reach and a small motion alarm was placed at the base of the remaining large plant. Obedience training was also recommended.

Progress was slow. Barney enjoyed his new toys but still managed to destroy several more household items. The owners were justifiably upset but resisted the temptation to punish Barney when he was not actually caught in the act. After four weeks of therapy, the owners were exhausted but the situation had improved such that Barney now rarely got into trouble.

DESTRUCTIVE CHEWING AND DIGGING

A. Choose the right toys

1. Make certain to choose toys that are appealing to your dog. This may vary from dog to dog as some may be most attracted to texture or appearance, while others may be more attracted to a food inserted or stuffed into the toy.
2. Choose toys that are durable and safe. Dogs that enjoy chewing should be given toys that take as long as possible to destroy without losing interest. If rawhide is given, the pieces should be large enough for the puppy to gnaw, without chewing off large pieces that can be swallowed. Rolled or thick, flat sheets may be preferable to sticks or pieces with knots.
3. Change toys, or rotate through them to keep up their interest.
4. Choose toys that are not overly similar to your possessions (e.g., old shoes, towels or clothes, child toys, etc.).

B. Encourage play

1. Reward correct chewing. Use praise, affection, or occasionally toss a small treat to the puppy for chewing on its toys.
2. Lace toys with food. Many toys are designed so that they can be coated or stuffed with food treats to attract the pet. Freezing the toys with food inside may extend the duration of play, chewing, or eating food or toys. Manipulation toys, such as Buster Cube™, Tricky Treat™, Crazy Ball™, etc., deliver small pieces of food which serve to reward the dog as it chews and may further increase the duration of interest in the toy.

C. Provide a regular regime of exercise and play

1. An overabundance of energy and lack of acceptable activities can lead to exploration and chewing. Provide enough exercise, interactive play, and training to calm and settle the dog before leaving it alone or unsupervised.
2. A number of interactive play toys have been designed to combine play and social interaction with family members or other pets. These toys include balls, pucks, and floating toys for chase and retrieval and some for tugging and pulling.
3. Tug and pull toys may not be appropriate for all dogs. As long as you are the one to initiate the play, can stop the game on command, and the dog does not have a problem with aggression or overly exuberant play, then these toys may be an acceptable means of directing play and chewing to an appropriate outlet.

D. Preventing and deterring undesirable chewing

1. Even though your dog has a number of appealing toys and has received plenty of interactive play, training, and exercise, he or she may be attracted to chew and investigate some of your household possessions. Therefore, supervision or confinement to a crate or pen when you are unable to supervise should prevent any inappropriate chewing.
2. If you are not available to supervise and you wish to avoid confinement training, it might be possible to move potential targets out of your dog's reach (dog-proofing), use aversive tasting substances (e.g., Ropel™, Chew Guard™, Bitter Apple™), or use avoidance devices (Snappy Trainer™, Critter Gitter™, Scraminal™, Spray Barrier™, Ssscat™) to keep your dog away from items that might be chewed.
3. If you catch the dog in the act of chewing something it shouldn't, immediately interrupt it with a sharp noise or a pull on a leash if one has been left attached. Then, give a proper chew toy to the pet and praise it as soon as it begins to chew. However, even if you consistently catch and interrupt your pet when it is chewing on inappropriate items, this may only teach it to avoid chewing these items in your presence.
4. Never punish after the act and never use physical punishment.

E. Chewing and anxiety

1. Chewing and destructiveness may also arise in response to anxiety and should not be considered as an attempt to 'get even with you.' Treatment requires correcting the underlying anxiety and this often requires a consultation with your veterinarian or a behaviorist to determine the cause of the problem and develop an appropriate treatment program.
2. Separation anxiety: some dogs become extremely distressed when they cannot be with their owners (separation anxiety), and may respond with destructive, housesoiling, or barking behavior. These dogs need to be taught that they cannot receive attention on demand, but rather for spending progressively longer periods of time away from the owner. Prior to departures the owners should ignore the dog and try and keep it distracted with some food-stuffed toys when they leave.

Figure 15.3   Destructive chewing and digging (handout #6 – printable from the CD).

F. Digging
1. First determine why the dog is digging. Dogs may dig to bury or retrieve bones and toys, to find a cool place to lie down, to escape from confinement, to dig for rodents or prey, and as a form of play and exploration. You'll need to know why your dog is digging in order to develop a treatment program.
2. Supervise your dog while outdoors and interrupt the behavior if you catch the pet in the act.
3. Use booby traps to deter digging of a particular area, such as placing balloons that pop or water in the hole or a motion detector device next to the hole.
4. Prevent access to the area by using chicken wire or hardwire over the area, rocks in the hole, paving or placing gravel in the area, by confining to a pen away from the area, or by using avoidance devices such as the citronella spray collar avoidance units.
5. Dogs that dig as a form of play or exploration will need increased stimulation in the form of training and exercise and outlets for play and chewing (see above).
6. Dogs that dig to flush out prey and those that dig cooling holes will need to be prevented from digging by confinement or avoidance devices, or by providing them with an acceptable area for digging. Digging in this area can be ensured by supervision and reinforcement of desirable digging or by confinement to the area.

Figure 15.3 (*continued*)

After two months, there had only been two incidents when Barney took one of the owner's shoes. However, instead of chewing it, he just played with it in the bedroom and did no real damage. The owner got Barney's attention, gave him a 'sit' command, and then rewarded him with a treat. He then offered Barney a chew toy to replace the shoe, which Barney gave up without incident. After six months, the owners felt they could truly trust Barney and he was given the run of the house while they were out. No further incidents were reported.

DIGGING

Digging may be a nuisance, but it is an innate trait for many dogs. Sled-dog breeds such as Siberian Huskies and Alaskan Malamutes dig holes that provide a cool place for them to lie. Terriers and Dachshunds were bred to flush out prey or to locate rodents in underground areas where digging is required. Other dogs may dig because their acute senses of smell and hearing inform them that there is something interesting beneath the ground. Since dogs may bury bones and toys, it is not surprising that they should also dig to locate them again. Some dogs use digging as a way to escape confinement. Digging may also be an activity similar to destructive chewing that occurs when young

dogs are left alone without sufficient stimulation.

When dogs become house pets, they often need to leave natural tendencies behind, such as digging, if they are to be good home companions. Most dogs have little problem with this compromise, as long as they have sufficient stimulation elsewhere in their lives. However, there are some dogs that are resistant to change and continue to dig despite other adequate outlets. They may dig because of lack of stimulation, to escape, or because digging is fun. For a client handout see Figure 15.3 (handout #6 on the CD).

Diagnosis and prognosis

Dogs dig for a number of reasons and, so it is important to determine the underlying cause. If the cause is not determined, you are only left with treating the signs, which may not provide a satisfactory conclusion. Carefully interview the owner as to the circumstances surrounding the digging. If the digging is along the fence or near a gate, the dog may be digging to escape from the yard. An intact male may do this if he is stimulated by a female in estrus. If prey animals are available, they may be the stimuli for digging. If the pet is young, understimulated, and underexercised, it may occur as a recreational event. If the digging occurs near an outdoor cooking area, then spilled food may be the stimulus.

The prognosis varies considerably with the underlying cause. Understimulated young dogs and intact males with a strong motivation to roam that have learned that digging provides freedom can be very frustrating to control. For these cases, keeping the dog indoors in a safe, destruction-proof area or providing a confinement area where the pet is unable to dig to escape may be the only viable solution. Discovering the underlying etiology, and having practical solutions available, significantly improves the chances for successful resolution.

Management

Digging can be suppressed in the owner's presence. However, unless the cause is identified and dealt with, the digging will continue in the owner's absence. If the pet is digging to catch rodents, some thought should be given to capturing and removing them from the yard. For dogs that are digging to escape, the motivation for the behavior should be elucidated and dealt with if possible. For example, if the dog is not getting enough exercise or social attention, this should be provided. If the escape behavior is motivated by sexual attraction (e.g., to roam), neutering may help to reduce the urge.

Environmental enrichment is most indicated for those dogs that dig because they have no acceptable alternative. Whenever the pet is left outdoors unsupervised, it is important to attempt to provide an appealing alternative activity to distract and occupy it. This distraction might include large balls to push around, or wooden boxes and ramps on which to crawl and explore. Large rubber toys can be stuffed with treats, tied to ropes, and suspended from tree limbs for some dogs. The success in enriching the environment is variable and may be negligible for some pets. Increased activity, such as vigorous physical exercise (fetch, jogging, speed walking) provided two or more times daily, may help reduce the amount of time spent digging.

Another option is to provide a sand/soil digging pit with partially buried toys and 'chews' to encourage digging in one area instead of many. Adding another pet may help, but the owner might also end up with two pets that dig and therefore twice the damage.

When dogs are digging to create a cool respite, they may stop if given a cool, shaded area or a wading pool is provided where they can cool off. Dogs that are digging as a response to fearful stimuli may enjoy the comfort and security of a doghouse or other forms of shelter. Anxiolytic medication may also help. If the digging escape behavior is due to separation anxiety, behavior modification and medication may be necessary (Ch. 11). For some dogs, confinement in a secure pen or run may be the best treatment plan.

Digging can be interrupted in the owner's presence by a variety of ways. This is best done by remote means so the dog does not associate the interruption with the presence of the owner. It can be accomplished by monitoring the dog and responding with a spray from a hose, turning on a lawn sprinkler, activating a remote spray collar, pulling on a long leash, or installing a motion-activated sprinkler. Close supervision, consistent interruptions, and providing the dog with alternative activities will resolve the digging problem in most cases. If the dog digs in only one or two specific areas, these areas can be protected by placing chicken wire or heavy fencing over them and anchoring the wire to the ground, or by placing rocks in the hole.

For some dogs, the best option is prevention. Building a dog run can serve two purposes. If it is sufficiently secure, the floor of the run is either gravel, patio stones, or paved, and the dog is properly trained to remain in the run (e.g., play toys, shelter), the dog run can serve as an inescapable den area. The second option is to allow some portion of the run to remain unpaved so that the dog can use it for digging (e.g., cooling holes, play, etc.). It is important to keep pets properly vaccinated and parasite free so that the area does not become contaminated and potentially infectious.

Certain common practices must be discouraged absolutely. These include delayed punishment; physical punishment; and filling the hole with water or feces and holding the pet's head in it.

Prevention

Dogs should be closely supervised when outdoors during the first 12–18 months of their lives so that the owner can quickly interrupt digging behavior every time it is exhibited. A shake can (tin can filled with six to eight large coins) may be tossed next to the pet each time it starts to scratch the ground in order to discourage the behavior. Adequate exercise, training, toys, and social stimulation are all very important. Young pets that are in the yard alone and allowed to entertain themselves by digging each day can be a challenge to correct.

If there is an acceptable area where the dog may dig in the garden, the owner might consider teaching the puppy to dig in that area soon after it has been brought into the home environment. Toys can be buried in the acceptable area to encourage the pet to dig there. Food or social praise can be used to reinforce the behavior. To accomplish this, the owner must always be with the pet when it is outdoors so that the correct behavior can be rewarded and digging in undesirable areas can be consistently interrupted. Timely interruptions are very important, because if the owner only uses positive reinforcement for digging in an appropriate area to condition the dog, it may never entirely cease digging in the inappropriate areas in the garden or yard (for more details on prevention of destructive behaviors see Ch. 3).

Case example

Sonic, an intact male Border Collie, was presented for digging under the gate to run in the neighborhood when the owner was at work during the day. Upon arriving home, the owner would see Sonic, call him, grab him by the collar, and punish him for escaping.

The owner was told that punishing the dog when he arrived home at the end of the day, long after the pet had performed the escape behavior, was counterproductive. In fact, Sonic was starting to avoid the owner when he came home and was more hesitant to come when called. Neutering was recommended to decrease the possibility of sexually motivated escape and roaming behavior. More exercise by way of jogging and fetch was suggested. The owner purchased several inexpensive soccer balls and encouraged the pet to play with them by throwing and kicking them around the yard. The owner anchored a double thickness sheet of chicken wire along the ground in front of the gate. Whenever he found the dog investigating the ground near the gate, a shake can was tossed near him.

Sonic did extremely well as long as the owner remained attentive to him in the evening. He came to anticipate the playtime and was eager for the owner's return home. However, Sonic did have relapses when the owner missed playtime for a few days in a row, and once when the owner was out of town for two days on business. The owner, upon realizing the situation, came up with a satisfactory solution for all concerned. He paid several of the neighborhood children to play with Sonic for at least one full hour on those days when he could or would not spend the time himself.

FURTHER READING

Borchelt PL 1983 Separation-elicited behavior problems in dogs. In: Katcher AH, Beck AM (eds) New perspectives on our lives with companion animals. University of Pennsylvania Press, Philadelphia, PA

Borchelt PL, Voith VL 1982 Diagnosis and treatment of separation-related behavior problems in dogs. Veterinary Clinics of North America, Small Animal Practice 12:625–636

Hunthausen WL 1988 Avoiding chewing problems. Intervet 23(6):23–24

Hunthausen WL 1991 The causes, treatment, and prevention of canine destructive chewing. Veterinary Medicine October:1007–1010

Patronek GJ, Dodman NH 1999 Attitudes, procedures, and delivery of behavior services by veterinarians in small animal practice. Canadian Veterinary Journal 215(11):1606–1611

Voith VL 1975 Destructive behavior in the owner's absence. Canine Practice 2(3):11

Voith VL, Borchelt PL 1996 Separation anxiety in dogs. In: Voith VL, Borchelt PL (eds) Readings in companion animal behavior. Veterinary Learning Systems, Trenton, NJ, p 124–139

16

Feline destructive behaviors

Destructive behavior is a very common complaint of cat owners. This type of problem can occur for a variety of reasons. In many cases it is simply a matter of normal behavior by a young cat being directed toward an unacceptable object or occurring in an unacceptable area.

Preventive counseling can help the family avoid these types of problems in young pets. Some problems involving destructive behavior can have more serious and complex underlying etiologies, such as compulsive chewing disorders. Other causes of undesirable chewing and scratching include chewing objects with an interesting odor or taste, inadequate stimulation, marking, and attention-getting behaviors.

DESTRUCTIVE ACTIVITY AND EXPLORATORY BEHAVIORS

Young cats that climb drapes, jump onto counters, knock over objects, or chew on household objects (e.g., string, electric cords, plants) are usually exhibiting play and exploratory behaviors. Most destructive behaviors by young cats can be corrected by providing appropriate outlets for play, investigation, and chewing, as well as by preventing or deterring access to problem areas and problem items. Exploration and investigation should be channeled toward proper toys at acceptable locations. Toys and frequent interactive play sessions can give the cat an opportunity to satisfy some of its innate needs for activity and play. The owner can provide high places for perching, as well as play areas for climbing and scratching. Owners must also identify and remove any rewards that might encourage the behavior. For example, cats that jump onto counters or tables and find a few morsels of food will keep coming back.

Supervision and timely interruptions (e.g., water gun, whistle) will usually discourage these behaviors in the owner's presence, but most cats will continue when the owners are not around. When owners are out of the home or cannot supervise, problems can be prevented by confining the cat to a cat-proofed area or by booby trapping areas with devices like motion-activated alarms. (See Fig. 5.4).

FELINE SCRATCHING

Cats scratch upright objects for claw maintenance by pulling off exterior layers of nail, and as a form of territorial marking. This type of marking provides both a visual (the behavior itself and the marks left on the object) and a pheromonal signal. During scratching behavior, the pheromones are liberated on the surface of a vertical object by the footpads. On occasion, the behavior is directed toward horizontal objects, such as the top or seats of furniture and carpeting. This normal behavior becomes a problem for the owner when walls, furniture, and carpets are destroyed.

When household scratching cannot be managed or resolved, it can be a major source of owner anxiety and one of the primary reasons for relinquishment. In a study in Germany (where declawing is illegal) of 1177 cats, the second most common owner behavioral complaint, second only to states of anxiety, was scratching (15.2% of cats). For 125 of these cats the owners had attempted to correct the problem, and 60% had partial success with environmental management or aversion conditioning, but only 10% were able to completely resolve the problem. Similarly, in a US study, it was found that 20% of pet owners have a problem with household scratching in their cat and an additional 4% have problems with scratching of family members.

Diagnosis and prognosis

In most cases, the owner has observed the cat scratching or has found evidence of damage in the home. Some cats that have been harshly punished by the owner when they were scratching may subsequently only scratch when the owner is out of sight. If the scratching is due to marking, the owner may notice some of the following sequence of behaviors: the cat approaches the surface to be scratched, the surface is sniffed, this is followed by flehmen, the limbs are stretched with extension of the body, and it scratches the site using both its forepaws alternately. Scratching that is due to marking usually occurs at a higher frequency than what is required for claw maintenance.

The duration of the behavior and the individual cat's inherent drive to scratch directly influence the prognosis. Cats that have been scratching frequently for a long period and individuals with a strong drive to scratch can be a challenge to correct.

Management

The first step is to find a scratching post that is acceptable to the cat. The owner may need to offer several different types until a suitable one is found. Sisal-covered posts and upright fireplace logs are generally well accepted. Scratching posts should be placed at the cat's favored locations, and perhaps even placed directly in front of (or mounted on) the door, wall, furniture, or object that the cat has chosen to scratch. During training, the pet should be under constant supervision and covertly interrupted whenever it scratches an unacceptable surface. When the owner cannot watch the cat, it should be confined to a room or area of the home where the only acceptable surface to scratch is its post. A small treat should be given to the pet whenever it approaches the post and a larger one should be given whenever it actually scratches it. More freedom can be allowed once the pet shows a preference for scratching its post and no interest in household items.

If the cat only scratches a few areas, it could have freedom in the home but the appeal of the scratched objects and areas could be reduced. This can be done by draping a loose covering over the scratched area, attaching double-sided tape to the surfaces, applying aversive scents, or by using humane booby traps (e.g., motion detectors, upside-down mousetraps, balloons set to pop). Frequent nail trims, or soft nail coverings that can be glued over the claws, may be helpful during the training period.

When the scratching occurs as a marking behavior, some attention should be given to controlling the stimuli for marking. Possible causes include cats visiting in the yard, a new pet added to the home, social problems within the home, major environmental changes (e.g., new furniture, new plants, remodeling, moving). For these cases, the pheromone spray Feliway™ may be helpful. Feliway™ should be sprayed over the scratched area once per day for 21 days on each area where the cat is scratching, as well as on other similar, prominent vertical areas in the home. Although stress-induced scratching is likely to be reduced, for cats that scratch as a form of territorial marking, Feliway™ may be useful at inhibiting the cat at specific sites, but untreated sites will likely still be used or selected. Feliway™ is also available as an electronic diffuser for more generalized room application.

Physical punishment of any type or even loud scoldings are not indicated as these techniques can cause fear of the owner and increased anxiety for the cat. When the owner needs to interrupt the behavior, a device used at a distance often works best. An air horn, handheld alarm, ultrasonic pet trainer, water rifle, or a can of compressed air can be used. The interruption will be more effective if the owner says nothing and makes very little movement while administering the interruption. When the owner remains out of sight while interrupting the pet, it is more likely to associate the unpleasant consequence with the behavior and not with the owner. More technically inclined owners may want to consider plugging an alarm, hair dryer, Water Pik™, or tape recording into a remote control

switch and placing it in the area where the pet misbehaves. Then as soon as the pet enters the area or begins the inappropriate behavior, the aversive device can be triggered by remote control while the owner remains out of sight.

Some owners are unable to train their cats to stop furniture scratching, despite attempts at scratching post training and behavioral modification techniques. These owners may then be faced with the undesirable options of removing the cat from the home, allowing the cat to go outdoors, or constant confinement. In North America, scratching is a major reason for cat relinquishment. Another alternative, which is performed relatively frequently in North America but is condemned and even illegal in some countries, is declawing. Recent estimates are that 25% or more of cats kept as house pets in North America are declawed, and that perhaps as many as 50% of pet owners that have their cats declawed would not otherwise have kept their cat.

While the humane and moral implications of declawing are open for discussion, the fact is that the surgery is being regularly performed in some countries. In addition to whether declawing is a humane act and whether the benefits, including being able to retain the pet and avoid relinquishment, are sufficient justification for the surgery, opponents of declawing claim that there are numerous adverse effects. However, with millions of declawed cats successfully homed across North America, there appears to be no increased risk of complications above what might be expected with any other surgery. In fact, other than the initial postsurgical pain (which must be addressed as discussed in Ch. 9) there have been numerous studies to show that declawing does not cause measurable adverse effects on behavior or physical health. It has been suggested that tendonectomy might lead to less short-term pain than declawing; however, pain assessment studies have indicated that the pain may only be increased for 24 hours and that this can and should be controlled with careful attention to pain management. However, in one study there was 96% owner satisfaction with declawing, while the satisfaction with tendonectomy was between 70% and 87%. After tendonectomy, 30% of owners had difficulty trimming their cats' nails and 55% reported that their cats could still scratch. Declawing, on the other hand, successfully met the owner's objectives in all cases and many owners of declawed cats felt that they had a better or healthier relationship with their pet (Fig. 16.1). Another consideration is that declawing by laser surgery or radio wave surgery may further reduce pain and speed recovery, but only with respect to the first day or two postsurgically.

Prevention

Prevention is accomplished by methods similar to those used for treatment. Owner instruction should include a thorough discussion of normal kitten behavior, how to provide for the pet's needs, how to humanely interrupt behaviors, as well as the judicious use of confinement and supervision. The family should be counseled to avoid allowing cats to scratch old pieces of furniture, since the pet will probably transfer the scratching to new pieces when the old ones are replaced.

Case example

Kermit was a seven-month-old neutered male cat that had been scratching the owner's living room sofa for the past two months. The owner was planning to replace the furniture but wanted to stop the scratching behavior first.

The sofa was covered with plastic while the owner trained Kermit to use a scratching post. A fire log mounted upright on plywood was selected because the cat showed some interest in it and it was dissimilar to the fabric on the sofa. A small amount of catnip was sprinkled on the post to attract the cat. When it approached the post it was given a modest semi-moist cat treat; when it made contact with the post it was given a larger treat. Eventually, treats were only reserved for times at which the cat made contact with its paws or actually scratched the post. After four weeks, the plastic cover was

DECLAWING STUDIES

Study	Reference	Findings
Borchelt and Voith (1987): aggressive behavior in cats	Compendium of Continuing Education 1:49	Declawed cats no more likely to bite, bite more times, or bite more seriously
Bennett, Houpt, and Erb (1988): effects of declawing on feline behavior	Companion Animal Practice 2:70	No change in behavior after declawing. Owners of declawed cats reported higher number of good behaviors than owners of clawed cats
Morgan and Houpt (1989): feline behavior problems; the influence of declawing	Anthrozoos 3:50	No difference in behavior problems (housesoiling, biting) between declawed cats and clawed cats
Landsberg (1991): cat owners' attitudes toward declawing	Anthrozoos 4:192	Declawing met the objectives of all owners. 70% of cat owners indicated an improved cat–owner relationship. No adverse behavioral consequences noticed by owners
Landsberg (1991): declawing is controversial but still saves pets	Veterinary Forum October:67	50% of cat owners may not have kept their pets if not declawed. As many as 50 000 cats' lives saved per year in Ontario alone
Halip J (1998): a descriptive study of 189 cats engaging in inappropriate elimination behaviors	Feline Practice 26(4)	In cats referred for elimination problems, declawed cats were at no increased risk

Figure 16.1 The effects of declawing.

removed from the sofa when the owner was at home and could watch Kermit. The owner was instructed to toss a key chain near the cat or squirt it with a water gun if it was caught in the act of attempting to scratch the furniture. Within two months the owners bought new furniture, supervised closely for the first few weeks, and had no further complaints.

DESTRUCTIVE CHEWING AND INGESTIVE BEHAVIORS BY CATS

Cats that chew or suck on objects may cause costly damage to the household or serious injury to themselves (see also Ch. 8). Kittens are highly investigative and tend to chew or ingest many household objects. At five to six weeks of age, some kittens may even begin to eat their own litter. Kittens given freedom to wander through the home and explore unsupervised can damage many of the owner's possessions. They can become obstructed or seriously injured when they chew on string, thread, latex, rubber, and electric cords. Indoor cats with little or no access to grass or other vegetable matter may chew houseplants.

Fabric chewing by some cats may also be a form of compulsive behavior (see also Ch. 10). Although sucking or chewing on fabrics can occur in cats of any lineage, there appears to be some genetic predisposition for this type of activity. Siamese and Burmese cats are especially prone to this type of behavior. Wool is most commonly chewed, followed by cotton and then synthetic fabrics. Rubber, plastic, wood, and cardboard may also be chewed. The damage done by these cats can be quite extensive. The behavior usually arises during the first year of life, commonly between four and 12 months of age. Some cats will show an increase in pica between six and 18 months, and about two months after rehoming.

Diagnosis and prognosis

Most destructive chewing by young cats is attributable to their desire to play and investigate. Adult cats that frequently engage in uncontrol-lable destructive chewing are likely afflicted with a compulsive disorder. A familial disorder is suspected in individuals of some breeds that are compulsive chewers, and for those cats the prognosis is guarded.

Management

Treatment for young cats with destructive chewing problems involves keeping the chewed objects away from the cat, teaching the cat to avoid areas where it might find objects to chew, making target objects taste bad, and providing the pet with its own chewing alternatives. Cat activity centers and interactive play toys can keep some cats distracted.

Cats that chew on plants may find them particularly appealing because of their taste or texture. Supplying the pet with lettuce, catnip, or access to a herb garden may reduce chewing on houseplants. Providing alternative oral stimulation in the form of dog chew toys, rawhide, bulky, dry, or chewy foods might satisfy the desires of some cats. Applying a little meat spread, cheese, or fish oil to the toys might help pique the pet's interest. Feeding sessions can be made more natural if the cat is provided with a means of searching for food. By offering small meals in a variety of locations, or requiring some form of manipulation to obtain food (feeders that deliver food when the cat interacts with them, toys or play centers with food inside), feeding can become a much more active and productive part of the cat's day.

Environmental punishment using taste aversion or booby traps may be necessary to deter cats that develop fixations for household items. A plant's leaves can be lightly sprayed with water, and then sprinkled with cayenne pepper. Commercial sprays with an adverse taste can also be used to coat objects to discourage chewing. Motion-activated alarms can be placed near the plants to chase the cat away when it approaches, or hidden under fabric items the pet chews. Balloons can be tied around the base of larger plants or trees, so that when the cat plays with them they pop. (See Ch. 5 and client handout #21 on the CD, Fig. 5.4, for examples of booby traps and their use.) For wool sucking by oriental and other breeds that is a manifestation of compulsive behavior, treatment with clomipramine, paroxetine, or fluoxetine might be helpful. See Chapter 6, Chapter 10, and client handout #4 on the CD, Figure 10.4, for more details on compulsive chewing and drug therapy.

Prevention

The best chance of preventing destructive chewing in cats is to provide them with acceptable chew toys and interactive forms of exercise when they are kittens.

Case example

Fred, a one-year-old neutered male domestic short-haired cat, was presented for chewing holes in the owner's clothing and other fabric objects found around the home. Since both owners worked long hours, Fred spent quite a lot of time alone in the apartment. He had intermittently chewed on a variety of objects since he was adopted at eight weeks of age, without causing a significant amount of damage. In the two months previous to the consultation, the chewing had escalated quite considerably. The primary objects that were chewed were fabric items, although on rare occasions he would chew on wooden chair legs, pencils, and plastic pens. Yelling at the cat served to distract it temporarily but did not stop the behavior. Physical examination, fecal examination, and routine hematological and biochemical tests failed to reveal a medical reason for the problem. The cause was thought to be behavioral.

The owner was told to keep all fabric items out of Fred's reach, except for two or three pieces that had been coated with a commercial antichew spray. Several times a day the items were moved to new positions around the house. Every few days, the type of items was changed. This was done to teach the pet to expect that all fabric items, no matter where they are located or what the shape, have an unacceptable taste. The owner was also encouraged to provide a variety of food-filled toys, as well as some dog chew toys and some catnip cat toys, and to spend more time playing with chase toys with Fred. A 'kitty condo' was purchased which had crawl spaces, perches, and hanging toys to keep him entertained and occupied.

Fred seemed to be doing well until he managed to get into the guest bedroom and discovered the drapes there. To stop this behavior, a light cotton fabric was pinned to the curtains to protect them and a bitter spray was applied to teach the cat to avoid them. After this minor setback, the entire process was recommenced and Fred finally relented and became an acceptable house pet. The owners did report that he had the occasional relapse, but the damage was not nearly as bad as with previous episodes.

FURTHER READING

Beaver BV 1992 Feline behavior: a guide for veterinarians. WB Saunders, Philadelphia
Bennett M, Houpt KA, Erb HN 1988 Effects of declawing on feline behaviour. Compendium of Animal Practice 2(7)
Bradshaw JWS, Neville PF, Sawyer D 1997 Factors affecting pica in the domestic cat. Journal of Applied Animal Behavioral Science 52:373–379
Carroll GL, Howe LB, Slater MR, Haughn L et al. 1998 Evaluation of analgesia provided by postoperative administration of butorphanol to cats undergoing onychectomy. Journal of the American Veterinary Medical Association 213(2):246–250
Franks JN, Boothe HW, Taylor L, Geller S et al. 2000 Evaluation of transdermal fentanyl patches for analgesia in cats undergoing onychectomy. Journal of the American Veterinary Medical Association 217(7):1013–1019
Gellasch KL, Kruse-Elliott KT, Osmond CS, Shih ANC, Bjorling DE 2002 Comparison of transdermal administration of fentanyl versus intramuscular administration of butorphanol for analgesia after onychectomy in cats. Journal of the American Veterinary Medical Association 220(7):1020–1024
Halip JW, Vaillancourt JP, Luescher UA 1998 A descriptive study of 189 cats engaging in inappropriate elimination behaviors. Feline Practice 26(4):18–21

Heidenberger E 1997 Housing conditions and behavioral problems of indoor cats as assessed by their owners. Applied Animal Behavioral Science 52:345

Jankowski AJ, Brown DC, Duval J et al 1998 Comparison of effects of elective tenectomy or onychectomy in cats. Journal of the American Veterinary Medical Association 213(3):370–373

Landsberg GM 1991a Feline scratching and the effects of declawing. Veterinary Clinics of North America, Small Animal Practice 21:265

Landsberg G 1991b Cat owners' attitudes toward declawing. Anthrozoos 4(3):192

Landsberg GM 1994 Declawing revisited. Controversy over consequences. Veterinary Forum September:94

Martin P, Bateson P 1988 Behavioural development in the cat. In: Turner D, Bateson P (eds) The domestic cat; the biology of its behaviour. Cambridge University Press, New York, p 9

Mison MB, Bohart GH, Walshaw R, Winters CA, Hauptman JG 2002 Use of carbon dioxide laser for onychectomy in cats. Journal of the American Veterinary Medical Association 221(5):651-653

Morgan M, Houpt KA 1989 Feline behaviour problems. The influence of declawing. Anthrozoos 3(1): 50

Pageat P 1996 Communication et territoire chez le chat. Cours de base du Groupe d'Education du Comportement des Animaux Familiers, Conference at Toulouse.

Patronek GJ 2001 Assessment of claims of short- and long-term complications associated with onychectomy in cats. Journal of the American Veterinary Medical Association 219(7):932–937

Patronek GJ, Dodman NH 1999 Attitudes, procedures, and delivery of behavior services by veterinarians in small animal practice. Canadian Veterinary Journal 215(11):1606–1611

Patronek GJ, Glickman LT, Beck AM et al 1996 Risk factors for relinquishment of cats to an animal shelter. Journal of the American Veterinary Medical Association 209(3):572–581

Robinson I 1992 Behavioural development of the cat. In: Thorne C (ed) The Waltham book of dog and cat behaviour. Pergamon

Yeon SC, Flanders JA, Scarlett JM et al 2001 Attitudes of owners regarding tendonectomy and onychectomy in cats. Journal of the American Veterinary Medical Association 218(1):43–47

17

Canine housesoiling

CANINE INAPPROPRIATE ELIMINATION

Overview

The main purpose of micturition and defecation for the young puppy is to rid the body of wastes. While this is also true for adult dogs, elimination behavior can serve a number of additional functions including communicating information about sexual status, individual identity and territories, and, possibly, social rank. It may also occur in young or adult dogs in a variety of situations as a component of submissive responses, fear, separation anxiety, and excitement.

At about three weeks of age, most puppies have begun eliminating away from the nesting area on their own. By five weeks of age, a general area for elimination is chosen and by nine weeks the area chosen for elimination becomes more specific. Most housetraining strategies involve taking advantage of the dog's innate proclivity to avoid eliminating in its den area and combining this inclination with operant and classical conditioning. The main techniques involve rewarding and shaping desired behavior, controlling the feeding schedule, and controlling the pet's environment in order to prevent elimination in undesirable areas. With patience and consistency, most owners are able to train the pet to eliminate outdoors and avoid eliminating indoors within a few months.

This tendency to keep the home area clean of wastes can be overcome in a number of circumstances. For instance, a dog that is confined for long periods will soil its living areas if not given the opportunity to relieve itself in a more appropriate area. Also, dogs with some medical problems may be unable to control elimination for entirely physiological reasons.

Housetraining

Most dogs are house pets, so it is very important that they are quickly and dependably housetrained. A pet may be abandoned or destroyed if it fails to learn this lesson early and continues to soil in the home. Housetraining is a simple process but one that should be explained in detail to new owners. They must understand and work with the dog's natural elimination patterns rather than waiting for the dog to eliminate in inappropriate areas and punishing it. Training that is based on positive reinforcement is far superior to punishment as a means of housetraining. Yet, most owners are quick to punish inappropriate elimination without giving proper credit (reinforcement) when a puppy does what is wanted. It is important for the family to understand that teaching a pet the correct location for elimination, through repetition and reward, is far more practical than trying to punish it at each of the thousands of locations where it might try to eliminate indoors.

Teach the desired behavior

The first step is to teach the pet where it is acceptable to eliminate. To accomplish this, the owner must regularly accompany the pet to the chosen elimination area to ensure that the pet relieves itself and to give a timely reward.

Young puppies (seven to eight weeks of age) should be taken outdoors to eliminate as often as is practical. Training should begin with a schedule of going to the elimination area every one to two hours when the puppy is awake and a family member is available. Within a short time, the family will learn to predict the interval at which the puppy actually needs to be taken out-

doors. The pet should also be taken to the elimination area after eating, drinking, playing, sleeping, and just prior to confinement. A direct route to an easily accessible outdoor location works best. Using the same area allows odors to accumulate and should increase the likelihood that the pet will return to eliminate there. The dog should be praised lavishly or given a small food reward as soon as it eliminates in the appropriate place. The owner should not wait until the pet is back indoors to give it a food reward since this teaches it to anticipate rewards on returning to the home, and not for elimination. If the puppy wants to play, this can also be used to reward it as soon as it has completed elimination. By pairing a verbal cue with each elimination (e.g., saying a cue word just prior to elimination) and then providing the reward, many dogs learn the concept of eliminating on command.

Provide a consistent feeding schedule

Controlling the feeding schedule will provide some control over the pet's elimination schedule. When puppies and adult dogs are fed on a regular schedule, rather than ad libitum, they tend to develop fairly regular elimination habits. Most young dogs will eliminate within a somewhat predictable time postprandial. While young puppies tend to eliminate shortly after eating, drinking, playing, waking, and being released from confinement, the interval between eating and eliminating tends to be longer for adults, as well as more variable. Food should be offered at the same time(s) each day for 20–30 minutes maximum. The last meal should be finished three to five hours prior to bedtime. The time during which most of the housesoiling occurs will have some bearing on the feeding schedule that is established. If the pet is more likely to housesoil during the day, the morning meal should be very small, or feeding should be limited only to the early evening. Adults with a high propensity to defecate indoors during the day can be fed a lower-fiber diet to reduce the amount of stool produced. Water should be available all day and taken up just prior to bedtime unless there are medical reasons for which restriction of nocturnal water intake would be inappropriate.

Confinement/supervision to prevent inappropriate elimination

The next important consideration is to provide close supervision or confinement until the dog is fully trained to eliminate in its appropriate area and no longer eliminates in inappropriate areas. This may take anywhere from several weeks to many months depending on the duration of the problem, the consistency of the family members, and whether or not the pet was ever house-trained. In general, the puppy should not be considered housetrained until it has gone for at least four to eight <u>consecutive</u> weeks without eliminating in an inappropriate area. Adult dogs that have been housesoiling for many years may take several months before they are dependably trained. Until this has been accomplished, the pet should be within eyesight of a family member 100% of the time. When it cannot be watched, it should be confined to a small area or placed outdoors. A leash can be a handy tool to keep the pet from wandering out of eyesight when the owner might be distracted.

A wire or plastic crate provides a safe area in which to confine the pet when it cannot be observed, but it has some limitations. It should not be used for longer than the pet can physically control elimination or for more than four to five hours during the day on a continuous schedule. Older pets sometimes have difficulty adapting to a small confinement area if this was never used when they were younger. These dogs should be introduced to confinement very gradually. Feeding in the crate, tossing toys in the crate, and hiding treats for them to find in the crate should all help adjust the pet to confinement. If the confinement area will be a small room or run in the home, the same techniques can be used, and the owner might also spend some time in the area playing with the pet or simply reading or doing paperwork as the pet rests in the area. If the pet eliminates in inappropriate areas while the owner sleeps, but

vocalizes excessively when crated at night, the owner might try tying the pet to the side of the bed on a length of leash that is just long enough to allow it to comfortably get up and turn around during the night. See the crate training client handout #5 on the CD, reprinted as Fig. 3.25, for details.

Transition

With careful observation and consistent training techniques, it soon becomes clear to most owners what is the minimum time after elimination before the pet may again need to 'relieve' itself. If there has been no inappropriate elimination for at least four weeks the owners may begin to provide short periods without confinement or supervision immediately following elimination (provided the puppy does not require supervision or confinement for other behavior problems such as chewing). If the dog continues to maintain a proper elimination pattern with no housesoiling for these short periods of time, the length of time out of the crate unsupervised can be very gradually increased over the next few months. The owners will need to determine their dog's limit for how long it can retain urine and stool without elimination so that they always return to allow the dog to its elimination site well before this limit is reached.

Owners who must leave their dogs for periods longer than those during which they can control elimination might have to consider keeping the dog confined to a room, pen, or indoor run, with paper or litter for elimination. At first, the entire floor (other than the dog's water and bedding area) may need to be covered with paper, but the area can gradually be made smaller as the dog begins to use a specific location. Dogs that have been conditioned to eliminate on paper may have a hard time understanding that outdoor elimination is also acceptable. Litterboxes and dog litter are another option for dogs that live in high-rise apartments or cannot be given access to the outdoors sufficiently often.

Another consideration is to provide a doggie door so that the pet has access to the outdoors and a fenced yard when the owner is not home.

For dogs that soil indoors even when a doggie door is available, the owner should build a small confinement pen around the inside door flap that is just large enough for the pet to rest. Most dogs will then use the door to go outside in order to avoid soiling the small indoor area.

Mistakes happen

If the owner sees the pet eliminating or beginning to eliminate in an inappropriate location, it should immediately be interrupted with a sharp 'no!' or hand clap given with enough intensity to stop the behavior and elicit a mild startle response without frightening the pet. The tone or volume of the interruption should not be strong enough to elicit a fear response. An appropriately timed verbal correction is helpful, but by itself will not ensure that the pet will refrain from further elimination indoors. If the puppy is properly supervised, the owner should soon learn to identify pre-elimination signs (sniffing, squatting, circling, sneaking away) and be able to anticipate and predict when the puppy needs to eliminate so that punishment is not necessary. In this way, the owner can get the puppy's attention before elimination begins and direct it to the appropriate location where praise and reward can be given for appropriate behavior.

Any area in the home where the puppy has eliminated must be thoroughly cleaned and treated with an effective odor neutralizer. Carpeting should be soaked with the deodorizer, since merely spraying the surface is not likely to be efficacious. Access to previously soiled areas can be controlled by closing doors or moving furniture over those areas. The pet can be taught to avoid an area by using various environmental devices. Booby traps such as upside-down mousetraps, balloons set to pop when disturbed, and motion-activated alarms are often successful in conditioning a pet to avoid an area. Most pets prefer to avoid eliminating in areas where they eat, sleep, or play. Therefore, food, water bowls, bedding, or toys can be placed in previously soiled areas in order to discourage elimination at those spots.

Punishment

This is the least important and most overused approach to housetraining as well as correcting housesoiling problems. The use of punishment is not necessary to train desired elimination behavior. It must be discussed with owners, since most owners attempt to incorporate the use of punishment into housetraining. Using harsh or delayed punishment may slow down training or cause other behavior problems. Physical punishment, strong scoldings, and rubbing the pet's nose in urine or feces must be prohibited.

Harsh punishment during the act of elimination may teach the dog to:

- Avoid further elimination in that location.
- Avoid further elimination in that location when the owner is present.
- Avoid all elimination in the presence of the owner.
- Become fearful of the owner.

Signaling

Many owners indicate that their dogs do not give any sign or 'ask' them to go outdoors. Some dogs learn to signal because of owner interruption techniques. This happens when the owner supervises the dog indoors and startles or disrupts the dog as it shows pre-elimination signs or as the dog begins to eliminate. The consequence of these actions is that many dogs attempt to sneak away to eliminate when the owner is watching; however, when the dog cannot sneak away it may begin to show signs of conflict and anxiety (whining, circling, barking, pacing), since it has learned there will be an unpleasant consequence associated with elimination in front of the owners. The key to training the dog to signal is to identify these signs and take the dog immediately to its elimination site where it is immediately rewarded for elimination. Over time the dog will learn to signal in some manner (whining, pacing, barking, or even going to the exit door) when it feels the urge to eliminate.

CANINE HOUSETRAINING

A. Choose the desired location and teach the puppy where to go
1. Ensure that the location is practical and easy to access (e.g., a short walk from the back door).
2. Go out with your puppy every time and enthusiastically praise elimination in the desired area.
3. Take the pet out when it is most likely to need to eliminate:
   - Following play, exercise, meals, naps, and being released from confinement. Feeding and drinking may stimulate elimination. Therefore, supervise well after feeding and plan to take the puppy out to eliminate within 30 to 60 minutes after it eats.
   - Prior to confinement or bedtime.
4. Consider teaching your puppy to 'go' on command by saying a command word, such as 'hurry up,' in a positive tone as it squats to eliminate.

B. Maintain a consistent schedule
1. Offer food two to three times each day at the same time.
2. Only leave the food down for 20 minutes or until your puppy walks away. However, you should also discuss with your veterinarian how to assess your puppy's body score (i.e., whether it is too heavy, skinny, or normal) so that food quantity can be adjusted according to your pet's needs.
3. Take up the water bowl about one to two hours prior to bedtime.

C. Confine/supervise (small room, crate, or tie-down)
1. Until the puppy has completed four consecutive weeks without soiling in the home, it should be within eyesight of a family member or confined to a safe puppy-proofed area.
2. The room, crate, or pen used for confinement is intended to serve as a safe, comfortable bed, playpen, or den for the puppy. The puppy should not be confined to this area until after it has eliminated and had sufficient exercise and social interaction (i.e., when it is due for a sleep, nap, or rest) and should not be confined for any longer than it can control elimination, unless paper-training techniques are being used.
3. Most puppies can control elimination through the night by four months of age. During the daytime, puppies four months or less usually have a few hours of control, while puppies five months and over may be able to last longer between eliminations.
4. If the puppy eliminates in its cage, it may have been left there longer than it can be confined without eliminating, or the cage may be large enough that it sleeps in one end and eliminates in the other; in this case a divider might be used temporarily. Also, if the puppy is anxious about being confined to its crate or left alone, it is unlikely to keep the crate clean.
5. Use a leash indoors to help supervise the puppy. By observing the puppy closely for pre-elimination signs, the puppy can be trained to eliminate outdoors without the need for punishment and may soon learn to signal when it has to eliminate.

D. Handling mistakes
1. Punishment is generally not indicated as part of a housetraining program. The goal is to interrupt your puppy if it is caught in the act of eliminating indoors, and direct it to the appropriate location so that it can be rewarded when it eliminates there.
2. If you catch your puppy in the act of eliminating indoors, quickly say 'no' and clap your hands or pull on the leash to interrupt the behavior (you have one to two seconds to catch it in the act). Then take the pet outside and praise it enthusiastically upon completion.
3. If urine or stool is found on the floor after the puppy has eliminated, do not consider any form of correction since the puppy will not associate the correction with the elimination. You can prevent resoiling in the home by closing doors or moving furniture to prevent access to the location, booby trapping the location with a repellent or motion detector, constant supervision of your puppy, and by consistently rewarding elimination outdoors.

(continued)

Figure 17.1   Housetraining (client handout #14 – printable from the CD).

E. Odor elimination

Clean up any odors from indoor elimination. Be certain to use enough odor neutralizer to get to the source of the odor. Use one of the products that have been specifically designed to eliminate pet urine odors (chemical modification, enzymes, bacterial odor removal), and follow the label directions.

F. Paper training

While it is best to skip paper training and immediately train the pup to eliminate outdoors, this approach is sometimes necessary for apartment dwellers or when it is not practical to take the puppy outside frequently enough. For paper training, the puppy should be confined to a room or pen with paper covering the floor except for a sleeping area. The puppy should be confined to this area while you are out, or when you cannot supervise. Paper training can be combined with outdoor training so that the puppy learns that there are two appropriate places to eliminate. The crate could be used for confinement for shorter departures and the papered area for longer departures. Another option is to train the pup to use an indoor litter product.

In some households and in some communities, it might also be practical to house the dog in an outdoor run, or provide a dog door with outdoor access if the owner cannot be home to let the dog outside when it needs to eliminate.

Figure 17.1 (*continued*)

HOUSESOILING PROBLEMS

Eliminating in the home can be due to a variety of reasons. The most common causes in young dogs are inadequate training, submissive urination, and excitement. During adulthood, marking and separation anxiety can result in inappropriate elimination in the home. Medical problems can occur at any age, but tend to occur with higher frequency in the older pet (see Chs 4 and 12 for details). Occasionally, you may see a housesoiling problem that occurs rather spontaneously and may be due to situations such as an abrupt change in the owner's schedule, failure of the owner to allow the pet access to the elimination area in a timely fashion, a change in the pet's feeding schedule, or a change in the pet's diet. When the problem is allowed to persist, it is likely that the pet will develop strong new location or surface preferences for eliminating within the home.

Diagnosis

When working up a housesoiling problem, some initial consideration should be given to the possibility of an underlying medical problem. Once medical problems have been ruled out or treated, a complete history must be obtained in order to sort through the various behavioral causes of elimination in the home (Fig. 17.2).

Medical workup

A medical workup should be done to ensure that there is not a physiological reason for the problem (Figs 17.3, 17.4). This is particularly true when working with older pets that have a relatively high incidence of medical problems. The patient should receive a thorough physical exam, including attention to the pet's state of mental awareness. Special consideration should be paid to the gastrointestinal and urinary systems. The medical history should include information about water consumption, diet,

Differential diagnosis for housesoiling
- Inadequate training
- Submissive urination
- Excitement urination
- Marking
- Separation anxiety
- Medical problems
- Management-related problems
- Location or surface preferences

Figure 17.2

Urination problem	Defecation problem
Urinalysis	Fecal sedimentation/saline smear
Complete blood count	Complete blood count
Creatinine/urea/glucose	Trypsin-like immunoreactivity
Alanine transaminase, calcium, phosphorus	Serum alanine transaminase
Serum alkaline phosphatase	Amylase/lipase
Urine creatinine: cortisol ratio or dexamethasone suppression if indicated	Serum alkaline phosphatase
	Bile acids
Water consumption measurement	Urinalysis
Water deprivation test if indicated	Thyroid evaluation (if indicated by history or other signs)

Figure 17.3 Laboratory tests that might be indicated for dogs with elimination problems.

pica, the volume and frequency of elimination, the appearance of the stool and urine, and a description of the act of elimination. Lab tests may include a fecal exam for parasites, urinalysis, serum chemistry panel, hemogram, and thyroid function evaluation. Ancillary testing and procedures might include a neurologic exam, radiographs, adrenal function tests, trypsin-like immunoreactivity, and water deprivation testing.

Medical causes of housesoiling

Any medical problem that causes an increased frequency of elimination can trigger a housesoil-ing problem if the pet's access to its elimination area is not concurrently increased. Urinating in the home is often one of the first signs noticed by owners of dogs that have conditions such as renal disease, hyperadrenocorticism, diabetes, or pyometra. Lower urinary tract infections, inflammatory disease, and irritation caused by cystic calculi typically lead to an urge to urinate more frequently. Anything that decreases the volume of the urinary bladder can also increase the need to urinate more frequently. Problems such as urinary bladder tumors, large calculi, or abdominal masses can compromise filling of the bladder and result in an increased frequency of urination. Urethral incompetence that results

Medical causes of fecal housesoiling
- Problems that cause increased volume of feces
  - Maldigestion disorders
  - Malabsorption disorders
  - High fiber diets
- Problems that cause increased frequency of voiding
  - Colitis
  - Diarrhea
- Problems that influence control
  - Compromised neurologic function
    - Peripheral nerve impairment
    - Spinal cord impairment
    - Cranial disease (tumors, encephalitis, infection, degenerative disorders)
  - Arthritis
  - Sensory decline
  - Cognitive dysfunction

Medical causes of urinary housesoiling
- Problems that cause polyuria
  - Renal failure
  - Hyperadrenalcorticism
  - Diabetes
  - Pyometra
  - Hepatic disease
- Problems that cause increased frequency
  - Lower urinary tract infection or inflammation
  - Urinary calculi
  - Urinary bladder tumors
  - Prostatitis
  - Abdominal masses
- Problems that influence control
  - Compromised neurologic function
    - Peripheral nerve impairment
    - Spinal cord impairment
    - Cranial disease (tumors, encephalitis, infection, degenerative disorders)
  - Urethral incompetence
  - Cognitive dysfunction

Figure 17.4 Medical conditions that might cause or contribute to inappropriate elimination habits.

in incontinence can be another cause of house-soiling.

Conditions that result in an increased frequency of defecation or cause inflammation and pain to be associated with the act can lead to housesoiling. Diarrhea, maldigestion, malabsorption, constipation, and colitis are all problems that can result in the pet defecating in the home.

Anything that compromises the neurological control of elimination can cause incontinence and result in housesoiling. Neurologic causes of housesoiling include peripheral nerve damage, spinal cord disease, and cephalic problems such as tumors, trauma, infection, inflammation, and age-related degenerative disorders. Impaired cognitive function in some elderly pets can cause confusion, disorientation, poor perception, and loss of learned behaviors, which can lead to housesoiling (see Ch. 12).

Besides gastrointestinal and urinary problems, anything that makes it difficult for the pet to get to its elimination area can result in it voiding in the home. Arthritis or weakness can cause the pet to avoid using stairs to the outdoors. Sensory loss can make ambulation difficult, lead to confusion, and cause the dog to urinate and defecate indoors. Intolerance to extremes in heat (obesity) or cold (hypothyroidism) may make the pet reluctant to leave a comfortable indoor environment to eliminate outdoors.

Behavioral history

Once underlying medical problems have been ruled out or treated, some time must be spent gathering sufficiently detailed historical information in order to formulate an accurate diagnosis, prognosis, and treatment plan. You will want to know where the pet is housesoiling, whether it is urine, stool or both, as well as a description of the act of elimination. Any information the owner can provide concerning the initial appearance of the problem may prove helpful in understanding the cause of the housesoiling as well as deciding what to do to prevent recurrence. You will want to find out if there were any major changes in the pet's environ-

ment, in the owner's schedule, or in its relationship with the owner that preceded the appearance of the housesoiling. An assessment should be made of the pet's appetite and eating habits. Some pets are relatively intolerant of diet changes, so switching food can cause diarrhea, increased frequency of defecation, and housesoiling. Changing an obese dog to a high-fiber diet can cause an increase in the volume of stool produced and a need to defecate more frequently. If the pet is not allowed outdoors more often, it may subsequently defecate in the home.

Information about the home environment, family members' schedules, and individual relationships with the pet will be helpful. If the family schedule results in the pet being left alone for longer than it is able to control elimination, a doggie door or paper training should be considered. Confinement, supervision, and reinforcement of desired behaviors are important parts of the correction program and may need to be assigned to individuals depending upon availability and dedication to the pet. Another reason to explore the relationship between the pet and family members is to investigate the possibility of separation anxiety triggering a housesoiling problem. A history of housesoiling that started after a change in the amount of time spent with the pet by a family member who has a very close relationship with the pet may suggest an underlying separation anxiety problem. Anxious behavior when the owner departs and the absence of housesoiling when the pet has access to the owner are suggestive signs.

Marking should be a strong consideration if there are specific territorial or anxiety-provoking stimuli that typically precede incidents of urination by the pet, especially if it is intact. Visits by other pets, visits by owners of pets, or visits that are disruptive, such as overnight visits by guests and holiday celebrations, may trigger marking behavior.

It is always important to ask if the housesoiling has taken place in front of a family member. In most cases, you will find that the pet eliminates out of sight of the owner. If the pet is housesoiling directly in front of the owner, there are several possibilities: the owner has not provided sufficient correction during the behavior; the pet tried to signal, but the owner was distracted; a medical problem has compromised the pet's control; or senile changes resulting in disorientation and mental confusion have compromised voluntary control. Another important consideration is what type of medication the pet might currently be taking, since some medications can cause polyuria or changes in the characteristics of the stool.

Prognosis

For dogs with elimination problems of a behavioral nature, the prognosis for a full recovery is generally good. For those dogs with physiological reasons for their problems, the prognosis varies with the ultimate diagnosis and chances for curing or managing the underlying medical problems.

Discerning the duration of the housesoiling, how often the problem occurs, the number of areas soiled, and the mental state of the pet is pertinent to determining the prognosis for successful treatment of a dog that is housesoiling. The prognosis is good for a pet with no cognitive problems and no untreatable medical conditions, and if the problem is of short duration, occurring infrequently in a limited number of areas in the home. The prognosis is also improved if the pet has already been accustomed to a crate or confinement room and the owner is available throughout the day to take the pet outdoors frequently to eliminate. The ages, maturity, consistency, and commitment of family members are other important considerations.

GENERAL PRINCIPLES FOR TREATING HOUSESOILING PROBLEMS

For the most part, housesoiling due to a training problem is addressed using the same principles as outlined above for housetraining. Dogs that relieve themselves in inappropriate locations

Treatment of housesoiling problems
- Rule out medical problems
- Remove triggers for the behavior if applicable
- Reinforce the desired behavior
- Control the feeding schedule
- Confinement/supervision
- Prevent resoiling
  - Odor elimination
  - Prevent access to areas
  - Avoidance conditioning
- Interrupt elimination in unacceptable areas
  - Use a mild auditory correction
  - Timing and intensity are important
- Avoid punishment

Figure 17.5 Summary of treatment for canine housesoiling problems.

over a long period of time have most likely developed the pattern because the behavior in itself is self-reinforcing and the owners have not intervened in a timely manner to prevent or correct the problem. When dogs relieve themselves, they do not perceive that eliminating in the area is unacceptable since there are no untoward consequences associated with the behavior, and in fact, the net effect is one of reinforcement (relief from discomfort). The behavior may then become conditioned as the pet may be stimulated to eliminate whenever they return to the area. Thus, an important key to effective housetraining is constant supervision. This allows the owner to prevent inappropriate elimination, redirect the pet to more suitable locations, and interrupt the pet if it is observed eliminating in an inappropriate location. The owner can then reinforce more acceptable behavior with lavish praise and a food treat given immediately after the pet completes the act. If the owner waits until the pet returns indoors, then returning indoors is reinforced, not eliminating outdoors. This can actually have a negative effect on the housetraining process (Fig. 17.5).

SUBMISSIVE URINATION

Submissive urination is a behavior related to social status. Although this problem can be seen in dogs of any age, submissive urination is most commonly seen in puppies and young female dogs. Urination occurs when the pet is presented with certain facial expressions, movements, or body postures by a person or another animal that it perceives to be socially dominant or threatening. Triggers for submissive urination can include approaching, standing over the pet, reaching for it, patting it on the head, strong eye contact, excited talk, deep or harsh tone of voice, and attempts to punish it.

Diagnosis and prognosis

The pet voids urine as it shows signs of submissive signaling. These may include ears laid back, horizontal retraction of the lips, avoidance of eye contact, and lowered body posture. Some dogs will lower into a recumbent position on their sides or backs while urinating. Submissive displays are typically used by subordinates to turn off dominant social threats. There may also be a component of conflict in that the pet is motivated to approach and greet the owners or visitors when they arrive but also responds submissively to the body language, postures, and reaching of the owners or visitor. A complete medical workup is required if the dog is also displaying signs suggestive of a medical problem such as inadequate urethral sphincter tone, ectopic ureters, or lower urinary tract disease.

In young dogs with no concurrent medical problems, the prognosis is good, but when the problem persists into adulthood, resolution may be more difficult. Fortunately, most puppies outgrow this behavior if family members and visitors change their method of greeting in order to reduce behavior that the pet perceives to be dominant or threatening.

Treatment

The first step is to identify all stimuli or situations that trigger the behavior. Then, the owner must do whatever is necessary to discontinue those movements and interactions so that all urination-eliciting stimuli are removed. It is important that the owner and all visitors interact with the pet in a less dominant or threatening manner. Instead of approaching and standing over the pet, the pet should be allowed to approach the greeter. Kneeling down, speaking softly, avoiding direct eye contact, and patting the chest of the pet instead of the head may help reduce submissive responses. Physical punishment and even the mildest verbal reprimands should be resolutely avoided. In fact, owners who attempt to punish the pet for urinating submissively will make things worse since punishment tends to intensify fearful and submissive behavior. When greeting a submissive or fearful dog, the owner and visitors should completely ignore it at the initial greeting, and wait till later when the pet is relaxed to calmly greet it.

Differential reinforcement or response substitution techniques can be very helpful in treating submissive urination. Using this approach, the dog is taught to perform a behavior that is not compatible with urinating, such as sitting for food or retrieving a toy when it greets someone. Clicker training for acceptable responses is another excellent option. When the owner enters the home, the dog can often be distracted from urinating by offering a toy or treat as it is requested to respond to a previously trained command given in a very calm, friendly tone. If the pet anticipates food or play at each greeting, it is less likely to eliminate submissively. The desired greeting response can gradually be shaped. Initially, the pet is given food on greeting, then only when it sits during greeting in a relaxed fashion, and finally only when it sits and is petted.

Submissive dogs require patience and confidence building in general. Obedience training that is based on positive reinforcement is an excellent way for owners to build a non-threatening rapport with their dogs. Shared physical exercise, such as long walks in parks, fetch, etc., can also be helpful. Punishment or scoldings of any type must be avoided. Drugs that might help to increase sphincter tone are discussed under excitement and conflict-induced urination below.

Prevention

Submissive urination reflects a perceived inferior social status or threat on the part of the pet. A very submissive dog can sometimes be identified with puppy temperament testing (see Ch. 3). Although selection tests are not very specific in their assessment, dogs that are exceptionally submissive or fearful can usually be identified. Advise owners to avoid selecting puppies that are overly anxious or exhibit avoidance behaviors. Calm, positive social interactions with young puppies should be encouraged, while harsh, threatening, and overly assertive social interaction should be discouraged.

EXCITEMENT AND CONFLICT-INDUCED URINATION

This problem may appear similar to submissive urination, but accompanying submissive behaviors are typically absent. The dog may lose bladder control because it is so highly aroused or when it is in a state of conflict (i.e., two competing emotions). Conflict may arise when the dog is excited to approach or greet the owners or visitors but also feels the urge to withdraw due to fear (e.g., previous punishment for jumping up, fear of the stranger) or submission. The treatment is basically the same as for submissive urination. For excitement urination, those stimuli that trigger the behavior should be avoided. During greetings, owners and guests should refrain from eye contact, and verbal or physical contact until the pet calms down. Greetings should be very low-key and words spoken in a low, calm tone. Counterconditioning, response substitution and distraction techniques are used and drugs might occasionally be useful. Caution must be taken only to reward appropriate competing behaviors at greetings (e.g., sit up and beg, stand-stay, retrieving a ball). Inappropriate use or timing of rewards might further excite the dog and serve as a reward for the excitement urination. The use of alpha-adrenergics (such as phenylpropanolamine) or a tricyclic antidepressant (such as imipramine) might also be considered as an adjunct to behavioral therapy to increase sphincter tone for refractory cases or frustrated owners.

MARKING

In most cases, this type of problem involves an intact male urinating on an upright object in response to a territorial stimulus or a stressful situation. It is likely to occur on or near odors and pheromones left by other dogs. The volume of urine voided is usually less than what is typically voided during normal micturition. Confirming the diagnosis involves associating specific territorial or anxiety-eliciting stimuli with the act. For example, the owner may have noted that immediately after barking at a stray dog or visitor in the yard, the pet went to the corner of a couch or side of a plant, lifted its leg and voided a small amount of urine. Anything that causes the pet to become anxious or thwarts a highly motivated behavior may also trigger marking behavior. For example, the dog that is denied access to the owner by a closed door inside the home or is unable to accompany the owner outdoors might urine mark indoors.

Consideration should be given to castrating the intact male, preventing exposure to stimuli that elicit urine marking, and avoiding situations that make the pet anxious. Spaying is recommended for female dogs that mark during estrus. Castration will reduce male marking behavior in 70–80% of dogs. Preventing the territorial pet from watching other dogs through windows in the home may be helpful. Urine residue must be removed from around doors, windows, or other areas where stray dogs have been marking. A stake can be driven into an appropriate area of the yard where marking is permitted. The owner should give food rewards to reinforce marking at the stake, and the dog should not be permitted to mark anywhere else. New upright objects that are brought into the home should not be placed on the floor until the pet is familiar with them. Spaying a resident female dog at home may be helpful if the male pet marks when the female is in estrus. Tricyclic antidepressants, selective serotonin re-uptake inhibitors, or D.A.P.™ may be helpful for raising the response threshold of exceptionally reactive dogs.

Setups involving remote punishment may be attempted. An object, such as a suitcase or grocery sack, can be placed in an area where the owner can observe from out of sight. When the dog attempts to lift its leg to mark, the owner can provide remote punishment by setting off an electronic alarm, tossing a tin can containing pebbles near the pet, or activating a remote citronella spray collar. The aversive stimulus should be strong enough to stop the behavior without causing fear and should not be associated with the owner's presence. During training, the owner should closely supervise the pet and confine it to a small area when it cannot be watched.

SEPARATION ANXIETY

When a dog has a very close relationship with a family member, it may become anxious when it suddenly loses access to that person. Anxiety-based problems, including separation anxiety, tend to occur with increased frequency and intensity in the older pet dog population. Situations such as changes in the family members' work schedule or returning to work after a long stay at home can lead to this type of problem. The dog with a separation anxiety problem may show signs of either increased activity and anxiety (pacing, restlessness, whining) or depression (lying around, reluctance to move or eat) as the owner prepares to leave. These behaviors often begin as the pet becomes aware of pre-departure cues, such as putting on a coat, reaching for keys, or picking up a briefcase. When the owner returns home, the dog usually exhibits high levels of arousal and may show exaggerated greeting behaviors. Separation anxiety can also occur when the owner becomes involved in an activity or relationship that takes a significant amount of attention away from the pet at home. This can occur when there is a new baby or spouse in the home. The anxiety then becomes a driving force for excessive vocalization, self-mutilation, destructive behavior, or housesoiling. An important clue that differentiates separation anxiety-related housesoiling

from other causes is that these pets will often eliminate in the home every time the owner leaves, even when the absence is of very short duration, and in spite of the fact that the pet has eliminated in an appropriate area just prior to the owner's departure.

Treatment involves desensitization to pre-departure cues and gradually accustoming the dog to separation from the owner. If the owner can provide a dramatic increase in daily exercise, this will usually have a calming effect. Enriching the pet's environment (rubber toys stuffed with treats) or distractions (another pet, radio) may help, although some dogs experience such high anxiety that food and distractions are ignored. During the early stages of treatment, a small confinement area, a pet sitter, or boarding may be necessary and general principles of housetraining should be followed. Drug therapy with tricyclic antidepressants (clomipramine, amitriptyline) and benzodiazepines (clorazepate, alprazolam) may be helpful when the anxiety is intense (see also Ch. 11).

THE GERIATRIC DOG

In general, geriatric dogs require access to an elimination area more frequently than younger dogs. Access to a doggie door, a pet sitter, or closer observation by the owner may help prevent housesoiling problems from developing. Problems in older pets, such as arthritis, muscle atrophy, and weakness make navigation of stairs more difficult. Ramps and carpeted stairs should make the dog less reluctant to take a trip outdoors. Medication may be necessary to reduce pain and stiffness and make it easier for the pet to get to its elimination area.

Housetraining requires voluntary control of the detrusor reflex at a cortical level. As the dog ages, physical and physiologic changes occur in the central nervous system that result in a general decrease in cerebral function. Impaired cerebral function can affect the geriatric pet's housetraining by influencing voluntary control of the emptying reflex and by reducing awareness. Loss of voluntary control can result in urge incontinence (the dog has a warning that micturition is about to occur but cannot stop it) or unconscious urination (there is no awareness or control). Reduced awareness may also result in the pet being less cognizant of its external environment, making it less likely to signal to the owner when it has to eliminate.

Selegiline will help some of these dogs that have problems with cognitive dysfunction as an underlying cause of the housesoiling. Establishing a frequent, regular schedule of guiding the dog to its elimination area will help ensure that the pet voids in a timely manner. A fixed diet and feeding schedule can also be helpful in preventing problems. Stress should be kept to a minimum, and when the owner expects a schedule change or an extended absence from the pet, steps should be taken to gradually prepare the dog. This will help prevent problems such as separation anxiety. Cold intolerance can be a problem for some older pets. Those dogs should be checked for underlying circulatory problems and hypothyroidism. For the pet with extensive mental deterioration, confinement to a safe, easily cleaned area may be the only way to manage the housesoiling problem (see Ch. 12 for more details on senior care).

MISCELLANEOUS CAUSES OF HOUSESOILING PROBLEMS

There are a variety of other factors that can lead to housesoiling. Changing the time when the pet is fed such that the dog has to eliminate when no one will be available to let it out (moving the meal closer to bedtime or confinement) can lead to housesoiling. Inappropriate punishment that results in fear of the owner can make the dog reluctant to approach the owner to signal when it needs to go outdoors to eliminate. A frightening incident that occurred in the area where the pet eliminates (abuse by a neighbor, severe thunderstorm), or intolerance of inclement weather (rain, wind, snow, heat), may make the dog hesitant to go outdoors and may result in it eliminating indoors. Failure to ensure that the dog eliminates just prior to bedtime or confinement can cause a well-housetrained pet

to urinate or defecate indoors. For example, if the owner was not paying attention when the dog was let out into the yard to eliminate just prior to bedtime, and the dog spent the allotted time chasing rabbits instead of eliminating, it is likely that the dog will eliminate in the home during the night.

SUMMARY

Medical reasons for a break in housetraining should always be considered when working up the dog that is housesoiling. Unresolved medical problems will cause any attempts to correct the behavior problem to fail. The basic approach to treatment involves correcting the factors that initiated the problem, rewarding the desired behavior, and preventing the undesirable behavior from occurring for a long enough period of time until the habit of eliminating in a desired location is well established, and eliminating in the home becomes extinct. Treatment of pets with housesoiling problems that have no underlying organic problems generally has a high rate of success. Housesoiling due to untreatable medical problems, such as advanced renal failure or senile mental changes that result in cognitive impairment, is not likely to be corrected, but merely managed.

CASE EXAMPLES
Case 1

Herman, a four-month-old Dachshund puppy, was eliminating in its crate and throughout the house, but never in the presence of the owner.

The puppy would eliminate outdoors in the yard and the owner would give appropriate rewards. The puppy would not eliminate indoors as long as a family member was closely supervising, but would occasionally sneak away and eliminate in another room. When the owners found the soiled area, they would immediately take the puppy to the spot, put its nose in the feces or urine, and verbally reprimand it. The puppy had also recently begun to eat its own feces. Herman slept in the bedroom with the owners during the night. On occasion, the owners would find that he had gone downstairs to eliminate while they slept. On weekdays, Herman was left in a cage in the laundry room, from about 8:30 a.m. to 4 p.m., and on most days the owner would find urine or stool in the cage. Whenever the owners found urine or feces in the cage, they would yell at the puppy and put him outdoors in the yard where he was ignored for 30 minutes. The owners were convinced that Herman knew that he was misbehaving because he would act guilty and fearful whenever they arrived home and found that he had eliminated in an inappropriate location.

The puppy had been forced to eliminate in its cage because it was being left for seven and a half hours (too long for this puppy to control itself). It had learned that it was safe to eliminate in other rooms provided the owner was not in view. The puppy seemed to act guiltily only because it had learned that it would get abused each time the owner found a soiled area. It was explained to the owners that if the puppy is to understand that the punishment is for elimination, it can only make this association if it receives the unpleasant consequences during elimination. Although it was unlikely that the puppy was eating its stools because the owners were forcing its mouth into the soiled areas, this practice was irrational and unsuccessful.

Since it was necessary to provide the puppy with an opportunity to eliminate within four to five hours, the owners either had to arrange to allow the puppy outdoors a few hours earlier or provide him with an elimination area while they were out. The owners chose to arrange for the dog to have an additional walk at lunch hour. Since the owners wished to continue to confine the puppy to its crate while out, a cage training guide was provided. The cage was relocated to the corner of the bedroom where the puppy normally slept, and the door was kept closed so that the puppy could not wander downstairs at night. The owners continued to reward the puppy for outdoor elimination and provided diligent supervision when indoors. With the additional walk at lunch hour and the relocation of the cage, the problem was immediately cor-

rected and by seven months of age the owners attempted to cut out the noon walk. Although the puppy no longer eliminated when left in the cage from 8:30 a.m. to 4 p.m., after further consultation the noon-time walks were resumed to ensure that the puppy had ample opportunity to exercise.

Case 2

An 11-month-old Bichon Frise would eliminate indoors whenever the owner did not supervise the dog. Even if the dog had been outdoors recently it might sneak away to eliminate. When the owners were away from home, the dog was left in the kitchen where it eliminated on paper. While the owners were outdoors with the dog, it would not eliminate in their presence. During the first two months of ownership the owners would supervise the dog and scream or hit it when it began to eliminate indoors. They would then throw the dog outdoors unsupervised. On occasion, the dog had managed to sneak away from the owners and eliminate in other rooms.

The dog had learned to eliminate indoors on paper and had never learned that it was supposed to eliminate outdoors. Because of the way punishment had been used, the dog was fearful of eliminating in the owners' presence, regardless of whether it was indoors or out.

The first step was to teach the dog that it would receive valuable rewards (food treats, ball playing) whenever it eliminated outdoors. This would be extremely difficult and time-consuming since the dog was fearful of eliminating in the owners' presence. Rather than send the dog outdoors at each scheduled elimination time, the owners were instructed to go outdoors with the dog and ignore it until it eliminated (regardless of how long it took). On the first occasion, after a long walk and a half hour of play, the dog would not eliminate so the owners returned indoors and continued to supervise the dog diligently. An hour later, the dog was taken out again to its favorite elimination site and with the owner several yards away the dog finally eliminated. As the dog eliminated, the owner quietly and calmly said 'go pee,' and rewarded the dog with a piece of meat and a game of fetch. When the dog was indoors, it was constantly supervised or left in the kitchen with paper. The only setbacks were when the dog sneaked away from the owners. This problem was resolved by leaving a 10-ft leash attached to the dog so that it could be kept in sight and directed quickly outdoors when pre-elimination signs were seen. At each scheduled elimination time the owner took the dog outdoors and used a 'go pee' command followed by a food reward and game of fetch whenever the dog complied. In time the dog responded quite well to elimination on command and was not reluctant to eliminate in front of the owners. As outdoor supervised elimination became more successful, indoor paper elimination became less and less frequent.

Case 3

Maggie was a six-month-old Labrador Retriever that held her ears back, looked away, squatted, and urinated whenever the owners reached to pet her as they entered the home. If their hands were full so they could not pet her when she was greeted, the urination did not

occur. A diagnosis of submissive urination was made.

The owners were told to avoid reaching for her at greeting during the first week of training. Maggie was first taught to sit in response to happy, verbal commands and hand signal cues using food lures. She learned to sit on command by the end of the first week. At that time, the owners were instructed to begin counterconditioning exercises. They were told to wait to start the exercises until she had calmed down following their arrival. Then, they would ask her to do several sits for food rewards in the family room. Next, they moved the exercises to the front door. During the last segment of the conditioning exercises, the owners exited through the door, immediately returned, and asked her to sit for a food reward. This was repeated six more times. The exercise was performed once or twice daily until the end of the second week. Each time the pet took the food, the owner calmly patted her on her chest with the other hand. During the third week, the owners started the exercises closer and closer to their initial arrival, and gradually moved the physical contact from her chest to her head. By the end of the third week they could enter, ask her to sit, and pat her without eliciting submissive urination. The food that was given for sitting when greeted was gradually withdrawn.

FURTHER READING

Beaver BV 1994 Differential approach to house soiling by dogs and cats. Veterinary Quarterly 16(Suppl 1):S47
Ewer RF 1973 The carnivores. Cornell University Press, Ithaca, NY
Hart B, Hart L 1985 Canine and feline behavioral therapy. Lee & Febiger
Hopkins SG, Schubert TA, Hart BL 1976 Castration of adult male dogs: effects on roaming, aggression, urine marking and mounting. Journal of the American Veterinary Medical Association 168:1108–1110
Hunthausen W 1994a Identifying and treating behavior problems in geriatric dogs. Veterinary Medicine 89(9):688–700
Hunthausen W 1994b Collecting the history of a pet with a behavior problem. Veterinary Medicine 89(10):954–959
Hunthausen W 1995 Housesoiling and the geriatric dog. Veterinary Medicine August(Suppl):4–15

Korefsky PS 1987 Letter to the editor: 'Identifying source of urine on rugs.' Journal of the American Veterinary Medical Association 191(8):917
Marder AR 1991 Psychotropic drugs and behavioral therapy. Veterinary Clinics of North America 21(2):329
Melese-d'Hospital P 1996 Eliminating urine odors in the home. In: Voith VL, Borchelt PL (eds) Readings in companion animal behavior. Veterinary Learning Systems, Trenton, NJ, p 191–197
Mosier JE 1989 Effect of aging on body systems of the dog. Veterinary Clinics of North America, Small Animal Practice 19(1):1–12
O'Brien D 1988 Neurogenic disorders of micturition. Veterinary Clinics of North America, Small Animal Practice 18(3):535
Oliver JE, Lorenz MD 1993 Handbook of veterinary neurology. WB Saunders, Philadelphia, p 74–75

Overall KE 1997 Clinical behavioral medicine for small animals. Mosby, St Louis

Overall KE 2001 Dealing with inappropriate elimination in an aging dog. Veterinary Medicine June:431–434

Ross S 1950 Some observations on the lair dwelling behaviour of dogs. Behaviour 2:144–162

Scott JP, Fuller JL 1965 Genetics and the social behaviour of the dog. University of Chicago Press, Chicago, IL

Voith VL 1991 Treating elimination behaviour problems in dogs and cats: the role of punishment. Modern Veterinary Practice December:951–953

Voith VL, Borchelt PL 1985 Elimination behaviour and related problems in dogs. Compendium of Continuing Education 7(7):538

Vollmer PJ 1977 Inappropriate elimination in an older dog. Veterinary Medicine Small Animal Clinics October:1577–1578

18

Feline housesoiling

Housesoiling is the most common behavior problem for which cat owners seek assistance, and a major reason why some cats are abandoned or euthanized. Medical disorders, litterbox avoidance, unacceptable elimination site preferences, territorial marking, and stress can all cause a cat to eliminate away from its litterbox. Because of the numerous and varied reasons for housesoiling, successful management requires collecting sufficient information to uncover the underlying cause(s).

You must be sure the cat presented for the problem is the one that is actually housesoiling. Multi-cat households can pose a challenge since it may not be immediately evident which cat is soiling the home. Separation for a few days or weeks may be necessary to find the perpetrator. Another method is to give fluorescein orally (0.5 ml of a 10% solution or the ends of six fluorescein strips in gel caps) or by injection (0.3 ml of a 10% solution SC) in order to trace urine stains to the individual with the problem. The soiled areas should be inspected frequently using a Wood's lamp since the urine will fluoresce for about 24 hours.

LITTERBOX TRAINING

Training most kittens to use a litterbox is a relatively simple procedure. Since most cats prefer to dig and scratch prior to elimination and perform a burying type ritual after elimination, providing a material that is clean, easily accessible, and has a texture amenable to digging (e.g., clay litter, clumping litter) is all that is usually necessary. Of course, the kitten must be prevented from accessing other similar substrates, such as plant soil, and the litter should be scooped daily and changed weekly. Kittens that do not use their litterboxes consistently should be assessed for any medical problems and if there are no abnormalities and there appears to be no abnormality with respect to the urine or stool, then thorough cleaning of the soiled sites, preventing access to these areas (or booby trapping the areas), and improved litterbox hygiene might be sufficient to re-establish litter use. However, if the kitten still does not use its box, it should be determined what surface and area the kitten does utilize and if there are any factors associated with the litter that might be deterring its use. For example, if the litter does not have easy access because of its location, the height or size of the box, or the lighting, then the kitten may select another location. The presence of another cat or dog in the home may be a factor in preventing or denying access to the litter – see Figures 18.1 (client handout #15 on the CD) and 18.2.

DIAGNOSIS
Medical considerations

The first step is to perform a thorough medical workup. There are a number of medical problems that can lead to housesoiling problems, including lower urinary tract disorders, diarrhea, arthritis, renal failure, diabetes, and constipation. A thorough physical examination and appropriate laboratory tests should be performed on all suspect cats. If the cat is urinating away from the box, a urinalysis, assessment of water intake, and urine frequency should be the minimum workup. Since some feline urinary conditions may occur intermittently and cause transient signs, repeat urinalyses may need to be performed. If a cat is showing signs of dysuria, but has a normal urinalysis, interstitial cystitis should be suspected. Additional diagnostic tests (e.g., serum chemistries, CBC, thyroid evaluation, radiography, ultrasonography,

endoscopy, biopsy) may also be necessary, depending on the results of the preliminary examination.

For inappropriate defecation, a stool evaluation, along with an assessment of eating, drinking, and elimination habits, would be the minimum workup. The owner should be questioned about signs of diarrhea, blood/mucus in the stool, hard stools, and discomfort while defecating (Fig. 18.3).

History

Once underlying medical problems have been ruled out or treated, the next step in working up a housesoiling problem is to find out whether the cat is spraying vertical surfaces or eliminating inappropriately on horizontal surfaces. Spraying occurs when a cat backs up to an upright surface and directs a stream of urine toward it. The amount is usually smaller than what is voided when a cat empties its bladder during normal urination. This is a marking behavior that may be triggered by territorial or stressful situations.

If the cat is eliminating inappropriately on horizontal surfaces, the reason is commonly due to either an environmental issue that causes the cat to avoid the box or one that attracts it to an area away from the box that is unacceptable to the owner. In a small number of cases, a cat will urinate on horizontal surfaces as a marking behavior.

Some of the important information you will want to unearth includes when and where the problem began; if there were any changes in the cat's environment associated with the commencement of the problem; whether the soiling involves urine, stool or both; what surfaces are being soiled; how frequently the problem occurs; if the appearance of the problem has changed; and what has been done to try to correct the problem.

The object is to elucidate the factors that lead to the undesirable elimination behavior. If you don't do a housecall consultation, ask the owner to diagram the house with litterbox placement, feeding stations, and soiled areas noted. Eval-

LITTER TRAINING YOUR KITTEN

In order to avoid litterbox problems in adult cats, it is extremely important that you get your kitten off to a good start. Fortunately, most kittens are attracted to an area where they can scratch, dig, and perhaps bury their urine and stool, so that dirt, clay, or any other substrate that allows for digging will usually be effective. Of course, if there are other appealing areas, such as plants with soil or a fireplace hearth, your kitten may be tempted to choose those areas instead. By choosing a suitable litter, placing it in an appropriate location for the kitten, keeping it clean and dry, and encouraging its use, most kittens can easily be housetrained. If you have more than one cat, add at least one litterbox for each new cat to ensure that there are enough clean litterboxes available at any one time, and to reduce the possibility of confrontation or conflicts at the litterbox.

To get your kitten off to a good start, it is a good idea to keep the pet within eyesight at all times or to confine it to a room with its litter when you cannot supervise. If your kitten stops playing and begins purposely sniffing around, there is a good chance that it needs to eliminate. Gently pick the kitten up, carry it to the litterbox, and place it inside. Praise any sniffing or scratching and give it loads of praise or a small food treat for eliminating. Do this for at least the first two weeks until it has established a regular pattern of using the box.

1. **Litter (substrate)**
   a) Choose an appropriate litter material. Studies have shown that more cats may prefer clumping litter and you may find it easier to keep clean. However, any other commercial litter material may prove to be equally or even more appealing to your particular kitten. Clumping litter may lead to tracking of material outside the box, and kittens that eat litter should not be given clumping litter.
   b) If the litter you have chosen is not being used by your kitten, try other types. Some kittens may prefer a different texture or type, while scented products may deter others. Traditional clay litter, recycled newspaper litter, a plastic litter pellet (pearls), cedar shavings, or even a little potting soil or sand added to the litter may prove to be more appealing.
   c) If your pet won't use the litterbox, try to determine if there is anything about the litter that is deterring your kitten. For example, you may find that scented litter, the texture of the litter, insufficient cleaning of the litter, or litterbox liners are leading to avoidance.

2. **Litterbox**
   a) Choose an appropriate litterbox. The box should be big enough that an adult cat can stretch and scratch. Some kittens prefer a litterbox with some privacy so that a hooded box may be preferable. Some kittens find the self-cleaning litterboxes highly appealing, while the product may frighten others.
   b) If the litterbox is not being used regularly by your kitten, try other types. A larger box may be more appealing, such as an underbed storage container or even a child swimming pool may be considered if you have multiple cats. Some kittens may prefer a deeper litterbox with more litter while others may prefer lower sides so that they can be more easily accessed. Some kittens may prefer a ledge on which to perch surrounding the litterbox.
   c) If your pet won't use the litterbox, try to determine if there is anything about the litterbox that is deterring your kitten. For example, you may find that a hood on the box, sides that are too high, a litterbox that is too small or cramped, or a motorized self-cleaning litterbox may lead to avoidance.

3. **Location**
   a) You may have a particular location where you prefer to locate the box, but this must also be acceptable for your kitten. The box should be easily accessible to the pet, especially when it wakes from a nap, or after eating or playing.
   b) If the litter is not being used regularly by your kitten, consider other locations. Is the litterbox located in an area that is inconvenient or hard to access? If you occasionally use the room for other functions (e.g., lavatory) it may be inaccessible to the kitten when it needs to be used.

(*continued*)

Figure 18.1   Litter training kittens (client handout #15 – printable from the CD).

c) If your pet won't use the litterbox, try to determine if there is anything about the location that might be deterring the kitten. If the litterbox is in an area that might be unpleasant or anxiety-evoking for your kitten (e.g., a dark basement, next to a furnace or air vent, next to a washing machine, or near a toilet or bathtub), it may be necessary to relocate the litterbox. In addition, some kittens will avoid the area if they are chased, cornered, or bothered by another cat or dog in the home. If this is the case, then additional locations or more privacy may be needed (e.g., a cat door to a secluded area).

Spraying

Some cats, especially intact males that have reached puberty and females in estrus (heat), may begin to mark their territory by spraying urine on vertical objects and surfaces. Neutering will stop spraying in most but not all cats. If neutering alone is not successful you will need to seek advice to determine why your cat is continuing to spray. Treatment may involve finding and resolving the source of territorial stimulation, addressing anxiety or conflict in the home, eliminating urine odor, using a pheromone spray (Feliway™), and perhaps prescribing drugs.

What to do if your kitten does not use the litterbox

You will need to seek veterinary advice to help design a program to correct the problem. The first step is to determine whether your kitten is housesoiling with urine, stools or both, as well as the surfaces and locations that are being used. Medical problems that might cause these signs must then be considered, since painful elimination, more frequent elimination, or loss of control may drive the kitten away from its box. If the pet has no medical problems that are causing the housesoiling, a behavior program needs to be implemented.

Sometimes it can be successful if you remove the odor thoroughly from flooring and carpets with an odor counteractant, and change the function of the area to one where the kitten plays, eats, or uses a scratching post. Another option is to block access to the area that the kitten is soiling or to make the area unpleasant with a motion detector alarm or a sheet of upside-down vinyl carpet runner with the nubs pointing up. If there is more than one cat, additional litterboxes, or preventing the sharing of boxes (e.g., by cat doors or confinement) can be successful.

Often, the best indication of what can be done is determined by finding out where and when the kitten is eliminating. Try to determine what might be deterring the kitten from using its litter (see above) and what the kitten might prefer about the new area. It might be possible to move the litter or change the litter or box to better suit the kitten.

Figure 18.1 (*continued*)

uating the information provided in this way can be very helpful. For example, if the cat is urinating in the house in response to visits by neighborhood cats, you may discover clusters of soiled areas around windows or doors in the house near the areas where outdoor cats call.

You need to keep in mind that the factors that contributed to the initiation of the housesoiling may be different than the factors that are maintaining the behavior. For example, a sudden change to a brand of litter that was unacceptable to the pet may have caused it to avoid the box and eliminate on the living room carpet. After a certain amount of time, the cat may develop new surface or location preferences and continue to eliminate in the living room even though the owner switches back to an acceptable brand of litter. In this case, the initiating factor was a litter

brand change; the maintaining factors are new elimination preferences. It is important to know the maintaining factors in order to curtail the problem. Uncovering the initiating factors will help the owner prevent the problem from recurring.

URINE MARKING

Overview

Urine spraying is a sexually dimorphic behavior, occurring with a higher frequency in male than female cats. During the spraying behavioral sequence, the cat will back up to the target, stand with its rear end held high, tail erect and quivering, and squirt a stream of urine. During or just prior to the release of urine, the cat may

TYPES OF FELINE HOUSESOILING

Urine marking	Inappropriate elimination
Generally vertical surfaces, but may be some cases where urine or stools on horizontal surfaces is due to marking	Horizontal surfaces but elimination on vertical surfaces may be a form of non-marking inappropriate elimination
Marking behavior – may be territorial signaling or an anxiety- or conflict-induced response	Elimination behavior – in rare cases may be a social or anxiety-induced behavior (marking)
Most common in intact males and females in heat	Males or females, intact or neutered
Adults	Any age
Urine (in rare cases, may be stool)	Urine and/or stool
Doors, windows, new objects, owners' possessions, or frequently used furniture	Elimination in a variety of areas

Figure 18.2 Comparison between marking and inappropriate elimination in cats.

alternately tread the ground with its rear paws. The behavior appears to be facilitated by sexual hormones because the incidence of spraying behavior is higher in intact animals, but it is not completely dependent on sexual hormones since 10% of intact males and 5% of intact females will continue to spray urine following neutering. For intact or castrated male cats, the appearance of an intact female cat in the territory will increase the likelihood of urine spraying. The total number of cats in the home territory can also have a strong effect on a cat's propensity to spray urine. Skeritt and Jemmett (1980) noted that the incidence of urine spraying in the home is directly related to the density of the cat population, and that the incidence of this behavior increased from 25%

in single cat households to 100% in those with 10 or more cats.

While urine spraying is readily recognized as a type of urine marking because of the conspicuous deposition of urine on upright surfaces, some cats may urine mark on horizontal surfaces. This type of urine marking can be more difficult to diagnose, especially when the eliciting stimuli are not readily apparent. This horizontal marking may be more likely to be performed by female cats. Conversely, some cats may spray urine as a form of litterbox avoidance. In fact, for some cats all urine elimination is by spraying urine on vertical surfaces.

The purpose of urine marking by cats is not well understood but it probably serves a

Housesoiling (urine)
Conditions causing polyuria (diabetes, renal, hyperthyroidism)
Conditions causing pollakiuria (feline lower urinary tract disease, calculi, feline interstitial cystitis)
Conditions causing incontinence (neurological disorders, anatomic problems)
Conditions affecting locomotion (arthritis, disc disease, muscle atrophy, weakness)
Miscellaneous conditions (hyperthyroidism, neoplasia, cognitive dysfunction)

Housesoiling (feces)
Conditions causing soft stools/poor control
Conditions causing increased frequency/urge (inflammatory bowel disease, colitis)
Conditions causing painful or difficult defecation (anal saculitis, obstipation, constipation)
Conditions causing incontinence (neurological disorders)
Conditions affecting locomotion, positioning (arthritis, disc disease, muscle atrophy, weakness)
Miscellaneous conditions (hyperthyroidism, neoplasia, cognitive dysfunction)

Figure 18.3 Medical causes of housesoiling in cats.

communicative function among conspecifics. Communication via chemical signals is used by many social as well as solitary species of mammals. It is likely that, as an environmental tag, urine marks provide information about the presence of the individual, as well as its reproductive status, to other conspecifics in the area. This may facilitate mating by making other cats aware that a sexually intact male or an estrus female is available. An increase in the incidence of spraying behavior occurs seasonally in coincidence with the appearance of estrus females during the mating season. Testosterone levels also increase during the mating season, as does the presence of the urinary amino acid, felinine. Although still a matter of speculation, it is possible that felinine may function as a pheromone or as a precursor to a pheromone with some sexual significance.

It has also been suggested that urine marking may serve to coordinate movements and territorial use, thus limiting contact between individuals in a given area that might be antagonistic. While this may be the case, there is no indication that discovering a urine mark causes the investigating cat to actively avoid or retreat form the marked area. Information about the time during which a cat passed through an area may be provided, since it has been observed that the sniffing and flehmen response to deposited urine varies depending upon the age of the urine.

While cats have been observed to overmark the urine marks of other cats, Verberne and de Boer (1976) found that urine marking does not always appear to be an immediate releaser for subsequent spraying by other intact male cats. In their study, they found little indication that cats are strongly motivated to cover recently posted markings of preceding animals with their own urine. The age of the urine mark may play an important role in influencing whether a cat will overmark, since cats are more likely to overmark older urine marks.

In some situations, urine spraying appears to reflect the affective state of the animal. It has been noted that some cats will spray urine during socially stressful situations, such as adding new pets or family members to the home, visits by animals or humans, absences by the owner, and tension between pets or with a family member. The actual reason why some cats spray urine during stressful situations is unknown. While it has been suggested that spraying urine might allow the cat to be more self-assured, it is just as likely that urine spraying during situations of stress, anxiety, and conflict is a form of displacement behavior. It is still open to interpretation whether the behavior is actually a coping mechanism or simply a sign of stress.

Besides marking with urine, cats also use secretions from skin glands for chemocommunication. The most well known example of this involves facial marking during which a cat rubs its head along an object from the side of the cheek up toward the ear. Both urine and skin secretion pheromones appear to function in social as well as sexual contexts. This is strongly suggested by the interest exploring animals demonstrate in such chemicals. Indeed, intact males show an oscillating interest in female urine and skin gland secretions that reflects the female's estrous cycle. Information collected by Pageat has demonstrated an antagonistic relationship between urine marking and facial marking. In two studies involving 99 cats, he observed that a cat was very unlikely to spray urine in areas where its cutaneous cheek secretions had been applied.

When taking the history of a cat that is spraying, close attention must be given to anything that might elicit a territorial response or make the pet anxious. The tendency to spray is influenced by factors pertaining to the individual (hormones, temperament), environmental stimuli that are upsetting to the cat (new room mate, new cat in the neighborhood, remodeling, moving), and its relationship with the owners (change in the work schedule, absences from home, spending less time with the pet, inappropriate punishment).

Sometimes, the slightest indication that another pet has invaded its territory can cause the pet to spray. For example, if a visitor has cats at home, a cat may spray the visitor's coat when it smells the odor of non-resident cats. Also, a cat may start spraying around the living room fireplace if fire logs are brought inside the home that have been sprayed by neighborhood cats (Fig. 18.4).

Treatment

Pertinent environmental changes or stimuli that trigger the marking must be discovered to determine the protocol required for treatment. New pets or humans in the cat's environment, major changes in its home environment, changes in the owner's schedule, and virtually any stressful situation may be underlying causes. The targeting of furniture containing another animal or family member's odor, such as the horizontal surface of specific furniture and clothing, may be a tip off that the urination is performed as a marking behavior.

The main approaches to eliminating urine marking involve altering the cat's exposure to triggering stimuli and altering the cat's response to the stimuli. Traditional methods have included environmental management, surgery, behavior modification, and medication, used together or in combination. A more recent approach involves the application of feline facial pheromones to the pet's environment. Conventional behavior modification involving desensitization and counterconditioning is generally not practical, and punishment is usually contraindicated, especially if anxiety is the underlying cause of the problem (Fig. 18.5).

Factors that might influence a cat's tendency to spray include:
- Hormones
- Temperament
- Feline population density (new cat in the neighborhood or household)
- Indirect signaling from other cats (scent on visitor's clothes)
- Changes in the environment (new room mate, remodeling home, new furniture, novel objects brought into the home)
- New work schedule for owner
- Owner absences from the home
- Owner spending less time with the cat
- Inappropriate punishment

Figure 18.4

If outdoor cats are the stimulus for spraying, then the owner should consider discouraging their visits with a water hose, motion-activated water sprinkler, or audible motion detector, or have the cats humanely removed from the property. Ultrasonic motion detectors are also available but do not appear to be effective for most situations (Fig. 18.6). Anything in the yard that might attract roaming cats should be removed (bird feeders, garbage, food, etc.). Besides removing the stimuli, the owner can prevent access to the stimuli. The spraying cat should be kept away from windows or out of rooms that permit it to view outdoor cats. Drapes can be closed. Windowsills can be modified so that the cat can no longer sit on them. Chairs near windows on which the cat perches can be moved. Urine odor should be cleaned from around doors and windows, indoors and outdoors. If other cats in the household are contributing to the problem, they should initially be separated, and existing social problems should be addressed and treated. In some cases, the number of cats in the home may need to be reduced. Another variable that can be controlled is the time the pet spends outdoors. Some individuals will spray less indoors if they have more access to the outdoors. Others do better if kept inside more.

Neutering is the most commonly used surgical method for controlling urine spraying. The procedure is very successful in curbing spraying behavior at any age: 90% of male cats stop spraying following castration and ovariohysterectomy successfully reduces the behavior in approximately 95% of female cats. Although rarely used, extreme methods such as olfactory tractotomy and ischiocavernosus myectomy have been used successfully in a small number of cases to control urine marking.

Environmental management has traditionally been reserved for cases of inappropriate elimination, but recent studies seem to support the need for this intervention. Whether some cases of spraying are due to litterbox avoidance or whether increase in odor and waste accumulation lead to anxiety-induced marking is open to conjecture. Regardless of the cause, cleaning

Goal	Approach
Control the stimulus	• Eliminate the stimulus if possible. For example, if outdoor cats are the stimulus for spraying, discourage their visits with water hose, booby traps, or humane removal • Move birdfeeders and rubbish bins that attract cats. Remove stray cat urine from around windows and doors • Reduce the number of pet cats in the home. Prevent children from teasing the pet
Remove access to stimuli	• Keep the pet away from windows or other vantage points where it can view outdoor cats • Use window shades and close doors to prevent the pet from seeing stray cats • Separate indoor cats • Confine the pet in an area of the home where visitors will not make it anxious
Surgery	• Neutering is very effective for curbing urine spraying. Efficacy has been reported at 90% for males and 95% for females • Olfactory tractotomy and ischiocavernosus myectomy have been used with varying success. These are extreme measures which should be considered as a last resort when all other approaches have failed and euthanasia is being considered
Confinement	• When the cat cannot be supervised, it should be kept confined away from areas that have been sprayed • Relapses may be reduced by ensuring that the cat is allowed back into previously soiled areas gradually and with constant supervision
Punishment	• Punishment should be avoided. Noise devices and water sprays can help deter a cat from marking when applied during the behavior. Use of an interruptive stimulus that is not associated with the owner is preferred. Booby traps, such as motion-activated alarms, can also be considered when indoor cats cannot be monitored or kept away from problem areas
Change the function of location that is sprayed	• If a cat only marks certain areas in the home, consider moving its sleeping, feeding, or play area there as a deterrent
Access to the outdoors	• Some cats will spray less indoors if they have some access to the outdoors, while others will do better if kept indoors all of the time
Provide marking area	• Cats that mark in only one or two particular areas or those that spray in or around their litterboxes could be provided with an indoor marking area (e.g., a high-sided litterbox or a tiled area or plastic sheeting placed around the litterbox
Environmental and litterbox hygiene	• Increasing the appeal of the litter by daily scooping and weekly cleaning or by switching to a more appealing substrate, box type, or area and cleaning of the sprayed areas may reduce urine marking in some cats
Drug therapy	• Useful when the stimuli for spraying cannot be eliminated and when the pet has a low threshold for spraying. None are approved for cats except clomipramine in Australia. There is significant individual variation in efficacy and side effects. Pretreatment lab tests should help identify cats that may not tolerate medication due to poor hepatic or renal function. Medication may not be an option if the owner is unable to get the pet to take the medication, although transdermal preparations are now available for some drugs. If the pet responds, a decrease in spraying is often seen within two to four weeks. After four to eight weeks the drug can be gradually reduced to the lowest effective dose. If the pet becomes anxious or resumes spraying as the dose is reduced, return to the previous level and either maintain at this level or reduce more slowly
Pheromone therapy	• Safe, no side effects • Applied once daily for at least four weeks on areas that have been sprayed with urine, as well as nearby, similar upright objects • Also available as a room diffuser • Cats that respond will usually decrease spraying behavior within seven to 10 days • Can be used in multi-cat households even if the individual that is spraying cannot be identified for certain

Figure 18.5   Treatment of urine marking.

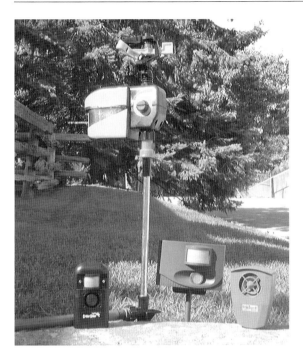

Figure 18.6 Outdoor deterrents. These products have been designed for keeping animals off the property. Audible motion detector (left), ScareCrow™ motion detector sprinkler (left center), and two ultrasonic deterrents (right center, right). For more details see Chapter 5 and client handout #21 on the CD (Fig. 5.4).

litter marks daily, scooping waste from the litterbox daily, and changing the litter and cleaning the box weekly has been shown to reduce spraying without any concurrent treatment for spraying. Therefore litterbox avoidance issues and surface preferences should also be considered in spraying cats (see inappropriate elimination treatment below).

Medication is often necessary to control urine spraying. None of the currently used medications are approved for use in cats except for clomipramine in Australia. Owners should be informed of extra label use. Pretreatment lab tests are important for identifying cats that may have metabolic problems, such as hepatic or renal disease, that might be a contraindication for the use of drug therapy. Since individual responses to psychoactive drugs may vary considerably, owners should give the initial dose when they can be at home to observe the cat's behavior. The dosage may be adjusted up or down by 25% increments until the behavior is controlled without causing undue sedation. Response to treatment may take from a few days to a few weeks depending on the drug used. Two to four weeks after a cessation in spraying, an attempt should be made to slowly decrease the dosage by about 25% every two weeks. Some cats can be successfully weaned off medication, especially if the behavior program has been effectively implemented, while others may require long-term maintenance with the lowest effective dose. Some cats maintained on long-term reduced dose therapy may ultimately show recurrence, perhaps associated with an increase in environmental stressors. Owners should be informed of all potential side effects and that none of these drugs are approved for behavior modification in cats. Cats that are maintained on long-term medication should be monitored regularly for any drug side effects and for any emerging medical problems that might lead to drug contraindications. Progestins, benzodiazepines, tricyclic antidepressants, azapirones, and selective serotonin re-uptake inhibitors have all been used with varying degrees of success.

Recent success has been shown with either clomipramine or fluoxetine at 0.5 mg/kg per day. In a small study of 17 cats, the cats on fluoxetine showed a significant improvement over placebo-treated cats. Although there were no control groups, two studies have shown a significant improvement with clomipramine. In one study of 25 cats, 84% showed an improvement of 75% or better over a four-week period, and in a second study of 25 cats, 80% showed a reduction of 75% or better over a one-week period. In countries where a 5 mg dog tablet is available, this is a practical treatment option. Another option, because of its small tablet size, might be paroxetine (0.5 mg/kg PO q 24 hr). However, like clomipramine it is mildly anticholinergic and might lead to urine or stool retention and a mild calming effect. Amitriptyline (5–10 mg per cat PO q 24 hr) has also been reported to be effective for treating urine marking, but is extremely bitter and hard to dose. Selective serotonin re-uptake inhibitors and tricyclic antidepressants may take up to four weeks to show significant improvement. If a dose of 0.5 mg/kg is not effective and there are no untoward side effects, a gradual increase to 1 mg/kg per day might be considered. Buspirone (2.5–7.5 mg/cat PO q 12 hr) is another good choice for spraying, with a reported efficacy of 55%. Buspirone is effective within the same range as diazepam, and greater than that for the progestins. Buspirone has a wide margin of safety and does not cause the adverse effects of sedation and ataxia commonly seen with most benzodiazepines. Buspirone may take up to two weeks to demonstrate significant improvement. It is a good choice to use cautiously in cats that are old, obese, or may have medical problems. Diazepam is an effective drug in a significant number of cats at a dosage of 1–2 mg/cat PO q 12 hr. Studies have shown that after cessation of diazepam, however, 90% of cats resumed spraying while only 50% resumed spraying when buspirone was discontinued. A small number of cats will become hyperactive when given diazepam, but the hyperactivity will usually decrease within three days. Another, more serious, side effect that has recently been reported is acute, fatal hepatopathy. This problem has been documented in a very small number of cats. Pretreatment lab work was not done on most of the reported cases, and the pathophysiology of this problem is not well understood. The use of oxazepam may be a safer alternative, since there are no active intermediate metabolites, and it is therefore preferred in humans when there is hepatic compromise. Selegiline has also been utilized in urine marking and horizontal elimination related to cognitive decline, and in some European literature has been reported to be effective for emotional disorders in cats. Progestins are not as effective as the above medications, except perhaps in neutered males. Due to their side effects they should only be considered if other alternatives fail. Some of these drugs have been formulated as transdermal preparations, but at present efficacy is unknown, much higher doses may be required, and there may be variability in absorption between cats. In addition, some drugs may not be absorbed or metabolized properly in transdermal form.

A relatively recent approach to the treatment of urine spraying involves the use of the environmental application of feline facial pheromones. Work done by Dr Patrick Pageat in France has appraised the use of feline facial pheromones to curb spraying behavior. He demonstrated a significant reduction in the incidence of spraying by cats when their own facial pheromones were collected on gauze pads and applied to areas in their environment that were being sprayed. His work was the basis for the development of a spray containing synthetic analogs of naturally occurring feline facial pheromones (Feliway™, CEVA). Several studies have demonstrated the efficacy of Feliway™ in a majority of cats for reducing or eliminating reactional-type urine spraying triggered by changes in the cat's surroundings such as moving, new occupants in the home, stress, remodeling, etc. It may also help settle a cat into a new environment, reduce social tension between resident cats, and reduce scratching behavior. If either Feliway™ or medication alone has not been entirely effective at controlling spraying, then a combination of drug and pheromone therapy might be another alternative. In fact, the use of Feliway™ in conjunction with drug therapy might help to minimize the possibility of relapse when the drug is withdrawn or decreased.

Drug therapy for urine marking in cats

Drug	Dosage	Comments
Clomipramine	0.3–0.5 mg/kg q 24 hr (2.5–5 mg/cat q 24 hr)	Mild anticholinergic; 80% or more of cats improved; no placebo trial; > 50% recurrence when drug withdrawn
Amitriptyline	0.5–1 mg/kg q 24 hr (app. 2.5–5 mg/cat q 24 hr)	Anticholinergic; highly bitter; no published trials
Fluoxetine	0.5–1 mg/kg q 24 hr (2.5–5 mg/cat q 24 hr)	Significant improvement over placebo in small trial
Paroxetine	0.5–1 mg/kg q 24 hr (2.5–5 mg/cat q 24 hr)	Mild anticholinergic effects
Buspirone	2.5–7.5 mg/cat q 12 hr	Expensive; minimal side effects; twice daily dosing; 55% improved, 50% recurrence on withdrawal
Diazepam	1–2.5 mg/cat q 24/12 hr	Potential for hepatotoxicity; up to 75% improvement; up to 90% recurrence on withdrawal; may cause ataxia, sedation, appetite increase
Oxazepam	0.2–1 mg/kg q 24/12 hr	No clinical trials; may be less potential for hepatotoxicity than diazepam
Selegiline	0.5–1 mg/kg q 24 hr	May be useful in cognitive dysfunction or for more generalized emotional disorders
Megestrol acetate	5 mg/cat q 24 hr for two weeks then wean slowly to lowest effective maintenance dose	Poor efficacy (50% neutered males; 10% spayed females); potential for numerous side effects (see Ch. 5)
Medroxyprogesterone	5–20 mg/kg subcutaneous q 4 or more months	May be less effective than megestrol; injectable formulation; potential for numerous side effects (see Ch. 5)

Figure 18.7

Prognosis

Factors affecting the prognosis of resolving a urine marking problem:
- Cause of the problem
- Duration of the problem
- Frequency of marking incidents
- Number of areas soiled
- Number of different surfaces soiled
- Number of cats in the home
- Ability to control the arousing stimuli
- Temperament of the pet
- Owner commitment to modifying the behavior
- Cost of treatment
- Health of the pet
- Ability of behavioral consultant/veterinarian to diagnose, explain, and treat the problem

Figure 18.8

FELINE INAPPROPRIATE ELIMINATION

Overview

Inappropriate elimination involves squatting to defecate or urinate on horizontal surfaces outside the litterbox that are unacceptable to the owner. Housesoiling that occurs as a squatting behavior occurs with an almost equal incidence in females and males. Horizontal surfaces may be soiled in a variety of areas, or the pet may develop specific location and surface preferences. In one study of inappropriate elimination it was found that a history of previous infection, the use of a scented litter, and cats that did not cover their elimination were the only statistically significant risk factors for inappropriate elimination and that there was no association with increased anxiety.

There are many causes of inappropriate elimination. If the cat suddenly starts urinating <u>and</u> defecating outside the box, then it is highly likely that something about the litterbox is unacceptable to the cat. The physical accumulation of waste, organic odor, disinfectant odor, unacceptable litter, or a negative experience associated with the litterbox may cause the pet to avoid it. The box may be in an area the cat does not like. There may be too much traffic through the area, or the area may be associated with something aversive that happened to the cat. Perhaps it was medicated, disciplined, or frightened in the vicinity of the box. If the pet has been severely punished for any reason, it may start eliminating in secluded areas in order to avoid family members. Some cats will eliminate outside the litterbox simply because they have found another area or surface that is preferable.

If the cat consistently defecates in the box, but urinates elsewhere, or vice versa, then the problem probably isn't caused by an undesirable litterbox, substrate, or box location. Likely causes include medical problems (lower urinary tract disease, constipation, diarrhea, diabetes, renal disease, arthritis, senility), new surface preferences, or new location preferences. Be suspicious of constipation or colitis if an older pet suddenly stops defecating in the litterbox, but continues to use it for urination.

For some cats, the act of eliminating on horizontal surfaces can be a marking behavior caused by the same stimuli that cause spraying. As mentioned earlier, the most common cause is increased cat density. Emotional problems, such as a stressful relationship with a family member, separation anxiety, or fear can trigger housesoiling. If the cat is urinating on top of specific items, such as the owner's clothing, bed, or favorite chair, you will want to be sure to explore an anxiety-motivated problem. This type of problem can be difficult to diagnose, especially if the behavior is only manifested intermittently. If emotional factors are influencing the housesoiling, you may see related changes occurring, such as hiding, avoidance, aggression, or an alteration in the pet's general temperament. Keeping a diary may help the owner identify the stimuli that trigger intermittent marking behavior (Fig. 18.9).

Treatment

Treatment involves three major considerations: (1) remove the cause, (2) re-establish the habit of litterbox use, and (3) prevent the cat from returning to previously soiled areas. If the housesoiling is due to litterbox or location aversion, the box may need to be moved, medical problems must be treated, an acceptable brand of litter must be found, and the box may need to be cleaned more often. Aversive handling in the box must be stopped. Changing the depth of the

Litterbox aversion	• Aversive odor (deodorant, ammonia)
	• Box is not cleaned frequently enough
	• Discomfort during elimination (lower urinary tract disease, constipation, diarrhea, arthritis)
	• Unacceptable litter (depth, texture, odor, plastic liner)
	• Unacceptable box (too small, sides too high, covered)
	• Disciplined, medicated, or frightened in the box
Location aversion	• Too much traffic
	• Traumatic/fearful experience in the area
Location preference	• Another area is more appealing to the cat
Surface preference	• Another surface is more appealing than the litter substrate
Anxiety	• Owner absence, high cat density, moving, new furniture, inappropriate punishment, teasing, household changes, remodeling in the home
Need for privacy	• Nervous or fearful pet
Geriatric problems	• Senility, arthritis, polyuria/polydypsia, constipation

Figure 18.9 Possible causes of inappropriate elimination.

litter or removing a plastic litterbox liner may help in some cases. Switching to a sand/potting soil mix or one of the fine-textured clumping litters may also be helpful. The results of a study of feline litter material preferences suggest that important factors contributing to establishing preferences for litter material are texture, granularity, and coarseness. The cats in the study showed a definite preference for a finely textured clay litter. Any new substrate should be introduced in an additional box in case it happens to be one the pet dislikes. As a rule of thumb, you should recommend that at least one box per cat be available. The boxes should be scooped once or twice daily and emptied at least once each week. Scalding hot water should be used instead of harsh-smelling disinfectants. If disinfectants are used, the box should be thoroughly dried and out of operation for at least 24 hours.

If the cat prefers hard surfaces, try using an empty litterbox or a food tray. Gradually add litter to the container. Some cats appear to need privacy. For these cats, the owner should place an open-ended cardboard box over the litterbox or purchase a covered box. Another solution is to put a cat door in the door to a closet or storeroom. This will also protect the pet from being bothered by children or the pet dog.

To re-establish a consistent habit of using the litterbox, the cat should be temporarily confined to a small area with the box and only allowed out when it can be supervised 100% of the time. When confined to a relatively small area, most cats seem to prefer to eliminate in the box rather than soiling the floor. It is then a matter of confining the cat long enough for a consistent habit to become established. As a rule of thumb, one week of confinement is usually recommended for every month of soiling. The ratio may be decreased for soiling problems in existence for more than six months. The owner should be advised to remove the pet from the confinement area as much as possible for socialization and play, but never allow it out of sight. Food rewards may help when given immediately after the cat finishes eliminating in the box.

If the cat refuses to use the litterbox when confined to a small room, the confinement area should be changed to a large cage. A perch or shelf should be added inside the cage to provide a place for the cat to rest. The floor should be covered with litter, forcing the pet to use it for elimination. The litter should gradually be removed and replaced with a litterbox. Once the cat has used the litterbox in a confined area for an appropriate amount of time, the owner can begin to gradually allow it to have more freedom in the home.

Previously soiled areas can be safeguarded by changing the behavioral function of the area. This can be done by placing food bowls, bedding, or toys in the area. The area can also be made unacceptable for the cat by placing a motion-activated alarm or lemon-scented room deodorant in the area. Plastic carpet runners can be placed upside down with the 'feet' facing up. Plastic, foil, or double-stick carpet tape can be used to protect specific areas. You may need to experiment. Each cat is an individual in regard to surface preference for elimination, as well as what will deter it. While some cats will avoid eliminating on plastic-covered surfaces, others will be drawn to these areas to eliminate. An inch of water can be left in the bottom of a bathtub or sink to curb elimination there. Access to the soiled areas can be denied by moving furniture or closing doors. In some areas, such as the corners of the basement, it may be prudent to place a litterbox where the cat has been soiling.

Removing urine and stool odor is important. Products that are specifically formulated to work on these types of odor should be used. Products that chemically neutralize the odor and those that break down the odor using enzymatic products or bacteria/enzyme combinations should actually remove the odor rather than just masking the scent. These products need to make contact with the organic material. In most cases, an ample amount should be poured on carpeting and porous surfaces to allow penetration into deeper layers rather than just spraying the surface.

Some cats are extremely sensitive to changes in their environment. They housesoil in response to minor changes. Owners need to realize this and do their best to keep the home environment as constant as possible. When situations occur that are likely to upset the cat, the owner may want to consider confinement, closer supervision, and the use of anxiolytic medication. Desensitization and counterconditioning may help reduce undesirable responses to anxiety-evoking stimuli.

Punishment is the least effective tool for correcting housesoiling problems and may make the problem worse. Punishment is especially contraindicated if anxiety or fear is an important component of the problem. Under no circumstances should the owner carry the pet back to the soiled area to scold it, swat, or physically rub its nose in urine or stool. If the owner catches the pet in the act of eliminating in an inappropriate area, the cat may be interrupted by squirted it with a water gun, or an object can be tossed near the cat. The owner should make as little movement as possible, avoid eye contact, and say nothing when interrupting the pet. It is very important that the cat does not associate the interruption with the owner or the bond between the pet and the owner may quickly deteriorate. Care must be taken so that the type or intensity of the interruptive stimulus elicits no fear (Fig. 18.10).

Prognosis

The chances of success depend on a number of factors including whether the pet was ever trained to use a litterbox; the duration of the problem; the pet's environment; the number of areas soiled; the number of different surfaces soiled; the ability to control the arousing stimuli; the temperament of the pet; and the patience, ability, and willingness of the family to commit to working with the pet. For a cat with physiological reasons for housesoiling, the prognosis may depend a great deal upon the medical diagnosis and the likelihood for curing or managing the medical disorder (Fig. 18.11).

SUMMARY

The steps in correcting a feline housesoiling problem include:

- Identify the soiling cat(s).
- Rule out medical problems.
- Remove the cause for housesoiling.
- Modify the pet's response to arousing stimuli.
- Re-establish the habit of litterbox use with confinement, supervision, and rewards.
- Prevent resoiling by using booby traps, remote punishment, or changing the function of the areas.

Figure 18.12 is a form (form #8 on the CD) that can be used as a treatment guide for housesoiling cases.

CASE EXAMPLES
Case 1

History

Morticia, a six-year-old spayed female cat, suddenly began to urinate in inappropriate locations. Although she continued to use her litterbox occasionally, she had also eliminated on a pile of clean laundry, on the owner's bedspread, and in the bathroom sink on three or four occasions. She was taken to her veterinarian who performed urinalysis and found marked hematuria, pyuria, and struvite crystalluria. She was placed on a canned prescription diet for struvite crystalluria and an antibiotic. Four weeks later the owner reported a marked improvement, but there were still occasional 'accidents,' usually in the sink or on the floor just outside the litterbox. A repeat urinalysis at the time revealed a moderate number of red blood cells, but no crystals and an acid pH. Three months after the initial onset of the problem, the cat was referred to a behavior clinic because the inappropriate elimination continued intermittently.

Diagnosis and management

It was the owner's impression that the cat occasionally vocalized during urination and that

Goal	Approach
Condition the desired behavior	• Food rewards and play may help reinforce the desirability of litterbox usage. • Cats can be followed into the litter area and rewarded for successful use
Remove the cause	• All medical problems contributing to the problem must be addressed • If the problem is due to litterbox aversion, the box may need to be moved, cleaned more often, or the litter brand changed. Harsh-smelling chemicals and detergents should be avoided in the litterbox. Avoid scented litter which might deter some cats • Identify potential deterrents in the litterbox area (noisy central heating boiler, laundry equipment, temperature extremes)
Remove access to soiled sites	• Move furniture over the soiled areas • Close doors to frequently soiled rooms • Re-establish normal litter use • Confine the cat to a small area and only allow it out when it can be supervised 100% of the time • Confinement should continue for a long enough time for a reliable habit to become re-established. This period should be from one to eight weeks depending on the duration of the problem. The pet should gradually be allowed to have more freedom and less supervision
Decrease desirability of inappropriate sites	• Change the surface at previously soiled areas by removing carpet, placing a sheet of plastic, aluminum foil, upside-down plastic carpet runner (nubs up), or double-sided tape in the area • Place food bowls, bedding, toys, or a play center in the area • Use environmental devices (upside-down mousetraps, motion alarms) that are aversive. A lemon-scented room deodorizer will deter some cats
Remove the odor	• Use chemical or enzymatic/bacterial odor eliminators. Be certain to use a sufficient amount of the product to saturate the entire area
Increase desirability of the litterbox	• Determine favorite litter by providing a few additional boxes with different substrates (clay, soil, sandy clumping, sand/potting soil) • Determine favorite box by providing a few different boxes (covered, lower sides, open, larger) • Determine favorite location by locating boxes in a number of locations • It may also be helpful to increase the total number of litterboxes, and clean them more frequently
Behavioral modification	• Desensitization and counterconditioning may help reduce undesirable responses to anxiety-producing stimuli • Litterbox use can be shaped by placing it at the soiled area and gradually moving to a more appropriate location
Punishment	• Punishment should be avoided. The cat should never be physically punished or have its nose rubbed in a mess • If the owner catches the pet in the act of eliminating in an inappropriate area, it can be interrupted with a hand clap or squirt from a water sprayer. The owner should remain quiet and non-threatening during the maneuver
Drug therapy	• Cats that eliminate on horizontal surfaces are unlikely to respond to psychotropic medication unless an underlying anxiety or territorial etiology exists

Figure 18.10   Treatment of feline inappropriate elimination.

there was an increased frequency. A subsequent urinalysis revealed the presence of moderate hematuria, proteinuria with no bacteriuria. Both scout and double-contrast radiographs were unremarkable. At this point the owner declined referral for cystoscopy or exploratory surgery. No environmental or stressful changes could be identified. Because the cat continued to use its litter for all defecation and most urination, it was unlikely that there was a litterbox aversion. However, to rule out the possibility, behavioral therapy was initiated. In an attempt to increase the appeal of the litter, the owner tried a variety of additional litterboxes and litter types, without improvement. The owner confined the cat to the washroom with its litterbox

Factors affecting the prognosis of resolving inappropriate elimination:
- Cause of the problem
- Litterbox experience
- Substrate experience
- Duration of the problem
- Frequency of housesoiling incidents
- Number of areas soiled
- Number of different surfaces soiled
- Number of cats in the home
- Temperament of the pet
- Owner commitment to modifying behavior
- Health of the pet
- Ability of behavioral consultant/veterinarian to diagnose, explain, and treat the problem

Figure 18.11

when it could not be supervised, but the cat continued to use the sink or the floor in front of the litterbox a few times each week. Confinement in a large cage was successful but when the cat was released from the cage after three weeks, the problem recurred every few days. Over a period of another three months a number of urinalyses were performed (free flow into a non-absorbable litter) and mild to moderate hematuria was seen on most but not all of the urinalyses. Based on the clinical history, lack of response to behavioral therapy, and the recurrent hematuria, feline idiopathic (interstitial) cystitis was considered to be a likely diagnosis. The cat was subsequently placed on 5 mg of amitriptyline daily and after four weeks there had been a marked decrease in the problem with only two recurrences.

Amitriptyline has been reported to correct some behavioral causes of inappropriate urination and may help to control feline interstitial cystitis. Over the next year the owner reported that there was infrequent inappropriate elimination (approximately once or twice a month), but when amitriptyline was discontinued for about a month, there were multiple weekly recurrences.

Case 2

History

Jasmine, a three-month-old female kitten that had been obtained at two months of age, was using the owner's benjamina plant for elimination. The kitten slept in the bedroom at night on the third floor and the litterbox was located on the first floor in the laundry room. The kitten had used its litterbox for the first few weeks but would no longer use it. The owner had tried a number of litter types and litterboxes with no apparent improvement.

Diagnosis

Physical examination revealed a healthy and very alert kitten. Urinalysis and fecal evaluation failed to suggest any organic cause for the elimination problem. The kitten had apparently developed a preference for using the soil in the benjamina plant and had perhaps developed an aversion for the area where the litterbox was kept. Since the kitten exhibited fear of loud noises, it was suspected that the sounds of the washer and dryer could have caused it to avoid the laundry room.

Treatment

The owner was advised to prevent the kitten from eliminating in the benjamina plant by covering the surface of the soil with chips of marble. The pet was confined to a small bedroom with its litterbox when it could not be closely supervised. This was carried on for two weeks to reestablish desirable litter habits. At that time, the litterbox was relocated to a quiet room away from the laundry facilities. The kitten used the litter consistently and there were no further problems.

FELINE HOUSESOILING THERAPY WORKSHEET   Consultation location: Housecall/Office/Phone

Owner: _____   Pet: _____   Date: _____

Medical:
_____ Consult family veterinarian about _____
_____ Lab tests _____
_____ Medication _____
_____ Feliway™ _____

General:
_____ Reduce anxiety/conflict stress _____
_____ Avoid punishment (No hitting, rubbing nose, yelling) _____ Increase playtime _____ Black light
_____ Remove odor _____ Reward elimination in box _____ Keep a diary
_____ Interrupt with a water gun, citronella spray, noise _____

Supervision/Confinement:
_____ Length of time: _____ weeks Area of house: _____ Cage _____
_____ Close off frequently soiled rooms for _____ weeks/months/forever
_____ Place a bell on the cat to aid supervision _____ Place a harness on the cat to aid supervision
_____ Prevent access to soiled areas or objects (e.g., keep clothing off floors/doors closed/shoes in closets)
_____ Prevent access to stimuli that trigger housesoiling _____

Safeguard previously soiled areas:
Change the function of areas:
_____ Food bowls _____ Bedding _____ Play area (leave toys) ____ Scratching post
Alter desirability of areas:
_____ Double-stick tape _____ Irish Spring soap bar _____ Citrus product _____ Potpourri
_____ Snappy Trainer™ _____ Upside-down mousetraps ____ Balloons set to pop ____ Home-made booby traps
_____ Motion-activated alarm ____ Scat Mat™____ Motion-activated spray
_____ Cat repellents ____ Moth balls ____ Mothball-impregnated blocks
_____ Move furniture ____ Take up rugs
_____ Cover furniture or floors with: ____ upside-down vinyl carpet runner ____ plastic ____ foil ____ other ____
_____ Fill bathtub ____ sink ____ other _____ with water
_____ Other: _____

Litterbox:
_____ Clean frequently _____ Self-cleaning litterbox
_____ Don't change brand of litter
_____ AVOID: _____ Scented litter _____ Deodorants _____ Litter liners _____ Covered box
_____ Increase number to _____ boxes _____ Change placement – offer additional locations: _____
_____ Use empty litterbox or food tray _____ Use litter on only one side of litterbox
_____ Offer different type of litter: ____ clumping ____ sand ____ dirt ____ paper ____ sawdust ____ cedar
_____ carpet ____ clay ____ peat moss ____ crushed leaves ____ plastic pearls
_____ Offer different boxes: ____ covered ____ uncovered ____ low sides ____ higher sides ____ larger

(*continued*)

Figure 18.12 Feline housesoiling therapy worksheet (form #8 – printable from the CD).

Miscellaneous:
_____ Discourage animals from visiting ___ yard ___ house ___ other _____
_____ Booby traps outside ___ windows ___ doors ___ fence ___ deck ___ other _____
_____ Take up ___ food ___ water ____ hours prior to bedtime
_____ When stressful situations are anticipated ___ confine ___ supervise ___ medicate ___ increase playtime

Assessment: Initiating factors:

                    Maintaining factors:

Diagnosis/Prognosis:

Figure 18.12   (*continued*)

Case 3

History

Mephistopheles, a three-year-old neutered male cat, was presented to a veterinary behavior clinic for urine marking of two months duration. Household diagrams were submitted with the history and it was determined that all urine sites were found in front of doors or windows on the first floor. The problem had begun in the early spring, and the owner was aware of the sight and smell of new cats on the property outdoors.

Diagnosis

Although the cat had been urinating primarily on horizontal surfaces, urine marking due to outdoor stimuli was tentatively suspected as the likely cause of the problem. The medical workup, including physical examination and urinalysis, was unremarkable. Although the cat resented abdominal palpation, there was no evidence of distended bladder or pain in the area. The history and lack of any physical reason for the problem supported the tentative diagnosis.

Treatment

The owner confined the cat in the master bedroom where it slept most nights and had never previously eliminated. The litterbox was relocated to the adjacent washroom and double-sided tape was placed on the windowsills to keep the cat from sitting there and watching outdoor cats. The cat used the litterbox for all elimination when confined to the bedroom. When the owner was home, the cat was allowed out of the bedroom and was supervised at all times by the owner. All soiled locations had been treated with a commercial odor eliminator. While supervised, the cat did not attempt to eliminate in the previous spots. After two weeks, the owner began to reduce supervision and a new spot was found in front of a sliding door. The owner cleaned the spot and placed vertical blinds on the door to reduce the cat's view of outdoor cats. This successfully stopped further elimination at the location but the cat continued to urinate by the rear doorway. Cat repellents and a motion detector were placed on the back porch to keep outdoor cats away and food bowls were placed at the indoor sites of housesoiling. For two months the owners continued to confine the cat when they were not at home and release it when they were. At a six-month follow-up there had been no further incidents of inappropriate elimination.

FURTHER READING

Bateson P, Turner DC 1988 Questions about cats. In: Turner DC, Bateson P (eds) The domestic cat: the biology of its behavior. Cambridge University Press, Cambridge, p 193–201

Beaver BV 1989 Housesoiling by cats: a retrospective study of 120 cases. Journal of the American Animal Hospital Association 25(6):631–637

Beaver BV 1992 Feline behavior: a guide for veterinarians. WB Saunders, Philadelphia

Beaver BV 1994 Differential approach to house soiling by dogs and cats. Veterinary Quarterly 16(Suppl 1):S47

Borchelt PL 1991 Cat elimination behavior problems. Veterinary Clinics of North America, Small Animal Practice 21:254–265

Borchelt PL, Voith VL 1981 Elimination behavior problems in cats. Compendium of Continuing Education for Practicing Veterinarians 3(8):730–738

Borchelt P, Voith VL 1982 Diagnosis and treatment of elimination behavior problems in cats. Veterinary Clinics of North America, Small Animal Practice 12(4):673–680

Borchelt PL, Voith VL 1996 Elimination behavior problems in cats. In: Voith VL, Borchelt PL (eds) Readings in companion animal behavior. Veterinary Learning Systems, Trenton, NJ, p 179–190

Buffington CAT, Chew DJ 1995 Idiopathic lower urinary tract disease in cats – is it interstitial cystitis? In: Proceedings of the 13th ACVIM forum, p 517–519

Center SA, Elston TH, Rowland PH et al 1995 Hepatotoxicity associated with oral diazepam in 12 cats. In: Proceedings of the 13th ACVIM forum, p 1009

Cooper LL 1997 Feline inappropriate elimination. In: Houpt KA (ed) Progress in companion animal behavior. Veterinary Clinics of North America, Small Animal Practice 27(3):569–600

Cooper LL, Hart BL 1992a Comparison of diazepam with progestin for effectiveness in suppression of urine spraying behavior in cats. Journal of the American Veterinary Medical Association 203:254–258

Cooper LL, Hart BL 1992b Comparison of diazepam with progestin for effectiveness in suppression of urine spraying behavior in cats. Journal of the American Veterinary Medical Association 200:797–801

Crowell-Davis S 1986 Elimination behaviour problem of cats, I. Veterinary Forum November:10

De Boer JN 1977 The age of olfactory cues functioning in chemo-communication among male domestic cats. Behavioral Processes 2:209–225

Dehasse J 1996 Retrospective study on the use of Selgian[R] in cats. In: Askew HR (ed) Treatment of behavior problems in dogs and cats. Blackwell Science, Cambridge, MA

Dehasse J 1997 Feline urine spraying. Applied Animal Behavioral Science 52:365–371

Ewer RF 1973 The carnivores. Cornell University Press, Ithaca, NY

Halip JW, Vaillancourt JP, Luescher UA 1998 A descriptive study of 189 cats engaging in inappropriate elimination behaviors. Feline Practice 26(4):18–21

Hart BL 1980 Objectionable urine spraying and urine marking in cats: evaluation of progestin treatment in gonadectonized males and females. Journal of the American Veterinary Medical Association 177:529–533

Hart BL 1981a Olfactory tractotomy to control objectionable urine spraying and urine marking in cats. Journal of the American Veterinary Medical Association 179:231

Hart BL 1981b Olfactory tractotomy to control objectionable urine spraying and urine marking in cats. Journal of the American Veterinary Medical Association 179:231–234

Hart BL 1985 Urine spraying and marking in cats. In: Slatter SH (ed) Textbook of small animal surgery. WB Saunders, Philadelphia, PA

Hart BL, Barrett RE 1973 Effects of castration on fighting, roaming, and urine spraying in adult male cats. Journal of the American Veterinary Medical Association 163:290–292

Hart BL, Cooper L 1984 Factors related to urine spraying and fighting in prepubertally gonadectomized cats. Journal of the American Veterinary Medical Association 184:1255–1258

Hart B, Hart L 1985 Canine and feline behavioral therapy. Lee & Febiger

Hart BL, Leedy M 1982 Identification of source of urine stains in multi-cat households. Journal of the American Veterinary Medical Association 180:77

Hart BL, Eckstein RA, Powell KL et al 1993 Effectiveness of buspirone on urine spraying and inappropriate urination in cats. Journal of the American Veterinary Medical Association 203(2):254–258

Hendriks WH, Moughan PJ, Tarttelin MF et al 1995 Felinine: a urinary amino acid of Felidae. Compendium of Biochemical Physiology 112B(4):581–588

Horwitz D 1997 Behavioral and environmental factors associated with elimination behavior problems in cats: a retrospective survey. Applied Animal Behavioral Science 52:129–137

Hunthausen W 1993 Dealing with feline housesoiling: a practitioner's guide. Veterinary Medicine August:726–735

Hunthausen W 1994 Collecting the history of a pet with a behavior problem. Veterinary Medicine 89(10):954–959

Hunthausen W 2000 Evaluating a feline facial pheromone analogue to control urine spraying. Veterinary Medicine February:151–155

Komtebedde J, Haupman J Bilateral ischiocavernosus myectomy for chronic urine spraying in castrated cats.

Korefsky PS 1987 Letter to the editor: 'Identifying source of urine on rugs.' Journal of the American Veterinary Medical Association 191(8):917

Kroll T, Houpt KA 1995 A comparison of cyproheptadine and clomipramine for the treatment of urine spraying in cats. In: Overall KL, Mills DS, Heath SE et al (eds) Proceedings of the third international congress on veterinary behavioral medicine. Universities Federation for Animal Welfare, Herts, UK, p 184–185

Landsberg GM 2001 A study to assess the effects of clomipramine therapy on urine spraying in cats. In: Overall KL, Mills DS, Heath SE et al (eds) Proceedings of the third international congress on veterinary behavioral medicine. Universities Federation for Animal Welfare, Herts, UK, p 186–189

Leyhausen P 1979 Cat behaviour: the predatory and social behavior of domestic and wild cats. Garland STPM Press, London

Marder A 1989 Feline housesoiling. Pet Veterinarian September/October:11–15

Marder AR 1991 Psychotropic drugs and behavioral therapy. Veterinary Clinics of North America 21(2):329

Mathews SL 1984 A different approach to the litterbox problem. Feline Practice 14(3):7–11

Melese-d'Hospital P 1996 Eliminating urine odors in the home. In: Voith VL, Borchelt PL (eds) Readings in companion animal behavior. Veterinary Learning Systems, Trenton, NJ, p 191–197

Natoli E 1985 Behavioural responses of urban feral cats to different types of urine mark. Behaviour 94:234–243

O'Brien D 1988 Neurogenic disorders of micturition. Veterinary Clinics of North America, Small Animal Practice 18(3):535

Oliver JE, Lorenz MD 1993 Handbook of veterinary neurology. WB Saunders, Philadelphia, p 74–75

Olm DD, Houpt KA 1988 Feline house-soiling problems. Applied Animal Behavioral Science 20:335–345

Overall K 1993 Diagnosing and treating undesirable feline elimination behaviour. Feline Practice 21(2):11–13

Overall KE 1997 Clinical behavioral medicine for small animals. Mosby, St Louis

Pageat P 1996 Functions and use of the facial pheromones in the treatment of urine marking in the cat. Interest of structural analogue. In: Proceedings of the 21st congress of the World Small Animal Veterinary Association, Jerusalem, p 197–198

Pryor PA, Hart BL, Cliff KD et al 2001a Effects of a selective serotonin reuptake inhibitor on urine spraying behavior in cats. Journal of the American Veterinary Medical Association 219(11):1557–1561

Pryor PA, Hart BL, Cliff KD et al 2001b Causes of urine marking in cats and effects of environmental management on frequency of marking. Journal of the American Veterinary Medical Association 219(12):1700–1713

Skeritt GC, Jemmett JE 1980 The spraying problem. Results and analysis of the Glaxovet/FAB survey. Bulletin of the Feline Advisory Bureau 18(2):3–4

Verberne G, de Boer 1976 Chemocommunication among domestic cats, mediated by the olfactory and vomeronasal senses, I. Communication. Zeitschrift fuer Tierpsychologie 42:86–109

Voith VL 1991 Treating elimination behaviour problems in dogs and cats: the role of punishment. Modern Veterinary Practice December:951–953

White JC, Mills DS 1997 Efficacy of synthetic feline facial pheromone (F3) analogue (Feliway) for the treatment of chronic non-sexual urine spraying by the domestic cat. In: Mills DS, Heath SE, Harrington LJ (eds) Proceedings of the first international conference on veterinary behavioral medicine. Universities Federation for Animal Welfare, Herts, UK, p 242

Wright JC 1988 Do cats with elimination problems need privacy and escape potential? Animal Behaviour Consultant Newsletter 5(2):2–3.

as well as a public danger. Pet owners with aggressive dogs are thus urgently in need of help in assessing the extent of danger present in their situations, and legitimate advice on how to correct the aggression. However, until they receive appropriate counseling and understand the risks, they should be cautioned to provide safe management of the pets and to avoid situations that are likely to trigger aggressive encounters (Fig. 19.1).

In general, aggression refers to threatening or harmful behavior directed toward another individual or group. Aggression encompasses a wide variety of behaviors, from subtle body postures and facial expressions to explosive attacks. It is not unusual for dogs to be presented that are exhibiting more than one type of aggression. Although there is some controversy concerning the classification of types of aggressive behavior, this chapter will examine several different types of aggression, defined according to function. A functional classification approach takes into account the circumstances in which the aggression occurs as well as the organization of behavior patterns involved. This allows for inferences concerning the motivation for the behavior as well as aiding in uncovering the factors leading to the behavior, thus facilitating the development of a prognosis and solid treatment plan (Fig. 19.2).

The best way to ensure an accurate diagnosis is to combine a physical examination and appropriate diagnostic tests with a complete behavioral history, and view the dog during a typical aggressive display either directly or by video observation. Since direct observation or video taping are not always practical or safe, the behavioral consultant may need to rely

• Dominance-related
• Conflict-related
• Possessive/food-related
• Fear-related
• Territorial/protective
• Pathophysiological
• Predatory
• Pain/medical/irritable
• Play
• Maternal/hormonal
• Redirected
• Idiopathic
• Learned
• Redirected
• Intraspecific (interdog)

Figure 19.2 Types of aggression.

entirely on the behavioral history to make the diagnosis. There are a number of criteria that are used for differentiating one type of aggression from another, including the aggressor's traits and behavior, characteristics of the target, and the conditions during which the aggression occurs (Fig. 19.3).

In formulating a treatment plan, consideration must be given to the type of aggression, the pet's temperament, and the mental and physical competence of individuals in the pet's environment. It is important to note that a pet may have a single type of aggression or there may be a number of forms of aggression in the same pet. In addition, each aggressive display may have components of more than one type of aggression, such as dominance and defensive, territorial and fear, or chase predation and defensive. There may also be learned and conditioned components in each display. Many types of aggres-

Owner concerns about an aggressive pet that need to be addressed:
• Why does my pet bite?
• Can anything be done to change the behavior?
• Will it bite again?
• Should I euthanize the pet?
• How can I avoid this with future pets?

Figure 19.1

Criteria used for diagnosing aggression:
• Type of vocalizations
• Postures and behaviors
• Context or situation in which the aggression occurs
• Stimulus or trigger for aggression
• Target of the aggression
• Temperament of the pet
• Signalment
• Health of the pet
• Location where the aggressive behavior is likely to occur

Figure 19.3

sion can be corrected using controlled exposure to the stimulus during desensitization and counterconditioning sessions. During exposure, the dog must be under complete owner control so that it cannot escape or cause injury. Oftentimes owners yell, scream, shock, choke, prong, or hit their aggressive dogs, yet they should be instructed that these techniques are not only ineffective but counterproductive. Punishing the aggressive dog increases its fear and anxiety, increases the general level of arousal, and increases the risks for family members. Dogs that are consistently punished during the warning phase of the aggressive behavioral sequence may learn to bite without warning (Fig. 19.4).

Exposure techniques are used to reduce the pet's response to stimuli that elicit fear or aggression. Counterconditioning exercises condition a calm, positive emotional state when exposed to the stimulus, and differential reinforcement exercises are intended to train the pet to display an alternative, acceptable behavior when exposed to the stimulus. The owner and counselor must determine all stimuli that cause aggression and formulate an appropriate treatment plan, complete with training sessions (Fig. 19.5).

Although the many individual forms of canine aggression are described below, aggression is often multifactorial or of multiple causes. For example, in cases of possessive or territorial aggression, fear may be a contributing factor. An underlying medical problem may lead to increased irritability, which might further aggravate an existing dominance-related aggression problem. Learning can also be an important component of many aggressive behavior problems. Owners may mistakenly reward their

I.	Educate the family
II.	Environmental intervention
	• Manage the pet and its environment
	• Remove or modify stimuli that trigger aggression
	• Remove targets
III.	Modify the pet
	• Behavior modification
	• Surgery
	• Drugs
	• Euthanasia

Figure 19.5 Treatment of aggression.

aggressive dogs, albeit unintentionally. They do this by patting and reassuring the dog when it is acting aggressive, even offering food rewards in order to try to calm it down and lessen the aggression. The situation can be further complicated when the dog learns that it can get its way by being aggressive. Growling and snapping may very well become an effective way for the dog to avoid an unwanted stimulus or situation (e.g., brushing teeth, trimming nails).

The manifestation of aggressive behavior may be appreciably influenced by the environment, situation, or people present. For example, a pet exhibiting territorial aggression at home may be friendly with strangers when at the park. Fear may be exhibited at the veterinary hospital, but not at a hardware store. A dog may show dominance-related aggression toward one family member, but not others. The health of the pet can also influence the display of aggressive behavior. Pain can lower the threshold for aggression. A pet that is normally friendly may bite when someone reaches to pat its head when it is suffering from a painful otitis condition. Diagnosing and treating aggressive behavior problems therefore requires an understanding of all the factors contributing to the problems.

The role of arousal in aggression

Dogs that are highly aroused are at higher risk for aggression, since their emotional state can interfere with the ability to respond 'consciously' or 'rationally' to stimuli. When

Use of pain to treat aggression can:
- Escalate aggression
- Lower the threshold for aggression
- Cause redirected aggression
- Destroy the bond between the owner and the pet
- Lead to fear aggression
- Cause conflict
- Result in injuries

Figure 19.4

exposed to a novel or startling stimulus, the dog that is highly aroused (whether excited or fearful) may respond impulsively, reflexively, and defensively. On the other hand, the dog that is calm and under owner control can assess and process stimuli so that they make a conscious and predictable response to the stimulus. Of course, this may still be a defensive reaction if the stimulus is fear evoking. Thus, the correction techniques for many forms of aggression require calming and controlling the dog before it can begin to be exposed to stimuli for retraining. See handout #23 on the CD (Fig. 5.13) for settle and calming exercises. Drugs may also be used to help some dogs be calmer and more focused for the retraining program.

ASSESSING THE RISK OF INJURY OF AGGRESSIVE DOGS

One of the most crucial aspects of working up a case of canine aggression is assessing the risk of injury that the dog poses to those in its environment. In order to accomplish this, a very complete history must be taken from all family members and others involved with the pet. Sometimes, it is not possible to get all of the pertinent details. No adults may have been present to see what triggered the bite of a very young child. Owners may know how the pet interacts with young children and adults, but since the pet has never been around teenagers, the danger the pet might pose to them is unknown. When little is known about the pet's social behavior around different types of people in a wide variety of situations, questions exist about its potential to act aggressively in specific circumstances. Therefore, conservative, safe management will be required. The consultant must evaluate predictability, potential to cause damage, characteristics of the family, and complexity of the whole situation in order to determine risk. Before consulting on cases of aggression, it might be prudent to consider having a release form signed, although this may not be sufficient to protect against liability depending on the case, your level of expertise, and the jurisdiction in which you preside. Therefore it

might be advisable to check with your lawyer to determine the type of release that might be most suited to your practice. A printable release form can be found in Appendix C, Fig. 12, form #1 on the CD.

In order to determine predictability, you first must determine the situations or stimuli that trigger aggression. If these are completely unknown, then it must be assumed that the pet could be aggressive at any time and the pet will need to be muzzled at all times or locked in a safe confinement area. Once triggers for aggression have been ascertained, it must be determined if the pet's responses to the triggers are consistent. For example, if you have identified that touching the pet's head causes it to bite, but not all of the time, danger increases because people tend to let down their guard when the pet is not consistently aggressive. The type of stimulus that causes the pet to be aggressive is also important. Most people realize that a strong stimulus, such as kicking a dog, will likely cause aggression and will avoid doing this. On the other hand, many would not expect a dog to bite if they calmly bent down, eye-to-eye to a dog, and patted it on the head. So, danger increases when 'benign' stimuli trigger aggression. The absence of warning signals also increases the risk of injury. A person is unable to avoid a dog that is being stimulated to aggressive behavior when there are no signs. Another issue is the latency from presentation of the stimulus to attack. It doesn't help the victim if the pet gives a warning, but attacks a millisecond after the warning begins.

The physical aspects of the dog are certainly important in assessing the potential for damage. It is obvious that large, young, strong dogs can cause the most damage, but the degree of bite inhibition the animal exhibits is also important. If a large pet has bitten a variety of people in a variety of situations many times and has caused nothing more than light contusions, it is probably a safer pet than a small one that has caused severe injuries, such as deep tears or broken bones. The intensity of focus and level of arousal of the dog during aggressive situations is important. If it is weak, then the pet can be more easily distracted and controlled. When the focus is exceptionally strong, interrupting a developing aggressive situation will be less successful and an injury will be more likely. The target of the aggression is another consideration. Young children and babies are more easily injured with less effort than are adults. The type of aggression being displayed can determine the amount of damage done. Predatory aggression is the most dangerous type, since the intent is to kill and ingest. Also, territorial aggression is usually more dangerous than fear aggression because a territorial dog will go after the target, while a fear aggressive dog may avoid interaction if off its own property.

Characteristics of the family can be very important variables influencing the danger of the situation. Some owners are in denial about their pet's behavior. In other cases, the owners may not have the cognitive ability to grasp the danger that is present, safely manage the pet, or understand treatment protocols. The amount of activity and complexity of schedules in some households makes safe control and management of the pet difficult. Homes with many family members or young children often have difficulty providing safe supervision or confinement of the pet. Doors are left open, locks on gates are forgotten, supervisory duties are not consistent, and families with many children often have visiting children in and out without adults knowing. Homes with young children or cognitively impaired adults have family members who are more likely to put themselves at risk without realizing it. And, importantly, the experience of the family with dogs in general is important. The more experience family members have living with dogs, the more they know about what to expect from them and how to appropriately interact with them. They are also more likely to be aware of danger signals and dangerous situations.

Finally, the complexity of the behavioral situation has an effect on the danger that is present. If there are many types of aggression being displayed by the pet, and if there are a wide variety of stimuli that will trigger aggressive behavior, the danger increases. The presence of other concurrent behavior problems also increases the risk that aggression might occur. For example, if the owner of a pet with a fear-related aggression problem is upset about destructive behavior or housesoiling, the person might be likely to react impulsively in a way that will elicit an aggressive response from the pet. The main concern regarding the factors just mentioned is that they tend to increase the likelihood of confrontations with the pet.

Factors relating to the risk of injury the pet poses, and whether the owners can control the opportunity for interaction with target people or animals, will determine if the pet should stay in the home, be rehomed, or euthanized. A large, strong dog that bites children unpredictably without inhibition in a busy home with many small children, and poor supervision by adults who cannot comprehend the danger of dog aggression, will pose an extremely high risk for a serious injury (Fig. 19.6).

In one recent study by Guy, Luescher and Dohoo, of biting dogs in a general veterinary caseload in three eastern Canadian provinces, 15.6% of 3226 dogs were reported to have biting behavior. Risk factors for biting in this study included small female dogs, the presence of teenage children, a history of skin disease, aggression over food in the first two months of ownership, sleeping on an owner's bed in the first two months of ownership, and a high ranking for excitability during the first two months of ownership. Biting dogs were more likely to be fearful of children, men, and strangers. While these results might vary between geographical regions, they tend to indicate that there are signs such as possessiveness and excitability that arise in the first two months of ownership that might be predictive of aggression, and that fear and a high level of reactivity appear to be significant risk factors. On the other hand, this study looked at a population of dogs that had been retained by their owners despite aggression, and does not therefore include those dogs that might have been sufficiently aggressive to be removed from the home.

CONSIDERATIONS FOR ASSESSING DANGER AND RISK OF INJURY

Factors	Essential points
Predictability	• Identifiable stimuli and situations • Consistent response to aggression-eliciting stimuli • 'Benignness' of stimuli that trigger aggression • Existence of warning signals • Latency to attack • Availability of pertinent historical info
Potential to cause damage	• Size and strength of animal • Degree of bite inhibition • Intensity of focus/level of arousal • Target for aggression • Type of aggression

The human element	• Comprehension of danger
	• Ability to understand management and treatment
	• Ability to provide safe control
	• Verbal control of pet
	• Dependability
	  – History of compliance and consistency
	  – Family size, lifestyle
	  – Ages of family members
	• Experience with animals

Complexity of the situation	• Number of types of aggression • Number of situations/stimuli that trigger aggression • Number of concurrent behavior problems • Opportunity for confrontations

Figure 19.6 Assessing danger and risk of injury.

CANINE DOMINANCE-RELATED AGGRESSION

Dogs have evolved from wolves and exhibit social behavior and organization similar to that of wolves. Wolf social structure involves a leader animal at the top of the hierarchy and subordinates with lower status. The existence of a hierarchy provides certain advantages for a social group. By using dominant and submissive signaling and expressions to communicate social status, the group can reduce serious aggressive encounters among members. Social communication also facilitates cooperative behaviors such as care of the young and hunting.

The determinants of dominance within the hierarchy include size, weight, sex, hormonal status, and previous experience. The status of members is maintained through an interplay of dominant and submissive behaviors and signals (Figs 19.7, 19.8). Dominant postures include direct eye contact (dominant stare), ears erect and rotated forward, vertical retraction of the lips, head and body held high, tail held above the horizontal, piloerection, and a tense rigid posture. Dominant behaviors include head or paws placed over the subordinate, grasping the muzzle or neck, pushing, bowling over, and mounting. These may also be accompanied by a threatening growl. Communication is a two-way street, and a proper submissive response by a subordinate is important to the maintenance of social relationships. Submissive signs include avoidance of eye contact, ears rotated back, lowered body posture, and tail held low. The use of this type of appeasement communication helps avoid more serious, dangerous confrontations.

Most concepts concerning canine hierarchies and dominant–submissive relationships are based on studies of the social interactions of wolves. Although it is tempting to make direct comparisons and extrapolations, the domestication of the dog for thousands of years may make absolute comparisons somewhat inaccurate and not totally reliable. Hierarchies do appear to

CANINE SOCIAL SIGNALS

Dominant postures and behavior:
- Maintained eye contact
- Ears rotated forward
- Vertical retraction of lips
- Head held high
- Increased height
- Tail above horizontal
- Tense, rigid posture
- Piloerection
- Standing over
- Head or paws over neck or body of subordinate
- Body slamming
- Grabbing the muzzle or neck of the subordinate
- Pushing, bowling over
- Mounting

Submissive postures and behavior:
- Avoidance of eye contact
- Horizontally retracted lips
- Lowered head and tail
- Ears rotated back
- Crouched body position
- Lateral recumbency
- Submissive urination

Figure 19.7   Dominant and submissive expressions and signals in dogs.

exist among domestic dogs and perhaps to some extent with family members with whom they live. An understanding of why they occur and how they are maintained is important when assessing aggression.

The condition in which a member of the social group consistently controls resources or the behavior of others in the group is referred to as dominance. The most dominant animal, the one at the top of the hierarchy, is the one that exercises the most influence or control over other members, social situations, and desired resources. Dominance-related aggression may be exhibited when an individual dog perceives that it is being challenged or is losing control of a resource or situation to a subordinate (other dog or human). A number of factors determine whether aggression is exhibited. These include the dog's temperament, the relative dominance of the individuals (i.e., near-equal individuals may have more conflicts), the effects of age (behavioral development through maturity) and health (including the effects of aging) on each pack member, the type of threat displayed, the motivation of the dog to protect or maintain a particular resource, and the behavior of members with which it interacts. Dogs that exhibit dominant displays toward a particular person may become aggressive if the person approaches when the dog is resting or eating, or in response to dominant social signals or handling (maintaining eye contact, owner-initiated petting, trying to move or lift the dog). The dog may initially signal its dominance with postures, facial expressions, and vocalization (see Figs 19.8, 19.9). If the person does not retreat or defer, or responds with threats or anxiety, the aggression may escalate to lunging, biting and attacking. The dog thus learns that aggression is successful at maintaining its status or holding onto a resource, and may also become increasingly defensive and anxious depending on the owner's response. If

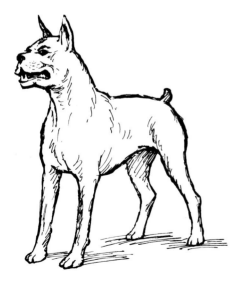

Figure 19.8   A dominant dog may stand with its ears forward and its hackles raised.

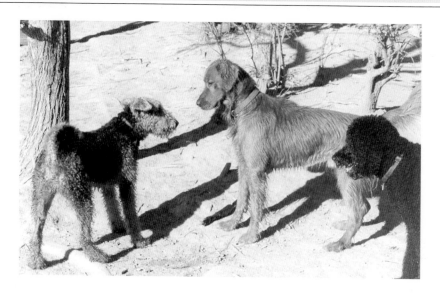

Figure 19.9   An assertive Golden Retriever postures toward an Airedale. The body posturing and positioning of the Golden Retriever in relationship to the Airedale indicates a position of dominance. Contributed by Wayne Hunthausen.

the owner then continues to defer to the dog when it desires food, affection, or play, this will further perpetuate the problem. Since these dogs can be either friendly or aggressive in somewhat similar situations, they may be unpredictable to the owners and at high risk for causing injury. The dog's dominant status with respect to family members is not predictive of whether it might be friendly or aggressive to people outside of the dog's social group (i.e., strangers).

Dominance-related aggression is most common in males and purebreds. Most cases emerge at between one and three years of age. In North American studies, English Springer Spaniels are the most frequently referred breed for aggression directed toward owners, although not all cases are for dominance-related aggression.

Diagnosis

Dominance-related aggression is diagnosed when historical information or direct observation of pet–owner interactions reveals a consistent pattern of owner-directed aggression in situations where the dog's control of resources or perceived position at the top of the hierarchy is challenged. The condition itself has three characteristic elements: assertive temperament, dominant signaling, and aggressive behavior directed toward family members. Therefore, the diagnosis is made based not only on family-directed aggression (growling, snapping, biting), but also that the dog must have an assertive personality and demonstrate a number of body postures suggestive of dominance (ears directed forward, elevated tail, staring, mounting, pushing, trying to stand above family members). The dominant dog may initiate sequences to which the owner defers, such as petting, play, treats, or going outdoors, and can be quite demanding. The dog may attempt to control the movements of family members by pushing, grasping with the mouth, or blocking their path. Evaluation of body postures and social behaviors of family pets is not always straightforward, because they are sometimes inadvertently reinforced by pet owners, so that they occur out of normal context. The temperament of the individual is very important, and if it does not exhibit overall confident behavior, something other than dominance may be causing the aggression problem.

It is not uncommon for attacks to occur suddenly with little warning and seemingly unprovoked. They may appear unprovoked because the owner does not recognize subtle dominant signals that usually precede the attack. Also, the owner's interaction with the pet can occur too quickly to give the dog a chance to signal. The pet's dominant stare or glare may make the dog appear to have a 'glazed' look before or during the attacks.

Problems occur when the owner has attempted to approach, handle, or move the dog, or when the owner performs a gesture that the pet interprets as a dominant signal that is inappropriate coming from a subordinate human. These pets are likely to be aggressive if disturbed while resting, disciplined, hugged, groomed, patted, or stared at. They may be overly possessive of their food, toys, and anything else they consider their own.

Although it is generally considered that dogs displaying dominance aggression are overly bold and domineering, there is no need for dominance aggression if the dog's position in the hierarchy is stable. Therefore, it is the mid-ranking dogs or dogs whose dominance status with another pack member is not well established that are more likely to exhibit dominance aggression. Similarly, inconsistent signals, actions, and attitude on the part of the owner may set up a situation of conflict in which the dogs do not have a clear understanding of their role/position in the family. This state of conflict can lead to aggression, even when the challenge seems to be relatively benign (e.g., owners attempting to pat a resting dog). In fact, many cases of dominance aggression have components of conflict and anxiety, which are more likely to be the actual cause of the aggression. Aggressive displays are often reinforced since the owner is most likely to back away from the threat, which teaches the pet that aggression is a successful strategy for avoiding being pulled off the couch (Fig. 19.10).

The use of aggression to control resources is not, by itself, sufficient to make a diagnosis of dominance-related aggression. Dominance aggression is arguably one of the most misdiagnosed types of canine behavior problem, because the diagnosis has either been based on too few criteria, other possible causes have not

Situations during which aggression might occur:
- Approached or disturbed while resting
- Protecting resources (food, toys, family members)
- Physical punishment, verbal discipline
- Staring, prolonged eye contact
- Handling by family members (lifting, patting, hugging)
- Restraining, pulling, pushing
- People trying to leave the room
- Family members entering the home
- Alpha roll – physically forcing into a subordinate position (e.g., side, back)

Figure 19.10

been ruled out, or are a result of learning how to achieve control.

Some forms of dominance-related aggression are so severe or dangerous that they have been labeled 'rage syndrome' (e.g., English Springer Spaniels). Dogs that are considered to be afflicted with 'rage syndrome' exhibit aggressive behavior that appears quite impulsive. Attacks occur very acutely with little warning and are very uninhibited in their intensity. Since the problem is often observed in certain breeds with common lineages, such as some lines of Springer Spaniels, there is likely a genetic component to the aggression. Although the pathophysiology of this and other forms of dominance-related aggression is poorly understood, preliminary studies have found that there may be identifiable neurochemical changes in these dogs involving serotonin pathways. Dogs with an assertive personality can become problems for owners who lack the ability or knowledge to assert enough control to become the leader. Young children are at high risk living with a dominant-aggressive dog.

Cases of dominance-related aggression must be differentiated from other forms of aggression. In fact, some behaviorists are now re-evaluating whether dominance challenges are truly the prime motivating factor in these cases. At the very least, many cases of dominance aggression have a component of fear, anxiety, or conflict, as it is the dog's anxiety related to inconsistent signals or an unstable position in the hierarchy that would lead to the aggressive displays. Some cases may have learned and conditioned factors so that the dog's response is a result of previous experience. Therefore it is critical that the situation in which the aggression first arose and how the problem progressed to the present point in time are assessed in determining the diagnosis. For example, the overexuberant puppy may use biting or grasping of the owner to gain attention or to initiate play sessions. By complying with the dog's demands, the owner's response reinforces the behavior. On the other hand, the owner's anxiety, anger, or attempts to punish the behavior could lead to conflict, fear, and defensive forms of aggression. In fact, some forms of handling, especially those that are sudden, unfamiliar, or cause discomfort (such as physical punishment, muzzle grasps, pinning, grabbing the collar), may lead to defensive responses that are often 'misdiagnosed' as dominance challenges. Similarly, dogs that are possessive of food, treats, toys, or stolen items (high resource-holding potential) and those that are painful or irritable may challenge when approached or handled and soon learn that the aggression is successful at removing the threat while owner anxiety or retaliation may aggravate fear.

Diagnostic criteria for dominance aggression:

- Assertive temperament.
- Dominant signaling is an integral part of the pet's behavioral profile.
- Resistance to dominant signaling and behaviors exhibited by family members.
- Aggression used to control social situations with family members.
- Aggression used to compete for resources with family members.

Dominance aggression or behavioral pathology?

It has also been suggested that underlying pathology may be a factor in some dogs with 'apparent' dominance-related aggression. Some cases have been likened to episodic dyscontrol (rage), a form of epilepsy. These dogs may respond to antiepileptic drugs such as phenobarbital or primidone. Other dogs may have syndromes similar to attention deficit hyperactivity disorder (ADHD) in people. Dogs with true 'hyperactive syndrome' show a paradoxical calming response to amphetamines. The rationale for the use of amphetamines is that they may mimic the action of noradrenaline or block its re-uptake, thus prolonging its effect. It is believed that the condition might result from a neurotransmitter imbalance that can be alleviated with amphetamine administration. These particular dogs thus have a pathophysiological reason for their aggression and are probably best not grouped into the category of dominance-related aggression. However, this diagnosis is rarely made because neurotransmitter evaluations are rarely if ever done in clinical practice. It is imperative that a full diagnostic evaluation be conducted before considering these diagnoses or administering experimental drug regimens that could make the situation worse. There are also a number of diagnoses of behavioral pathology by European behaviorists where aggression is a component of the problem (see Ch. 21).

Prognosis

The consultant must take into account the breed, age of onset, duration of the problem, sex of the dog, familial history (if available), the degree of danger to family members, and the ability of the family to cope with the pet with a dominant personality. Dominance-related aggression has been identified in certain lines and within certain breeds. An underlying genetic component to the problem may make safe resolution more difficult.

When evidence of dominance-related aggression appears in the lineage, when infants, the elderly, or infirm are at risk, when dominance-related aggression emerges prior to a year of age, when aggression is unpredictable, when bites are severe, or when the owner is not capable of instituting a safe and effective correction program, dominance-related aggression may be difficult or impossible to resolve safely. In a study in the USA, it was determined that dogs over 18 kg were more likely to be euthanized, as were dogs that reacted aggressively to benign dominance challenges by the owner and those reacting unpredictably to stimuli. Family safety has to be the first concern. In some cases, removing the dog from the home is the best solution. Giving the dog to someone else is risky. Although that person may be more authoritative and dominant to the dog, someone may still end up getting hurt. The option of euthanasia should be discussed. Owners must be made aware of all these factors before undertaking behavioral modification efforts.

Management

Situations and stimuli that elicit aggressive behavior from the pet must be identified. Although the owner must take a position of leadership with respect to the dog, confrontations that might lead to injury (and further success on the part of the dog) must be avoided. When the stimuli are identified, they can be eliminated or the pet can be taught to display an appropriate acceptable response when exposed to the stimulus. For example, the pet should be avoided when eating or chewing on toys and prevented from resting on furniture or other potential problem locations. In fact, the environment should be modified to prevent further problems. Barricades or a motion alarm can be used to keep the pet from getting into areas where problems might arise, such as on or under furniture. Rawhide or toys might have to be removed if the dog is possessive. A head halter can be left on the pet when the family is at home for more control.

Goals of treatment:

- Prevent further aggression and injury.
- Gain control of the pet.
- Train the dog to defer.
- Stop deferring to the dog.
- Teach the pet to respond acceptably in situations that formerly elicited aggression.

Family members must be consistent in their interactions with the dog, keeping in mind that gaining control must be done in a gradual and safe fashion and without physical confrontation. If too many major changes are attempted too quickly, aggression could potentially increase.

Using a trainer or family member whom the dog will not challenge is the safest way to begin to gain control of the pet, so that behavioral modification can proceed. Safe control can be achieved if the dog is taught to wear a head halter. Then if the dog must be placed in a situation where aggression or defiance is a possibility, the leash and head halter (or a basket muzzle – Fig. 13.4) should be applied so that the situation can be safely and successfully managed (Fig. 19.11). Leadership exercises that involve using obedience commands to control resources, ignoring pushy behavior, and controlling the pet's movements with stay commands are helpful. Counterconditioning and desensitization exercises can be used to change the pet's behavior in aggression-eliciting situations. Surgery, behavior products, and drug therapy may all be useful (Fig. 19.12).

It is important that the dog with dominance-related aggression has regular re-evaluations. The initial consultation will typically take about two hours, and rechecks will need to be planned based on the individual patient. Do not lose touch with these clients; the risks of injury and liability are too great. If after six to eight weeks of counseling, progress is poor or unacceptable, the chances for further rehabilitation may be poor.

Prevention

From the time the dog is obtained, the owner's responses to the dog's actions and demands can communicate to the dog who defers to whom. From the outset, the owner should teach the dog that rewards can only be earned for responding to the owner's control in the form of obedience training and handling. By training the dog to defer to the owner before any rewards (attention, play, walks, treats, food) can be obtained, the dog learns that the owner controls all resources and that responding to obedience training and physical handling exercises leads to rewards. In addition, undesirable behaviors are not inadvertently reinforced. Identifying dominance challenges as soon as they emerge and dealing with them promptly and effectively is essential. Dogs that

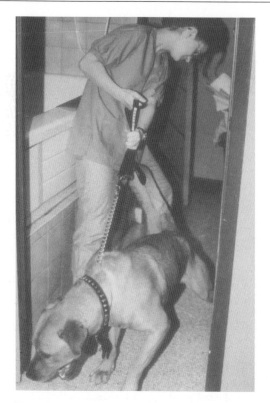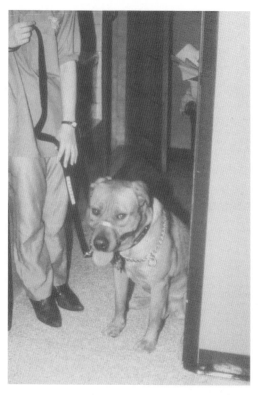

Figure 19.11 Left: Dog that is unruly and uncontrollable in the presence of a stimulus (in this case a cat), while wearing a choke collar. Right: This photo, taken 60 seconds after the one on the left, demonstrates how the dog can be effectively controlled in the presence of the stimulus using head halter training.

are too assertive to be trained effectively are unlikely to be suitable pets.

Puppy selection tests (see Ch. 3) may be useful in identifying problem puppies before they are welcomed into a home, but dominance-related aggression does not often emerge until long after testing is performed. These tests can provide an idea of the puppy's existing temperament and what the new owner might initially expect in gaining control and training. Below three months of age there is no evidence that puppy testing can actually predict adult behavior, although as the puppies age and mature the testing likely becomes predictive.

Case example

William, a 16-month-old Old English Sheepdog, was referred for aggression toward the hus-

band of the young couple that owned it. The dog frequently growled and snapped at the husband when he grabbed its collar to pull it away from rubbish. Recently, the dog had begun growling at the husband whenever he approached when it was lying near the wife. When the husband was on the floor watching television, William would occasionally stand over him, stare, and growl. The dog's personality was described as 'aloof, independent and irritable.'

The owners were instructed to review obedience training with the dog, require it to sit or lie down before receiving anything it wanted, and request it to 'stay' for a short period whenever it was about to move from one area of the house to another. Feeding was switched from free choice to a regular schedule and the dog had to perform a 'down-stay' for at least 60 seconds before getting the food. In order to ensure that the owners could control and handle the dog in any possible confrontational situations, it was trained with a head halter and leash, and the leash was left attached during training sessions. A pull on the leash was used to correct undesirable

responses and it was relaxed or released as soon as the dog complied and showed no threats.

After two weeks, the owners were instructed to begin daily exercises to condition the dog to accept and enjoy having the collar grasped.

Step	Comments
Remove all opportunities for the dog to injure or control	• Identify all situations that might result in aggression and discuss how these situations and interactions should be avoided. For example, pets that are aggressive when resting on the owner's bed or on furniture should not be permitted to have access to these areas • Confining the pet to its own bed, crate, or pen prevents the dog from gaining control of resources or gaining access to locations or resources that it might protect • When the dog is out from confinement and has access to the owners, a leash and either a head halter or basket muzzle can be used to ensure control, prevent the dog from controlling the owners, and reduce any possibility of injury • Safety is an overriding concern. All training exercises should be initiated by the family member who has the most control and is least likely to be challenged or with the aid of an experienced trainer
Who's controlling whom?	• Do not allow the dog to take control by confining the dog away from resources and from family members as needed, and by ignoring all demands for attention or other rewards • The owners should ensure control by training the dog with command–reward training and ensuring success by keeping a leash attached
Training	• Obedience training is needed to gain control. This should begin with the family member who has most control or with the aid of a qualified trainer • The dog must be taught to respond immediately to simple commands (heel, sit/stay, follow, settle – Fig. 5.13) by all family members using reward training techniques • The use of a leash and head halter (Fig. 19.11) or leash and muzzle can help to ensure immediate, consistent, and safe control
Establish a dominant attitude	• The owner must be in a position of leadership with the dog. This is initially accomplished by using obedience commands, consistency, and reward-based training techniques to control the pet • Family members should make the pet defer before it acquires anything it desires (attention, food, walks, toys, play) by first responding to a command • Owners must avoid submitting to any of the dog's demands as this serves to reward the dog's leadership and control over the owner. When the pet nudges or barks for play, affection, or food, it should be ignored. In fact, any behavior initiated by the dog should be ignored, as it is the owner who must initiate and control resources and not the dog • Once the pet has learned to do a dependable 'stay,' the owner should command it to 'stay' for a short period and then release it before it is given play, affection, walks, treats, or even its food. The dog should also be taught to follow/heel when going through doorways or on walks
Rewards	• Rewards should be used to retrain the dog to respond to the owners in all aspects of the relationship. Rewards can be used to shape desired responses including obedience to commands and tolerance of all forms of handling • A formal program of 'nothing in life is free' should be initiated so that the owner is consciously aware that each reward is under their control • Conversely, if the dog is successful at getting rewards on demand (controlling the owner) the problem is further reinforced

(continued)

Figure 19.12   Approaches taken during the management of dominance aggression in dogs.

Step	Comments
Desensitization and counterconditioning	• These measures may be dangerous because of the temperament of the pet, the gravity of the problem, and the assertiveness of the owner. They should only be attempted under the close supervision of an experienced behaviorist • A dominant dog should be desensitized and counterconditioned to stimuli, handling, and approaches that elicit aggression, thereby reducing the aggressive response to the stimuli and conditioning an alternative, acceptable response • For example, if the pet is aggressive when the owner pats its head, exercises should begin with the owner giving a piece of food with one hand and moving the other hand toward the pet's head, stopping at a distance at which no growling would be elicited. During subsequent exercises, the second hand is moved closer to the pet's head until contact is made. Eventually, the dog should associate hand movements and contact on the head with food, and the aggression during patting should cease • Progress should be slow enough that no aggression is elicited during training sessions. If aggression results, cease the exercise immediately and resume training on the next day at a more conservative stage and proceed more slowly
Surgery	• Neutering should be considered in all dogs with dominance-related aggression. This type of aggression has been shown to be sexually dimorphic (approximately 90% of cases are males), with testosterone perhaps acting as a modulator or facilitator of aggression in dogs with a propensity for aggression. While castration will not eliminate dominance-related aggression without concurrent behavioral modification, it may increase the chances of successful behavioral therapy and prevent the possibility of passing on the trait
Drug therapy	• Serotonergic drugs (fluoxetine, paroxetine) may be useful for dogs that have aggression that is impulsive, very intense, and uninhibited. These drugs may require several weeks to take effect and are unlikely to provide significant improvement without concurrent behavioral management • Anti-anxiety drugs such as benzodiazepines, buspirone, and even propranolol may also be indicated if there is a fear or anxiety component to the problem • Unless drug therapy is combined with behavioral modification techniques, the aggressive behavior usually returns with the cessation of drug therapy • There appears to be little effect of diet on aggressive behavior, although one study with a reduced protein diet and concurrent tryptophan supplementation may have led to some improvement (see Chs 7, 8 on diet and natural therapeutics) • Megoestrol acetate or medroxyprogesterone acetate may occasionally help some individuals (perhaps neutered males), but for the most part are contraindicated due to the potential for excessive side effects unless all other therapeutic options have been unsuccessful • Antipsychotics such as lithium carbonate or respiridone might also be a consideration for some forms of aggression in dogs, especially when behavioral pathology is considered
Physical control and punishment	• Although it is important that the owner has complete control of every interaction, and that the dog does not control the owner, this must be done without confrontation. Physical punishment, choke and shock devices, and confrontational techniques, such as alpha rolls or scruff shakes, are potentially dangerous as they could lead to dominant or defensive reactions from the dog • The owner should ensure control with commands, rewards, and physical devices such as a leash and head halter, which can gently but firmly ensure the desired response

Figure 19.12   (continued)

Using the head halter to ensure control, they began by lightly touching the collar as they gave a very tasty meat treat and said 'good boy.' As the weeks went by, they very gradually began touching the collar more forcefully, grasped it and, finally, pulled it as food was given, thus teaching the dog to look forward to having the collar handled.

To stop the growling when the husband approached his wife, she was told to use a shake can or other loud, aversive noisemaker to interrupt the growling as the husband approached. The leash and head halter were used to ensure that if any aggression or threats were exhibited, the dog could be immediately interrupted. The approach exercise was repeated on multiple occasions until the husband could approach without any growling from the dog. Once the dog did not growl when the husband entered, it was told to sit for a very tasty meat reward as the husband approached. This last phase was then repeated at least 10 more times before the exercise was finished.

CONFLICT-RELATED AGGRESSION

Conflict-related behaviors are seen when there are competing states of motivation (conflict and frustration are discussed in further detail in Ch. 10). The resultant behavior can vary with the situation or the stimulus but might be a displacement behavior (one that is out of context with the stimulus such as tail chasing), a redirected behavior (e.g., aggression that is directed at the handler rather than the stimulus), aggression, or retreat. Conflict-related aggression is often associated with heightened levels of arousal. One common example is the pet that is excited and sociable but suddenly frightened by a movement or gesture. The response is often one that is reflexive; the stimulation of an autonomic fear response that might include aggression. Defensive, anxiety, and fear-induced aggression are usually a component of conflict-related aggression. Calming the dog with a controlled heel, or a calm sit-stay before introduction to the stimulus may be all that is needed for a safe introduction (as long as the stimulus itself is not a threat). Similarly, reaching quickly for, or moving quickly around a dog that is excited, even if it appears to be friendly and sociable, may lead to aggression.

Diagnosis and prognosis

If the dog exhibits mixed signals such as social approach mixed with fearful withdrawal or suddenly reacts aggressively when it is excited, these may indicate conflict-induced aggression.

Management

Before introducing pets to situations that might be startling or fearful, it must be sufficiently calmed and controlled. Training the pet to heel calmly on walks and to settle down immediately on command provides a means for safe and successful exposure to the stimulus (see Fig. 5.13, handout #23 on the CD for details). Although desensitization and counterconditioning may also be necessary to ensure that there is a positive emotional response to the stimulus, often the dog is immediately calm as soon as it observes that there is no 'real' threat.

Prevention

Most important are basic training commands, so that the dog can be exposed to new stimuli when it is calm. Harsh training methods should be avoided. Fair rules should be in place when the pet is first brought into the family, and consistently enforced. Reinforcement and correction should be fairly and consistently applied in all situations by all family members. Situations that cause anxiety should be addressed in a timely manner. Greeting of an excited or aroused pet should be calm, with the hand displayed before slowly reaching to offer a treat or affection.

Case example

Honey, a three-year-old spayed female Border Collie cross was extremely sociable and excited when visitors came to the home. With other dogs she was also sociable and highly aroused if the dogs were small or familiar. However, Honey also showed fear and territorial behavior when she was tied on her front porch or when she was looking out the window as strangers passed by the home. Her behavior with large dogs and strangers who were large, wearing uniforms, or boisterous was to approach playfully with her tail wagging, but when she reached a certain critical distance or when the stranger or dog moved closer she tucked her tail, her ears flattened, and she began to crouch and retreat. However, if she was on her property or could retreat no further (e.g., on leash or on her porch), she would lunge and snap.

Honey's aggression appeared to be defensive. However her signals were confusing to the owners because she seemed to want to play and greet excitedly until she reached a certain threshold and then would immediately become fearful. Because of Honey's level of arousal, her generally social nature, as well as what appeared to be fearful and territorial responses, Honey was diagnosed as having conflict-related aggression. The owner was instructed to use a head halter and teach Honey to sit calmly when the front door was open, to follow the owners out the door calmly, and to heel calmly on walks. Greetings were then practiced with family members where Honey was taught to sit calmly and take a favored food reward before proceeding to greet. Similarly on walks Honey was taught to approach and greet friendly small dogs by heeling calmly beside the owner and by sitting and receiving food rewards before being allowed to play. Honey's improvement was remarkably quick. As soon as Honey could be controlled with a head halter she could quickly and successfully be taught to sit and take a reward when strangers or large dogs approached or arrived on the property. Training was practiced with friends of the family and large, friendly unfamiliar dogs owned by friends and the trainer. As soon as the stranger or other dog arrived, Honey was taught to sit and settle, given a favored reward, and when entirely calm allowed to slowly approach. For the most part, she would then remain friendly and sociable and enjoy friendly stroking or take treats from the strangers and would play with the large dogs. From that point on whenever she met a new person or dog and began to get excited, all it took was a sit command and an occasionally gentle pull upward on the head halter to get

Honey to sit and settle down. She was then given a favored food reward and allowed to interact with the person or other dog as long as she remained calm and showed no signs of overexcitement or fear.

POSSESSIVE AGGRESSION

Possessive aggression may be directed at humans or other pets that approach the dog when it is near or in possession of something it values. This could be a food bowl, chew toy, or even a person, pet, or place, but is often some food or item that is novel (highly motivating). Possessive aggression may be associated with dominance aggression but this is not always the case. A dog that is highly motivated to retain a possession (resource-holding potential) may exhibit possessive aggression, regardless of its hierarchal status with respect to the person attempting to remove the object. In a sense, the drive to maintain possession 'trumps' the need to defer.

Diagnosis and prognosis

The dog barks, growls, lunges, snaps, and/or bites when a person or animal approaches it while it is in possession of or near something it does not want to relinquish. This problem can occur in puppies but is more common in adults. It occurs with equal frequency in both males and females.

Defensive aggression shown by a dog that has frequently been beaten for stealing the owner's possessions may appear to be possessive aggression. A detailed history and close attention to body postures during the behavior should differentiate the two. The pet that is exhibiting defensive aggression will show behavioral and postural signs of fear.

Prognosis is guarded for dogs that show this type of aggression frequently from the first few months of life or have exhibited the problem for many years. The situation will also be more difficult to safely resolve in cases where the pet has a very confident, assertive temperament, where family members are non-assertive, or where there are children or the infirm at risk. The prognosis is good for a problem of short duration where aggressive incidents are predictable and can be prevented or are mild and infrequent. Dogs that are possessive of a few types of items may be more easy to train than those that are possessive of a large variety of objects.

Management

Behavioral modification techniques are the cornerstone of treatment (Fig. 19.13). A verbal correction that is sharp enough to stop the behavior without eliciting any sign of fear may be suitable for puppies but is rarely suitable for adult pets and advanced cases.

It is important to identify all situations in which aggression might occur. The owners are then instructed to avoid these situations or prevent them from occurring until they have more control of the dog and the situations in order to handle them safely. Leadership exercises, teaching the pet to relinquish objects on command, and exposure exercises to reduce aggression when the pet is approached while near an object it guards may all be important for treatment.

Prevention

As soon as the pup is adopted, the family should begin obedience training, leadership exercises, and handling exercises. Teaching a young puppy to drop objects while playing fetch is a nice way of training object relinquishment (Fig. 19.14, handout #7 on the CD). If family members are clearly in control, they should be able to take food, toys, or any other items away from the pet. It is best to build this tolerance while it is still a puppy rather than trying to convert an already possession-aggressive adult dog.

Food bowl guarding can be avoided if the puppy is not ignored when it is fed. The family should take steps to allay the pet's apprehension that it may lose its meal. This can be done by gently stroking the non-aggressive puppy while it is eating and periodically handling its food (Fig. 19.15; Appendix C, Fig. 13, handout #11

on the CD). Visitors might also be asked to handle the food while the puppy is eating. The pup will look forward to having humans present at dinner time if they occasionally add small meat or cheese treats to the bowl. The dog then learns to associate the food handling with receiving treats, not with the meal being taken away.

Case example

At nine months of age, a Cocker Spaniel named Jamie began growling at family members who approached when it was chewing on a rawhide bone.

The owners were instructed to take up all rawhide bones and teach the pet to fetch a ball and to drop it on command using food lures. Once this was accomplished, a variety of objects were used in the fetch game. After about two weeks, a new rawhide bone was introduced into the game. After Jamie fetched and retrieved several toys for small meat rewards, the rawhide was tossed a few feet, retrieved, the dog was asked to 'drop it,' and it was put away. In subsequent games of fetch, the rawhide was used more and more frequently. The owner was able to establish verbal control of the dog and take objects from it on command. By frequently giving and taking the rawhide away from Jamie, the owner maintained ownership of the rawhide, reducing the likelihood of an aggressive challenge from the dog.

FEAR-RELATED AGGRESSION

Fear aggression is triggered by a stimulus that appears threatening to the dog. It is sometimes referred to as defensive aggression, although there might be aspects of defensive aggression where the pet does not appear to be fearful. For example, aggression in response to ear cleaning or physical punishment might be examples of defensive aggression where the fear component is minimal. Fear aggression may be displayed when a dog is the recipient of assertive posturing or facial expressions, or is approached by another dog or person that is unfamiliar, unfriendly, or in some way threatening to the

Step	Comments
Avoid confrontations and make situations safe	• Feed in a separate room with the door closed • Take away all guarded objects. Keep highly favored toys, treats, and other objects out of reach • Prevent access to rooms or areas of rooms where problems occur. Control the dog's activity with a leash, baby gate, exercise pen, or training crate • Use a head halter, long leash, or muzzle during problem times • Do not physically punish the dog. This will likely make the situation worse • A remote spray collar or ultrasound device can sometimes be safely used to interrupt undesirable behavior • If a safe and effective correction cannot be found when the pet acts aggressively, it is better to ignore it than to risk injury
Discourage the pet from obtaining objects that are off limits	• Use booby traps, such as motion-activated alarms • Spray objects that are stolen and guarded with aversive-tasting substances
Reinforce the owner's leadership position	• Review obedience training using a method that does not require physical force • Make the dog respond to a command before getting anything it wants • Do not allow the pet to successfully solicit attention on demand • Frequently ask the pet to stay before it is allowed to follow family members around the home
Teach the dog to drop objects on command	• Teach the 'drop' command with reward training (see handout #7 on the CD, Fig. 19.14) • The family member who is the most confident, assertive, and in control of the dog should be the first to begin working with it • To insure owner control and prevent injuries, the dog can be trained with a leash and head halter • The exercises should be performed with a variety of objects in a variety of locations to foster dependability in all situations
Desensitization and counterconditioning	• Use repeated, controlled, safe exposures to teach the pet to be relaxed when approached when in possession of something it guards • Refer to handout #11 on the CD (Appendix C, Fig. 13) for specific details on treating food bowl guarding
Treat underlying problems	• Any underlying factors that are contributing to the possession problem, such as dominance aggression or fear, must be addressed • Owners sometimes inadvertently reward undesirable behavior by offering a more acceptable toy while the dog is misbehaving. This only reinforces the bad behavior and should be avoided • The bond between the pet and owner is often weakened in these situations. Strengthen the bond with shared, enjoyable activities, such as long walks, visits to parks, play, etc.
Drug therapy	• Medication is generally not warranted unless the aggression is severe and impulsive or there are other coexisting causes of aggression that might warrant a drug trial. Selective serotonin re-uptake inhibitors may be of some help for serious cases

Figure 19.13   Steps in the management of canine possessive aggression.

dog. It usually occurs when the dog is unable to avoid the stimulus that brings about a fear-aggressive response.

Inadequate socialization, traumatic experiences, punishment, and genetics can all contribute to the development of fear aggression. For more details on why and how fear might develop, see Chapter 11. Fear aggression may be aggravated when the owner responds with punishment, if the owner displays fear or anxi-ety, when the stimulus (e.g., other dog) shows fear or aggression, or when the stimulus retreats (negative reinforcement). It is also possible that the owner's attempts to settle the dog by offering a toy or treat may reinforce the behavior.

Genetics can play a role in determining the threshold for a fear response. There is considerable variation in the canine population regarding the types of responses that are generated by fear-provoking stimuli. Some dogs require a

TEACHING THE PET TO FETCH AND DROP OBJECTS ON COMMAND

'Fetch' and 'drop it' are excellent commands to teach a young dog. Fetch is a great game that most dogs love. It is mentally stimulating, wonderful for wearing the pet out, an acceptable type of play for children and dogs, and can provide a means for social interaction between visitors and shy dogs. Teaching the pet to drop things on command reinforces the idea that the owner has control over the dog, and comes in handy when the pet has something in its mouth that it shouldn't.

Teaching fetch

Pick a time when the pet is in an energetic mood and there are few distractions. Toss an interesting toy a short distance. As the pet picks it up and turns to look at you, lower your body, take several quick steps in the opposite direction, wave your hand and wiggle your fingers in an animated way, and say 'fetch' in a very upbeat tone. This should catch the attention of the pet and prompt it to come toward you. Continue to repeat 'fetch' as the pet approaches.

If the pet runs the other way with the toy, lies down and chews it, or does not come all the way up to you, simply walk away and end the play session. You must avoid chasing after the pet, walking toward it to take the toy, or attempting to coax the pet to return.

Drop it – first step

The first step involves luring the pet to drop the toy and teaching a cue word. As the pet approaches with the toy, place a piece of food between your forefinger and thumb. When the pet reaches you, move your hand and the food toward the pet's mouth with a bit of a flourish. Hold the food in front of the mouth without saying anything. When the pet opens its mouth to take the food, the toy will fall out. As this is happening, say the cue words, 'drop it,' and pick up the toy with the other hand as you allow the pet to take the food. Repeat until you notice that the pet is starting to drop the toy as your hand just begins the downward movement toward it.

Use a small piece of food that is more interesting than the toy, but not so interesting that the pet will forget the toy and only focus on the food. Each time the pet takes the food from your hand, say 'good dog.' If the pet is not interested in food, you can use a second toy in place of food to lure it to drop the fetched toy.

Drop it – second step

The next step is to turn the cue words into a command. Instead of putting the food in front of the pet's mouth and waiting until it opens to say 'drop it,' you will say 'drop it' as you begin to swing your hand down toward the pet. Pick up the toy, give the food, and say 'good dog.' Repeat this at least 12 times before advancing to the next step.

Drop it – third step

The last step involves gradually phasing out the food. Hold your hand like you have food in it, swing it down toward the pet, and say 'drop it.' When the pet drops it, say 'good dog' and give it loads of praise. As you continue to practice, alternate between a food reward and praise, but vary the ratio of praise rewards to food rewards so the pet doesn't know exactly which reward it will get each time it drops the toy. As the training progresses, you should be using more praise and less food. When combining the drop and fetch exercises, your dog may also learn that by dropping the toy, it gets the opportunity to chase and fetch it again. End the session on a positive note with your dog dropping the toy and getting a final reward.

Give it

If you prefer to have a 'give' command, you would proceed exactly as with drop it, but in each case you would place your second hand under or on the toy and reward the dog when it is released into your hand.

(continued)

Figure 19.14   Teaching the pet to fetch and drop objects on command (handout #7 – printable from the CD).

Having problems?

If the dog will not drop the toy, you can first increase the value of the lure while using a toy to fetch that is of less interest to the dog.

If your dog is overly distracted or playful and will not focus on you or the reward during training, you could keep a leash and head halter attached. If the toy is large or long enough and the dog will not bring it back, you can pull the dog into a sit position with the leash and head halter, offer the reward, and if the dog does not drop the toy, pull it gently from the mouth while applying light pressure on the leash and head halter to keep the dog in position.

Drop it – other items

Once the pet learns the 'drop it' command during play, it can be used whenever it has anything in its mouth. The transition from dropping toys during fetch to dropping more desirable items, like rawhide or food wrappers, should be made very gradually. Rank the pet's toys from the most desirable to least desirable. When you notice that the pet has the least desirable toy in its mouth, ask it to drop it using a command and hand signal. Praise it or give a small food reward, then ask it to sit and return the toy to the pet. When you find that it drops that toy readily, move to the next toy in the rank, and so forth. Be sure to always use an upbeat tone of voice and make the training fun. Practice is very important. The pet needs to drop something on command at least several times each day if you expect to be able to get to the point where it will drop special items like food wrappers and dead birds on command.

Figure 19.14   (*continued*)

very strong stimulus to elicit fear, while others become extremely anxious in response to mild stimuli or any auditory or visual stimulus that is only the least bit unusual.

A dog that has a low threshold for becoming fearful and that encounters multiple, strong, fear-inducing stimuli with little chance for escape has a high likelihood of biting, especially if biting has caused the stimulus to move away during past encounters (Fig. 19.16).

Diagnosis and prognosis

Fear aggression is manifested by fearful facial expressions and body postures (tail down, ears rotated back, crouched body, weight shifted away from the fear-eliciting stimulus) accompanied by aggressive signs such as piloerection, barking, growling, snarling, and biting. Dilated pupils, increased respiratory rate, and a rapid heart rate generally accompany an overwhelming fear response. The pet might also defecate or urinate if it is exceptionally fearful.

Factors that might suggest a good prognosis include:

- The duration of the problem is short.
- The fearful behavior was acquired as an adult.
- All fear-eliciting stimuli are well defined.
- Fear-eliciting environmental stimuli can be controlled.
- The pet has a relatively high threshold for responding to fear stimuli.

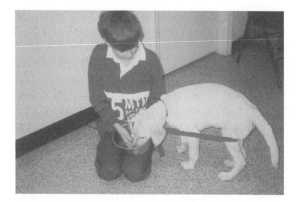

Figure 19.15   Hand feeding: 'enjoyable' handling of a puppy during meal times can help prevent the possibility of food bowl associated aggression in the adult dog.

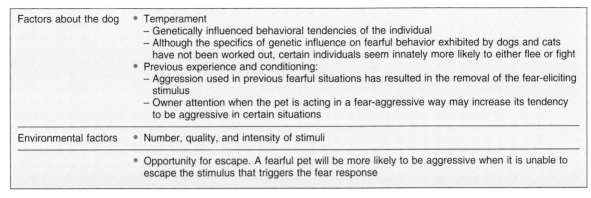

Factors about the dog	• Temperament
	  – Genetically influenced behavioral tendencies of the individual
	  – Although the specifics of genetic influence on fearful behavior exhibited by dogs and cats
	    have not been worked out, certain individuals seem innately more likely to either flee or fight
	• Previous experience and conditioning:
	  – Aggression used in previous fearful situations has resulted in the removal of the fear-eliciting
	    stimulus
	  – Owner attention when the pet is acting in a fear-aggressive way may increase its tendency
	    to be aggressive in certain situations

Environmental factors	• Number, quality, and intensity of stimuli
	• Opportunity for escape. A fearful pet will be more likely to be aggressive when it is unable to escape the stimulus that triggers the fear response

Figure 19.16   Factors that affect the risk of biting in a fearful dog.

- The pet can be protected from strong stimulus exposure during treatment.

The prognosis for safe resolution of fear aggression is generally more favorable (particularly if all potential stimuli can be identified) than for dominance-related aggression, but adequate care must still be taken. The owners, as well as others, are at risk handling a dog with fear aggression and must be counseled accordingly.

Management

Early recognition and intervention lead to the most effective cures. Fear aggression is best managed with gradual exposure techniques involving desensitization and counterconditioning exercises (see also Ch. 11). It is crucial that all fear-eliciting stimuli and situations are identified before behavioral modification begins. The goal is to replace the pet's fear response with another response, such as anticipation of food or play. Safety is very important. Injuries should be prevented by taking precautions and by proceeding with patience. Family members must be cautioned to avoid consoling the pet or giving treats to calm it down when it acts in a fear-aggressive way, or they may inadvertently reinforce the behavior (Fig. 19.17). Punishment is contraindicated. See Figure 11.8 (handout #9 on the CD) for a client handout on desensitization and counterconditioning and Figure 5.13 (handout #23 on the CD) for settle exercises.

Prevention

Socialization and protection of the puppy during the early, sensitive months of development are extremely important. The young dog should meet many different types of people in controlled, pleasant situations as often as possible during the early months of life. Food treats given by the people the dog meets can help facilitate socialization. Owners should be encouraged to concentrate on using positive reinforcement rather than punishment for training.

Case examples

Case 1 Sammy, an eight-month-old Chow Chow, was presented for growling at visitors who reached to pat him. He had been adopted from a neighbor who kept him chained in the backyard and who frequently struck him on the side of the head for barking. Whenever a stranger reached for his head, his ears went down and he growled as he backed away. If he was on a leash or in a chair when reached for, he would snap. When left alone during visits by the owner's friends, he stayed by himself and rested quietly. Although he occasionally cowered when the owner reached for him, he showed no signs of aggression toward her. Traumatic experiences had caused this dog to be fearful of hands extended toward him.

The owner was counseled about gestures and behaviors that visitors should avoid during the

Step	Comments
Safety	• Completely control the pet's environment in order to prevent exposure to fear-provoking stimuli or situations that occur outside training sessions • Review obedience training, concentrating on positive reinforcement and owner control • Use a leash and a muzzle or head halter as needed so that the dog can be successfully controlled and exposed to the stimuli without escaping and without causing injury
Identify all fear-provoking stimuli	• All stimuli that might evoke fear-related aggressive responses must be identified to determine the focus for desensitization and counterconditioning exercises
Identify the threshold for the fear response	• The amount, intensity, or proximity of the fear-provoking stimulus that is required to elicit signs of fear should be established in order to set a subthreshold starting point for behavioral modification
Modify the behavior	• Use desensitization and counterconditioning • It is helpful to use highly motivating rewards such as food, social attention, or a favorite toy to reward a 'sit-stay' or 'down-stay' command during training sessions. Later, the commands and reinforcers can be combined with low-level exposure to the fear-evoking stimuli • Train to settle on command in the absence of stimuli (Fig. 5.13, handout #23 on the CD) • When the pet responds well to commands, begin desensitization by exposing the pet to a stimulus intensity just below the threshold that would evoke fear. Distance is the variable that is typically used to control the intensity of the stimulus. When the pet shows no fear or anxiety give immediate reinforcement • Gradually increase the intensity of the stimulus • Controlled flooding with a stimulus intensity above the threshold for a fearful response can sometimes be used for pets with very mild problems and good owner control • Remember the goal is to calm the pet and change the association with the stimulus to one that is positive. Therefore the owner must be calm, as anxiety and punishment will increase fear and the stimulus used for retraining must be non-threatening/non-fearful
Avoid reinforcing or punishing fear-related behavior	• If the fearful pet is consoled when it is acting aggressive, the behavior may be reinforced • If the pet is punished, the state of fearful arousal may increase during subsequent exposures to fear-eliciting stimuli
Drugs	• Selective serotonin re-uptake inhibitors may be helpful for reducing panic and extreme fearful states • Benzodiazepines or buspirone may be better at reducing fear and anxiety but are not useful for long-term therapy and may disinhibit so that aggression may increase

Figure 19.17 Management of canine fear aggression.

initial therapy because they may appear threatening, such as prolonged eye contact, quick movements, loud noises, cornering the dog, and sticking a hand in its face for it to sniff at the initial greeting.

The owner was instructed to use food lures (cooked chicken was used because it was determined to be the most highly valued food) to teach the dog to come and sit on command. Every time Sammy took the food from her hand, she said 'good boy.' This caused the words to become a secondary reinforcer that could be used to alter the dog's mood when

encountering an anxiety-provoking situation. This was the initial step in easing the fear associated with an outstretched hand. The next step was to have a visitor toss the food reward to the dog following each response to the owner's obedience request. Each time the food was given, the owner and visitor would say 'good boy.' The following step involved having the visitor ask for a command response and then flip the food to the pet as the words 'good boy' were spoken.

Once Sammy showed no sign of fear or anxiety when a visitor entered the home, he was conditioned to accept patting. The owner began this part of the therapy by patting the dog on the head and saying 'good boy' at the same time as he took the food from her hand. After a few weeks an adult friend of the owner took part in working on the handshyness. Each time the dog took food for an obedience response, she would slowly move her other hand an inch or two toward him. As the weeks went by, she was able to slowly move closer and closer until she could pat the dog as it took the food from her hand. The exercises were then repeated with other adults, with an attempt being made to include people of varying size and appearance.

Case 2 Maxie, a three-year-old, intact, male Cocker Spaniel mix, was presented by his owners for aggressive behavior toward family members. The pet had no history of aggression to visitors and was friendly during the consultation and exam. The owners complained that Maxie growled and snapped when he was resting on the couch and they attempted to sit beside him, and when they grabbed him by the collar to pull him away from the window where he barked excessively. The owner had been told to grasp the collar and either shake or pin the dog when it misbehaved. Physical discipline of this sort or yelling at the pet escalated the aggression. Otherwise, he was a very obedient pet that generally did what the owners desired and rarely caused problems.

Although there were components of dominance aggression in that Maxie was aggressive when confronted while occupying a favored resource, aggression at other times was generally related to times of high arousal and to punishment. Therefore it was most likely that Maxie also displayed redirected aggression when grabbed while barking at the window and defensive aggression when being punished. In addition, Maxie had become defensive and fearful of having his collar grasped and had learned that aggression led to withdrawal of the owner. Therefore, as with many clinical cases of aggression, Maxie's threats, growling, and biting were due to fear and defensiveness, situations of arousal and con-

flict, with possible dominance-related aggression components.

The owners were advised to review obedience training with the pet so they could begin leadership exercises that involved the use of obedience commands to control resources. A motion-activated alarm was suggested to teach the pet to stay off furniture. This suggestion was declined because the couple liked having the pet on the furniture with them, but they just wanted to be able to get Maxie off when they told him to get off. In order to accomplish this, the owners were taught to train their pet to immediately get off the couch on demand using food lures. For the first two weeks of training, Maxie was not allowed to be on the couch unless a family member was present. A leash was left attached to ensure control without having to reach for or grab Maxie. Access was prevented by placing cardboard boxes on the couch. When a family member sat on the couch, the boxes were removed and Maxie was called up. Shortly after getting on the couch, the person showed him a small piece of chicken meat, and with an obvious hand movement, tossed the meat to the floor. As Maxie was about to jump off the couch for the chicken, the owner said 'off.' This was repeated 10 to 20 times each day during the first week. By the end of the week, the pet was anticipating the maneuver and quickly jumping off the couch. Next, the owner began saying 'off' and moving the hand toward the floor, but did not toss the food until the pet had been on the floor for at least one second. A gentle pull on the leash was to be used if the dog did not immediately jump down. After the second week, the owner began phasing out the food, as the pet would jump to the floor every time a family member said 'off' and pointed to the floor. The family also used desensitization and counterconditioning exercises to teach the pet to look forward to having its collar grabbed. The problem at the window was solved by having the pet wear a citronella spray antibark collar. The leash was left attached when the owners were at home and supervising for several weeks until the dog consistently responded to the owner's verbal commands.

TERRITORIAL AND PROTECTIVE AGGRESSION

These types of aggression are directed toward a person or another animal that is not a member of the group or pack, or is unfamiliar to the dog. Aggression may be exhibited toward people or other animals that approach family members or the pet's perceived territory, while the very same dog may be non-aggressive or even friendly when meeting unfamiliar people and dogs off the property. When the dog guards the home or family members aggressively, a dangerous situation results. Anxiety and fear may also play a role in the development of territorial aggression since threats and aggressive displays are more likely to be exhibited to novel, unfamiliar, or fear-eliciting stimuli. Dogs that also exhibit signs of fear or anxiety when meeting new people or animals off their property are more likely to be exhibiting fear-induced aggression either alone, or in combination with territorial aggression. Dogs that are allowed to frequently exhibit aggressive behavior toward passersby at windows, fence lines, or along the boundaries of the property progressively get worse. The reason for this is that the end result of the dog's territorial behavior is movement of the person or animal away from the home. Thus, the dog's aggressive behavior is reinforced.

Diagnosis and prognosis

Aggressive behaviors are seen when a person or animal approaches an area (e.g., home, yard, car), person, or animal toward which the dog is protective. This is manifested by aggressive postures (ears up, tail held with stiff wagging, assertive stance with weight forward, lunging, and biting), and vocalizations (growling, barking). The behavior can be seen in both males and females and usually first appears at less than three years of age. The initial signs are typically noted toward the end of the first year of life.

The prognosis is good provided the owner has good control over the dog, and approaching the dog can be avoided in the owner's absence. The prognosis for safe resolution is worse for dogs over which the owner has little control or in situations where it is confined in a home or garden without supervision and frequently allowed to exhibit territorial aggression without any owner intervention to correct the behavior.

Management

An owner with good control over a dog can usually suppress the behavior with firm commands and appropriate rewards for compliance (Fig. 19.18). A bark-activated citronella spray collar may be an effective tool if it will suppress the barking that precedes the aggression. Unwary owners may inappropriately reward the aggressive behavior by offering food or attention to the dog in order to distract it or try to calm it. This can be corrected by effective owner education.

The first important step is to immediately take complete control of the pet and its environment. The pet should never be exposed to anything that triggers aggressive displays without a family member being present to control its behavior. Aggressive barking and lunging at passersby through windows and doors must not be permitted. The owner can close drapes, move furniture in front of windows, or use a motion-activated alarm to keep the pet away from window areas. The pet should never be allowed to be in the backyard unless it is wearing a head halter and controlled with a leash by a family member. Vigilance is very important, because a dangerous situation could arise should the owner become distracted. The owner who does not have sufficient control over the dog should seek additional obedience training guidance and should follow the steps needed to gain control of the dog. A head halter and leash provide an excellent means of ensuring control while progressing through the exposure program. A pull on the leash can be used to ensure that the dog remains in place without attacking or retreating. Release of the leash provides reward for compliance.

This problem can best be managed by desensitization and counterconditioning. Retraining should begin by gradually exposing the dog to

Step	Comments
Prevent all territorial and protective displays	• Confine to an area where the pet cannot see passersby • Block visibility through doors and windows • Do not leave the dog in the yard unattended
Control the pet	• Use a muzzle or head halter and leash as needed • Review obedience training, concentrating on the use of positive reinforcement and owner control • Confine the pet when unfamiliar people or pets are in the home • Do not depend on electronic fencing to keep the pet in the yard
Identify all aggression-provoking stimuli	• All stimuli that might evoke territorial aggression must be identified to determine the focus for desensitization and counterconditioning exercises
Identify the threshold for the territorial or protective response	• The amount, intensity, or proximity of the territorial or protection-evoking stimuli that are required to elicit signs of aggression should be established in order to set a subthreshold starting point for behavioral modification
Modify the behavior	• Use desensitization and counterconditioning. However, to be successful the dog must first be trained or controlled with a head halter so that it will immediately settle on command (Fig. 5.13, handout #23 on the CD) • Use a highly motivating reward such as food, social attention, or a favorite toy to reward a 'sit-stay' or 'down-stay' command during training sessions. Later, the commands and reinforcers can be combined with low-level exposure to the territorial-evoking stimuli • When the pet responds well to commands, begin desensitization by exposing the pet to a stimulus intensity just below the threshold that would evoke fear. Distance can be the variable used for desensitization. Reinforcements are only given when the pet shows no sign of aggressive behavior • Gradually increase the intensity of the stimulus by increasing the proximity to the pet or exaggerating the behavior of the person that approaches the pet • Besides desensitizing the pet to people and animals that elicit a territorial response, it will also help to desensitize the pet to environmental cues associated with visitors, such as door bells and cars entering the driveway • Controlled flooding with a stimulus intensity above the threshold for an aggressive response can sometimes be used for pets with very mild problems and good owner control
Avoid reinforcing aggressive behavior	• If an attempt is made to calm the pet down with soft talk when it is acting aggressive, the behavior may be reinforced
Avoid punishment	• It may increase the level of aggressive arousal • It may suppress warning behaviors, such as growling and snarling, without actually making the pet less likely to bite • It may cause redirected aggression toward the owner • Harsh corrections with choke collars, pinch collars, and shock collars generally make the problem worse by associating pain with visitors or other animals
Interrupt aggressive behavior	• A leash and head halter, air horn, shake can, ultrasonic device, water gun, or bark-activated citronella collar might be helpful
Surgery	• Castration or spaying may help, but is usually not successful in completely suppressing this behavior
Drugs	• Selective serotonin re-uptake inhibitors may be helpful

Figure 19.18 Steps in the management of canine territorial and protective aggression.

stimuli and situations that previously evoked aggression. However, training should not proceed until the owner can successfully calm and control the dog on command with or without the aid of a head halter (see Fig. 5.13, handout #23 on the CD). The stimuli and situations should be controlled and muted so that they are recognized by the dog, but are not strong enough to elicit an aggressive response. Non-aggressive behavior during exposure to the stimulus should be associated with its most favored food treats. The dog should gradually be exposed to progressively more difficult situations and stimuli at closer distances. By withholding special food rewards from all situations except training sessions, happy anticipation of treats should replace aggressive arousal.

Sometimes, training may be accelerated by using an interruptive auditory stimulus or distraction device during conditioning sessions. An effective approach for the dog that is aggressive at the front door is to have the owner and dog inside with the pet on a leash with a head halter or muzzle. A person who is unfamiliar to the dog is asked to approach the front door from the yard, knock, and enter. As soon as the pet begins to show any sign of aggression, the owner stops the behavior with the sound of a shake can, air horn, or ultrasonic device. A bark-activated citronella spray collar should also provide immediate interruption for many dogs. At this point, the visitor stops and returns to the starting point. The visitor should continue making approaches until he can enter the home without the dog showing any sign of aggression. When this occurs, the owner should happily request that the dog sit for a very tasty food treat. This stage should be repeated several more times until the dog seems relaxed and looks forward to sitting for food as the visitor enters the home. At this point, the visitor should request the obedience response and toss the food to the pet. While this approach works well for many dogs, aggressive arousal could potentially increase if the owner does not have good control over the pet or if the stimulus is too strong. This method should not be used if there is any sign that the use of an interruptive device actually increases the arousal and aggressive behavior of the pet.

Punishment may help suppress the behavior in some dogs, but often has just the opposite effect. Harsh corrections with choke collars, pinch collars, and shock collars generally make the problem worse by associating pain with visitors or other animals. Also, the use of punishment may only suppress warning behaviors, such as growling and snarling, without actually making the pet less likely to bite. Castration or spaying is usually not successful in significantly suppressing these types of aggression.

Prevention

Adequate early socialization and early obedience training can reduce or eliminate territorial and protective aggression in dogs. Owners should be encouraged to take control over their dogs by establishing a strong leadership position for themselves when the pet is young. Veterinarians should strongly recommend obedience training, puppy parties, and other ways for dogs to interact with people in an appropriate manner during the early months of life. However, it is true that some breeds and certain individuals are genetically more territorial and more difficult to control. These dogs require even more socialization and training, not punishment. Dogs, especially those from guard dog breeds, have a high likelihood of developing territorial aggression problems if they are inadequately socialized and left for long periods unattended in the yard behind a fence or on a tie down.

Case example

A five-year-old, neutered male German Shepherd Dog named Rufus was presented for aggressively barking and lunging at visitors who entered the home. Rufus had not bitten anyone because the owner always had firm control with a leash. After the visitor entered, Rufus was banished to the basement or backyard. When the owner was at work, he was confined in the backyard where he spent most of the day lunging and barking at passersby at the fence line.

The owner was told to keep Rufus indoors to eliminate the daily displays of territorial aggression, and to review obedience training using tasty food rewards. A distraction/counterconditioning exercise was set up to discourage undesirable aggressive displays and replace them with acceptable social behavior. The exercises involved having a visitor approach the front door, knock, and enter. The owner had Rufus under control in the entryway, using a leash and head halter. Each time the visitor approached and the pet responded with any aggressive behavior, it was interrupted with a loud blast from a compressed air horn, at which time the visitor would go back to the starting point in the front yard. Each time the exercise was repeated, the dog waited longer before starting the aggression, and the intensity of the aggression gradually decreased. Once the visitor was able to enter the home and stand for 60 seconds without any sign of aggression from the pet, Rufus was asked in a happy tone to sit for a tasty food reward. This stage of the exercise was repeated until the dog appeared relaxed and automatically sat and looked to the owner for food as the visitor entered. The next stage involved having the visitor give the command to sit and the food reward after entering. Following this, the exercise was repeated with a wide variety of people of differing appearance.

PREDATORY AGGRESSION

Predation is a normal instinct in dogs. It is in their nature to chase and hunt prey. However, when this instinct is directed toward people and domestic animals, it causes problems that need to be corrected.

Predatory behavior involves stalking, chasing, catching, biting, killing, and eating. Domestic dogs may go through the whole sequence or may stop at any stage. Predatory behaviors may be stimulated by the movement of joggers, cyclists, playing children, or moving automobiles. The strongly inherent desire of some breeds to chase and herd may also be a component of the predatory drive. Auditory stimuli, such as the cries and screams of babies or young children, may also elicit a predatory response. Predation is not preceded by threats because it represents a normal instinct to hunt and kill, during which the performance of warning or threat behavior would be counterproductive. This aspect, along with the fact that killing and feeding are parts of this behavior, can make it an extremely dangerous problem.

Diagnosis and prognosis

Predatory aggression may be exhibited by dogs of either sex and any age. A quickly moving stimulus is the usual target. The response of the dog is to chase, bite, and potentially kill its perceived prey. Pre-attack vocalization by single dogs is rare, but is not uncommon by a group of dogs. Dogs that show an extremely unwavering focus directed toward the movements or vocali-

zations of a baby should be suspect and watched very closely. In some dogs, counterconditioning, punishment, and aversion therapy are effective, but not in others. Dogs in a group may exhibit intense chasing and predation in situations where they may have done little or no chasing when on their own (e.g., to children).

The prognosis is quite variable. The manifestation of a high arousal level, a strong focus on the prey object, and difficulty in distracting the dog during the behavior all suggest a poor prognosis. Since this is an instinctive behavior, it is difficult to override in many cases. Correcting dogs that chase and kill game animals is typically more difficult than correcting dogs that chase cars. Regardless of the chances for eventual correction, if a dog attempts to prey upon people or pets the prognosis for safe correction should be considered guarded to poor.

Management

Punishment, desensitization, and counterconditioning techniques are considerations for therapy of dogs that chase moving targets, including joggers, cyclists, and playing children (Fig. 19.19). An owner with very good control may be able to prevent or interrupt the behavior with training commands, distraction, or punishment devices. To be effective, the punishment must be considered aversive and the dog must associate the punishments with its predatory actions. Do not underestimate the extent of punishment necessary to curb this instinctive behavior. Dogs will repeatedly attack porcupines and skunks, regardless of the consequences, because this trait is so strongly instinctive and difficult to

> **Managing predatory aggression:**
> * Identify all stimuli that elicit the behavior
> * Deny exposure to any stimuli that elicit the behavior, except during training
> * Keep confined or under complete owner control
> * Obedience training, concentrating on reward cues and owner control
> * Use desensitization and counterconditioning to change the pet's response to prey stimuli
> * Consider remote punishment

Figure 19.19

override. In some cases, the predatory instinct is so strong that it cannot be suppressed, regardless of the training technique. Although remote shock collars may be more successful than other corrections, their use can cause other problems and should be avoided if at all possible.

For some dogs exhibiting predatory aggression, the only sure way to prevent the behavior is to keep the animal strictly confined. Walks should only be taken with a lead and halter. The use of a muzzle should also be considered. Continuous outdoor supervision under full control is obligatory. The owners must understand that if the dog gets loose, it may cause injuries for which they have full liability.

Prevention

Predatory aggression is difficult to prevent because it is an instinctive behavior. The fact is that some dogs are born with more predatory drive than others. Obedience training is a must, and may be sufficient for the dog with mild to moderate predatory instincts. These dogs should always be on a lead when outside. Young dogs should not be encouraged to chase squirrels and other small animals.

Case example

Emma, a three-year-old, female mixed breed dog, was presented for attacking a young female cat which had recently been adopted by the family. The cat was about one-third the size of Emma, who had a history of frequently chasing and occasionally killing small wild mammals in the backyard. The first attempt to introduce the two pets to each other resulted in Emma immediately rushing to the cat without warning, grabbing it in her mouth, and shaking it. The owners intervened without delay to save the cat. They attempted to reintroduce the two on the following day by carrying the cat into the room with the dog. As soon as Emma saw the cat, she immediately lunged and attempted to grasp the frightened cat out of the owner's arms.

Because of the dog's history of predatory behavior, the quickness of intense attack beha-

vior and lack of warning, the owners were urged to place the cat in another home. Although they were hesitant to do so, after another attack (and a large bill from the veterinary emergency clinic), they agreed.

PAIN-INDUCED AND IRRITABLE AGGRESSION

All veterinarians are aware of pain-induced aggression, even in the most sociable and docile animals. Any handling that elicits pain or discomfort can lead to this type of aggression. A similar problem is irritable aggression, which refers to any medical condition that might not cause pain but does increase irritability and therefore aggression (or retreat) during approach or handling. Metabolic disorders such as liver disease or renal disease, endocrine disorders, CNS disorders, sensory decline, or perhaps even a lack of sleep might lead to irritable aggression. Because pain monitoring is such a subjective assessment, it may be difficult to accurately separate irritable from pain-induced aggression (i.e., does the dog have dental pain, arthritis, or even a headache, or is it more irritable due to its illness?). Handling or the anticipation of handling (approach, reaching) might lead to this type of aggression. This can happen when an individual attempts to manipulate a painful area, even if that manipulation is just patting, grooming, or applying medication. This problem may also occur if a dog's ear is pulled or when its tail is stepped on. The presence of pain may lower the threshold for the manifestation of other types of aggression, such as fear or dominance-related aggression.

The use of physical punishment can also lead to pain and discomfort and any resultant aggression could be pain-induced aggression, fear or defensive aggression, dominance aggression, or any combination of these types. Therefore, physical punishment should not be used as it may lead to a conditioned fear response, which may manifest itself as aggression during similar types of handling or approach in the future.

Diagnosis and prognosis

The diagnosis is usually not difficult. When the dog with a painful area is touched or anticipates being hurt, it reacts aggressively. The dog might growl or bite people who seem intent on causing it pain, or may redirect its aggression to a more subordinate individual or the person restraining the pet. Similarly, pets with a variety of medical conditions from endocrine imbalances to infections may display irritable aggression when approached or handled. Therefore a medical workup would be the first step for most aggressive cases. If the dog perceives that biting accomplished its goals (i.e., stopped the pain or interaction), it might use aggression when similar situations arise in the future, whether or not the pain is still present. Thus, the situation must be corrected so that routine care such as nail trimming, home dental care, medicating, and grooming can be accomplished without triggering aggressive episodes.

Management

Ideally, if the dog is in pain or ill, it would be best not to manipulate the area and cause further pain and to use appropriate pain management and medical therapy to treat any underlying problems. However, this is not always possible, especially when medications may need to be applied to a painful area, or physical therapy utilized. Thus, the approach must be to treat the pain, avoid eliciting further pain, and employ desensitization and counterconditioning exercises to increase the dog's tolerance to being handled (Fig. 19.20).

Prevention

The best way to prevent pain-induced aggression is to anticipate it and handle the dog in such a way that pain does not occur or is minimized. Handling exercises that are performed when the pet is a puppy may help increase the individual's tolerance to being handled when it is experiencing pain. These can be done at dinner time. While the puppy is being hand fed, the

> **Managing pain-induced aggression:**
> * Eliminate, reduce, or control the pain, illness, or disease
> * Adjust the treatment approach so it is more tolerable
> * Be patient and gentle when handling the dog and consider muzzling for protection
> * Promote owner control with training
> * Desensitization and counterconditioning to gradually accustom the dog to handling the sore area
> * Avoid any type of painful punishment

Figure 19.20

owner can handle all parts of its body. As days go by, the intensity and variety of handling should increase. Grooming and nail trimming should occur during these exercises. Although it is not possible to anticipate the effects of all painful stimuli, the dog that is trained to be handled, have its claws trimmed, its teeth brushed, and its anal sacs expressed (without complaint) will also be more likely to tolerate handling when it is in more severe pain.

Case example

Babe was a five-year-old Labrador Retriever with recurring painful ear problems. Over the past year, she had progressively become more and more irritable when treated at home by the owner. Two days ago she had bitten the owner who had lifted Babe's ear to instill medication.

Recommendations were made to address the problem on two fronts. Babe was sent to a dermatologist for further evaluation of the recurrent ear problem and the owner was instructed in behavioral modification techniques for allowing access to the ears.

The owner was counseled about paying closer attention to the ears so that cleaning and treatment were begun before the problem reached a painful stage. She was told to say 'hold still' in a happy tone and give a meat reward many times each day. Between treatments, she was instructed to touch the ears frequently in a very gentle manner, and say 'hold still' in a very happy tone as she gave the food reward. Eventually, 'hold still' became a secondary reinforcer that could be used to reduce the pet's apprehension during ear treatments. The handling exercises gradually changed from simple, gentle handling to handling that closely approximated actual ear treatments until the owner was able to treat the ears with no problem.

PLAY AGGRESSION

Play aggression is a normal behavior in young dogs that needs to be constrained because of potential danger to family members and other pets, and because it can be downright annoying when the pet is out of control. A very large portion of canine play involves aggressive behaviors, such as growling, biting, bumping, and attacking. If the dog is rowdy, engages in a lot of heavy physical contact, and bites without inhibition, it becomes a problem for the family and visitors. Uncontrolled play poses significant danger to young children and adults with fragile skin. While play can be very vigorous and physical, young pups usually learn at an early age that hard bites and overwhelmingly exuberant play with littermates cause play to stop. The same rules must be taught to the house pet. Puppies without training that do not get adequate amounts of exercise and mental stimulation are the most likely to become a problem.

Diagnosis and prognosis

Play aggression is typically seen in puppies and young dogs and is accompanied by playful postures and behaviors. A classic play-soliciting behavior is the *play bow*. The dog will present its front end or side toward the person or animal with which it wants to play. The front part of the body is down and low to the ground, the rear end up and the tail wagging rapidly in a relaxed manner. The dog may quickly dart forward and back, barking and thrusting its muzzle toward the target. Vocalizations tend to be higher pitched than the growls and barking associated with more serious types of aggression. Play attacks can involve very spontaneous attacks and hard bites which can be quite disconcerting, as well as damaging. Mouthing and biting that achieve a goal of soliciting play or maintaining

control of a resource can escalate into an aggression that is akin to dominance-related aggression. However in these dogs the puppy has learned through play that aggressive displays can successfully achieve goals which have desirable consequences.

This behavior can mimic dominance-related, conflict-related, possessive, protective, and predatory forms of aggression. Prolonged, deep-tone growling associated with staring and stiff body postures may indicate that the behavior is more serious than simple play aggression, especially when this occurs in competitive situations or when the pet does not want to be disturbed. While play attacks can be very spontaneous, almost all other types of aggressive attacks occur in response to specific stimuli that are provoking to the dog. If anything other than play-related aggression is occurring, quick intervention is extremely important to prevent the emergence of a dangerous behavior problem.

The prognosis for correction is good for a puppy living with a family that will provide consistent training and implement a program that will satisfy the pet's needs for mental stimulation and sufficient physical exercise. Prognosis for safe resolution is guarded for active, assertive puppies that get little exercise or training, who also live with families that have young, active children and poor adult supervision.

Management

Play aggression can be effectively managed with exercise, obedience training, and behavioral modification (Fig. 19.21). The more exercise the puppy receives, the less energy it will have to expend on rowdy behavior. Long walks and games of fetch should be provided several times daily. Setting up regular play sessions with another social, active young dog may be helpful. Puppies can learn obedience commands as early as seven to eight weeks of age, so training should begin shortly after the puppy is brought into the home. The puppy should be enrolled in a formal puppy class at eight to ten weeks of age, and then in adult classes during adolescence. When the owner has trained the

Step	Comments
Satisfy the pet's needs	• Provide plenty of vigorous exercise • Provide interactive toys for mental stimulation • Use toys and games, such as fetch and soccer, to channel the puppy's energy in a positive direction
Promote owner leadership and control	• Enroll in socialization and training classes as early as eight to ten weeks of age. Enroll in a second class before one year of age • Begin leadership exercises early (sit before getting anything, stay before following the owner, avoid pushy attention-soliciting behaviors)
Training and physical control	• The puppy should be command trained to a point that it will settle down on command (see Fig. 5.13, handout #23 on the CD) • Head halters will give all family members, even young children, control over the dog • Have the pet wear a leash in the home that it can drag around so that the owner can grab it for quick control when necessary • In the yard, the pet can drag a 20-ft line so a family member can quickly grab it for control • Muzzles may be helpful in some situations
Avoid	• Tug of war and teasing • Wearing gloves and allowing the pet to bite hard
Playbiting	• Correct playbiting by using a quick, short, startling verbal reprimand followed by redirecting the pup's attention to other types of play
Interruptions and distractions	• A shake can, water gun, or sharp 'no!' may be helpful • Toys stuffed with biscuits and frozen food items (cheese and kibble, mashed potatoes, etc.) may help keep the pet's mouth on appropriate items instead of family members
Time out	• Confine the pet away from family members during periods when they cannot effectively deal with the behavior • Toys stuffed with food may work to keep it quiet in time out
Punishment	• Don't do it • Hitting, thumping the nose, scruff shakes, ramming a fist into the mouth, harsh alpha roll overs, or other forms of physical punishment may make the play problem worse or cause other problems

Figure 19.21 Steps in the management of canine play aggression.

puppy to respond to commands reliably, it can be controlled in a variety of situations.

Hitting the puppy on the nose, squeezing the gums against the teeth, scruff shakes, harsh alpha roll overs, or other forms of physical punishment that the owner might use in an attempt to gain control should be discouraged. These techniques are generally not successful and may lead to other problems such as handshyness and fear aggression.

Prevention

Play aggression can be effectively prevented by providing adequate exercise, mental stimulation, appropriate socialization, and early obedience training. Exercise is very important, and vigorous exercise should be encouraged several times during the day. On bad weather days, the puppy can be exercised at its dinner time. Two family members can go to opposite ends of a long hallway, each taking half of the pet's dinner. The pup is then called back and forth between the family members to sit for a piece of dinner kibble. This is a great game for the pet because it provides exercise, social interaction, obedience training (sit and come), and teaches the pet to come up to people and sit instead of jumping up on them. The more opportunity the puppy has to burn off excess energy, the less likely it will be that the owner will have problems with play aggression. See Chapter 3 for more information on working with new puppies and kittens, as well as socialization and habituation. For a client handout on the control of play biting, see Figure 19.22 (handout #20 on the CD).

Case example

Simon was a four-month-old Standard Poodle presented for biting his owners. Both of the owners spent long hours at work. Simon's only opportunity to exercise was when he was let out into the backyard. The husband would often tease the puppy with a towel and Simon would respond by lunging at the towel and occasionally at the owner's hand. In the evening, the puppy would come up to the owners, bark, lunge, and nip at any available body part. Attempts at verbal and physical discipline only seemed to aggravate the situation.

Puppy training and socialization classes were suggested. Daily long walks were advised and the owners were taught how to teach Simon to play fetch. The husband was told to stop engaging the puppy in all biting games. Any attempts at nipping and biting were to be treated by ignoring the puppy or walking away until he calmed down. A variety of toys were kept on hand at all times to distract the puppy into acceptable behavior. The owners were not happy with what they considered a slow rate of progress, but with some encouragement they persevered in their efforts. Although they resented having to change their approach to satisfy Simon, after three weeks they were happy with the results.

MATERNAL AGGRESSION

Maternal aggression refers to aggressive behavior directed toward people or other animals that approach the bitch with her puppies. All mothers have protective instincts concerning their offspring. The amount of aggression that is shown may be quite variable. Some exhibit only mild growling and threatening, while others may attack and injure without warning. Bitches that experience pseudocyesis (false pregnancy) may also display maternal aggression despite the lack of puppies. The well trained and socialized bitch is most likely to allow her puppies to be handled, especially by trusted family members.

Diagnosis and prognosis

The diagnosis is not difficult. The animal is a newly whelped bitch or one with pseudocyesis. She barks, growls, or attempts to bite humans or other animals that approach the puppies, puppy surrogates (e.g., toys), or nest area.

The prognosis is good and there is usually spontaneous remission as the puppies age. Behavioral modification can be used if the puppies need to be handled while the mother is still very protective.

Management

Some bitches are more protective than others, and gentle handling by trusted family members is the best way to allay apprehension. It is best to minimize handling of the puppies during the first few days when the bitch tends to be most protective.

Since the problem usually is self-limiting, avoidance may be the safest and most practical strategy. Muzzling the bitch before the puppies are approached and handled may be necessary when she is most likely to be aggressive. Desensitization and counterconditioning should be helpful for future pregnancies, but may not be successful soon enough when conditioning does not begin until after the pet gives birth (Fig. 19.23).

Prevention

The best way to prevent maternal aggression is to have bitches ovariohysterectomized (spayed) before their first heat. This prevents actual maternal aggression as well as that resulting from pseudocyesis. In breeding animals, extensive socialization, handling, and obedience training starting at an early age are the best ways to minimize the risks of maternal aggression.

PUPPY MOUTHING, NIPPING, AND BITING – BITE INHIBITION AND TEACHING OFF

Bite inhibition
1. No hard bites or pressure.
   (a) When the puppy is calm, place your hand in its mouth and praise it when it mouths softly.
   (b) Give an immediate, loud 'ouch!' whenever the puppy applies too much pressure, and stop playing with it. Once the puppy ceases, you can give it an alternative form of play or attention (e.g., chew toy, exercise session, training session) or a settle exercise (see our settle exercise handout), and reward the desirable behavior.
2. Mild attempts at deterring the puppy and physically discouraging the puppy can actually serve to increase the intensity of play and biting.
3. Gentle mouthing as a form of play is OK, but it should not be initiated by the puppy, and the family must be able to stop it on command. Any hard biting or overexuberant play must be discouraged.
4. Avoid tug of war if the pet becomes too excited, aggressive, or out of control. Tug of war games should only be allowed when you have initiated them and when you can quickly stop the game on command with an ouch, give, or drop command.
5. If the puppy is constantly demanding attention through mouthing and biting or is overexuberant in its play, then it is likely not receiving sufficient stimulation. You should consider additional or longer periods of play, training, and exercise, and more outlets for chewing to pre-empt the puppy's unacceptable play biting.
6. If the puppy cannot be quickly calmed and settled, then confining it away from the target (e.g., children, visitors) until it settles may be necessary. When the puppy is calm it can then be released, and encouraged to play in an appropriate manner.
7. For those problems that cannot be quickly and effectively controlled with bite inhibition techniques, a leash and head halter can be left attached when the puppy is with the family. Mouthing or biting can be immediately stopped with a pull on the leash, with tension released as soon as the puppy settles. The leash and head halter can also be used to teach the off command by first giving the command and if the puppy does not immediately cease, pulling the hand back and guiding the dog into the proper response with a pull on the leash.
8. For some puppies in some homes, all forms of hard mouthing and play biting may be unacceptable. This may be the case when there are elderly or young children in the home.

Teaching off
The purpose of this command is to get the puppy to stop mouthing or playbiting on command.
Procedure:
1. Present a piece of food to get the pet's attention, say 'OK' in a friendly tone of voice and give the food.
2. Present another piece of food and say 'off' in a firm tone of voice, but don't yell.
   (a) If the puppy doesn't make contact with your hand or the food for two seconds, say 'OK' and give up the food.
   (b) If the puppy touches your hand before the two seconds pass and before you say 'OK,' immediately yell 'off' loud enough to make the puppy back away without frightening it. Be dramatic, lean toward the pup, make eye contact, and give a forceful command.
   (c) Repeat, gradually increasing the time the puppy has to wait.
3. Once the pup learns to back away from food on command, practice the above exercise using only your hand. Later, repeat the exercise when the puppy is in more excited moods.
4. Work toward the puppy not taking food, or touching your hand, no matter how tasty the treat or how your hand is moving, once you have said 'off.'
5. You must practice every day to attain a dependable response

Figure 19.22 Bite inhibition and teaching off (handout #20 – reprintable from the CD).

Step	Comments
Prebirth preparation	• Provide adequate socialization, training, and handling experiences. Begin when the female is a puppy • Discourage excessive territorial displays • Address any behavior issues that involve guarding behavior • Don't use punishment
Control the environment	• Provide a quiet, low-stress environment with a door that can be secured when visitors are in the home • Postpone remodeling, home repairs, parties, and other situations that might be upsetting for the mother • Minimize the number of visitors • Avoid eliciting the aggression by minimizing approach and handling of puppies
Take control of the mother	• Review obedience training using reward training
Desensitization and counterconditioning	• Use controlled conditioning sessions to teach the pet to be comfortable with people approaching it
Safety	• Use a leash and head halter, or muzzle as needed
Drug therapy for pseudocyesis	• Mibolerone, megoesterol acetate, cabergoline (see Ch. 6 for details)

Figure 19.23   Steps in the management of canine maternal aggression.

Case example

The owner of Helga, a two-year-old intact female Rottweiler, reported that her dog had been acting aggressively when visitors were present since giving birth to six healthy puppies three weeks ago. Helga showed mild signs of agitation when the doorbell rang, then growled and barked when she saw the visitor. Prior to this she had been friendly to visitors and never exhibited any sign of aggression. This was the pet's first litter.

The owners were told to keep the dog's environment as quiet as possible and limit the number of visitors. Desensitization and counterconditioning exercises were recommended to change the response to the doorbell. First, the doorbell was muffled until it was barely audible and elicited no aggressive arousal from the pet. Then, the owners would ring the bell and give Helga a small chunk of canned dog food. The exercise was repeated until the dog showed signs of happily anticipating food whenever the bell was rung. Gradually, the loudness of the bell was increased. The next step was to have friends quietly visit in an area of the home that was farthest from the dog. During the visit, a family member would accompany the dog and give a small portion of canned food every time it was alerted by visitors' voices at the other end of the house but did not act aggressively.

REDIRECTED AGGRESSION

Redirected aggression occurs when aggressive behavior is directed to a person or object that is not the stimulus for the aggressive arousal. The most common example is the situation in which a person is bitten while trying to break up a dog fight. In this case, the aggression becomes redirected from the original target to a person who did not initiate the aggression. The target is therefore an 'innocent bystander' who gets caught up in an aggressive act.

Diagnosis and prognosis

The diagnosis of redirected aggression is usually not difficult. The history suggests victim interference when the dog was threatened or fighting. The dog growls or bites a nearby person or pet who was not the original target. Males or females may exhibit this type of problem and it is more common in adult pets.

The prognosis is good for cases in which there have been few incidents, bites have been inhibited, and the underlying motivation for aggressive arousal can be controlled. Prognosis is generally guarded to poor for dogs that manifest an exceptionally high level of aggressive arousal in social or territorial situations, and where the owner has very little verbal control. These are usually dogs that become so focused on the stimuli that it is next to impossible to distract them or get their attention.

Management

It is important to educate owners in detail about the nature of the problem so that they can avoid interfering with the pet when there is a realistic chance of getting bitten (Fig. 19.24). Treatment requires a clear understanding of the problem, and identification of all stimuli that might arouse the dog and lead to aggression. It is important to treat underlying causes of aggressive arousal such as territorial aggression, fear-related aggression, social aggression, and predatory aggression. The use of desensitization and counterconditioning to change the pet's response to stimuli that elicit aggression is the behavioral modification approach of choice. Owner control of the pet is important, as is anticipation and avoidance of stimuli that arouse it.

Prevention

The best ways to prevent redirected aggression are to socialize the pet adequately when it is young, establish control through early obedience training, and treat any type of aggression as soon as it appears. Owners should be cautioned not to intervene in aggressive situations. Good handling and training skills should allow the owner to control the dog safely before an aggressive episode occurs. In early cases, situations that lead to high arousal states can be prevented from getting worse by using desensitization and counterconditioning (see Ch. 5).

Case example

A young couple owned a neutered, male German Shepherd Dog cross that weighed 35 kg. The dog spent each day in a fenced backyard while the owners were at work. Their home was on a corner lot and the dog spent most of the day barking at various noises and movements in the neighborhood. He charged the fence line and lunged aggressively at most of the passersby just outside the fence.

One day, the husband was talking to a friend who was standing on the other side of the fence when the dog charged out of the house, ran to

Step	Comments
Avoid the problem	• Prevent exposure to stimuli by confinement or avoiding situations that elicit aggressive arousal • Avoid physical contact with the pet when it is aroused
Treat underlying problems	• Identify stimuli and situations that trigger aggression • Desensitize and countercondition the pet's response to these stimuli
Training, calming, and controlling the pet	• Review obedience training until the owner has complete control of the pet in all situations and in the presence of all strong distractions • The dog should be trained to settle and focus on the owners on command (see Fig. 5.13, handout #23) independent of the stimuli before being exposed to the stimuli • Place a leash and head halter or muzzle on the dog when stimulus exposure is likely • Use a muzzle as necessary
Distract	• Sometimes, a pet's attention can be diverted away from the stimulus with an auditory stimulus (e.g., horn, whistle, shake can)
Drug therapy	• Depends on underlying cause – anxiolytic drugs or selective serotonin re-uptake inhibitors may be a consideration

Figure 19.24   The management of canine redirected aggression.

the fence, and aggressively lunged toward the neighbor. The owner reached for the dog and grabbed it by the scruff of the neck. The dog turned and bit the owner's wrist, causing two deep lacerations. Prior to this incident, the pet had no history of exhibiting aggression toward either of the owners.

The cause of the bite was redirected aggression. The stimulus for the high state of aggression was the visitor. When the attack was thwarted, the pet's aggressive energy was directed to the owner's arm. The underlying problem was territorial aggression. Since territorial aggression is somewhat of a self-reinforcing behavior, it was desirable to stop the frequent displays of aggression that occurred throughout the day. The owners were instructed not to allow the dog in the backyard unsupervised and to confine it to the basement when they were not at home. The owners were encouraged to enroll in obedience training to give them more control of the pet. Desensitization and counterconditioning exercises were recommended to decrease the pet's high arousal state when it saw someone (see section on territorial aggression). A head halter was used to reduce the likelihood of an injury occurring during training exercises and to ensure control of the dog during periods of high arousal. A decrease in territorial aggression was noted within two weeks, and within six months the territorial aggressive displays could be controlled or minimized in the owner's presence.

INTRASPECIES AGGRESSION

Dogs can be aggressive toward other dogs for many of the same reasons that they exhibit aggression toward people. Aggression toward unfamiliar dogs might be fear induced (perhaps related in part to inadequate socialization), territorial, possessive, redirected, etc., and these are discussed under these headings in the text.

Within a household, dogs generally work out their hierarchy with a minimum of injury. However, with some forms of aggression and when there is a size or strength disparity

between dogs, injuries may occur and behavioral modification is necessary. Dogs that have not received adequate social contact with other members of the species during early sensitive periods of development may never reliably get along with other dogs.

Situations in which fights are most likely to occur are usually either competitive in nature (e.g., food, toys, resting area, access to a family member) or ones in which there is high arousal (e.g., greetings, territorial barking, running through the home, exiting through a door into the yard).

Diagnosis and prognosis

Intermale aggression

Male–male aggression often results from hormonally driven competition, but dominance issues or fear may also play a role. The behavior is usually first evident in males at one to three years of age and they may respond by barking, growling, and attempting to bite other male dogs they encounter. Dominant, submissive, or fear postures may be exhibited, depending on the motivation for the aggressive behavior. The prognosis is fair and treatment may involve surgery, behavioral modification, and drug therapy. The prognosis is guarded for males that will not be neutered and for males that show the problem after they are neutered.

Interfemale aggression

Female–female aggression problems usually involve two females in the same home. Typically, the behavior is first seen in intact bitches between one and three years of age. Females show the same posturing and vocal responses as described for male–male aggression. In most cases, the problem results from an unstable social hierarchy. The condition is sometimes hormonally driven and may worsen during estrus and pseudocyesis, but that is not always the case. Fighting between female dogs in the same household can be very difficult to safely correct. Fights are often very intense, bites may be completely uninhibited, and severe injuries are common.

The prognosis is guarded to fair and treatment may involve behavioral modification, drugs, and sometimes surgery. In general, female–female aggression among pets in the same household is more difficult to resolve than male–male aggression.

Social status aggression

Another form of intraspecies aggression is seen when two or more dogs inhabit the same house and have nearly equal social status. This competition is usually resolved without injury as the dogs sort out the social hierarchy through social posturing and minor skirmishes, but not in all cases. The problem may also result when clear differences in the social status of two dogs exist, but the dominant animal is inappropriate and excessive in using aggression to socially control the other dog. Similarly, the submissive animal may respond with overly fearful displays that cause the more dominant dog to proceed further with the aggression.

Competitive aggression is usually most intense when food, resting areas, highly desirable chew items, or owner attention is involved. Competitive rivalry can be successfully resolved if a stable dominance hierarchy can be established amongst all the dogs in the household. A very strong leadership role for the owners in respect to all dogs is extremely important.

Social status among dogs can change when:

- A new dog is introduced to the household.
- A family dog returns from surgery, boarding, or vacation.
- A dominant animal becomes ill, aged, or dies.
- A younger dog matures and challenges a dominant individual.
- A human family member leaves the home.

Management

Advanced cases of intraspecies aggression can be very difficult and frustrating problems to control. The owners need to be sufficiently educated about canine social behavior and committed to training (Fig. 19.25). The goal of training is for the owners to gain sufficient control over both dogs that they no longer exhibit any inappropriate behavior toward each other. This can be achieved through reward-based training as well as desensitization and counterconditioning to stimuli and situations in which aggressive displays might arise. In addition, it may be necessary to help support the pack hierarchy so that the dogs can interact appropriately even when the owner is not present. This would involve identifying which dog is the most likely to be dominant in the relationship and then discouraging the subordinate from challenging the dominant and encouraging it to defer. Coming to the aid of, or supporting, the subordinate member of the relationship may encourage challenges to the dominant dog if it knows that it will receive the aid and attention of the owners. In some cases it is the more dominant dog that does not recognize or properly respond to subordinate and deference signals, and these dogs must be taught to cease their challenges or aggressive displays as soon as the other dog submits. A leash and head halter or a basket muzzle may be necessary to properly supervise and control the interactions of one or both dogs awhile avoiding any possibility of injury.

Choosing which dog to support may be obvious from observation of the dogs when they interact with each other (especially when away from the owners). Entering and leaving the home through doorways, body postures and positioning during play and eating, and determining whether one dog defers to the other can be helpful in determining which position to support for each dog. In some cases it may be necessary to support the younger dog

Method	Rationale
Neuter	• Neutering males may reduce intermale fighting • Spaying may eliminate hormonally driven interfemale aggression
Re-establish stable hierarchy with family members in control of both dogs	• Dogs usually coexist peacefully within their own hierarchy. If the problems only occur in the owner's presence, the owner's actions that incite or reinforce the problem must be identified • The initial goal is for owners to have sufficient control of both dogs when they are at home so that the dogs respond appropriately when the owners are present. Each dog should be trained separately to respond immediately to commands to settle or focus on the owners. Then training should progress to a point where each pet will sit, stay, and settle reliably so that attention can be given to each dog individually while the other remains in place • Family members should control access to everything the pets want by first requiring a response to an obedience command. The pets should also be required to stay and wait for a release command before being allowed to follow family members around the home. During retraining, the dogs are not allowed to obtain social attention by being pushy or assertive with family members • Once the family members have sufficient control of each dog, the interdog relationship should be reaffirmed by determining which dog is most likely to be able to maintain dominance and teaching the subordinate to defer to the dominant and follow the dominant. Any owner actions that encourage or support the subordinate to challenge the more dominant must be discouraged. Owners must also ensure that the dominant dog ceases its aggression as soon as the subordinate signals are given • If accurate determination of the dominant dog is not possible, then both dogs should be treated as subordinate to all family members, effectively bumping them both down the hierarchy a few notches. Consistent leadership exercises, command responses, and control of resources tend to focus the pets more on family members and less on each other. This also tends to reduce reactivity and impulsivity
Separation and confinement	• If the risk of injury is very high whenever the pets are together, they will have to initially be separated as conditioning begins • Confinement areas should be set up so that the pets are unable to posture aggressively toward each other through windows, doors, or gates
Avoid all potentially aggressive situations	• Identify all situations in which the aggression occurs so that the possibility of conflicts and competition can be minimized • Feed the dogs in different parts of the house or on tie downs • Do not allow the dogs to greet visitors or family members excitedly together. Teach them to sit and stay quietly during greetings • Do not allow the dogs to run the fence line aggressively together. Block access to windows where the pets demonstrate territorial aggression • Deny free access to highly desirable objects for which the pets might compete (rawhide, bones) • The owner should have very strict control over the pets when giving them attention by using repeated sit, down, and stay commands so there is no nudging or posturing for position
Safety	• Use control devices such as leashes and head halters or muzzles to ensure that no family members or pets are injured
Exercise	• Large amounts of aerobic exercise can have a calming effect • Unless the problem is very severe, most family dogs are less likely to show aggression toward each other when walked on a lead, so this presents an optimum time to begin building the bond between the pets • Using head halters, two family members can walk the dogs with the people in between and the dogs on the outside. Next, they are walked with one dog on the outside and the other between the family members. Finally, the dogs are walked together between the family members. The dogs should be required to sit/stay at a safe distance when waiting to cross streets

Figure 19.25   Steps in the management of canine intraspecies aggression.

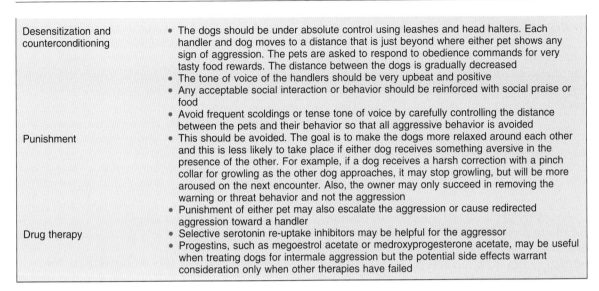

Desensitization and counterconditioning	• The dogs should be under absolute control using leashes and head halters. Each handler and dog moves to a distance that is just beyond where either pet shows any sign of aggression. The pets are asked to respond to obedience commands for very tasty food rewards. The distance between the dogs is gradually decreased • The tone of voice of the handlers should be very upbeat and positive • Any acceptable social interaction or behavior should be reinforced with social praise or food • Avoid frequent scoldings or tense tone of voice by carefully controlling the distance between the pets and their behavior so that all aggressive behavior is avoided
Punishment	• This should be avoided. The goal is to make the dogs more relaxed around each other and this is less likely to take place if either dog receives something aversive in the presence of the other. For example, if a dog receives a harsh correction with a pinch collar for growling as the other dog approaches, it may stop growling, but will be more aroused on the next encounter. Also, the owner may only succeed in removing the warning or threat behavior and not the aggression • Punishment of either pet may also escalate the aggression or cause redirected aggression toward a handler
Drug therapy	• Selective serotonin re-uptake inhibitors may be helpful for the aggressor • Progestins, such as megoestrol acetate or medroxyprogesterone acetate, may be useful when treating dogs for intermale aggression but the potential side effects warrant consideration only when other therapies have failed

Figure 19.25 *(continued)*

as it matures and becomes more dominant, and this can be difficult for owners to accept when the position of the long-time family friend is being usurped by the newcomer. On the other hand, there are cases in which the older dog is unwilling to yield its role as dominant and is still capable of maintaining its dominant position. It may be possible to re-establish the previous relationship if any underlying painful or medical problems can be controlled and when the owner is present the young dog can be discouraged from challenging the old dog. When the owner is not available to supervise, separation and prevention may be necessary.

The classical approach to treating intracanine aggression within the family by choosing an individual to promote can sometimes be problematic. The 'natural' or logical hierarchy may be difficult to accurately determine because of inadequate and misleading information from family members who are not accurate observers. Also, it is not uncommon for families to inadvertently reinforce social behaviors so that they occur out of context, making interpretation difficult. In some cases, the family may be reluctant to make a beloved older, longstanding member of the family defer to a young, assertive new addition. And lastly, care must be taken to avoid reinforcing 'bully dogs' that are assertive and hold their appropriate place at the top of the hierarchy, but are inappropriate and uninhibited in using aggression to maintain status or resources.

Prognosis

Although it has been suggested that most dogs work out their relationship without injury if the owners do not interfere, this may not always be the case. Inadequate early socialization with other dogs, marked differences in breed, size, and genetics between dogs, pain and medical conditions, and other forms of aggression (such as fear-induced and redirected) may prevent the dogs from being able to 'work things out without injury.' In these cases, it may be necessary to identify all possible interactions that might lead to aggression and prevent the problem when the owner is not around to supervise.

Prevention

Intraspecies aggression can, in part, be prevented by neutering dogs while they are not yet fully mature. This is most effective for intermale aggression but may also be helpful for interfemale aggression that is associated with estrous cycles. Some behaviorists believe that aggression may actually increase following ovariohysterectomy in a small subset of female dogs, but this is debatable and information needs to be collected from a larger number of animals to appraise this notion accurately.

The owner should begin developing obedience skills in puppyhood, so that all pets are under dependable verbal control. Care should be taken to ensure that all family pets are well socialized to other dogs throughout life, but especially during the first few months. Frequent social interaction with adult dogs and peers can help facilitate normal social communication. Dogs that have been well socialized and allowed to engage in a lot of interdog play as puppies are much less likely to do serious damage to another dog in a fight because they learn bite inhibition during play. They are very aware of the pain caused by a hard bite and are less likely to use excessive force in a hierarchical struggle. Taking a puppy away from its littermates and preventing interaction with other canids prior to six weeks of age may impede its ability for normal social interaction with other dogs throughout life. Owners should understand the concept of social hierarchies and be sure to be the dominant pack members.

Case example

Annie was a five-year-old spayed Dalmatian cross, adopted from the dog pound by her owner six months previously. The owner complained that although the dog acted fine with people, it became very aggressive every time it saw another dog of either sex. Aggressive lunges by the pet were so forceful that the owner was occasionally pulled off her feet.

To provide the owner with some control, Annie was fitted with a head halter and was taught to sit on command. Since the dog seemed to be able to recognize another dog at 45 m and became aggressive when it was within 22 m, the owner was told to take it for walks and look for other dogs that were at a distance of 22–45 m away. Every time it saw another dog at this dis-

tance and showed no signs of aggression, it was asked to sit for a very tasty food reward. The owner gradually performed the exercises closer and closer to other dogs until Annie was counterconditioned to be non-aggressive whenever she saw another dog. The owner was instructed to proceed sufficiently slowly in decreasing the distance between dogs during training, so that no aggressive responses would be elicited. If Annie did show any sign of aggression, the owner was instructed to give an immediate verbal correction, quickly turn around, and walk her pet away from the other dog.

OTHER FORMS OF AGGRESSION
Pathophysiological aggression

Pathophysiological aggressive disorders are those that have an underlying medical cause. These conditions may arise at any age, may have a sudden onset, and may not fit neatly into the other aggressive behavior categories already described. Many of these are described in Chapter 4, in the discussion of the medical examination, and some are reviewed under the French perspective in Chapter 21. Some of these are shown in Figure 19.26. In most cases, a combination of behavioral factors and medical problems is necessary for the aggression to be manifested clinically.

The treatment for pathophysiological aggression involves addressing and correcting the underlying problem. The prognosis for this type of aggression depends on response to medical treatment and is usually poorly managed by behavioral modification techniques alone.

Idiopathic aggression

A diagnosis of idiopathic aggression is reserved for those dogs that have had a complete medical workup and have been thoroughly assessed by a competent behavior consultant, with no identifiable stimulus or cause for the aggression found. Some cases of idiopathic aggression may represent unusual types of pathophysiological aggression for which the cause has not yet

Underlying cause	Example
Infectious agent	• Rabies
Endocrinopathy	• Hypothyroidism
Neurological disease	• Epilepsy, neurotransmitter/receptor alterations
Painful conditions	• Dental disease, otitis, arthritis, pancreatitis, wounds
Drug, toxic effects	• Undesirable effects of a therapeutic agent or toxicity
Neoplasia	• Effects of tumors on the brain region affected
Degenerative diseases	• Cognitive dysfunction
Other problems	• Sensory loss, fatigue

Figure 19.26 Some examples of pathophysiological causes of canine aggression.

been determined. Any cases of aggression for which a solid diagnosis cannot be made, or for which the stimuli for aggressive attacks cannot be ascertained, should be considered very dangerous. For most of these, euthanasia is the appropriate choice.

A specific category of idiopathic aggression, 'mental lapse syndrome,' was described by Dr Bonnie Beaver in 1980. A small number of cases have been reported in young adult dogs of popular breeds. Affected dogs seem to undergo a dramatic personality change between 18 months and two years of age, changing from amiable to aggressive. The aggressive incidents are sudden, dramatic, and seemingly unprovoked. Affected animals exhibit an abnormal electroencephalogram with a low-voltage fast activity pattern. The EEG pattern has been described to more closely resemble a wild animal than a domestic dog. It is a very dangerous type of aggression with no known treatment.

Learned aggression

Learned aggression can result from teaching dogs to be aggressive. However, it can just as easily result when other causes of aggression are unintentionally reinforced by the owner. For example, the owner who talks softly to the fearful dog that is growling is conditioning the growling behavior. A dog that growls and stops the owner from grooming it not only learns to control grooming sessions, but may generalize the behavior to control other interactions with the owner. In general, any time a dog's aggressive behavior results in removal or withdrawal of the stimulus, the behavior is further reinforced. In addition, dogs that are threatened or punished for aggressive displays can learn to associate pain or fear with the stimulus and become even more aggressive each time the situation recurs.

The problem is managed by first educating the owner about how to stop conditioning the behavior. Depending on the type of aggression, other considerations might include handling exercises, and desensitization and counterconditioning to correct the specific type of aggression that is being reinforced (e.g., fear, dominance-related, territorial, protective).

FURTHER READING

Beaver BV 1980 Mental lapse aggression syndrome. Journal of the American Animal Hospital Association 16(6):937–939

Beaver BV 1983 Clinical classification of canine aggression. Applied Animal Ethology 10:35–43

Beaver BV 1993 Profiles of dogs presented for aggression. Journal of the American Animal Hospital Association 29(6):564–569

Beaver BV 1994 Differential approach to aggression by dogs and cats. Veterinary Quarterly 16(Suppl 1):S48

Beaver BV 1999. Canine behavior: a guide for veterinarians. WB Saunders, Philadelphia, PA

Borchelt PL 1983 Aggressive behaviour of dogs kept as companion animals: classification and influence of sex, reproductive status and breed. Applied Animal Ethology 10:45–61

Borchelt PL, Voith VL 1996a Aggressive behavior in dogs and cats. In: Voith VL, Borchelt PL (eds) Readings in companion animal behavior. Veterinary Learning Systems, Trenton, NJ, p 217–229

Borchelt PL, Voith VL 1996b Dominance aggression in dogs. In: Voith VL, Borchelt PL (eds) Readings in companion animal behavior. Veterinary Learning Systems, Trenton, NJ, p 230–239

Cameron DB 1997 Canine dominance-associated aggression – concepts, incidence, and treatment in a private behavior practice. Applied Animal Behavioral Science 52(3&4):265–274

Christiansen FO, Bakken M, Braastad BO 2001 Social facilitation of predatory, sheep-chasing behaviour in Norwegian Elkhounds. Applied Animal Behavioral Science 72(2):105–114

Crowell-Davis SL 1991 Identifying and correcting human-directed dominance aggression of dogs. Veterinary Medicine 86(10):990–998

DeNapoli JS, Dodman NH, Shuster L et al 2000 Effect of dietary protein content and tryptophan supplementation on dominance aggression, territorial aggression, and hyperactivity in dogs. Journal of the American Veterinary Medical Association 217(4):504–508

Dodman NH, Miczek KA, Knowles K et al 1992 Phenobarbital-responsive episodic dyscontrol (rage) in dogs. Journal of the American Veterinary Medical Association 201(10):1580–1583

Feddersenpetersen D 1994 Reduction of aggressive behaviour in dogs. Praktische Tierarzt 75:104–108

Guy NC, Luescher UA, Dohoo SE et al 2001a Demographic and aggressive characteristics of dogs in a general veterinary caseload. Applied Animal Behavioral Science 74:15–28

Guy NC, Luescher UA, Dohoo SE et al 2001b Risk factors for dog bites to owners in a general veterinary caseload. Applied Animal Behavioral Science 74:29–42

Guy NC, Luescher UA, Dohoo SE et al 2001c A case series of biting dogs; characteristics of the dogs, their behaviour and their victims. Applied Animal Behavioral Science 74:43–57

Hopkins SG, Schubert TA, Hart BL 1976 Castration of adult male dogs: effects on roaming, aggression, urine marking and mounting. Journal of the American Veterinary Medical Association 168:1108–1110

Joby R, Jemmett JE, Miller ASH 1984 The control of undesirable behaviour in male dogs using megestrol acetate. Journal of Small Animal Practice 25(9):567–572

Landsberg GM 1990a A veterinarian's guide to the correction of dominance aggression. Canadian Veterinary Journal 31(2):121–124

Landsberg GM 1990b Diagnosing dominance aggression. Canadian Veterinary Journal 31(1):45–46

Luescher A 2001 Conflict-related aggression. Newsletter for the Society of Veterinary Behavior Technicians 1(1):8–9

Marder A 1989 Aggressive types. Managing canine aggression depends upon diagnosing the type involved. Pet Veterinarian November/December:8

Marder A 1990 Aggression Rx. Make a specific diagnosis and use specific management methods. Pet Veterinarian May/June:43–46

McKeown D, Luescher A 1988 Canine competitive aggression – a clinical case of 'sibling rivalry.' Canadian Veterinary Journal 29(4):395–396

Overall KL 1995 Sex and aggression. Canine Practice 20(2):16–18

Overall K 1997 Clinical behavioral medicine for small animals. Mosby, St Louis

Overall KL 1999a Understanding and treating canine dominance aggression: an overview. Veterinary Medicine 94(11):976–978

Overall KL 1999b Using avoidance and passive behavior modification to treat canine dominance aggression. Veterinary Medicine 94(11):981–982

Overall KL 1999c Teaching your aggressive dog deferential behavior. Veterinary Medicine 94(11):984–985

Overall KL 1999d The role of pharmacotherapy in treating dogs with dominance aggression. Veterinary Medicine 94(12):1049

Podberscek AL, Serpell JA 1998 Environmental influences on the expression of aggressive behavior in English Cocker-Spaniels. Applied Animal Behavioral Science 52(3&4):215–227

Polsky RH 1996 Recognizing dominance aggression in dogs. Veterinary Medicine 91(3):196

Reisner IR 1995 The biting dog: diagnosis, prognosis, and resolution of canine aggression: a case study. Presentation to the AVMA annual conference, July

Reisner IR 1997 Assessment, management, and prognosis of canine dominance-related aggression. Veterinary Clinics of North America, Small Animal Practice 27(3):479–496

Reisner IR, Erb HN, Houpt KA 1994 Risk factors for behaviour-related euthanasia among dominant-aggressive dogs: 110 cases (1989–1992). Journal of the American Veterinary Medical Association 205(6):855–863

Reisner IR, Mann JJ, Stanley M et al 1996 Comparison of cerebrospinal fluid monoamine metabolity levels in dominant-aggressive and nonaggressive dogs. Brain Research 714:1–2

Sacks JJ, Kresnow M, Houston B 1996 Dog bites: how big a problem? Injury Prevention 2:52–54

Uchida Y, Dodman N, Denapoli J et al 1997 Characterization and treatment of 20 canine dominance aggression cases. Journal of Veterinary Medical Science 59(5):397–399

Voith V 1982 Treatment of dominance aggression of dogs toward people. Modern Veterinary Practice 63:149–152

Voith VL, Borchelt PL 1982 Diagnosis and treatment of dominance aggression in dogs. Veterinary Clinics of North America, Small Animal Practice 12(4):655–663

White MM, Neilson JC, Hart BL et al 1999 Effects of clomipramine hydrochloride on dominance-related aggression in dogs. Journal of the American Veterinary Medical Association 215(9):1288–1291

Young MS 1982 Treatment of fear-induced aggression in dogs. Veterinary Clinics of North America, Small Animal Practice 12(4):645–653

20

Feline aggression

Aggression is the second most common feline behavior problem, next to housesoiling, referred to veterinary behavior consultants. In fact, most recently some behaviorists have reported that aggression may be surpassing housesoiling as the primary reason for referral, perhaps because practitioners are becoming more familiar with the diagnostic and treatment options so that housesoiling cases can be handled in their own practices. Aggressive cats are risky to have at home because they pose a significant danger to family and visitors. Problems can vary from the cat that hisses and avoids interaction to one that aggressively attacks. Owners with aggressive cats are thus in urgent need of advice on how to manage danger and correct this type of problem. Initially, they should be cautioned to avoid situations that are likely to trigger or exacerbate aggressive encounters until they receive appropriate counseling and fully understand the risks involved. Owners should be informed that

427

keeping an aggressive pet in the home always presents some risk. It should never be suggested that treatment will completely eliminate any chance for future injuries to occur.

In general, aggression refers to threatening or harmful behavior directed toward another individual or group. Aggression embraces a wide variety of behaviors from somewhat subtle body postures and facial expressions to violent attacks. This chapter will examine several different types of aggression, defined according to function, and how each can most successfully be prevented and managed. Although diagnostic considerations for each type of aggression may be clear-cut and straightforward, clinical cases of aggression may be multifactorial. As with every behavior case, it is essential that the veterinarian first assesses the cat's physical health to determine if there are any medical problems that might have caused or contributed to the aggression, as well as to decide the effect that these problems might have on treating the aggression. Painful conditions (e.g., abscesses, arthritis, anal sacculitis, dental disease), conditions affecting the central nervous system (e.g., brain tumors, encephalitis), sensory decline, and endocrine imbalances (e.g., hyperthyroidism) can all have a direct effect on behavior. Medical conditions can act in concert with environmental, genetic, and other health factors, to push the cat beyond the threshold at which aggression is exhibited. Cognitive dysfunction (brain aging) may also be a factor in older cats (see Ch. 12).

Combining a complete behavioral history with either direct or video observation of the cat during a typical aggressive display is the best way to ensure an accurate diagnosis. Viewing the behavior is ideal but not practical in most situations, so a detailed history is most important. It should include a description of the cat's facial expressions and body postures, and a description of all situations in which the aggression occurs. When formulating a treatment plan, consideration must be given to the type of aggression, the cat's temperament, and the mental and physical competence of individuals in its environment. The aggression release form

Appendix C, Fig. 12, form #1 on the CD might be modified for cats.

Factors of concern in determining the prognosis for safe resolution of aggression:

- Age at onset of the aggression.
- The length of time the problem has existed.
- Type of aggressive behavior.
- Predictability of aggressive behavior.
- The degree of intensity of the aggressive behavior.
- Presence of bite inhibition.
- Successful diagnosis and treatment of concurrent medical problems.
- Age and cognitive ability of family members.
- Ability of each family member to implement the treatment program safely, consistently, and effectively.
- Whether immediate steps can be taken to control the pet and avoid aggressive encounters.
- The availability of a safe and effective drug to improve the problem.

Desensitization and counterconditioning exercises are frequently used for treating many types of aggression by using repeated, controlled exposures to stimuli that trigger the behavior. During exposure, the owner must provide complete control of the cat so that it cannot escape or cause injury. Many owners yell, scream, and hit their aggressive cats. They must be instructed that this is not only ineffective but counterproductive. Punishing an aggressive cat increases its arousal and anxiety and increases the risk of injury for family members. Owners might also mistakenly reward their aggressive cat's behavior, albeit unintentionally. They do this by patting and reassuring the cat when they sense that it is aggressive, even offering food rewards in order to try to calm it down and lessen the aggression. The situation may also worsen when the cat learns that it can succeed by being aggressive, and that growling, scratching, and biting are effective ways for it to avoid an unwanted stimulus or situation (e.g., brushing teeth, trimming claws).

Exposure techniques are intended to change the cat's response to stimuli or situations that trigger aggression. It is important that the owner and counselor work together to determine all stimuli that cause aggression and formulate an appropriate treatment plan, complete with conditioning sessions.

During retraining, drug therapy may also be a consideration to reduce the intensity of the aggression or the number of aggressive displays. Drugs may alter the cat's threshold or tolerance of the stimuli, so that the number of aggressive events may be lessened or more easily prevented or controlled. Most commonly selective serotonin re-uptake inhibitors or tricyclic antidepressants such as clomipramine or amitriptyline are utilized in an effort to control impulsive, explosive, or excessive aggressive displays or for situations of excessive anxiety or fear. Buspirone may also be effective if there is mild anxiety but there appears to be a higher tendency to disinhibit and lead to increased aggression. Benzodiazepines have fallen into disfavor because they have the potential to sedate, cause incoordination, and increase appetite, and they may disinhibit leading to increased aggression. In addition, they generally need twice daily therapy, may have a rebound effect if not withdrawn slowly, may cause paradoxical effects such as increased agitation, and there is the potential in rare cases for hepatoxicity. However, for the most immediate and effective control of anxiety and to facilitate counterconditioning programs with food, benzodiazepines might be most effective. Although as yet unproven in cats, the use of oxazepam, lorazepam, and perhaps clonazepam should have less potential for hepatotoxicity since they have no active intermediate metabolites.

PLAY AGGRESSION

Play aggression is a common behavior in kittens and young cats. It is the most common type of aggressive behavior that cats exhibit toward their owners. Although the name implies a rather benign behavior, play aggression can result in a variety of injuries, and needs to be controlled to reduce the danger posed to family members and other pets.

Predatory-type play behavior directed toward family members can be quite intense and may result in serious injuries if biting and clawing are done without appropriate inhibition. The behavior can be quite alarming and frightening for family members who may think they have a 'mean' pet in the home.

Kitten play contains many elements of intraspecies aggression and predation. Play behaviors include: exploration and investigation; stalking, chasing, attacking, pouncing, and leaping sideways; fighting; wrestling; swatting and biting. Kittens typically 'play hard' with each other but quickly learn when they are actually causing pain. Since the bitten kitten will either stop playing or react with defensive responses, hard bites tend to become inhibited. Swatting is usually done with claws retracted. When a kitten grows up without appropriate social interaction that discourages hard biting, it may bite without inhibition into adulthood and be quite dangerous. The fact that vocalizations are rare during this type of behavior can help differentiate it from other types of aggression that involve biting and attacking (e.g., fear-related, territorial, redirected, pain-induced). Owners often contribute to the problem by playing with kittens in a way that encourages attacks toward hands and feet, or by allowing kittens to bite hard at a gloved hand. Unless encouraged, the behavior tends to wane as the cat grows into adulthood.

Situations that warrant treatment of play aggression include:

- Biting or scratching is deep and uninhibited.
- The play is directed toward the face.
- Targets are small children.
- The behavior is directed toward a family member with fragile skin.
- The target is someone with an immune-deficient disorder.
- Nocturnal play keeps family members from sleeping.
- The behavior is upsetting for a passive or fearful pet in the home.

Diagnosis and prognosis

Play aggression is typically seen in kittens and young cats (Fig. 20.1), and is accompanied by predatory or aggressive behaviors given in a playful context. The play usually involves inhibited biting and, occasionally, scratching. The amount of actual inhibition varies among individual kittens, with some biting quite hard. It is often associated with stalking, pouncing, and hopping sideways. The cat typically targets moving objects and attacks in response to hand movements, foot movements, and the owner moving through the home. Occasionally, the unwanted attention is directed exclusively toward one family member. In most cases, these problems are seen in single-cat households where the pet does not have the opportunity to engage in normal play with conspecifics. Problems with other cats in the home occur when the object of play is another cat that is passive, weak, fearful, or old and cannot tolerate the young cat's playful behavior.

The prognosis for correction is good, but if left unchecked or handled improperly, play aggression can develop into more severe forms of aggression that are less amenable to correction.

Management

Play aggression can be effectively managed by behavioral modification while cats are still young (Fig. 20.2). The most important consideration is to provide and encourage plenty of exercise that involves acceptable chase and attack behavior. Toys that bounce, flutter, or move in such a way that entices the cat to chase should be provided. Teasing and any interaction with the cat that encourages attacks directed toward the owner should be avoided.

Owners should be discouraged from using any type of physical punishment to correct the behavior because other problems, such as fear and defensive aggression, are likely to develop. If an aversive stimulus is required to stop a play bout, the hissing noise made by releasing compressed air from a canister used to clean photographic lenses, a water gun, or a citronella spray will generally work without being too disagreeable. For bolder cats, audible alarm devices (e.g., foghorns or battery-operated alarms) may be necessary. Owners should be taught to anticipate play attacks so they can be prevented by engaging the cat with toys (i.e., reinforcing the appropriate response) or interrupted with interruptive stimuli (no reinforcement for inappropriate behavior). This is one of the few behavior problems that might be corrected by adding another pet to the home. Adopting a young cat of the same size and temperament may immediately take care of the problem with little effort required on the owner's part.

Play aggression may be either a problem between the cat and a family member, or between two cats in the home. This is likely to be the case if the other cat is old, weak, or very passive. In those situations, the owner must keep the pets separated whenever they cannot be very closely supervised. Behavioral modification sessions should be set up during which the aggressor is squirted with a water gun each time it begins to direct any assertive or aggressive play behavior toward the other cat. Alternatively a leash and harness can be attached to the cat for control and interruption of undesirable behavior. During the same sessions, the kitten should receive a tasty food reward every time the other pet moves and the kitten exhibits no attempt to go after it. It is helpful to teach the attacking cat a few commands, so

Age of cat	The problem is more common in kittens and young cats
Play experience as a kitten	The pet was encouraged to chase and attack hands and feet
Number of cats in the household	The pet lives alone without other feline companions
Type of play with owners	Play frequently involves rough play and teasing the pet with fingers or toes
Amount of time spent alone	The pet is alone most of the day and spends little time with humans or other pets

Figure 20.1   Factors favoring feline play aggression.

- Owner should initiate play sessions using chase toys
- Avoid engaging the cat in aggressive play
- Redirect play toward appropriate objects (e.g., moving toys)
- Interrupt undesirable behavior (e.g., air, foghorn)
- Avoid all physical punishment (hitting, swatting)
- After the cat tires of chasing a play toy, try a novel toy since the cat may be tired of the toy but still in need of play
- Consider getting a second cat of similar age and temperament

Figure 20.2   Managing feline play aggression.

that its behavior in the presence of the other cat can be more easily controlled. Sometimes, the cat that is bearing the brunt of the play attacks becomes so stressed that anxiolytic medication (e.g., buspirone, selective serotonin inhibitors, benzodiazepines, tricyclic antidepressants) may be helpful to increase its confidence and reduce its fear.

Prevention

Play aggression may be prevented by routine socialization, appropriate exercise, and avoidance of inappropriate play with the kitten (see Chs 2 and 3 for more information regarding working with new puppies and kittens, as well as socialization and habituation).

Case example

Although the owners loved Cameron, a feisty little four-month-old kitten, they were about ready to get rid of him because of the intensity of his play. Their arms and ankles were full of scratches and teeth marks and they could hardly relax without him playfully attacking them. Swatting the kitten, or thumping it on the nose only served to increase the intensity of the attacks.

Treatment included a substantial increase in play with the kitten that involved tossing and dragging toys for him to chase. Play attacks were discouraged by directing a blast of compressed air at him from an air canister used to clean the owners' camera lenses. The owners were also told to stop using physical punishment. The problem quickly improved.

FEAR AGGRESSION

Fear aggression results when a cat is exposed to someone or something it perceives as being a threat, and escalates if there is no opportunity to escape. Aggression may also arise if the cat is frightened by inanimate stimuli such as sounds, but in these cases the aggression may be redirected to a nearby person or other animal (see redirected aggression below). The more threatening the stimulus is to the cat, the more heightened is the fear response. The behavior may be displayed when a cat is approached, touched, looked at, or stared at (Fig. 20.3). Fear aggression is sometimes referred to as defensive aggression.

Environmental influences and genetics can contribute to this problem. Punishment and inadequate socialization are common causes of fear aggression. Cats that have aversive experiences associated with humans or other cats may learn to be frightened of that individual or similar individuals, or a conditioned fear response to the stimulus might occur. Kittens that have not been adequately socialized are also very likely to be fearful of people and aggressive when approached or handled. Another important factor contributing to fear-related aggression is the genetic make-up of the cat. There is considerable variation in the feline population. Some cats require a very strong stimulus to elicit fear, while others become extremely anxious in response to mild stimuli, such as small movements or any noise that is the least bit unusual.

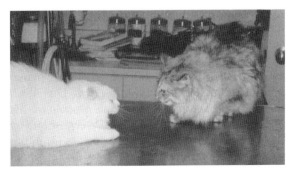

Figure 20.3   The cat on the right approaches with an offensive display while the cat on the left holds its ground and displays defensive aggression.

Aggressive behavior by a fearful cat can be aggravated by an anxious owner or by a fearful or aggressive victim. The behavior can also be self-reinforcing when growling, threatening, or biting drives away the stimulus that caused the fear reaction.

Diagnosis and prognosis

Fear aggression is typified by a variety of facial expressions and body postures. The cat usually displays a combination of defensive behavior (ears flattened against the head, tail tucked under the body, lowered body position, leaning away from the fearful stimulus) and aggressive behavior (piloerection, hissing, teeth bared, growling, swatting, biting, and scratching). Pupillary dilation is usually pronounced.

Defensive signals include:

- Hissing, spitting, growling
- Teeth bared
- Ears laid back, flattened against the head
- Crouched body position
- Body lowered, legs tucked under body
- Rolling to the side
- Tail tucked underneath.

The prognosis for fear aggression depends on a number of factors. If the problem is of short duration, initially occurred in adulthood, is mild in intensity, and the cat can be kept away from fear-evoking stimuli during treatment, the prognosis is favorable. The owner could be at risk handling a cat with fear aggression and must be counseled accordingly. The cat may attack the owner because of something about the owner (odor, sound, gesture) that elicits a fear response or it may attack due to redirected aggression when it is fearful of some other stimulus.

Factors suggesting a good prognosis include:

- Adult onset
- Problem of short duration
- Level of arousal is mild
- The threshold for fear responses is relatively high
- All fear-eliciting stimuli are well defined

- Exposure to fear-eliciting stimuli can be controlled
- The cat can be protected from strong stimulus exposure
- The owner is capable of controlling the cat for training sessions.

Management

Fear aggression is best managed with exposure techniques (Fig. 20.4) involving habituation, desensitization, and counterconditioning. Flooding may also be effective when the fear is mild or when the cat and the stimulus can be well controlled. Early recognition and intervention lead to the most effective cures. Full exposure to threatening stimuli that elicit a strong fear response should be avoided. The cat should repeatedly be exposed to modified or muted stimuli that are below the threshold that evoke a fear response until it is comfortable.

Formulating a treatment plan involves identifying fear-eliciting stimuli, identifying the threshold for arousal, and using controlled exposure sessions to reduce the pet's fear. Many cats that are fearful in certain situations can successfully be treated with exposure techniques involving food rewards for appropriate responses. Until the pet is successfully treated, it should be prevented from having any exposure to stimuli that cause the anxiety or might elicit fear-induced aggression.

For example, if women cause the cat to be fearful when they approach to 3 m or closer, then sessions should be set up so that a woman approaches at 4–5 m (desensitization) and the owner gives a very tasty food treat if the pet shows no sign of anxiety (counterconditioning). Using a wire crate may be beneficial in some cases because it will allow the owner to expose the cat to the fear-eliciting stimulus with no chance of the cat escaping or causing harm (Fig. 11.10). A leash and harness will also provide more control if the cat has been previously accustomed to wearing them. After each positive association, the woman can be very gradually brought closer and closer. It is advisable that the person initially avoids eye

Steps	Comments
Identify stimuli	• Identify all fear-eliciting stimuli and the threshold (intensity or distance) at which that fear is manifested. During treatment, it is important that the cat be insulated from anything that would cause anxiety or fear
Desensitization and counterconditioning	• If the threshold for fear is a man within 3 m of the cat, the man should be visible but further away than 3 m when desensitization exercises begin • A family member provides a reward (consider clicker training) when the cat is not fearful. Very gradually, the man moves closer. It may be helpful to use a halter or pet carrier for control • Patience is very important and this process must not be rushed
Flooding (controlled exposure)	• Use only when the fear response is mild • The cat is placed in a cage in a room with the person who triggers a fear response until all signs of fear or aggression have stopped • Exposure continues until the cat shows no sign of anxiety (habituates) • Once the pet habituates to the fearful stimulus, begin counterconditioning with favored food rewards (consider clicker training) • The fear may get worse if the person leaves before signs of fear or aggression have ceased
Drug therapy	• Clomipramine, amitriptyline, paroxetine, or fluoxetine may be effective at modifying the extreme states of anxiety, panic, arousal, or dyscontrol but may not calm and reduce anxiety sufficiently for some cats • Prescription agents such as buspirone or benzodiazepines may help to reduce fear and anxiety to a level that is low enough to allow behavioral modification to begin. These drugs may help to make the cat more bold and confident but may lead to disinhibition and aggression
Pheromones	• Felifriend™ applied to the individual introduced (cat, person, dog) to whom the fear is exhibited or Feliway™ room diffuser introduced into the environment

Figure 20.4 Managing feline fear aggression.

contact with the cat, and remains quiet and calm. Withholding the treats except during exposure training increases their motivation and ensures contingency. The goal is to develop a positive association with the stimulus by linking food with the fearful stimulus.

Patience is particularly important since the process must proceed very slowly. Some owners may begin by immediately asking a visitor to extend a hand with a food treat toward the pet's face. This does not usually work since the attractiveness of the food is initially not strong enough to overcome the close proximity of the fearful stimulus. If it fails, this approach usually makes the situation worse. Punishment must absolutely be avoided since it will likely increase the level of fear, strengthen avoidance behaviors, and cause the aggression to worsen.

Feline facial pheromones, in particular the F4 fraction, commercially available in a synthetic form known as Felifriend™, are associated with familiarization and allomarking in cats. Felifriend™ is designed to be applied

to the individual to whom the cat is being introduced to facilitate acceptance and reduce aggression (dog, cat, person). This product is presently available only in France, Belgium, and Japan. The F3 synthetic analog Feliway™ room diffuser may to a lesser extent be useful in reducing anxiety when Felifriend™ is not available.

Drug therapy may also be beneficial. Drugs such as buspirone, benzodiazepines, tricyclic antidepressants, or selective serotonin re-uptake inhibitors may be helpful in reducing fear and anxiety to a level that is low enough to allow behavior modification to proceed. Medication may be particularly important in situations where exposure to fear-eliciting stimuli is difficult to control on a daily basis. While benzodiazepines may be contraindicated for the most part because of the potential for hepatic toxicity, a drug such as oxazepam may help to reduce anxiety as well as stimulate appetite for counterconditioning. However, drugs that reduce anxiety, particularly buspirone and the benzodiazepines, may lead to disinhibition and an increase in aggression in some cats.

Prevention

Selecting a friendly, sociable kitten can be very important, as kittens that exhibit fear and aggressiveness may be difficult to socialize. Owners should be advised to adopt a kitten by seven weeks of age from a family situation that has provided an adequate amount of gentle handling and interaction. In most cases, fear aggression can be effectively prevented by encouraging owners to socialize their cats adequately. Veterinarians should educate owners about the concepts of socialization, habituation handling, and behavioral development, and how they can prevent such problems.

Case examples

Case 1 Brenda was a five-year-old, spayed female domestic long-haired cat adopted by her owner at eight weeks of age from a friend at church. The woman lived by herself and had only few visitors, most of whom were women or children. The cat was playful and confident when it was alone at home with its owner, but became nervous and usually hid when a visitor entered the home, especially when the visitor was a man. The owner had recently begun a relationship with a man named Ralph whom she met at work. She was disconcerted about the fact that Brenda had not taken to her new friend. In an attempt to facilitate the relationship, she encouraged Ralph to attempt to pick up the cat during each visit and give it a food treat. Each time he did this, Brenda would become very agitated, hiss, growl, flail her legs, and occasionally bite to get released. Instead of getting better, Brenda's behavior worsened. The cat became more nervous around Ralph and frequently hissed at him when he visited.

The owner was told that, while her intentions were good, she had tried to encourage a relationship between the cat and the new boyfriend too quickly. To make Brenda less anxious, Ralph was told to enter quietly, maintain a distance

from the cat, avoid eye contact, and not move toward it when he was in the apartment. Whenever the cat ventured out from hiding, Ralph was instructed to casually flip a very tasty piece of food toward it without looking directly at or reaching for the pet. Initially, Brenda ignored the treats, so food was taken up eight to 12 hours prior to his visits in order to increase her appetite. After one week, the cat was eating the food flipped to it, and Ralph was instructed to toss the food so that it would land closer and closer to him. Two to three weeks later, the pet was willing to take food from his hand. Next, the food was offered on the sofa at the end opposite to Ralph and then closer to him. Through subsequent visits, Ralph gradually moved the non-feeding hand closer and closer to Brenda until he was able to stroke the cat gently when he was feeding her. This last step took about five months.

Case 2 Elaine and Jerry lived in a large home with their cat Cosmo. When the children were grown up and had moved out of the home, Elaine and Jerry decided to take in a boarder named George. Although the boarder lived in the finished basement, he shared the kitchen facilities with Elaine and Jerry. If George entered the kitchen when Cosmo was present, the cat would fearfully back into a corner and begin to hiss. If George approached, Cosmo would lunge and swat with a paw. Attempts by George to talk reassuringly to Cosmo or to offer food did nothing but increase Cosmo's fear and threats.

Cosmo had an open wire cage that was used for travelling and where he was placed when company came over. Elaine and Jerry were instructed to place Cosmo in the cage near the kitchen table and to have George come to the kitchen after dinner to spend a few hours with Elaine, Jerry, and Cosmo. Cosmo was to be ignored and when there was no apparent fear or anxiety, the cage was to be moved closer to the table. After one hour, Cosmo was still anxious and fearful whenever George arose or moved in the cat's direction. After two hours, Cosmo showed no further anxiety, but the owners decided to call it a night, and requested an anti-anxiety drug for further retraining sessions.

Because alprazolam (0.125 mg/cat PO) had been used successfully on previous occasions (e.g., veterinary visits), it was redispensed.

The next evening George was invited up for dinner and drinks. Cosmo was not fed all day and was given the alprazolam one hour before George arrived. The cage was placed about a meter from the table. After about 30 minutes Cosmo showed no further anxiety. The cage was moved progressively closer to George throughout the evening so that after two hours the cage was situated at George's feet. At this point George was able to toss a few cat treats into the cage, which Cosmo ate willingly. By the end of the evening, Cosmo was taking the treats from George through the bars of the cage. On subsequent evenings, the exposure techniques were repeated without the alprazolam, and during the fourth session, Cosmo was released from the cage. Cosmo ate his dinner and showed no fear even if George left and re-entered the room. George was instructed to flip cat treats to Cosmo but not to approach him, and after a few more evening sessions, Cosmo would approach George and take food treats from his hand.

PREDATORY BEHAVIOR

Predation is a highly motivated, instinctive behavior for cats. It is in their nature to hunt, chase, and kill prey animals. The initial movements of this behavioral sequence are characterized by silent stalking. The body is held close to the ground during the approach and the attack is patterned to achieve a quick kill of the prey. Predation is not preceded by vocal or postural threats because it represents a normal instinct to hunt and kill that does not include threats or warnings. In cases where cats are kept for rodent control, the kitten might become a better hunter if it is kept a little longer with its mother until it learns to hunt, as there is also a learned component to hunting (and prey preference). When this behavior is directed toward family or other pets in the home, it may cause problems that need to be corrected.

Diagnosis and prognosis

This type of behavior can be found in cats of either sex and any age. A moving stimulus is the usual target. The innate response of the cat is to stalk, chase, and attack, and there may be a killing bite. The most severe danger is when the prey target happens to be an infant or a small pet. True predation directed toward humans is rare, but play predation is very common (discussed above). The behavior of chasing and catching prey, such as small mammals or birds, is to a great extent instinctive and therefore difficult to modify. The prognosis for complete resolution of this type of problem is generally quite poor. Pets that are most at risk are birds, rabbits, hamsters, gerbils, and the like.

Management

Owners may want to discourage wildlife from visiting the yard so that they do not succumb to their cat. Wildlife feeders should not be present to attract animals that will be at risk. Outdoor motion detectors that spray water may be successful at repelling potential prey that might wander into the garden. Since the predatory instinct is so difficult to suppress, the best approach is to prevent the cat's access to its intended prey. Although putting a bell on the collar may be sufficient for many cats, most require confinement indoors to guarantee that the predation will cease. Declawing seldom reduces a cat's ability to hunt or kill prey. Constant outdoor supervision may be the only practical course of action for cats that continue to go outdoors.

Many urban areas are at risk of losing song bird populations and other wildlife due to the hunting behavior of domestic cats. Veterinarians in those areas should strongly suggest that all pet cats be kept indoors.

Prevention

The development of predatory aggression is difficult to prevent because it is primarily an instinctive behavior. A portion of hunting behavior is learned from the queen, so that keeping a queen indoors with no access to hunting until after the kittens are weaned and adopted may prevent the learned component of hunting and killing from developing. Selecting a kitten from parents that do not hunt may also be helpful. The fact is that some cats are born with more predatory drive than others. These cats should either be kept inside if predatory behavior is a problem, or only allowed out when on a halter and leash.

Case example

Amos was a three-year-old neutered male Siamese cat. Whenever he could get into the children's room, he spent a large part of the day sitting next to the hamster cage, batting at the hamsters and trying to get into the cage. Although the children were repeatedly advised to keep the door to their room shut, this was extremely impractical as they played and did their homework in there, and were constantly coming and going with their friends.

The hamsters were temporarily moved to a different cage in the basement. This was done without the cat watching. An electronic mat was placed on the table next to the cage where the hamsters were kept in the children's room. When Amos jumped up on the table, he received a harmless but uncomfortable stimulus. The cat avoided the table top even after the hamsters were placed back in the original cage.

PETTING-INDUCED AGGRESSION

Some cats have the disconcerting habit of accepting their owner's attention only to respond by biting when they have had enough. In general, these cats seem to enjoy social attention. They may actually seek attention by crying, rubbing against people, or jumping into their laps. However, they seem to have a certain threshold for the amount of physical attention they will tolerate. When they have no more tolerance for stroking, they bite and run off. The observant owner may be able to tell when the bite is

about to occur as the pet usually will show typical behaviors that may include fidgeting, tail twitching, tenseness, leaning away, ears flattened against the head, retraction of the lips, and hissing.

Diagnosis and prognosis

The history will reveal a cat that is initially calm and comfortable with being petting, but bites after a period of time. The bites may be inhibited or they can cause significant damage. While vocalization may precede the bite, this is not as likely as with other types of aggression, such as fear-related, pain-related, redirected, or territorial aggression.

The prognosis for correcting this type of behavior is fair to guarded, depending on the duration of the behavior, the pet's threshold for physical interaction, and the patience of the owner. Young children are at a greater risk, as they do not 'read' the postural signs that a bite is imminent.

Management

The crux of treatment is to identify the threshold of tolerance for the cat and to gradually condition it to accept more stroking while avoiding the risks of attack. To do this, the owner must first determine how long the cat can always be stroked before it attacks.

Retraining sessions only take place when the cat is in the mood for affection. Petting should then take place for a short period of time and stop before the threshold is reached. The cat can then be given a food treat and placed on the floor before it shows any evidence of nervousness or aggression. The cat must not be held or confined in any way. It is more desirable for it to jump down on its own rather than become aggressive. The sessions can gradually be lengthened as the cat learns to tolerate longer and longer stroking sessions in anticipation of a food reward (desensitization and counterconditioning). The owner should have frequent petting sessions with the pet in the lap or next to the owner on the sofa. Conditioning can be facilitated by feeding on a schedule and holding the sessions just prior to meal time. Special food treats should be restricted to training sessions (Fig. 20.5). Clicker training might further help to improve the owner's timing of rewards. The owner must be instructed to be careful to avoid absentmindedly petting the cat between counterconditioning sessions. There may also be aspects of status-induced aggression and learning, so that all attention-soliciting behavior initiated by the cat should be ignored. On the other hand, the owners should initiate short play and affection sessions and stop the affection or play before the cat gets aroused or aggressive. Food rewards can then be given for each successful session.

Physical punishment and yelling at the cat should be avoided. Hitting the cat on the nose, swatting it, or forcefully tossing it to the floor invariably make matters worse.

Prevention

Early socialization, grooming, and frequent gentle handling of the young kitten may help to prevent this problem. Resistance to handling might be improved by associating food rewards with petting and handling.

Case example

Harry was a two-year-old, domestic short-haired cat who would rub against the owner's leg, jump into her lap, and purr as she stroked him. After about five to 10 seconds of petting, he would suddenly bite her and run off.

The owner was instructed to avoid absentmindedly petting the cat and to set up sessions of owner-initiated petting for rewards (provided the cat was 'in the mood'). She was cautioned to watch for pre-bite behaviors and to stop well before a bite might occur. She was instructed to stroke him only for four seconds and then give a very tasty food treat whenever he jumped in a chair beside her or in her lap for attention. Harry was then to be ignored until he voluntarily approached or sought attention again. The petting sessions gradually increased in

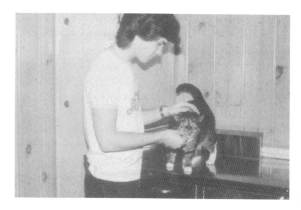

Figure 20.5 Desensitization and counterconditioning – petting is associated with favored food rewards and the time and intensity is gradually lengthened with each session.

duration as Harry learned to allow himself to be groomed in anticipation of getting a food reward.

STATUS AGGRESSION

Some cats may display aggression toward their owners or other cats when displaying assertiveness. This type of aggression is infrequently described in the veterinary literature but is a consideration for those cats that bite or attack their owners or other cats in order to control a situation. Expressions of the cat's assertiveness may be exhibited as biting during stroking, when the cat is lifted or approached, or when the owner attempts to remove the cat from a worktop or piece of furniture. Cats that solicit attention or play by biting may also be displaying assertiveness.

Diagnosis and prognosis

The diagnosis may be difficult as this condition is poorly described in the literature and the cats may actually be displaying other forms of aggression (fear, territorial, predatory, play, petting-induced) in combination with status aggression. Cats that have this type of problem usually display a confident temperament. They exhibit assertive or status aggression by biting or threatening when the owner attempts to approach or handle them. This bite behavior may be an attempt to control these situations. Assertive displays, pushy attention-seeking behavior, and attempts to control the environment by blocking access to doorways and refusing to be moved from perches or sleeping areas may be displays of social status. Although some cats exhibiting this behavior may be overly demanding, vocalizing or constantly soliciting affection from the owners, others may appear aloof and independent, preferring to be left alone when the owner attempts to initiate affection or attention. One sign that might signify this type of aggression is aggression toward members of the household that it can control, avoiding aggression with family members that control the cat and do not routinely give in to its demands. The prognosis is guarded as these cats may be dangerous and the problem may have both innate and learned components.

Management

The goal of management is that the owners gain control over the cat (Fig. 20.6). Much like the dominant aggressive dog, the owners can best gain control by identifying and avoiding those situations that might lead to aggression and training the cat that all rewards (play, food, affection, attention) must be earned. If the owner accedes to the cat's demands for affection or attention, the cat may become increasingly aggressive in its attempts to play or gain attention. On the other hand, if the owner attempts to initiate attention or move the cat from a favored sleeping area, the cat may become aggressive toward those that it feels it can control. If the cat cannot gain attention or affection on demand, the owners will demonstrate to the cat that they cannot be controlled and the resources can then be used to reward and motivate the cat for responding to the owner.

Cats can be taught to respond to a few basic commands such as 'come' with food reward training. Commands and rewards can then be used to overcome potential problems such as getting the cat off furniture. The owner holds a small piece of a very tasty meat, fish, or cheese treat in front of the pet's nose. The hand is moved away from the nose as the treat is tossed to the floor. As the cat leaps toward the treat and follows it to the floor, the command 'move' is given. The food is gradually phased out over time. Eventually, the owner will be able to get the pet to leap to the floor with just a hand sweep and command. The cat should not be allowed to gain any form of attention or reinforcement on demand. As rewards are withheld this not only ensures that the cat does not control the owner, but also increases the motivational value (desire) for the rewards. In fact, the cat should learn that the owner and not the cat will initiate affection, play, or treats of any type and that it must defer to the owner to gain these rewards.

Prevention

From the outset, the owner should never accede to the kitten's demands but should insist that all play, feeding, or handling be initiated by the owner. Hand feeding may be helpful since the cat can be taught to perform a command or accept some handling before any food or treat is given. Teaching a few basic commands or tricks (e.g., 'come,' 'sit up') to kittens can also help the owner gain control. Petting and handling should be practised regularly for short periods and play or food rewards can be given after each session. Any demanding or pushy behavior should be ignored and never rewarded. Also consider clicker training.

Case example

Napoleon was a 16-month-old, neutered, male domestic short-haired cat who would lunge and bite at the owners whenever they attempted to remove him from any chair, table, or worktop where he had 'parked' himself. Although he would growl and bite when the owners attempted to lift or stroke him, he would solicit and enjoy a few minutes of petting whenever he was in the mood. Napoleon's aggression had become so severe that the owners were afraid

Step	Comments
Make the situation safe	• Identify stimuli leading to aggression • Avoid confrontations and any stimuli or interactions that elicit aggression such as approaching, stroking, or handling
Training	• Teach simple commands such as 'come' or 'sit' by using food lures whenever the cat is receptive to food or play. Consider clicker training to improve success • Teach the pet to move off furniture on command
Withhold rewards unless earned	• The cat should be taught to defer to the owners for any treats, affection, or play • Play, affection, and treats must never be given on demand but can be given if the cat accepts a small amount of handling, holding, lifting, or responds to a command
Teach tolerance to handling, approach, etc.	• Use desensitization and counterconditioning • After a few weeks of teaching deference, the cat can be taught to accept stimuli that have triggered aggression • The owner begins by performing a behavior that has triggered aggression in the past, but in such a muted way that no aggression is elicited (approach, handling, touching). If no undesirable behavior is exhibited, the pet is given a very tasty food reward or play, or an immediate click and treat (if clicker training) • Once the pet is conditioned to accept a mild level of the stimulus, the sessions can progress with stimuli that very gradually become stronger
Interrupt or deter undesirable behavior	• Physical punishment must be avoided, but undesirable behavior may be interrupted with devices such as alarms, water guns, or a can of compressed air • This is best done without looking at the cat or saying anything • Care must be taken with this approach since some strong stimuli can make a cat more aroused and aggressive
Control devices	• A harness and long leash can be left attached to the cat to provide more control in some situations without the need for physical contact
Drug therapy	• Uninhibited aggressive displays that appear impulsive, explosive, or excessive may be reduced with selective serotonin re-uptake inhibitors such as paroxetine or fluoxetine • Amitriptyline, buspirone, or a benzodiazepine might be considered if there is concurrent anxiety, but these drugs may also disinhibit, leading to an increase in some forms of aggression

Figure 20.6 Managing feline status aggression.

to approach him when he was lying on their bed, sofa, or kitchen worktop.

Napoleon was fitted with a body harness and a 3-m lead was attached whenever the owners were at home supervising him. The leash was then used to remove Napoleon from his resting areas without confrontation or injury. The owners were instructed not to feed, play with, or stroke Napoleon except during training sessions. At scheduled feeding or play times, the owners were to hold out the food or toy, call Napoleon to come, pet him for a few moments, and then provide the reward. Each day, Napoleon was conditioned to be held, stroked, or lifted a little longer than the previous day before the rewards were given. Whenever Napoleon assertively approached the owners for play, food, or affection he was to be ignored. The owners were told to wait a few minutes, hold out a food treat or toy, give a command to come, and have Napoleon approach for a short handling session before the reward was given. The owners were also taught to identify any signs of impending aggression so that they could avoid the situation or use a small can of compressed air to distract the pet. After a week, Napoleon had learned to come when called and would tolerate a minute or more of handling before receiving his play or food. When he had to be moved from a piece of furniture he could either be enticed to leave with a command and food reward or, at the very least, removed with a leash and harness. Napoleon soon learned to tolerate approach and several minutes of handling without aggression, and would voluntarily get off the furniture without showing aggressive displays.

REDIRECTED AGGRESSION

Redirected aggression occurs when the target of the animal's aggression is not the stimulus that triggered the state of aggressive arousal. It is most common in adult cats, especially males. Intermale, territorial, fear-induced, and defensive aggression are the types of behaviors that are likely to be redirected. The aggressive attack usually occurs when a person or animal approaches or touches the aroused cat. But it is not always necessary for the target of the aggression to actually make contact with the cat. In some cases, the aroused cat will attack a person or another pet that is moving around the room 3–5 m away and paying no attention to it. The attacks are often very acute, intense, and may seem unprovoked. Multiple, uninhibited bites and severe injuries are common. Attacks may seem unprovoked to the family because the arousing stimulus was present earlier when they were not present, and the pet remained in a high state of arousal. The family is often quite unsettled about the apparent unpredictability and unprovoked nature of the aggressive displays, thinking that the cat has 'gone mad.'

Stimuli that can cause an aggressive state of arousal include the sight or sound of another cat, unusual noises, odors of other animals, unfamiliar people, and unfamiliar environments. The aroused cat may exhibit varying degrees of hypervigilance, agitation, nervous pacing, piloerection, fixed gaze, tail flipping, dilated pupils, or low vocalizations. During the attack, the cat usually exhibits very loud growling and yowling, vigorous lunging and attacking, and uninhibited biting, which result in serious, deep wounds. A common situation is one in which the pet becomes aroused upon seeing or hearing another cat while sitting in a window. When the owner attempts to pet it, pick it up, or nudge it away from the window, it attacks. It may also show aggression toward another pet when approached in similar situations. In another situation, an indoor cat that escapes to the yard may become frightened by another animal or by being in an unfamiliar environment. If the arousal level is high enough, it may bite when a family member attempts to pick it up to return it indoors. Another situation in which redirected aggression occurs is when a veterinarian gives an injection and the cat bites the nurse.

Redirected aggression is a common cause of the sudden appearance of aggression between cats in the same household that have been living together amicably for quite some time. Occasionally, a family member will have been present to see the situation develop. This is not always the case and owners are often perplexed about why their pets suddenly don't get along with each other. In cases where there is an unexpected appearance of intercat aggression for no apparent reason, historical evidence often suggests that one or both cats have exhibited high levels of fearful or territorial arousal, and unfamiliar cats have recently been visiting the pets' territory.

This type of aggression is probably the most dangerous type of aggression cats exhibit due to the uninhibited nature of the bites. Attacks are usually very frightening, vicious, and damaging, and might result in multiple, deep bite wounds and extensive damage that requires medical attention.

Stimuli that can cause redirected aggression include:

- Sight, sound, or odor of another cat
- Sight, sound, or odor of other animals
- Unusual noises
- Unfamiliar people
- Unfamiliar environments
- Pain.

Diagnosis and prognosis

In general, the history suggests victim interference or contact when the cat was threatened, territorially aroused, afraid, or fighting. Although medical problems are not common causes of sudden expressions of aggressive behavior, pathophysiologic etiologies should be ruled out through a good physical exam and appropriate lab tests. Medical rule-outs include abscesses, intervertebral disc disease, psychomotor seizures, feline ischemic encephalopathy, brain tumors, and virtually anything that might make the cat painful.

The diagnosis involves recognizing that a specific stimulus or situation has aroused the cat and resulted in a nearby person or animal being attacked. A thorough behavioral history is very important. The interviewer should get a detailed description of the problem, including all other incidents in the pet's past when it exhibited aggression or high levels of fearful arousal. Since a cat may stay in a high state of arousal for hours after stimulus exposure, it is possible that the owner may not know what stimuli resulted in the aggressive attacks. A history of all situations that resulted in high arousal may lead to a list of likely stimuli. It may also be helpful for the owner to keep a diary of aggressive events.

The prognosis is poor if the cat is frequently and easily stimulated to a state of aggressive arousal, the stimuli are difficult to identify or control, and the aggression is intense or prolonged. Family members who are unable to recognize when the cat is aroused are in particular danger.

Factors influencing the prognosis of redirected aggression include:

- Ability to identify arousing stimuli
- Ability to reduce exposure to stimuli
- Frequency of stimulus exposure
- The cat's threshold for becoming aroused
- Severity of the aggression
- Ability of all family members to recognize and avoid the aroused cat.

Management

Treatment involves identifying triggers for arousal and then removing the pet's access to the stimuli and/or modifying the response to the stimuli (Fig. 20.7). If the pet becomes highly aroused when it goes outdoors, it should be confined indoors. If it becomes aroused watching outdoor cats through windows, that opportunity should be removed by closing drapes, blocking access to windowsills, and keeping the pet off screened porches. Castration should be helpful for most cases. Medication can be beneficial for reducing the animal's response to environmental stimuli. Desensitization, counterconditioning, and timely distractions can occasionally be used to change the cat's response to stimuli that cause it to become aroused.

It is very important that the owners be educated about all aspects of the problem. They need to understand what causes the aggression, how to recognize signs of arousal, how to avoid problems, and how to handle the aroused cat. When the pet is in a high state of arousal, the ideal way to handle it is to leave it in a darkened room and close the door without touching it until it calms down. This can take several hours or several days. If it must be handled, thick leather gloves, a fish net, or a large towel can be used to protect the owner.

Since owners often respond to the aggression with behaviors that make things worse, such as screaming, hitting the cat, etc., you may have to treat the consequences of these behaviors. Cats that are treated this way may begin exhibiting avoidance or fear-related aggressive behavior. Fearful behavior can be treated with systematic desensitization and counterconditioning.

When the aggression is directed toward another pet in the home, the pets should be separated until the level of arousal entirely diminishes. The cats should be kept apart at least until the aggressor is entirely calm and will take food. Reintroduction should be gradual, closely supervised, and associated with positive interactions such as feeding, just as if new pets were being introduced to the home. In highly aroused cats this reintroduction program can take from a few days to a few weeks. Antidepressants (paroxetine, fluoxetine, clomipramine, amitriptyline) may be helpful to reduce overall arousal and perhaps reduce the possibility of future events. Anxiolytic medications, such as a benzodiazepine, might be another alternative as they may also stimulate appetite for a food counterconditioning program.

On occasion, if the victim cat has begun to display excessive fear to the aggressor, it may

Identify stimuli for aggressive arousal	• Explore all situations or stimuli that cause anxiety or aggressive arousal • Have the owner keep a diary
Prevent exposure to stimuli	• Close windows, drapes, or blinds • Don't allow the pet to perch on windowsills or visit the sun porch • Confine when visitors are in the home
Safety	• Teach the owner to recognize and avoid the aroused cat • Keep a heavy blanket, pillow, or fishing net available for protection • A leash and body halter can be left on the pet for control and to safely guide it into a quiet room when it becomes aggressively aroused
Carefully interrupt the behavior	• Use a device (whistle, air horn, water gun) to distract the pet • Avoid doing anything that makes the pet more aroused • Avoid eye contact or saying anything during the procedure
Carefully remove the cat from the situation	• Some cats cannot safely be moved when aroused • A blanket, towel, or gloves may provide some safety when moving the pet • Use a leash and body halter • Food lures may work if the cat is not exceptionally aroused • Confine in a darkened, quiet room until calm • If aggression has arisen toward another household pet, gradually reintroduce using desensitization and counterconditioning
Behavior modification for inciting stimuli	• Desensitize and countercondition the pet's response to anxiety or aggression-provoking stimuli
Medication	• Paroxetine is a good choice and can be used for the aggressor cat as well as the fearful cat that is the target of the aggression • Anxiolytic medications, tricyclic antidepressants, or selective serotonin re-uptake inhibitors may be helpful • Pheromone therapy may also help to reduce any anxiety associated with the stimulus

Figure 20.7 Managing feline redirected aggression.

also be helpful to consider drug therapy with an anxiolytic such as buspirone or a benzodiazepine. Antidepressants such as paroxetine, clomipramine, or amitriptyline might be another option. Feliway™, the synthetic pheromone product, might also be helpful.

Sometimes, the cat's behavior can successfully be interrupted by using a device such as an ultrasonic alarm, compressed air, or spray of water. This should be done without looking at the cat or saying anything. Interruption should be done very carefully because additional stimuli may actually increase the level of arousal in many cats. Desirable behavior in the presence of the other pet can then be reinforced. Physical punishment and yelling at the cat invariably make the situation worse and should be avoided.

The decision as to whether or not to keep the pet in the home should be based on the frequency and severity of the attacks, the ability of family members to recognize and avoid the aroused cat, and the owners' ability to recognize and control arousing stimuli. If there are people in the home who cannot avoid the aroused cat, serious consideration should be given to removing the pet from the home or euthanizing it.

Prevention

Prevention of redirected aggression involves early recognition of stimuli and situations that trigger aggression, followed by desensitization and counterconditioning to change the pet's behavior. Prevention of attacks involves knowing how to recognize and avoid the cat in a high state of arousal, as well as taking steps to prevent the cat from being exposed to these stimuli.

Case example

The owner was sitting in the living room one evening watching television when he heard a cat howl outside the apartment. B.G., his two-year-old, spayed, domestic short-haired cat, sprung to her feet, appeared very agitated, and hissed. As the owner quickly got up, the pet turned toward him, yowled, and viciously attacked his leg. Before the owner was able to shake the cat loose by striking it several times, B.G. had delivered a number of deep bite wounds. The cat ran off into the guest bedroom and hid under a chair where it hissed and growled every time the owner entered the room.

An animal control officer was called to pick up the stray intact male that was howling outdoors. As is often the case with redirected aggression, fear aggression developed due to the owner's response to the attack and it was very important that this be addressed. The cat was kept confined to the guest bedroom immediately after the incident and was placed on paroxetine (2.5 mg PO sid). For the first few days, the owner was instructed to leave a large bowl of food and water and two litterboxes for the cat in the room, keep things quiet around the apartment, and stay out of the room other than to occasionally check on the pet. After three days, the owner was instructed to enter the room numerous times during the day and casually toss pieces of chicken or tuna to the cat without looking at it. When the cat became calm and stopped showing signs of apprehension, the door was left open for the pet to leave at its own will. For the following week, the owner continued to limit his interaction with the cat, only tossing food when it approached. Within three weeks, the cat was back to acting normally. The paroxetine was continued for four more weeks, then gradually reduced.

Although desensitizing and counterconditioning the pet to the stimulus of a yowling cat

would have been ideal, it was not practical. The owner was educated about redirected aggression and made aware of signs of arousal so that he would know when to avoid the cat. It was suggested that the pet not be allowed out on to the balcony to observe outdoor cats, and that if the owner should ever hear a cat call outdoors and notice that the pet oriented toward the noise, but did not become aroused, he should praise it or reward it with food.

PAIN-INDUCED AND IRRITABLE AGGRESSION

Even the most sociable and docile animal may exhibit pain-induced aggression. A similar term is irritable aggression, which refers to any medical condition that might not cause pain but does increase irritability and therefore aggression (or retreat) during approach or handling. Metabolic disorders such as liver disease or renal disease, endocrine disorders, CNS disorders, sensory decline, or perhaps even a lack of sleep might lead to irritable aggression. Because pain monitoring is such a subjective assessment in cats, it may be difficult to accurately separate irritable from pain-induced aggression (i.e., does the cat have dental pain, arthritis, or even a headache, or is it more irritable due to its illness?). Handling or the anticipation of handling (approach, reaching) might lead to this type of aggression. This problem may also occur if a cat's hair is pulled or when its tail is stepped on. It can also happen when an individual attempts to manipulate a painful area, even if that manipulation is just stroking, grooming, or applying medication. Cats that are presented for aggression should be examined for underlying painful diseases such as fight abscesses, otitis, and arthritis.

Although painful forms of punishment have been employed to produce submission and facilitate restraint in some species, these are neither effective nor humane for gaining control of cats or modifying behavior, especially since the cat will quickly realize what people are the source of the pain. In most cases, the use of a painful correction will intensify the aggression that already exists or add aggression to the list of the pet's behavior problems. At the very least it is likely to lead to fear and avoidance behaviors.

Diagnosis and prognosis

The diagnosis is usually straightforward. The cat experiences pain and reacts aggressively. It might hiss, snarl, and growl, or bite people who seem intent on causing it pain. It is important to remedy the situation because if the cat perceives that biting accomplished its goals (i.e., stopped the painful interaction) it might use aggression when similar interactions arise in the future, whether or not the pain is still present. Thus, the situation must be corrected so that routine care such as claw trimming, home dental care, medicating, and grooming can be accomplished without triggering aggressive episodes. Degenerative disease, trauma, and illness that lead to pain or increased irritability may be more difficult to identify, so that a good history and medical workup is essential for all aggressive cats. If pain due to a medical condition is suspected, a trial with a pain control medication might be warranted.

Management

If possible, it is best not to manipulate the cat when it is in pain. However, this is not always practical, especially when medications may need to be applied, or physical therapy utilized. Thus, the approach must be to control the pet to reduce danger to the handler, avoid eliciting pain, treat the pain, and employ desensitization or counterconditioning exercises to increase the cat's tolerance of being handled (Fig. 20.8).

Prevention

Handling exercises performed with a kitten may help raise its threshold for pain-elicited aggression. These can be done at feeding time. While the pet is being hand-fed, the owner can gently handle all parts of the pet's body. As days go by, the intensity and variety of handling should

- Eliminate or reduce the source of pain or irritability (medical therapy/therapeutic diets/drugs)
- Modify treatment to make it more comfortable
- Handle the patient gently and consider muzzling for protection
- Promote owner control with training and rewards
- Desensitization and counterconditioning to gradually accustom the cat to handling
- Avoid painful punishment

Figure 20.8 Managing feline pain-induced aggression.

increase. Grooming and claw trimming should occur during these exercises. Although it is not possible to anticipate the effects of all painful stimuli, the cat that is trained to be handled, have its claws trimmed, and its teeth brushed without resistance will also be more likely to tolerate handling when it is in pain. The best way to prevent pain-induced aggression from a cat that has been hurt is to anticipate the problem and handle the pet in such a way that pain does not occur or is minimized. Veterinarians should also place increasing emphasis on pain control when pets have been traumatized by injury or surgery or are sick or ill.

Case example

Zeke was an 18-month-old, neutered, male domestic short-haired cat who received a painful bite wound over his right shoulder. As part of the treatment, the owner was instructed to cleanse the area gently three times daily. To make Zeke less anxious about having the shoulder treated, the owner gave him a small piece of tuna 15–20 times each day as she touched the opposite shoulder and said 'good boy.' When she treated the wounded shoulder, she gave him a large piece of tuna and repeated 'good boy' as she applied the compress.

MATERNAL AGGRESSION

Protective instincts to offspring are present in virtually all mothers. Maternal aggression refers to aggressive behavior directed toward people or other animals that approach the queen with her kittens. This type of aggressive activity is believed to be a function of the hormonal state of the female during lactation as well as the presence of the young. The queen can be quite aggressive in defending her young.

Diagnosis and prognosis

The diagnosis involves observation of a queen that hisses, growls, and attempts to bite humans or other animals that approach the kittens or nest area.

For well-socialized queens, the prognosis is good since there is usually spontaneous remission as the kittens age. The prognosis for quick resolution of the problem is guarded.

Management

Although regular handling of newborn kittens is regarded as beneficial for their development, it might be necessary to avoid handling them for the first few days, as this is when the queen tends to be most protective. Gentle handling by trusted family members accompanied by tasty food offerings is the best way to allay apprehension. Subduing the queen by gently wrapping her in a towel or applying a cat muzzle when she absolutely has to be handled, or enticing the queen to leave her kittens with food or toys, may be the most expedient way of minimizing the dangers during the short period when she is most likely to be aggressive (Fig. 20.9).

Behavioral modification can be attempted if the kittens need to be handled while the queen is still very protective, although the maternal behavior usually runs its course in perhaps the

---

- A quiet, low-stress environment should be provided
- Avoid approaching and handling of the kittens if the queen appears agitated
- Use a muzzle or gentle restraining device (blanket/towel) when the queen needs to be handled
- Distract or lure the mother to leave the litter before the kittens are handled
- Desensitization and counterconditioning

Figure 20.9 Managing feline maternal aggression.

same or less time than would be required to complete a desensitization and counterconditioning program. Simply avoiding the queen and kittens may be the most prudent and practical solution because of the relatively short duration of this type of aggression.

Prevention

Early socialization and handling of young, female kittens should reduce the likelihood of maternal aggression. For breeding animals, the owner should provide extensive socialization and handling from kittenhood into adulthood. Gentle handling of the queen and hand feeding throughout pregnancy and after parturition may also be helpful.

Case example

After giving birth to a healthy litter of six kittens, Sheba, a two-year-old queen, became very protective and hissed or growled at anyone who approached, except one teenage daughter in the family. Prior to this time, the cat appeared very social and exhibited no signs of aggression.

The family was told to provide a quiet environment and to keep visitors to the home at a minimum. The teenager fed canned food to the pet four to six times daily. Each time she entered the room with food, she rang a bell very softly. Within a few days the cat would leave the litter and approach the daughter when she heard the bell. After two weeks, other family members would accompany her into the room, ring the bell, and provide the canned food.

When the kittens were four weeks old, the family attempted to have a friend visit the litter. The mother hissed, so visitors were discouraged from entering the room with the litter for another two weeks, after which time the maternal aggression had abated.

It was a bit unfortunate in this case that socialization of the kittens with strangers had to be delayed until six weeks of age. Handling by visitors starting earlier is generally more effective in promoting socialization to humans.

TERRITORIAL AGGRESSION

Individuals of many species engage in aggression to expel or keep out other individuals from their territories. This can be a beneficial behavior in that it helps protect important resources. It is a very common type of aggression and occurs in both females and males, although males may defend a much larger territory. Territorial boundaries may vary greatly between cats, with some cats attempting to defend only their own property and others protecting a much larger part of the street on which they live. Aggression toward other cats in the neighborhood may also be due to status/hierarchical conflicts, fearful or defensive behavior, or hormonal/sexual influences. This latter form of aggression might be particularly noticeable during the breeding season. The cat may take a slow, steady approach as it stalks or it may immediately and aggressively chase the other cat. The focus on the intruder can be intense and the cat can be very determined in pursuing and attacking the newcomer. Defensive displays by the intruder or new pet in the home may include hissing, growling, yowling, and pilo-erection. Cats that are highly aroused by the arrival of another cat on the property (e.g., fearful, territorial) but cannot gain access to the intruder (e.g., a closed window) may be at risk of exhibiting redirected aggression if approached by a family member or other cat in the home. Territorial aggression may also be displayed toward visitors entering the home.

Territorial and fear aggression are two common types of aggression shown toward human visitors. They can be differentiated by noting the cat's behavior with respect to the visitor. Although there may indeed be fear components to the behavior, territorial aggression generally differs from fear aggression where the cat tries to avoid an encounter and is only aggressive when it cannot avoid the person or other cat. The territorially aggressive cat is bolder and typically approaches or lunges at the individual. This may be accompanied by growling and hissing. Batting with forepaws or biting may occur even if the visitor stands still or attempts to move away. On the other hand, the fearful cat generally growls and hisses at a safe distance or from a hiding place. It only attacks if approached, crowded, or handled. Determining the difference is important because fear-induced aggression is usually a safer situation with a better prognosis than territorial aggression.

AGGRESSION BETWEEN CATS IN A HOUSEHOLD

Territorial aggression, along with aspects of fear and anxiety, may be exhibited when a new cat is added to the home. Of course genetics and previous social experience with other cats play a role in how one cat may react to a new addition to the household. While cats often choose to avoid social altercations by maintaining social distance, some that are more bold, confident, or domineering may display offensive threats to the new cat. In the confined area and narrow hallways of a home, avoidance is not always an available solution so that aggression becomes more likely.

Another situation in which aggression might occur is between two or more cats already present in the household, where there had been little or no previous history of aggression. Relationships may change as cats mature and age. In addition, increased conflicts may arise when there has been a change in the social group (people or animals becoming a part of the household or leaving the household), or when there have been major changes to the environment like moving house, or more subtle changes such as where the cats sleep, eat, perch, or eliminate. Medical problems could lead to pain or irritable-induced aggression, or may alter the way the cat interacts with other cats in the household. Any event leading to redirected aggression could also lead to a change in the way that cats interact with other cats in the home. It is also not unusual for aggression to arise when a cat has been out of the home and then returns (e.g., from a groomer or veterinary hospital stay). This may be due to pheromonal alterations, anxiety or discomfort of the returning cat, or the response of one or more cats that remained in the home to some alteration in the way the cat looks, acts, or smells upon its return. There may also be territorial and status issues that need to be re-established, even if the departure has been relatively short. Many of these problems are mild and will resolve themselves over time, particularly if there is enough space, perches, and hiding places for the cats to avoid interactions while they again 'recognize' each other and re-establish a compatible relationship. This may take anywhere from a few hours to several weeks for some cats, while on rare occasions the problem may be sufficiently intense to require a formal reintroduction program of desensitization and counterconditioning in much the same way as a new cat is introduced into the household.

Diagnosis and prognosis

When confronted by an intruder or perceived intruder into the household or onto the territory (another cat, other animal, or perhaps even person), aggression displayed by the household cat is generally territorial in nature, although, as mentioned, there may be aspects of fear, defensive, and status-related aggression. The resident cat typically hisses, growls, chases, swats, and attacks the newcomer. This can quickly evolve into relentless pursuit. The likelihood of a favorable outcome depends on the duration of the problem, the social experience of the cat, its temperament, and its threshold for arousal in response to territorial stimuli.

Management

Territorial and fear aggression are best managed by desensitization and counterconditioning. Drugs may be necessary, not only to control the behavior of the aggressor cat, but also to decrease the defensive posturing and vocalizing of the cat that is being threatened. Defensive signaling and escape behaviors tend to elicit chasing and aggressive attacks from the bolder cat in these situations. Reducing the fear and anxiety, and increasing the confidence of the 'victim' cat is therefore an important aspect of

the therapeutic program. Providing sufficient climbing, hiding, and perching areas (three-dimensional space) may allow the victim the opportunity to prevent conflicts, and display less anxiety. Electronic cat doors, which are opened only by the cat wearing the collar that activates the door, are also a means of allowing the victim cat the opportunity not only to access the entire home but also to retreat to a safe, secure area. Another therapeutic tool involves the use of synthetic feline facial pheromones sprayed throughout the cats' environment. Unwary owners may inappropriately reward undesirable behavior by offering the aggressive cat food or attention to try to calm it down. This can be corrected by effective owner education. Instead, the owner should stop the undesirable behavior with a disruptive stimulus (such as a compressed air canister or water gun) and then reinforce the desirable response. It should be noted that these devices may help to suppress the undesirable behavior of some cats, but may lead to increased anxiety and aggression in others. Castration or spaying may also reduce intraspecific aggression.

Treating aggression toward another cat that is being introduced (or reintroduced into the household) should begin with isolating the cats in confinement areas where they are unable to see or hear each other. Synthetic feline facial pheromones should be applied once or twice daily to several prominent upright areas in several locations in all rooms where the cats spend time. In some situations, an electronic diffuser may be more effect for disseminating the pheromone throughout the environment. This should continue for at least four weeks. In North America, the F3 fraction, Feliway™, is available for the reduction of territorial marking, which may help to calm the cat during reintroduction. However it is the F4 fraction, Felifriend™, that would be preferable since it is associated with familiarization and allomarking in cats (see Ch. 7 for details). This product is presently available in France, England, Belgium, and Japan. The owner should alternately release one cat at a time to roam in the home. Once all signs of aggression, anxiety, or hypervigilance subside, desensitization and counterconditioning can begin. If there is no significant decrease in agitated behavior within a week, medication should be considered. Selective serotonin reuptake inhibitors, tricyclic antidepressants, or anti-anxiety medications may be helpful.

The cats should gradually be exposed to each other in very controlled situations. This can be done with the cats in carriers or controlled with a harness and leash at opposite ends of the largest room or longest hallway in the home. During the sessions, the cats are fed highly palatable food or engaged in play. During following sessions, the cats are slowly brought closer together. By withholding food and rewards except for training sessions, each cat may learn to associate the presence of the other cat with food and play, rather than fear and anxiety. Once the cats are showing no tension at close proximity to each other during the sessions, the owner can attempt to allow them to have freedom in the same room. A high-power compression water gun may be used to interrupt unacceptable behavior by the aggressor cat. Small treats can be tossed to reinforce non-aggressive behavior. They can also be used to distract the cats and lure them to safe distances away from each other when they are close and might begin showing undesirable signs of arousal. The owners can begin allowing the cats to have freedom together in the home when no signs of aggression are shown during supervised conditioning sessions for several weeks. Initially, this should only be allowed when the owner is present in the home. At least two feeding stations and litterboxes should be available when the cats are finally allowed to roam freely in the home. They should be placed so that a cat will not be trapped or surprised when using either.

Conditioning can take months and may require considerable patience and time on the part of the owner. Cats should not be allowed to 'fight it out' as these fights rarely settle conflicts and may make the situation worse. Holding the pets to introduce them is commonly attempted by owners and should also be discouraged. In some instances, the most expedient and safe way to end the conflict is to remove one of the cats from the household. For the poorly socialized cat that is extremely territorial, it may be more prudent to confine it when people visit or to avoid adopting another cat.

The aggression that occurs when a cat returns home from the veterinary hospital or groomer, and cases of redirected aggression involving two cats in the home, are treated in the same manner as described above. Client handout #10 on the CD (Fig. 11.9) describes fear in cats and its modification through desensitization and counterconditioning.

Prevention

Adequate early socialization can help reduce the occurrence of territorial and fear aggression in most cats. However, certain individuals are genetically more territorial or fearful and their behavior may be more difficult to shape. In all cases, it is best to have an initial separation period when introducing a new cat to a household. A useful way of doing this is to establish the cats in separate rooms and then, periodically, switch the rooms. This allows the cats to become familiar with the scent of each other before they are actually introduced. Next, one cat can be given freedom of the entire home, while the second is kept in its own room. The situation is then reversed. The cats should then be slowly introduced during meal times by being fed at opposite ends of the same room. They should be more intent on eating at that time than on fighting. A harness and leash may be used for control. If aggression is seen when the cats are placed together at meal times, it might be necessary first to place the cats in separate cages during meal times and switch cages at each subsequent meal. Another approach is to feed them on either side of a door that is only open a few centimeters. Feeding should start at the far end of the rooms and gradually be moved closer to the doorway. When there are no signs of aggression, the cats can be given more freedom to be together in the home. At least two litterboxes and two feeding stations should be made available in relatively open areas. This will allow one cat to see the other approaching without getting surprised. It may also be helpful to use feline facial pheromones in the home during the introductory period.

Case example

When the family's elderly male cat died, they decided to adopt a four-month-old female to keep the remaining five-year-old female cat, Carley, company. As the owner carried the kitten into the home, Carley immediately focused on the kitten, walked deliberately toward it, yowled, and jumped to attack it in the owner's arms. The owner turned and was badly bitten on her leg by Carley. The kitten was confined to a bedroom, and during the following two weeks Carley sat outside the bedroom door, hissing and rattling the door. Two attempts to introduce the cats resulted in Carley immediately hissing or growling and attacking the kitten. The kitten was becoming increasingly more anxious and exhibited some hissing and withdrawal when the owners entered the room in which she was confined.

Carley was given buspirone (5 mg every 12 hours) and the cats were separated in such a way that Carley was unable to get near the door to the kitten's confinement room. During the second week, each cat was allowed to roam in the house while the other one was confined. By the end of that week, both cats had started to settle down and acted much less anxiously. During the third week, the owners started desensitization and counterconditioning exercises. Body harnesses and leashes were placed on the cats and they were taken to opposite ends of a long hallway and fed pieces of chicken for 15 or more minutes, at least five times each week. Every few days, the distance between the cats was decreased by small increments. After four weeks, the cats could be fed a few feet apart on a leash without any sign of aggression or anxiety. The feeding exercises were carried out in various areas of the house over the following two weeks. Following this, the pets were fed and allowed to move about on their own while under close supervision for short periods after feeding for another two to three weeks. During that period, they were allowed freedom in the home and Carley was gradually taken off the buspirone.

INTERMALE AGGRESSION

Aggression between male cats is a common form of feline aggression. This evolves as male cats mature sexually and behaviorally. It is particularly common during the mating season. The aggressive interactions involve posturing, threatening, and fighting. Hissing and growling are common. The behaviors are facilitated by postpubertal androgen secretion and are largely prevented or eliminated by castration.

Diagnosis and prognosis

Male–male aggression often results from hormonally driven competition, but territorial interests or fear may also play a role. This problem usually develops shortly after sexual maturity in males. They may respond by hissing, growling, scratching, attacking, and biting when in the presence of other males. Elaborate and ritualized threat displays may precede the events. The prognosis for successful treatment is good for cats that respond to castration, but guarded for those that do not.

Management

Treatment may involve behavioral modification, surgery, and drug therapy (Fig. 20.10). Castration is the treatment of choice for intact males and is effective for about 90% of male cats. Neither the fighting experience nor the age of the cat seem to affect the success of castration. While desensitization and counterconditioning may be attempted, this approach is usually not practical and may not be successful. Drug therapy with selective serotonin re-uptake inhibitors, tricyclic antidepressants, buspirone, or progestins may be effective in some cases. Drugs may suppress the cat's motivation to engage in this behavior, but the pet may become aggressive again when taken off the medication.

Method	Rationale
Castration	• The most successful approach • Neutering reduces or eliminates intermale fighting in approximately 90% of cases • Neither the fighting experience nor the age at the time of surgery seem to affect the success rate
Avoid all potentially aggressive situations	• Minimize the possibility of conflicts and competition • Feed cats in different parts of the house in open areas • Provide multiple litterboxes in open areas
Confinement	• Confine cats in crates or separate rooms if there is a risk of aggression
Behavioral modification	• Desensitization or counterconditioning • Success rate is low when used by itself • Light punishment (water gun) may be effective at suppressing aggression by either cat. This should be done without saying anything or looking at the cat
Drug therapy	• Selective serotonin re-uptake inhibitors, buspirone, or tricyclic antidepressants may be helpful • Progestins may be useful when treating cats for intermale aggression but have a number of side effects • Effects tend to be temporary and the behavior may resume after the drug is discontinued

Figure 20.10   Managing feline intermale aggression.

For aggression that persists following castration, separation from other male cats may be the only successful remedy.

Prevention

Care should be taken to ensure that all family pets are well socialized during infancy. Cats that have been well socialized may be more likely to get along and less likely to injure other cats. Introducing new cats into the home should always be done gradually (see territorial aggression, above). Intermale aggression will be prevented in most cats by neutering.

Case example

Barney was a 13-month-old, male Persian cat that the owner, a part-time cat breeder, had been raising for breeding stock. Six months earlier the owner had purchased Fred, a one-year-old Himalayan male, also for breeding purposes. There were also two intact adult female Persians and one intact female Himalayan in her home. When the owner was out, the Himalayans were housed in one room and the Persians in another. Whenever the owner was home, the cats had always played and eaten together. Approximately one month earlier, the owners had noticed that one of the male cats had begun to urine spray on a few of the walls in the kitchen and family room. The owner started to separate the males so that most of the time only one of the males was allowed to roam freely at a time and this had been successful at reducing the spraying. However, with play times, feeding times, cleaning times, and many family members and visitors in the home, it was impractical to keep Barney and Fred away from each other at all times. Now, the cats had begun to fight whenever they saw each other, and even hissed and growled through the closed door at each other. Barney had just returned from the referring veterinarian for treatment of a deep abscess on the side of the face.

The owners were extremely reluctant to neuter either cat, so exposure and counterconditioning techniques were discussed. The cats were kept apart except during feeding times when they were placed in separate metal carrying crates where they could see each other. Although some aggressive displays were exhibited, the cats soon ate in their separate cages without incident, even if the cages were side by side. The owners then attempted to allow one cat out at a time during feeding and there was only the occasional threat that occurred when Fred was the one out of the crate. However, when both cats were allowed out (a harness and leash was attached to each cat to maintain control and ensure safety), threats and attacks resumed whenever the cats got within a few feet of each other. Toys, catnip, and food could be used to occupy the cats without aggression for very short periods, but as soon as the cats investigated or approached each other the aggression recurred. The owners decided that the most practical solution for their household was to have one of the cats neutered. It was likely that Fred was the instigator of the aggression and the one most likely to spray. Also, it was in the owners' best economic interest to attempt to neuter Fred first and to use Barney for breeding. If this was not successful, they would have Fred adopted out into another home. Within one week of the neutering, spraying stopped and aggressive displays between the two cats were almost entirely eliminated.

PATHOPHYSIOLOGICAL AGGRESSION

Pathophysiological aggressive disorders are those that have an unusual underlying medical cause. These conditions may arise at any age, may have either a chronic or an acute onset, and may not fit neatly into the other aggressive behavior categories already described. Many of these are described in Chapter 4 in the discussion of the medical examination; some are listed in Figure 20.11. In some cases, the medical problems alone may not cause the problem but a combination of behavioral factors and medical problems may be necessary for the aggression to be patent. Underlying medical problems need to be addressed for successful treatment of pathophysiological aggression. This type of aggression is occasionally drug-responsive but is often poorly managed by behavioral modification techniques. Neurologic disorders stemming

from such conditions as metabolic disease, infection, trauma, and infestation of parasites can all lead to abnormal behaviors.

IDIOPATHIC AGGRESSION

Idiopathic aggression is a catch-all category for aggressive behavior that appears unpredictably and for which the underlying cause is not known. The diagnosis is reserved for those cats that have had a complete medical workup and have been thoroughly assessed by a competent behavior consultant without revealing an identifiable stimulus or motivation for the aggression. In fact, many cases that fall into this category may have a discernible etiology. The problem is that all pertinent information is not available to the owner and consultant. Redirected aggression or fear aggression that has resulted from circumstances that the owner did not observe are likely to end up in this category. Whatever the case, owners must always be instructed to be cautious around a cat that behaves aggressively where the stimuli are unknown. Unpredictability, especially when associated with uninhibited bites, significantly increases the danger of the situation. Euthanasia may be appropriate for these cases.

LEARNED AGGRESSION

There may be a learned component with many types of feline aggression. Learned aggression may arise out of a single aversive event or out of multiple exposures to mildly threatening stimuli. Learned aggression can result from intentionally and repeatedly provoking cats to be aggressive. Pets that are threatened or punished for aggressive displays can learn to associate pain or fear with certain stimuli and become even more aggressive each time the situations recur.

In other cases, it may occur because the owner has unintentionally conditioned the aggression. When a family member attempts to soothe a cat exhibiting aggression, the aggression may be

Underlying cause	Example
Infectious agent	• Rabies
Endocrinopathy	• Hyperthyroidism
Neurological disease	• Epilepsy, CNS inflammation, infection
Drugs and toxins	• May be due to side effects or paradoxical effects of therapeutic agents or due to toxins, e.g., paradoxical increase in anxiety with benzodiazepines
Painful conditions	• Dental disease, arthritis, abscesses, musculoskeletal problems
Other medical problems	• Sensory loss, fatigue
Degenerative diseases	• Cognitive dysfunction
Neoplasia	• Effect of tumors on the brain tissue affected (e.g., limbic tumors)

Figure 20.11 Feline pathophysiological aggressive disorders.

reinforced. In addition, when an aggressive display successfully removes the source of fear, pain, or territorial intrusion, the cat learns to use the display in any future fearful or threatening encounters. Owners that are anxious or threatening in the cat's presence will further aggravate the cat's aggression. Behavioral modification is the treatment of choice.

FURTHER READING

Ackerman L, Landsberg G, Hunthausen W 1996 Cat behavior and training: veterinary advice for owners. TFH Publications, Neptune City, NJ

Anderson RK 1996 Feline aggression. In: Ackerman L, Landsberg G, Hunthausen W (eds) Cat behavior and training: veterinary advice for owners. TFH Publications, Neptune City, NJ

Askew HR 1993 The treatment of aggression problems in cats. Kleintierpraxis 38(1):35

Barry KJ, Crowell-Davis SL 1999 Gender differences in the social behavior of the neutered indoor-only domestic cat. Applied Animal Behavioral Science 64(3):193–211

Beaver BV 1989 Feline behavioural problems other than housesoiling. Journal of the American Animal Hospital Association 25:465–469

Beaver BV 1992 Feline behavior: a guide for veterinarians. WB Saunders, Philadelphia, PA

Beaver BV 1994 Differential approach to aggression by dogs and cats. Veterinary Quarterly 16(Suppl 1):S48

Blackshaw JK 1991 Management of orally based problems and aggression in cats. Australian Veterinary Practitioner 21:122–124

Blum SR 1979 Aggressive behavior. Feline Practice 9(2):9

Borchelt P, Voith VL 1982 Diagnosis and treatment of aggression problems in cats. Veterinary Clinics of North America, Small Animal Practice 12(4):673–680

Borchelt P, Voith VL 1987 Aggressive behavior in cats. Compendium of Continuing Education for Practicing Veterinarians 9(1):49–56

Borchelt P, Voith VL 1996a Aggressive behavior in cats. In: Voith VL, Borchelt PL (eds) Readings in companion animal behavior. Veterinary Learning Systems, Trenton, NJ, p 208–216

Borchelt P, Voith VL 1996b Aggressive behavior in dogs and cats. In: Voith VL, Borchelt PL (eds) Readings in companion animal behavior. Veterinary Learning Systems, Trenton, NJ, p 217–229

Chapman BL, Voith VL 1990 Cat aggression redirected to people: 14 cases (1981–1987). Journal of the American Veterinary Medical Association 196(6):947–950

Fitzgerald M, Turner DC 2000 Hunting behaviour of domestic cats and their impact on prey populations. In: Turner D, Bateson P (eds) The domestic cat: the biology of its behaviour, 2nd ed. Cambridge University Press, Cambridge, p 152–175

Hart BL 1977 Aggression in cats. Feline Practice 7(2):22

Hart BL 1985 The behavior of domestic animals. WH Freeman, New York

Hart BL, Barrett RE 1983 Effects of castration on fighting, roaming and urine spraying in adult male cats. Journal of the American Veterinary Medical Association 163(3):290–292

Heidenberger E 1993 Aggressive behaviour of household cats. Tierztliche Umschau 48(7):436

Houpt K 1998 Domestic animal behavior for veterinarians and animal scientists, 3rd ed. Iowa State University Press, Ames, IA

Marder AR 1991 Psychotropic drugs and behavioral therapy. Veterinary Clinics of North America 21(2):329

Marder AR 1993 Diagnosing and treating aggression problems in cats. Veterinary Medicine August:8–13

Matthews-Cameron S 1987 Diazepam treatment of fear-related aggression in a cat. Companion Animal Practice 14:4–6

Overall K 1994a Feline aggression (part 1). Feline Practice 22(4):25–26

Overall K 1994b Feline aggression (part 2). Feline Practice 22(5):28–31

Overall K 1994c Feline aggression (part 3). Feline Practice 22(6):16–17

Reisner IR, Houpt KA, Erb HN et al 1994 Friendliness to humans and defensive aggression in cats – the influence of handling and paternity. Physiology and Behaviour 55(6):1119–1124

Schwartz S 1994 Carbamazepine in the control of aggressive behaviour in cats. Journal of the American Animal Hospital Association 30(5):515–519

Turner DC 2000 The human–cat relationship. In: Turner D, Bateson P (ed) The domestic cat: the biology of its behaviour, 2nd ed. Cambridge University Press, Cambridge, p 193–206

The European approach to behavior counseling*

INTRODUCTION

The veterinary approach to the behavioral disorders of pets, and most noticeably of dogs, varies from one country to another. It can be simplified by considering that two major tendencies currently exist. The first, which we shall describe as Anglo-American, has relied on the behaviorist school. Here, unwanted behaviors are most often described as the result of involuntary or ill-conducted learning processes. The clinical approach therefore consists of seeking reinforcing elements, in order to suppress or redirect the behavior. The second tendency could be described as 'Latin,' since it groups French, Italian, and Spanish-speaking researchers. This approach is supported by ethology, physiology, and psychopharmacology. It approaches behavioral disorders from both a medical and ethological angle, seeking to highlight the level of disorganization in behavioral function. This means that each clinical case should be assessed with the consideration that the clinical signs could arise from an overriding disorder. This approach is based on the observations and findings from 11 052 clinical cases. Two French editions, one Spanish edition, and an Italian edition of a book entitled 'Pathology of the dog's behaviour' have been published. Of course, this chapter cannot describe the complete approach, just an alternative point of

*Adapted from the work of Dr Patrick Pageat.

view, including some techniques that may be helpful for veterinarians. Adapted from Pageat P 1998 Pathologie du comportement du chien, 2nd ed. Editions du Point Veterinaire, Paris.

Author's note: First, Dr Pageat describes some of the clinical scales that have been designed to be used as tools to standardize the clinical evaluation of dogs, followed by some common behavior disorders. He also describes the use of synthetic analogs of pheromones in clinical practice in Chapter 7, and his approach to senior pet behavior problems in Chapter 12.

SCALES

Clinical ethology consultations should be viewed as having the same objectives as consultations conducted within all other clinical medical fields. They are concerned with recognizing signs that will help us to identify the processes and pathological states that have caused the illness. The only specificity of our discipline lies in putting value upon the interview with the animal's owners with a view to establishing the diagnosis. This interview process is the point at which inexperienced clinicians frequently encounter problems, since owners have an unfortunate tendency to give redundant, unreliable, and even unbelievable histories. In addition, since the owners are not usually well versed in ethology, they give information that has been subjected to cultural or emotional interpretation. In order to simplify the task for novice clinicians, a number of scales have been developed for data collection and assessment. In addition, the most significant presenting signs for each condition will be discussed.

In the interview, there is a degree of unearthing a certain amount of emotional motivation and impulse. The behavior consultation can thus be considered as the first step in developing a treatment program, since it will help to understand the functional perspective of the dog's behavior within its own species, and within the family structure as the animal perceives it. This act of playing down the emotional and anthropomorphic aspects of the history, along with a

clear explanation of the facts, is essential to the therapeutic contract to be agreed upon with the pet's owners. This ensures the commitment and cooperation of the owners. The consultation is carried out in several stages, but the order may differ from what is discussed below. For example, the physical examination may either follow or precede the consultation process, and some stages may be simultaneous.

It is both reassuring and useful for clinicians to have objective clinical tools to help them confirm their patient's state. On the other hand, these evaluation systems do not replace a close attention to clinical signs. Their role is to help us identify the stage of development, assess the progression of the behavior problem, and thus objectively assess the effect of the treatment.

Currently, three scales are utilized that have been validated to confirm their reliability and sensitivity. The scale for assessment of old dogs, known as the ARCAD scale, has been discussed previously in Chapter 12.

Scale for evaluation of aggressiveness

For clinicians, monitoring aggressive dogs constitutes a serious problem, due to the complexity of a patient's clinical picture as well as the ethical and legal consequences of any errors in evaluation. This scale classifies aggression into three types of sequential organization. It measures the intensity with two types of measurement: a global aggressiveness index (Iag) and a social aggressiveness index (Ias), as well as the ratio of the two $(Ias/Iag) \times 100$ (expressed as a percentage). Three types of sequential organization are possible: type 1, growls; type 2, growls and attempts to bite; type 3, direct bite (without warning).

The global aggressiveness index (Iag) and the social aggressiveness index (Ias) are calculated from the scores obtained in Figure 21.1 using the following eight parameters:

A. Owner's attitude toward the dog
B. Use of the dog
C. Frequency of aggressive manifestations

D. Gender
E. Dog's age
F. Bite description
G. Reaction after owner's reprimand
H. Area occupied by the dog

The higher the score, the less favorable is the prognosis. Thus, the fact that a dog has displayed aggression, followed by a new threatening phase, is more unfavorable than withdrawing rapidly to hide, which leads to a score of 5 for the former and 1 for the latter. Each parameter should be determined by questioning the owner rather than allowing them to read the grid, to reduce the possibility of distorting the answers. People who are offered a questionnaire often tend to try to improve their image to the 'pollster' or create an empathy with them by supplying answers they think they want to hear.

The Iag global aggressiveness index evaluates the intensity and frequency of all a dog's aggressive behavior within a social group (pack, family, etc.) and its interactions with a given person. A measurement will therefore have to be carried out for each member of a group. Approximations of the group may lead to underevaluation of the seriousness of the problem and distort the initial evaluation as well as the patient's monitoring. The global index is calculated thus:

$$Iag = [(A + C) \times F] \times (D + E)$$

The Ias social aggressivity index helps evaluate the intensity and frequency of aggressive behavior that is connected with maintaining hierarchical rank or the acquisition of a higher status. It is calculated thus:

$$Ias = (B + G) \times H$$

Finally, the ratio $(Ias/Iag) \times 100$ provides an estimate of the role of social phenomena in the genesis of aggressive manifestations. For each age and sex group, it is possible to give 'normal' value ranges, i.e., corresponding to the values obtained from animals not displaying any affective behavioral symptoms and not living in a hierarchically unbalanced group.

It is also possible to compare the values obtained for a given patient with the norms of

its age and sex group (Fig. 21.2). These measurements help to simplify differential diagnoses of behavioral changes associated with an aggressive case:

- In primary hyperaggressiveness (idiopathic or caused by lesions), aggression is type 3. Iag is strongly increased (35–40%) while Ias remains unchanged or decreases slightly (10–15%). The ratio between the indices is strongly decreased. This type of aggression is abnormal in sequence, intensity, context, and/or degree of inhibition.
- In reactional aggressiveness (while this type may be normal, it is essentially stage 1 of sociopathies), only the Ias index is increased. It may then represent 70–90% of Iag. Aggressions are of type 1 or 2 form.
- In secondary hyperaggression (instrumentalization of the previous types), both indices are increased and aggression is type 3. The ratio between the indices is often quite close to normal values.

This scale was validated using 270 control dogs and 132 dogs suffering from behavioral disorders (Fig. 21.2).

Scale for evaluation of emotional and cognitive disorders (EDED scale)

This scale's objective is to measure emotional disruptions in all age groups. It is constructed using simple behavioral parameters that are modified by affective disorders. These parameters were selected following factorial analysis of the history associated with each type of complaint. The scale was then validated with a population of 190 controls and 215 dogs suffering from affective disorders. The result is an approach in four parts:

- centripetal behavior
- centrifugal behavior
- cognitive evaluation
- somatic examination

The presence of a behavior in the grid does not mean that it has to be pathological, but only that it is statistically associated with clinical pictures

EVALUATION GRID OF AGRESSIVENESS IN DOGS		Score
A: Attitude of the owner toward the dog		
Fright	4	
Apathetic, carefree	3	
Disappointment	2	
Anger	2	
B: Use of the dog		
Guard and defense	3	
Herd	2	
Company	2	
Breeding, show	2	
C: Frequency of aggressive manifestations		
Daily	5	
Weekly	4	
Monthly	3	
Very spread out	2	
Never *	1	
D: Gender		
Male	2	
Castrated male	3	
Female	2	
Spayed female	3	
E: Age of the dog		
<1 year	1	
1–5 years	3	
>5 years	5	
F: Description of the bite		
The dog holds assertively (not shaking and tearing)	3	
It releases but remains threatening	5	
It releases and goes away quietly	4	
It releases and hides	1	
G: Reaction after rebuke from the owner		
The dog defends itself	4	
It lets the owner punish it	1	
It tries to flee	2	
H: Degree of access of dog		
The whole house	4	
All rooms excepts the parents' bedroom	3	
The whole house except the bedrooms	2	
Limited to a few rooms	2	

*In this case, F and G should both receive a value of 1.

Figure 21.1 Evaluation grid of aggressiveness in dogs (form #18 on the CD).

		Iag	Ias
0 to 1 year	males	25 to 35	10 to 12
	females	20 to 35	8 to 10
1 to 5 years	males	20 to 25	10
	females	30 to 45	10 to 12
5 years and over	males	30 to 45	12 to 18
	females	30 to 40	10 to 12

The chi-squared test confirms that there are significant differences at the 5% threshold for the value of the indices according to sex and age.

Figure 21.2 Normal values of aggressiveness indices; results of 270 dogs.

of emotional disorders. With each category, some selected types of behavior are taken into account and the different configurations that they may take are assigned an arbitrary numerical score between 1 and 5. The highest score is given to the poorest prognosis. The final mark, called the EDED value, is the result of adding all the scores together (Figs 21.3, 21.4).

THE EDED SCALE – EVALUATION OF DOG'S EMOTIONAL AND COGNITIVE DISORDERS

	Behavior type	Specific behavior	Score	Date	Score
C E N T R I P E T A L	Feeding	Hyperphagia[1]			3
		Anorexia/hyporexia			4
		Dysorexia (moving from hyper to hypo)			5
		Normal appetite			1
		Hyperphagia with regurgitation and reingestion			3
	Drinking	Normal drinking			1
		High-frequency drinking (documented)			5
		Chews at water without swallowing[2]			3
		Carries empty water bowl around (ritual)[3]			2
	Autostimulatory	Normal cleaning behavior			1
		Excessive licking, nibbling[4]			4
		Stereotyped nibbling, dizziness, turning on itself (or other stereotypies)[5]			5
	Sleep	Normal (or no change)			1
		Increasing, hypersomnia[6]			2
		Insomnia during sleep (and hyposomnia)[7]			3
		Wakes up shortly after falling asleep, anxiety at time of going to sleep (and restlessness)[8]			5
C E N T R I F U G A L	Exploratory (scanning)	Normal			1
		Inhibited			2
		Increased, hypervigilant			4
		Oral			5
		Frequent avoidance responses			3
	Aggression (defense)	No aggression or aggression stable (no increase or decrease)			1
		Irritation-related aggression			3
		Fear-related aggression			4
		Displays both fear and irritation aggression			5
	Learned social behavior	Steals, will not let go of stolen objects			5
		Bites without growling			4
		No submission response			2
		No self-control when playing			2
		Unchanged			1
	Specific learned behavior	Same response capacity (allowing for disease or age)			1
		Arbitrary responses			3
		No response to previously learned behaviors			5
PHYSICAL EXAM[9]		Normal			1
		Periods of tachycardia and/or tachypnea			2
		Diarrhea, colic			2
		Dyspepsia (and ptyalism)			2
		Increased emotional micturition			3
		Acral lick granuloma (and extensive lick alopecia)			4
		Obesity			4
		High-quantity drinking and urination (PU/PD)			4
TOTAL					

Centripetal = internal factors; Centrifugal = external stimuli. (See p. 460 for notes 1–9.)

Figure 21.3 Evaluation of dog's emotional and cognitive disorders (EDED scale) (form #17 – printable from the CD).

EDED value	Interpretation
9 to 12	normal state
13 to 16	phobias
17 to 35	anxieties
36 to 44	emotional (thymic) disorders

Figure 21.4 Interpretation grid of EDED scores.

Certain behaviors referenced in the EDED grid (Fig. 21.3) are clarified below:

[1]*Hyperphagia with regurgitation and reingestion.* The dog eats rapidly, displays spasms, followed by vomiting. It then reingests what it has just expelled and resumes its meal. This behavior appears regularly (1 meal in 2).

[2]*Chews water without swallowing it (dipsomania).* The dog nibbles the water and spreads it around its bowl while swallowing very little.

[3]*Carries its empty bowl.* The dog moves or carries its bowl toward one or several family members. This behavior stops as soon as the bowl is filled.

[4]*Licking, nibbling.* A dog that is licking or nibbling itself, then spontaneously stops.

[5]*Stereotypic nibbling, dizziness.* When there is licking or nibbling that does not stop spontaneously (the owners must stop the dog or divert its attention) or else dizziness or any other stereotypy (licking of the face, jumping, wandering, etc.).

[6]*Increase in sleep, hypersomnia.* When the duration of sleep is longer than the age norm (+25%).

[7]*Insomnia, during sleep.* Awakenings appear more than 90 minutes after going to sleep.

[8]*Awakes a short time after going to sleep; anxiety at the time of going to sleep.* The dog awakes in the 30 to 45 minutes following going to sleep. Prior to going to sleep the dog may display moans, excitement, and a search for contacts, as if it is afraid of going to sleep.

[9]In order to take the physical examination into account, all the manifestations observed must be scored and counted.

Once clinicians have obtained this score, they can evaluate it using the interpretation grid (Fig. 21.4). As with the aggressiveness indices, the EDED score does not replace the semi-logical approach; it complements it, facilitates the differential diagnosis, and helps objectively evaluate the animal's progress during treatment. As with the other forms, the evaluator and not the owner should complete the form.

The ARCAD scale (age-related cognitive and affective disorders)

The calculation grid of the ARCAD score was constructed according to the same rules as the emotional and cognitive disorder scale (EDED) (see Ch. 12 for details). While the parameters that make up both scales are very similar, they can have different diagnostic meanings. Therefore, while the EDED scale helps evaluate dogs of all ages, the ARCAD measurement provides a better means of assessing problems that might be specific to the older dog. For example, old dogs can obtain an EDED score of the anxious type, while their ARCAD score suggests a temperament disorder. The EDED scale is not designed to assess thymic disorders, which have a more discreet symptomatology in old dogs. Moreover, the ARCAD scale helps discriminate affective disorders (emotional score) from cognitive disorders to determine if drugs such as selegiline might be indicated.

BEHAVIOR DISORDERS

It is always difficult to establish a classification for disease entities, whatever our conviction concerning the educational and instructive necessity of such an approach, since it is still somewhat arbitrary. Therefore, the classification we offer here is not the only one possible. The criteria we use are, first of all, of a clinical and progressive nature, as we are actually trying to follow the usual path of development of these disease entities. Many of these pathologies seem to depend on the animal's stage of behavioral development, so this is an important aspect of the classification process.

The description of these conditions is based on more than 10 000 cases. Although this is a considerable number, it does not protect us from possible mistakes. The classification, arbitrary but with a logical base, should not obsess clinicians. The main object is to have a correct symptomatic approach, which is the only means to understand the affection and put together a treatment. For each one of the affections described, the treatment generally requires both biological intervention as well as many of the behavioral techniques discussed throughout the previous chapters.

DISORDERS APPEARING DURING PUPPYHOOD OR ADOLESCENCE

Sensory homeostatic disorders

In this category, we shall group both clinical pictures dominated by a hyperreactivity concerning one or several sensory systems associated with a lack of control of motor responses, and affective disorders ranging from phobia to depression. This highlights how both hyperproductive and deficiency states may be observed in these cases. Passing from one clinical form to another is often the rule. This is why we will focus on those problems that are most often the source of diagnostic difficulty.

Hypersensitivity–hyperactivity syndrome (HS-HA)

Description: These dogs have motor activity that appears to be overdeveloped. They cannot keep still. They run, jump, and never stop playing. The activities have almost complete absence of structure. No sequential organization can be found and, in particular, the appeasement phase that follows the achievement of the consummatory act is rarely found. Even with apparently normal activities (ball play, predatory play), the comparison with 'normal' subjects of the same age helps establish that the consummatory phase is extended, which most often leads to a new appetitive phase. Everything happens as if there was no 'stop signal' at the end of the sequence. During play fighting, the lack of an 'inhibited bite' is observed in puppies aged

two months and over. In addition, the total duration of the wakeful periods appears considerably greater in the most developed cases. These dogs sleep on average seven and a half out of 24 hours, which corresponds to a deficit of 30–50% of what is considered normal. It seems likely that the basic element in this clinical picture is an extremely low reactive sensory threshold. The animals we observe in clinical practice display the peculiarity of responding to very weak stimulation, be it visual, tactile, or auditory stimuli. Each stimulus triggers a characteristic motor response (hypertrophied and ill structured). Oral exploration is often observed.

Diagnosis: Two stages can be defined based on the presence or absence of sleep disorders.

Stage 1:
- Absence of bite inhibition with pups aged over two months.
- Incapacity to stop a sequence after the consummatory phase, and reappearance of an appetitive phase.
- Almost normal dietary satiety.
- Hypervigilance associated with the production of a behavioral sequence in the presence of stimuli continuously present in the animal's environment.

Stage 2 (stage 1 symptoms plus the following):
- Absence of dietary satiety.
- Global decrease of sleeping time (<8/24 hours), without alteration of the cycles, nor pre-sleep anxiety.

Differential diagnosis: It is necessary to distinguish between this syndrome and stage 1 deprivation syndrome, primary dyssocialization and sociopathy.

Although the tendency to react excessively to stimuli may be common to HS-HA and deprivation syndrome, dogs with deprivation syndrome display behavioral responses of fear aggression or inhibited responses associated with displacement activities. In addition, dogs with deprivation syndrome acquire an inhibited bite and have normal mobility. These latter considerations must be taken into account to help differentiate deprivation anxiety from dogs with a hypersensitivity–hyperactivity syndrome and concurrent anxiety.

Differential diagnosis is based on two essential points that are characteristic of primary dyssocialization: the absence of an alteration in the total length of sleep and the existence of irritable and hierarchical aggression without the acquisition of a submissive posture. The bites inflicted by the pup on its owners are often the reason that the client seeks help, so it is necessary to assess all of the signs. During the hypersensitivity–hyperactivity syndrome, pups inflict bites during sequences that are not aggressive sequences.

This is very different from what is seen in reactive stage sociopathies, which are characterized by perfectly regulated aggressive sequences in response to specific triggers. The differential diagnosis with a sociopathy with secondary hyperactivity may be more difficult when the HS-HA has developed secondary hyperaggressiveness. It is possible to distinguish between the two by reviewing the development of the disorders, and by highlighting the existence of alterations in behavioral sequences in the HS-HA.

Prognosis: This depends on the stage of development and the duration of the clinical picture. But it is especially the age at which treatment is started that seems to determine the establishment of self-control. An analysis of therapeutic results from 120 dogs relates to the juvenile period, but no particular age within this period. Conversely, subjects treated after the start of sexual activity respond less well to treatment, and correct control of dietary behavior (dog continues to steal food) and activity level are rarely obtained. Stage 2 shows a greater resistance to the treatment. Usually, dietary disorders and sleep disorders require drug therapy for almost a whole year. Whatever the age when treatment is started, it seems necessary to warn owners of the handicap this illness constitutes for the learning of complex tasks (hunting, search and rescue, drugs and explosives detection, guide dog, hearing dog for the deaf, or dog for the disabled). An early diagnosis must therefore be

encouraged in order to recommend a quick return to the seller. In all cases, it is essential to warn the owners of the long duration of the treatment (five to nine months).

Treatment: This is based on the administration of psychotropic drugs aimed at controlling the overactivity and the establishment of a higher sensory homeostatic threshold. In addition, play therapy may help to stabilize all the animal's reactions. The possible ambiguities in the hierarchy between the dog and its owners have to be treated by a complementary behavior modification program to prevent the development of a sociopathy. During chemotherapy, different groups of psychotropic drugs may be used according to the clinical picture. Clinicians must refrain from resorting to sedative or anti-productive neuroleptics, which hamper the evaluation of the dog during therapy. But anti-productive neuroleptics might be used initially in order to facilitate the keeping of the dog in the family environment. We have used sultopride, an anti-deficient dose (200 mg/m^2), in two doses. Currently, selegiline is the reference treatment for this affection. Its dosage is 0.5 mg/kg taken in a single morning dose. In some stage 2 cases, establishing normal satiety and sleep duration necessitates the use of fluoxetine at 3–4 mg/kg in one morning dose. Unfortunately, the improvement may disappear very quickly after the drug is discontinued. Therapy combines elements of play therapy and the learning of social inhibitions in techniques derived from direct social regression. We insist that play sessions are carried out with a lot of care and rigor. At this point the problem may appear to get worse even though the behavior is partly destabilized by chemotherapy. Therapy must therefore be accompanied by practical advice, which aims to reduce the chances of recurrence. The main pitfall is that if the dog jumps when it has reached maximal excitement during play, it may seek to nibble its owner. In order to avoid these reactions, owners are advised to stop play as soon as the dog produces these acts, which are not strictly connected with the play offered (e.g., during ball play, very quick short running phases around the play area while the ball trajectory is straight). Moreover, when the dog starts to jump around its owners, they should avoid all interaction including waving their arms, which unfortunately is the spontaneous reaction of many people when a dog jumps on them.

Sensory deprivation syndrome

Description: Dogs suffering from deprivation syndrome may present three clinical pictures, which correspond to very different deficiency levels. We shall study them successively, in order of increasing seriousness. During stage 1 sensory deprivation syndrome (ontogenic phobias), dogs are presented for consultation because of their incapacity to withstand exposure to one or more types of stimuli. The most classic stimuli are cars, urban noises, crowds, children, and persons with walking sticks or crutches. When exposed to these stimuli, the animals display such behavioral responses as flight, the need to hide, irritation, or fear aggression. Anticipation phenomena appear and the number of triggering stimuli may increase so the problem may progress to a more serious clinical stage or to other pathologies (secondary hyperaggressiveness). A primary complaint might then be housesoiling if the dog refuses to go outside or stays outside for a time which is too short for it to do its business. This is the clinical picture of a phobia and its typical development and not that of an anxious state, as we used to believe a few years ago. The term 'deprivation anxiety' is therefore not suitable for stage 1, but for stage 2 which we shall now describe.

During stage 2 sensory deprivation (deprivation anxiety), the clinical picture quickly becomes dominated by inhibition signs and substitution activities. In the chronic state, activities may be permanently altered.

Exploratory behavior is deficient, with almost pathognomic postural signs such as static exploration (feet together, neck stretched, ears bent backward, and tail between the hind legs) or an expectation posture at the start of many activities. Feeding behavior is also modified. In particular it may be inhibited in the presence of or following exposure to new or unfamiliar stimuli. In a chronic case, night-time eating periods are short and ingestion is quick (sometimes followed by regurgitation and reingestion), and the dog lies with belly up, tail between the thighs, ears bent backwards. In fact, more than 75% of the dog's daily ration may be consumed at night. The other notable fact is the rigidity of behavior of these animals. They always follow the same route inside and outside the house and they always come for their food at the same time. Any change to their routine may provoke withdrawal or panic attacks. Similarly, the layout of their environment must not be modified. A new piece of furniture or any unusual item (garbage can, boxes) that they come across on their normal walking route may trigger an expectation posture usually followed by an attempt to flee or a trembling attack associated with immobility sometimes combined with somatosensory signs. Self-injurious behavior of the limbs, flank, or tail, which is produced as a result of these traumatic situations, is frequently the reason for consultation. We have especially observed them in deprivation anxieties to which a state of hyperattachment is associated. Other displacement activities are sometimes observed, the most frequent being polydypsia, whereas bulimia is extremely rare. Potomania is in itself exceptional since out of 230 cases of deprivation we only encountered it five times. As with all potomanias, there is very spectacular water consumption, which may reach over 10 liters per day, with a very active search for water. This behavior may prove to be very dangerous for the dog, if it were to drink polluted or toxic water. Potomania may then lead to a complaint of housesoiling since, as in stage 1, the dog may refuse to defecate and urinate outside the house.

Stage 3 sensory deprivation (depressed state) is largely dominated by the disappearance of exploratory behavior and play. Thus, this state is particularly easy to identify in a pup. Most often, the pup is lying down but does not sleep. It remains prostrate in a corner and only goes out at night. Eating happens exclusively at night. Elimination behavior is poorly controlled and may be observed at only a few meters from the normal sleeping place, or the dog may even exhibit encopresia and enuresis (elimination in the sleeping area). These clinical signs, although not pathognomic (we find them in attachment depression), are typical of a young age-onset depression, which will have the best prognosis if the clinician intervenes early. Very quickly (four to 10 weeks), sleep disorders complicate the clinical picture. Micturition is generally associated with these awakenings. Progressively, the pup displays excitement and worrying periods (anxiety) just prior to going to bed for the night. It gets up, whines, scratches the walls, and looks for dark corners before giving in to sleep. Awakening occurs sooner and sooner after falling asleep and is repeated several times a night, thus decreasing the total duration of sleep.

Diagnosis: The diagnostic criteria for stage 1 (ontogenic phobias) are as follows:

- Phobic responses whatever their stage of development.
- Appearance in the days following the pup's arrival in its new living environment.
- Strong tendency to anticipate.

The diagnostic criteria for stage 2 (deprivation anxiety) are as follows:

- State of permanent anxiety with strong anxiety.
- Very inhibited exploratory behavior with the emergence of static exploratory acts.
- An expectation posture that is inserted at the beginning of the behavioral sequences.
- Ingestion of food in short bouts, predominance of night-time eating.
- Incapacity to tolerate changes in the organization of space and time.

The diagnostic criteria for stage 3 (deprivation depression) are as follows:

- Chronic depressive state (sleep disorders are present).
- Enuresis and/or encopresia.
- Maintaining normal intra- or interspecific social behavior.

- Intermittent excitement and the appearance of somatosensory acts (e.g., self-injurious behavior).

Differential diagnosis: This is described according to the stage of sensory deprivation. During stage 1, it is necessary to mention post-traumatic phobias and hypersensitivity—hyperactivity syndromes (HS-HA) in the differential diagnosis. For post-traumatic phobias, the decisive differential criterion is the age when the disorders appear. These phobias occur suddenly in a subject that was initially indifferent to the recent phobic stimulus. In many cases, the sensitizing episode or the sensitization mechanism is easy to identify. The HS-HA syndrome and deprivation syndrome have an increase in vigilance in common (at least for stage 1 with a few weeks' evolution). However, in HS-HA syndrome there is an absence of specificity of the stimuli triggering uncontrolled responses, whereas dogs at stage 1 of the deprivation syndrome are responding to stimuli that are easily identified. During stage 2, the differential diagnosis includes separation anxiety and anxiety disorders in the young adult. When the separation anxiety is expressed as a permanent anxiety, the distinction between both diagnostic entities is difficult. Many deprivation anxieties progress favorably by having a hyperattachment relationship, which itself is the source of a separation anxiety. Only a precise analysis of the clinical data, especially the development of the disorder, helps achieve this distinction. In the case where the clinical history does not help to make a clear decision (dogs adopted after several owners), we fear that therapy using detachment might induce clinical signs of the deprivation syndrome to reappear. Whatever their origin (spontaneous development of a phobic disorder, deritualization anxiety, secondary anxiety due to thyroid or adrenal dysfunction), the anxieties of the young adult or adolescent may sometimes be mistaken for an untreated deprivation syndrome. Sequential analysis, the absence of expectation postures, and static exploration of these anxiety disorders, as well as the development and the causes of appearance of the clinical signs, generally enable differential diagnosis.

The differential diagnosis of stage 3 includes detachment depression and reactive depression in pups. In the latter case, the easiest differential character to identify is the existence of social behavior, which is typical for dogs suffering from stage 3 deprivation syndromes, but is never the case in detachment depression. In addition, the first clinical manifestations are much earlier since they appear from the first week of life. However, this characteristic is sometimes impossible to identify because the pup's buyers do not know about it. In the case of reactive depressions in pups, differential diagnosis relies on the existence of a range of behaviors, including social acts typical of the animal's age, as well as a normally developed exploratory behavior during the period preceding the appearance of the disorders. Moreover, the majority of reactive depressions in pups are characterized by a sudden appearance of anorexia, which leads owners to early consultation. Sleep disturbances, a permanent manifestation in stage 3 of the deprivation syndrome, are not found.

Prognosis: It depends on the stage of the illness and the age at which treatment is started. Those at stage 1 have the best chance of recovery, whatever the age at which they are treated. We have obtained more than 77% 'good' or 'very good' results with these patients. Conversely, those at stage 2 have less chance as the age at which treatment is initiated increases. Before puberty, it is possible to obtain a satisfactory recovery in almost 60% of cases, whereas the success rate of treatment does not exceed 50% when treatment begins after puberty. Those at stage 3 have the lowest rate of recovery after treatment. These animals later develop serious sequelae, since almost 57% of them display a clear playful, exploratory, and cognitive deficit one year after the end of the treatment. The clinician must therefore warn the owners of the risk of a deficient state being maintained which may prevent the use of the dog for more complex work, when a stage 2 or 3 deprivation syndrome is diagnosed.

Treatment: Therapeutic strategies vary considerably according to the stage of the illness. In all cases, drug therapy must be combined with behavioral or cognitive therapy. Some stage 1 cases may be subjected to a simple therapy with no drug support. In such cases the phobic responses must be only slightly developed and the owners very patient. Chemotherapy depends on the clinical stage.

Stage 1. When the response to exposure to the phobic stimulus is characterized by avoidance behavior or threats, the beta-adrenergic antagonists (beta 1/beta 2) are particularly recommended. Propranolol, at a dosage of 10–20 mg/kg spread over two daily doses, is of particular interest. In large dogs we prefer the prolonged release forms. On the other hand, when aggressive behavior is a component of the problem, normothymics such as carbamazepine at a daily dosage of 20–40 mg/kg divided into two daily treatments for the delayed release form helps control the unwanted responses.

Stage 2. The choice of psychotropic drugs is made according to the patient's reactive dominance, which helps identify the monoaminergic systems on which it is necessary to act. It is not unusual, in the most developed cases, to have to use several psychotropic drugs, which act on different neurotransmitter systems. In patients displaying strong manifestations of anticipation, it is indispensable to use neuroleptics with a strong affinity for the dopaminergic structures. But it may become necessary to search for dosages or drugs that do not inhibit exploratory behavior. This is why we prefer substituted benzamides. The clinical forms marked by strong inhibition and those characterized by the presence of the expectation posture and static exploration benefit from tetracyclic antidepressants such as mianserine (2–5 mg/kg divided into a morning and evening dose).

Stage 3. Firstly, we seek to stimulate the dopaminergic system in order to induce the appearance of exploratory behavior associated with a stronger tendency to ingest food. This behavioral modification can be accomplished with the aid of substituted benzamides at the anti-deficient dosage. Sultopride (200 mg/m^2) and sulpiride (25 mg/m^2) are the molecules we believe to be the most appropriate, given in two equal doses in the morning and evening. In the future, molecules such as selegiline may produce good results without the problems of dosage associated with neuroleptics.

The behavioral and cognitive therapies, for stage 1, are either therapies of habituation, or desensitization with counterconditioning. Habituation is only possible when the phobic stimulus is unique and can be produced at will, which considerably limits its practical application. Moreover, this is a laborious and delicate technique and we clearly prefer desensitization associated with counterconditioning which, in addition to its flexibility, rapidly modifies patient behavior and thus simplifies the daily life of owners.

The indications for behavioral therapies in stage 2 are not good. Techniques based only on the triggering and reinforcement of behavior are only partially effective in states of inhibition and in the absence of a degree of behavioral organization. This is why it is more useful to carry out a cognitive therapy aimed at triggering behavioral patterns that do not yet exist. Thus, we prefer to use play-structuring therapy. We associate it with a detachment therapy if necessary, in order to avoid the development of a separation anxiety. As for stage 3, it is necessary to proceed in two stages, along with drug therapy. First, when the dog receives neuroleptic treatment, it is necessary to enrich the environment in order to increase the sensory experiences initiated by the psychotropic drugs. It is necessary to make sure that these experiences are positive in order to sustain the tendency to explore. It may be effective to temporarily favor a state of hyperattachment of the dog to one of its owners, in order to increase the animal's self-assurance without having to increase the dosage of drugs prescribed. However, it is necessary to remain vigilant so that a significant emotional dependency is not established, which would prevent a move toward a second phase of treatment. Having let the patient make contact with a great variety of stimuli in optimal conditions, we can then move to a play-structuring therapy, as

in stage 2. This therapy is generally facilitated by serotonin re-uptake inhibitor antidepressants.

Disorders in the development of social behavior

Separation anxiety

Description: The dog is presented for consultation because of the production of behavior problems when separated from its owners, including furniture destruction, vocalization, micturition, and defecation spread throughout the home, and sometimes vomiting or an intense ptyalism. These signs may occur when the owners are absent, during the night if the dog sleeps in another room than their bedroom, or even during daytime when it cannot be beside them. These dogs are described as 'very clingy,' and they follow one or more family members very closely. It is usual to hear that the dog tries to enter the toilet with them, and cries behind the door when it is not let in. These manifestations can be observed while the dog is with someone other than the person it always follows, since solitude is not the triggering stimulus. Some dogs may develop a lick granuloma, bulimia, or polydypsia. Reunion triggers excited movements, which may last several minutes. However, the owners quite frequently describe a completely different sequence in which the dog is 'sheepish,' displays signs of 'guilt,' going away from its owners with head low, ears bent back, a 'tucked up' behind, tail wagging between the legs, with perhaps some whining. This response may be, according to the owners, due to the damage done during the separation period.

Diagnosis: This relies on highlighting the following five factors:

- An appearance of the disorders during the period preceding puberty;
- A state of hyperattachment, highlighted by all activities being organized around the attachment person, by the search for visual contact before starting any activity, and by

some excitement and occasional whines triggered by any attempt to move away;

- The existence of anxious manifestations triggered by separation and resulting in an intermittent anxiety (destruction of furniture in the whole area visited by the dog, fear micturition and defecation, vomiting, ptyalism, whines) or a permanent anxiety (inhibition of the exploratory activity, lick granuloma, polydypsia, whining);
- The persistence of infantile social behaviors after puberty (notably making contact with family members by nibbling; a very high frequency of play-eliciting postures);
- The existence of departure and return rituals.

Differential diagnosis: One must not forget that the appearance of a hyperattachment bond is one of the signs of spontaneous improvement for the clinical picture of stage 1 and 2 deprivation syndrome. When the symptoms of this affection are associated with separation anxiety or come before it, it is possible to diagnose both deprivation and separation anxiety syndrome. In sociopathy, the dominant subjects tend not to let the members of their group go outside their territory. As a result, during hierarchical confrontations such as those that are seen with sociopathy, the departure of the owners triggers aggressive behaviors against them. When they do manage to get out, the aggression tends to be directed at the exits they have used, or windows through which the dog sees them go away. Thus, furniture damage is extremely localized. Moreover, stains may appear on certain family gathering places (tables, chairs, sofa, etc.) due to social marking with urine or stool. As a result, differential diagnosis relies mainly on the locality of the damage (dispersion in separation anxiety), the locality and kind of stains in separation anxiety (dispersed on the floor, multiple and soft stools, urine in small and multiple amounts), and on the presence of aggression during attempts at going out, in sociopathy. The hyperattachment syndrome of the adult and separation anxiety present some clinical features, which are almost identical except for two details that are the sudden appearance of hyperattachment in a previously independent adult male and the existence of a normal social repertoire (absence of nibbling when making contact). The hyperattachment syndrome of the adult is always a secondary affection of another affective or mood disorder. Confusion with involutive (degenerative) depression can sometimes exist since animals suffering from both these conditions may soil the inside of the house and may produce whining and sometimes suffer from insomnia. However, in the case of involutive depression the sudden appearance of disorders after age five constitutes a sufficiently noticeable diagnostic factor to avoid diagnostic errors. Only the separation anxieties which, because of the absence of appropriate treatment, have evolved toward an involutive depression may pose diagnostic problems. The highlighting of the signs of degeneration, the fact that the housesoiling is not only made up of emotional micturition and defecation, but also of infantile elimination behaviors occurring even in the presence of the owners, and finally the value of the EDED and ARCAD scores help the clinician to come to a decision. The fact that a separation anxiety may appear in conjunction with involutive depression must guide clinicians in their therapeutic action, and particularly lead them to carry out a detachment therapy in order to decrease the risk of relapse after treatment has stopped. A hyperattachment of the adult may appear in the first stages of the development of involutive depression and complicate the differential diagnosis. It is the timing of when the disorders appear (sudden appearance in a dog over five years) that helps us distinguish them.

Prognosis: This is very favorable provided that the owners have understood what has happened and go along with the exercises. Any situation of affective distress in the family of the animal constitutes an important difficulty in establishing the therapy and must be taken into account in the prognosis.

Treatment: To be conducted properly, chemotherapy necessitates that the type of anxious expression has been identified properly. At the beginning of the illness, when hyperreactivity and anxiety coexist, beta-blockers, and particularly propranolol (10–20 mg/kg), are sufficient. But this stage may be missed with the owners seeking consultation when the dog is far more disturbed, when the damage done is more severe, and their patience has run out. Thereafter, chemotherapy must provide a rapid attenuation of the disorder. The molecule that helps, whatever the form of separation anxiety, to stabilize the anxious state and facilitate detachment is clomipramine at the dosage of 2–4 mg/kg per day. Different drugs might then be added to modulate other specific expressions of anxiety. Its anticholinergic properties help it to curb fear micturition and defecation very rapidly. These same properties, together with its effects on the serotoninergic system, also help to decrease and possibly suppress bulimia where it exists. When motor excitement, increased exploratory behavior, and destruction constitute one of the main aspects of symptomatology, neuroleptics, active at the level of the D2 and D3 dopaminergic receptors, are particularly useful. Among these, pipamperone (60 mg/m^2 divided into two daily doses) is the molecule that, associated with clomipramine, gives the best results. Because of the potentialization of sedative effects when these two drugs are used together, one needs to administer only 50% of the usual dose of pipamperone. Lastly, in the case where separation anxiety is mainly expressed by the appearance of lick granulomas, the use of alpha-2 agonist drugs such as clonidine (0.015 mg/kg divided twice daily) or etomidate (0.5–1 ml/5 kg divided twice daily), when administered on their own, suppress licking in eight to 14 days as well as decreasing the intensity of anxious manifestations.

Behavior therapy consists of two elements: a detachment therapy that aims at breaking the hyperattachment bond whilst establishing a link to the group; and a deritualization of departures and returns. In certain cases, the establishment of hierarchical markers is added, in order to stabilize and make durable the relations between the animal and its owners.

Primary dyssocialization

Description: These dogs could be described as 'canine delinquents.' These dogs are older than three months, in which irritable aggression and sometimes hierarchical aggression is observed, triggered by the owners' attempts to control the activities of the dog. Similarly, these animals are food 'thieves,' but these thefts are generally associated with aggressive behaviors. The dog has never initiated submission; they are described as 'preferring to be knocked out rather than give in;' as a result, the owners are used to no longer reacting. During aggression, the bites are violent, inflicted without any control, but always associated with threat signals that are generally produced simultaneously with the bite and sometimes continue while the dog is biting its opponent: this is a 'holding' bite. In some cases, micturition, defecation, and emptying of the anal sacs can be observed together with the aggression. When exposed to other dogs, these dogs are thought to be fighters and, in fact, they often initiate the attack and start serious and bloody fights. Since there is an absence in control of the aggression, when the opponent submits, this immediately re-triggers the fight. Similarly, confronted with a more powerful opponent, dyssocialized dogs are often the victim of deep wounds because of their incapacity to submit and thus to inhibit the aggressiveness of the opponent.

Diagnosis: This is based on highlighting the following four key symptoms:

- Irritable aggression and hierarchical aggression with a phase of intimidation simultaneous with the bite.
- A defect in the acquisition of the 'inhibited bite.'
- A defect in the acquisition of the capacity to submit (absence of submission posture).
- An absence of feeding hierarchy organization.

With age, other modifications of social behavior appear and, in particular, a strong tendency toward sexual behaviors in the presence of the owners, aggression when the animal meets fellow creatures of the same gender, particularly when the dog or bitch are with an owner of the opposite sex. These dogs are often in a situation of hyperattachment with one of the family members and thus may develop a separation anxiety. In this case, the diagnosis is primary dyssocialization with separation anxiety.

Differential diagnosis: Two behavioral affections that have some symptoms in common with primary dyssocialization match with very different pathological states: hypersensitivity–hyperactivity syndrome and sociopathies. It is easy to tell the difference between the HS-HA syndrome and primary dyssocialization. The bites from animals suffering from HS-HA syndrome do not result from aggression (there are no threat signals), but from motor responses during play. In addition, sleep disorders are observed in these patients but not in dyssocialization. In real sociopathies, the dog has a complete social repertoire, and hierarchical imbalance only develops because of the acquisition of prerogatives, as a dominant, at the time of puberty, or during the remainder of its adult life. It is possible to notice, in particular, with these patients a very good capacity to modulate bites (the owners often say that their dog 'grasps' more than bites), threat phases that are very distinct from the rest of the aggression, and these dogs do not 'steal' food. These dogs respond in an expected manner to the triggers of expression.

Prognosis: It is generally good. However, two factors may affect it: when the dog is large and when there are young children. Indeed, facing a large subject we must think of the danger such an animal represents when it is incapable of controlling itself and has no limitation to the satisfaction of its wishes. The dangerousness of such an animal, the risk that treatment poses, and the clinician's legal responsibility (both civil and criminal) in the case of an accident should lead them to be extremely careful and to warn their clients of all potential risks. In addition, the presence of very young children poses an important risk of accidental injury. These children, because they are attracted to the dog and because they are unaware of how to interact safely and appro-

priately with the dog, may trigger irritable aggression. Their sudden movements and the fact that they eat food at the same level as the dog all contribute to the risk of triggering serious bites, which often affect the face. In these cases practitioners must be very careful to discuss all aspects of the problem before deciding to proceed.

Treatment: This should be varied according to the clinical picture and the elements of prognosis. As a result, several protocols may be offered. The combination of clomipramine (1–4 mg/kg divided twice a day) and pipamperone (30 mg/m^2 divided twice a day) facilitates therapy for the less aggressive subjects, whilst facilitating the treatment of separation anxiety that is frequently present. However, a recurrence and a new wave of irritable aggression may appear very often after eight to 15 days. This modification is associated with a total increase in mobility. This worsening may be explained by a sensitization of the dopaminergic structures in response to the suppressive action of pipamperone. This hypothesis might explain the positive effect of an increase in the dosage of pipamperone (60 mg/m^2) from the eighth to the tenth day. However, this solution may prove insufficient in some subjects, especially if these relapses recur during treatment. The thymoregulators may then provide a useful response. This is particularly true of carbamazepine (20–40 mg/kg), whose regulating activity on the impulsiveness phenomena, and also suppressing effects of irritable aggression, help us treat the most excitable subjects. Selegiline, although it is usually not part of the normothymics in pharmacological classifications, offers interesting possibilities in the treatment of these disorders; however, these are still at the developmental stage. In the most dangerous patients, it is necessary to resort to the use of neuroleptics at a suppressive dose in order to restore contact that the owners can tolerate. These treatments, which may, at first, put the animal in a state of indifference that is not tolerated very well by the family, must be set up during hospitalization. The most appropriate drug is sultopride (1 g/m^2 divided bid), which is combined with pipamperone (30 mg/m^2 divided bid), and helps to control all the D1, D2, D3, and D4 dopaminergic structures. Therapy should be effective in about eight to 10 days.

Behavioral therapies must be part of the treatment, in association with chemotherapy. On the one hand, we use directed social regression and, on the other, a therapy of self-control by play. Both therapies are set up jointly. It is necessary to follow the progress of the families very carefully, in order to prevent any mistakes due to a feeling of fear or withdrawal, which might lead the owners to let the dog occupy a dominating position.

Heterospecific imprints

Description: These are animals whose disorders only appear after puberty, from the absence of courting behavior and attempts to mate in the presence of a receptive fellow creature of the opposite sex, to the production of typical sexual acts in the presence of subjects of the opposite sex of a different species. Secondly, other behavioral changes may appear later and be especially characterized by an appearance of the symptoms of sociopathy. The clinical picture is frequently complicated by the existence of a hyperattachment.

Diagnosis: This is simple and relies on the following symptoms:

- An absence of sexual behavior in the presence of a receptive conspecifics partner (in males, pheromones still trigger a state of excitement).
- Sexual behavior triggered by a heterospecific partner usually of the opposite sex belonging to the species with which the dog lived during the imprint period.

We may sometimes find the signs of a sociopathy; a sociopathy along with heterospecific imprint is then diagnosed. Similarly, in the case where a state of hyperattachment exists and is the source of a separation anxiety, a diagnosis of separation anxiety with heterospecific imprinting is proposed.

Differential diagnosis: We need to distinguish between the sociopathies, the sexual deviancies of owners perpetrated on their pets, and the normal sexual inhibition of subordinate individuals. In the sociopathies, we may find real, sexual manifestations and mounting connected with dominance that may confuse and lead to a worse prognosis (with the heterospecific imprint complicating the situation, the situation is often barely manageable). The distinguishing criterion in sociopathies is based on the existence of normal sexuality triggered by conspecific partners. In the very particular and delicate case of anthropophilia with dogs living with a zoophilic partner, the dog, if it seeks sexual relations with the human being, still displays a normal sexuality when in the presence of receptive fellow dogs. The admission to zoophilic practices by the owner simplifies the work of clinicians. It must be noted that this situation, which generally concerns male dogs, tends to increase the sexual fervor of the animal, which also displays a courting behavior even in the presence of a non-receptive bitch (outside estrus). We have seen that subordinate individuals display a normal sexual inhibition in the presence of a dominant subject of the same sex. This phenomenon concerns both males and females, but confusion with a heterospecific imprint is only possible with males. Indeed, even a subordinate individual, in the presence of a female in estrus, displays a phase of excitement followed by a series of appeasement signals toward the dominant present. As a result, we may receive for consultation dogs that, when introduced to a female for mating, in the presence of their owner, do not mount but turn to the owner, moaning, rubbing their neck on the owner's legs and wagging their tail, ears bent back on the neck. This is a normal sequence and the only way to achieve mating consists of putting the dogs into contact, outside the presence of the owners.

Prognosis: This is very poor. We have only in exceptional circumstances been able to redirect the specific identification and thus the choice of the sexual partner. Only with animals in which it is feared that imprinting disorders might occur, and for which immersion in a pack is set up, may normal sexual behavior be restored. It is important to recognize these factors in order to act very early on and especially to warn the owners who might want their animal for breeding purposes.

Treatment: Currently, this is almost impossible. It is however possible to avoid the development of disturbing sexual behaviors in subjects imprinted to the human species and in so doing, prevent the appearance of a sociopathy. When the developmental conditions of the male or female pup help us to predict the appearance of such disorders, early neutering may prevent the occurrence of sexual acts. Later, castration only provides a decrease in the frequency of sexual manifestations. Apart from cyproterone acetate (3–5 mg/kg divided twice daily for two to three weeks) in males, few preparations help at all. As a therapy, directed social regression is particularly recommended. By placing the dog or bitch in a subordinate position, the expression of its sexuality is also inhibited, which suppresses disturbing sexual behaviors. Conversely, when the result sought is the appearance of an intraspecific sexuality, immersion for at least 15 days with conspecifics of both sexes is necessary. As we have highlighted regarding the prognosis, only very young subjects or those in puberty are likely to respond positively to this therapy.

Thymic disorders of puppyhood and adolescence

Reactive depression in pups

Although reactive depression may occur at any time in the life of dogs, reactive depression in pups deserves to be treated separately, both because of the particularities of its symptomatology and because of its seriousness.

Description: Pups display a homogenous clinical picture, marked by a generalized state of inhibition. They are immobile, apathetic, no longer play, and may barely drink at all. The physiological state, as a result, deteriorates

rapidly and involves the rapid adoption of reanimation methods.

Etiology and pathogenesis: Any violent stress is likely to incite this type of state. Accident, violent punishment inflicted by a human or a fellow dog, painful stimuli (we have observed 11 cases in five years that resulted from tattooing with a pincher), or abandonment. This state results from an extreme emotional response. In pups a pathology need not be a consideration if the problem continues beyond 10 days, but this would be a limit that is significant in adult dogs. One might think that it is the age of the animals that plays a sensitizing role. An attachment bond seems to protect the pups, as found in the 44 cases we have studied. When the pups have developed a proper attachment bond with their environment, the stressful situation seems to be tolerated better; on the other hand, when this bond is associated with the stressful situation, the depression develops from the onset.

Diagnosis: The diagnosis is made following a clinical assessment for any underlying pathology and after a first therapeutic phase aimed at getting the pup to eat. However, the symptoms of reactive depression are easily identifiable:

- Sudden stop of any activity in a pup that had been normally active before.
- Sudden appearance of hypersomnia (average duration of sleep multiplied by 1.5 to 1.8).
- Anorexia and adipsia.
- Enuresis/encopresia.
- If there was reanimation and force feeding, an absence of resumption of activity is noticed despite the return to a normal feeding state and the worsening of enuresis and encopresia.

Differential diagnosis: An infection, parasitic illness, or a feverish state, etc., or a stage 3 deprivation syndrome, or an early detachment depression, or finally a separation anxiety must be considered. In pups, any morbid state is frequently accompanied by a restriction in activity, an indifference to stimuli, and a decrease, or possibly a disappearance, of appetite. This is why a comprehensive clinical examination is always necessary when assessing any behavioral problem. The differential diagnosis of stage 3 deprivation syndrome relies on the kinetics of the affection. In patients suffering from a stage 3 sensory deprivation syndrome, the disorders can be observed in the days that follow the arrival of the pup with its owners. Conversely, reactive depressions occur in animals that previously did not present any behavioral abnormality. In the case of early detachment depression, the incapacity of the owners to establish any contact with the animal and the absence of a period during which the animal might have shown some 'normal' behavior are major criteria in differentiating both illnesses. In the most severe cases of separation anxiety, during a prolonged separation, a clinical picture can be observed that is totally identical with reactive depression. In this case, we believe it is logical to make the diagnosis of reactive depression and of separation anxiety. Separation from the person to whom the pup is attached triggers the depressive state. It is important to take into account both morbid states, because lifting the depressive state may bring back the range of behavioral manifestations of separation anxiety, which may disturb the owners.

Prognosis: This is always positive at the behavioral level. However, very worrying situations may be encountered at the somatic level when the cause of anorexia has not been diagnosed and the animal has continued to fade because of lack of appropriate supportive care.

Treatment: The main element of treatment is drug therapy. It combines antidepressants and anxiolytics. The former help restore behavioral competence in the patient, whereas the latter immediately relaunch the activity of the animal whilst avoiding the appearance of anxiety that might accompany the first week of antidepressant treatment. The antidepressants used are essentially 5HT1A inhibitors whose specificity is more or less marked. Mianserine (2–5 mg/kg divided bid) with a mixed activity (alpha-2 antagonist, H1, H2) is interesting because it can be prescribed on its own in animals that have recently been affected. No specific forms of

behavior therapy are indicated, except in the particular case of reactive depression associated with a separation anxiety. Then, specific therapies of these anxieties are instituted as soon as antidepressants have helped the dog resume a state of anticipation. In the other cases, it is sufficient to make the dog play by attempting to vary the types of games in order to stimulate all the sensory channels. Clinicians will need to remain vigilant about the risk of food rituals and preferences that might have developed when the owners were trying to treat their anorexic puppy.

DISORDERS IN THE RELATIONSHIP WITH THE EXTERNAL ENVIRONMENT

This category currently contains one single clinical entity: the dissociative syndrome of dogs.

Dissociative syndrome

The statistical analyses we carried out on data from populations of dogs suffering from behavioral disorders have led us to identify a new clinical entity: the dissociative syndrome. One of the main characteristics of this consists of the progressive loss of relationships with the real world in favor of increasingly severe hallucinatory-type episodes. Hallucinatory episodes might be defined as repetitive behaviors that are not caused by underlying medical pathology and do not appear in response to an identifiable stimulus (e.g., snapping at air, circling, looking upward). This is a very crippling affliction whose treatment and/or monitoring must be maintained during the life of the animal. Moreover, some subjects may, during their hallucinatory episodes, constitute a danger to their family.

Description: The average age of the dogs affected, at time of first consultation, is between 12 and 20 months. The animals are presented because of the appearance or increase of the repetitive activities (circling, clicking jaws, jumping, etc.) which appear to be related to no identifiable stimuli. In most cases, owners describe an animal that appeared normal during the first six to eight months of life, then began to display an initial 'strange' episode often called a crisis. This first episode may have appeared spontaneously or in response to a highly stressful event. This distinction is important at the prognostic level. There may also be concurrent medical problems, such as demodicosis.

Etiology and pathogenesis: Although the etiology is unknown, all the clinical factors, both somatic and behavioral, suggest a disturbance in a number of neurotransmitter systems. Based on therapeutic trials, there appears to be a mixed serotoninergic and dopaminergic dysfunction.

Epidemiology: German Shepherds and Bull Terriers appear to be overrepresented (although this diagnostic category is not used in North America so this breed predisposition may prove to be regional). Other breeds may also be affected, including Irish Setters, Rottweilers, Dobermans, Pyrenean Shepherds, and some cross breeds of shepherds and spaniels. Family prevalence is important. Clinical signs first arise between seven and 31 months for the majority of subjects (88.5%), though we have observed in 9.7% of cases a first episode between four and seven months (mainly with German Shepherd bitches), and some cases may not appear until around the age of five years, when the history is somewhat more unusual (dogs living outside).

Development: Before the morbid phase, there is a 'pre-morbid phase,' during which many disorders in social behavior are observed. This pre-phase may appear from the age of six to nine weeks. In females, a tendency for withdrawal is mainly observed. The pup avoids taking part in games, with both its conspecifics and humans, without showing any fear or panic. Social communication is characterized by avoidance or may cease during execution, for no apparent reason. The family generally describes these animals as 'shy.' With males, a great impulsiveness is noticed which manifests itself mainly by 'brutality' during strong affective interactions (positive or negative depending on the anger of the owners). As with females, a tendency not to finish social interactions is also noticed.

Females represent 78.5% of the subjects having an avoidance-type pre-morbid phase, whereas males represent 69.3% of subjects with a pre-morbid impulsive phase. During the rest of their lives, in the absence of any treatment, dissociation worsens and leads noticeably to severe cachexia.

Diagnosis: This relies on highlighting three class 1 symptoms. The existence of a symptom of at least class 2 helps to confirm the diagnosis.

Class 1:
- Disorder appears between the pre-puberty period and five years.
- A growing loss of receptivity to the environment.
- The existence of hallucinatory episodes with constant themes.
- The production of stereotypies during hallucinatory phases.
- The existence of dumb-looking phases with somatosensory activity.
- The existence of a pre-morbid stage of the avoidance or impulsive type.

Class 2:
- Uni- or bilateral dilatation of the lateral ventricles.
- The presence of isolated peaks on the EEG (noticeably in occipital region).
- Demodicosis.

Differential diagnosis: As in all cases of developmental disorders, there can be many diagnostic possibilities, especially in the early stages when the signs are mild. However, six affections should be considered in the differential diagnosis: stage 2 and 3 deprivation syndrome, constraint stereotypies, recurrent hallucinations due to ketamine, hydrocephalus, hyperadrenocorticism, and primary or functional hypothyroidism.

Prognosis: The prognosis is poor. Almost 28% of animals do not seem to respond to treatment. To examine the prognosis, one should consider the circumstances of appearance of the first dissociative episode. Some dogs develop their first episode following a violent and objectional stress, whereas others enter into a morbid phase without any noticeable event. The former seem, after the analysis of 59 cases, to respond better to the first therapeutic protocol, at significantly lower doses and with a longer interval between outbreaks.

Pharmacological therapy: Therapy may help to stabilize the animal, and limit the risk of development of anxiety disorders. Two well-known therapeutic strategies can be used according to the context and the objectives. In cases where treatment is initiated very early after the appearance of the first dissociative episode, selegiline provides improvement, dominated by a reassociation with the environment and an emotional stabilization that delays future episodes. In cases with short stereotypies and impulsive components, fluoxetine provides some stability. However, the results obtained with these treatments are only transitory, with movement to more specific molecules necessary. In chronic cases, neuroleptics and the like are the preferred molecules. To date, after trying many molecules that are used for the treatment of schizophrenia, risperidone is our treatment of choice at a dose of 1 mg/m^2 once a day.

Conclusion: The dissociative syndrome is probably still an underdiagnosed affection, but appears to be an important condition because of its prevalence in some breeds. It is especially at the level of comparative medicine that we believe it to be important. It is clear that there are numerous analogies with schizophrenia.

DISORDERS OF SOCIAL INTERACTIONS

Social phobias

Description: This section groups disorders in which the animal proves unable to tolerate certain intra- and interspecific social interactions (gaze, physical and vocal contact). This phobic state bears no relation to the environment or the individual with which the interaction is happening; it only relates to the interaction itself. This is why we have described these phobias as 'social.'

It would be both overzealous and useless to draw up a catalog of all the social phobias that can be encountered in clinical medicine. However, some are more frequently seen than others in the canine species. These are noticeably interactions based on sight, sound, or touch. Whatever the individual, breed, or place where the social interaction takes place, the dog suddenly breaks the interaction and moves away from the participant. This systematic breaking of contact generally constitutes the reason for consultation.

Diagnosis: This relies on the following symptoms:

- A systematic avoidance of one type of social interaction.
- The existence of a normal social repertoire in other regards.

Differential diagnosis: This largely aims to exclude confusion with precocious detachment depression and primary dissocialization. In precocious detachment depression all communication functions are altered; i.e., these subjects have no social repertoire. In the case of primary dissocialization, in addition to the absence of social inhibition mechanisms, a search for contact is often noticed, even if it leads to aggression.

Prognosis: This depends on the age of the dog at the time of the diagnosis. Older subjects seem to necessitate a longer therapy, which is often difficult for the owners. The development of a secondary anxiety tends to worsen the condition, particularly when it manifests itself as an intermittent anxiety and includes aggressive manifestations.

Treatment: As with all social behavior disorders, this relies primarily on drug therapy. Drug therapy aims to suppress flight reactions and is focused on the regulation of noradrenergic activity. Beta-blockers are an important aid without facilitating aggression. Propranolol (10–20 mg/kg) is the drug of choice unless there are cardiac contraindications. In this case, the anti-productive phenothiazines used at a low dose helps these patients. Thioridazine (30 mg/m^2 divided bid) and especially fluphenazine (50 mg/m^2

divided bid) are the most reliable compounds. Behavior therapy uses play to induce positive interactions in a normally fearful context. This is a counterconditioning technique, which can be complemented by other techniques, noticeably cognitive therapies. These aim to show the dog that the interactions usually sought by the animal can only begin after the establishment of a contact that would normally lead to a phobic interaction. This pushes the animal to tolerate it. These cognitive techniques should not be applied from the onset because they can favor the establishment of a state of acquired distress and then depression. If the dog does not manage to overcome its aversion to the phobic stimuli, it may be deprived of other very important interactions at the hierarchical level as well as the affective level. Propranolol helps to decrease these risks.

Disorders of hierarchical organization

In any analysis, these disorders should be considered as attacks on the social group and not the individual. However, incoherent hierarchical markers rapidly disorganize the behavior of the dog, which explains their place in this category. However, in order to highlight the involvement of the whole social group in these problems, we have called them sociopathies.

Sociopathies in canine groups

Description: These are the most frequent complaints in veterinary behavior practice. These sociopathies appear in dogs living in groups of variable size (two dogs and more). Classic symptomatology is characterized by an increase in the frequency of hierarchical, irritable, or both territorial and maternal aggression. Besides these common clinical forms, sociopathies may also be encountered that mainly manifest themselves by hierarchical micturition or pseudocyesis. In some cases, the sociopathy may lead to one group member being put to death.

Diagnosis: This implies the existence of one of the following factors: behavioral disorders occurring after the introduction of a new subject into the pack or behavioral disorders occurring after the start of sexual maturity of one of the members of the pack. These factors are associated either with the animals being unable to carry out fights until submission of one of the opponents, or with the loser being unable to move away from the group.

There is also one of the following symptoms:

- An increase in the frequency of hierarchical, irritable, or territorial and/or maternal aggression that may be direct or redirected.
- An increase in the frequency of hierarchical micturition.
- An increase in the frequency of hierarchical mounting.
- Pseudocyesis with little mothering behavior but maternal aggression.
- An increase in the frequency of eating.
- Stealing of pups by bitches.
- Infanticide.

Differential diagnosis: This must consider primary dyssocialization and dysthymias. In the case of a primary dyssocialization, the trigger does not match the above description as the dog has always been aggressive toward its fellow creatures. Moreover, it does not possess a full social repertoire and, in particular, is unable to submit. The differential criterion with dysthymia is made up of the unpredictable and especially incoherent character of the aggression, which is only limited to irritable aggression.

Prognosis: This is variable according to the age of the disorder, and also the size of the pack. In our experience, packs of more than eight dogs prove difficult to reorganize, and it can then be simpler to divide the group whilst respecting the affinity of subgroups.

Treatment: This is mainly focused on behavior therapy. Biological treatments should be used with a lot of care. Drug therapy is limited to the control of impulsiveness. Thymo-regulators and in particular carbamazepine (20–40 mg/kg) are most interesting. Hormone therapy and castration usually complicate things by disturbing pheromonal communication. Therapy is systemic and aims at helping the group reorganize by using its own mechanisms. The work of the behaviorist mainly consists of informing the owners to stop as much as possible their attempts to intervene. We must also insist on spatial organization of the breeding areas by allowing the losers to withdraw from the sight of the victors. Kennels whose opening is turned toward the outside of the enclosure, or corridors that allow the making of sanctuaries, are simple practical solutions to help avoid serious accidents and conflicts becoming permanent.

Sociopathies in human–dog groups

Description: Hierarchical conflicts between humans and their dogs are undoubtedly the behavioral disorders most frequently mentioned by veterinarians and the public. Unfortunately, this has led to many trainers and veterinarians now trying to explain all problems as hierarchical disorders, but there are many other causes that must be considered. Sociopathies in human–dog groups are behavioral disorders that occur in a context of relational ambivalence. This diagnosis should not be made on dogs that completely dominate their owners, but with animals whose hierarchical situation has been made ambiguous by allowing privileges usually associated with a dominant status, while adopting a dominating attitude in other hierarchically significant situations. Many behavioral complications result from this: aggression, hierarchical micturition, pseudocyesis, and destruction of the furniture.

Etiology and pathogenesis: In essence, this is the same mechanism as sociopathies within a pack. Maintaining an ambiguous situation leads to the production of dominant communication signals, and aggressive behaviors that help to resolve the situation. Very rapidly, an increase in vigilance and the appearance of anxious behaviors are observed. The problem may arise with owners where ambivalence in their actions pervades their style of communica-

tion and leads to the ambiguity that characterizes their relationship with their dog.

Development: In more than 35% of cases, anxious development dominates. The first phase may be characterized by phobic behavior that leads the owners to seek help and may conceal other aspects of the clinical picture. The dog looks wary, always on guard, and reacts to any noise. At this point fear aggression is observed, while other types of aggression become less frequent. Most untreated sociopathies evolve toward a secondary hyperaggressiveness under the effect of instrumentalization (learning). At first there may be an appeasement phase, but over time this entirely disappears. Soon this phenomenon affects the intimidation phase and bite control disappears. The problem progresses with each successful event. Retreating and submission of the owners serve as reinforcements. This development of sociopathies justifies a distinction of two clinical stages:

- Stage 1 or reactive stage sociopathies, which are characterized by complete aggression sequences.
- Stage 2 sociopathies or secondary hyperaggressiveness, in which all the aggression sequences have been instrumentalized.

Diagnosis: This requires a compulsory condition, a dog enjoying one or several prerogatives associated with a dominant status. At least two of the symptoms from the following list must also be present:

- A triad of sociopathies (hierarchical aggression + irritation aggression + territorial aggression).
- An increase in eating by the dog in the presence of one or several family members.
- Hierarchical micturition (marking).
- Hierarchical mounting on one or several persons of the same gender as the dog.
- Pseudocyeses with little milk, no mothering near the substitution subject when the owners approach.

- Appropriation of the children and maternal aggression when the female owner approaches.
- Aggression with the female owner.
- Destruction of furniture around the exits by which the owners leave their home or around windows from which the dog sees them leave.

Differential diagnosis: This includes primary dyssocialization, hypersensitivity–hyperactivity syndrome (HS-HA), and separation anxiety. The distinction with primary dyssocialization relies on the fact that the dyssocialized dogs are unable to submit when they have lost a fight. In the case of the HS-HA syndrome, the only aggression is irritable aggression and the dog has not acquired an inhibited bite. If it really is a separation anxiety, there is extensive destruction, and micturition and defecation are of an emotive nature.

Prognosis: This must be precisely evaluated because of the risks that the dog may pose to the family. The first criterion is the developmental stage of the sociopathy. The reactive stage generally has a good prognosis. Conversely, at the secondary hyperaggressivity stage, the dog is dangerous and the owners must be warned. It is also possible that the veterinarian could be liable if clear and sound advice is not provided. At this stage, the prognosis is guarded. The behavior of the animal is completely disorganized, which implies an intensive and long treatment program. Another practical consideration is the size of the dog. Indeed, it is easy to understand that a sociopathy in a 1.5 kg Chihuahua is less of a concern than in an 80 kg St. Bernard.

We should also take into account when determining the prognosis, the hierarchical position of the dog in relation to its owners. This factor can easily be evaluated by a description of the way the dog carries out the bite during the sequences of hierarchical aggression. When the dog bites briefly, we have a dog that perceives itself as dominating its opponent. In this case, we can conclude that the position of the dog necessitates a much longer and more difficult therapy in order to invert the relationship.

Conversely, when the dog maintains its hold until it or its opponent submits, we are in a challenge situation. The dog is in an ambiguous hierarchical position and the balance may be easier to tip.

Treatment: The decision to resort to drug therapy depends both on the developmental stage of the sociopathy and the physical strength of the animal. In stage 1 sociopathies, drug therapy only becomes necessary if the animal is particularly strong. However, at stage 2, it becomes compulsory.

The feelings of the owners must also be taken into account. Indeed, if they fear interactions with the dog, resorting to psychotropic drugs might help facilitate the behavioral techniques. The objective of drug therapy is to decrease the transition to the biting phase and not to completely suppress aggression. Suppression might only be achieved with treatments that deeply alter the learning capacity of the animal and render the behavior therapy inoperative. Therefore these types of drugs also have the inconvenience of demotivating the owners who no longer see the need to modify their behavior. The treatments most used generally combine carbamazepine (20–40 mg/kg divided bid) and cyproterone (3–5 mg/kg divided bid). But it is also possible to use the combination of tiapride (600 mg/m^2 divided bid) and pipamperone (30 mg/m^2 divided bid). In recently developed sociopathies, risperidone (1 mg/m^2) produces excellent results. In the more developed cases, when the mood of the animal has destabilized (EDED > 20), selegiline provides rapid stabilization.

The treatment of stage 2 sociopathies involves more complex strategies. For the safety of the owners, the first eight to 15 days of treatment must be carried out under hospitalization in order to obtain a stable and reliable state. The objective is the reappearance of growling in all aggression sequences. Until this objective has been reached, the dog must be kept hospitalized. Currently, the most useful treatment is the combination of sultopride (1 g/m^2 divided bid) at an anti-productive dose and pipamperone (30–60 mg/m^2 divided bid). However, alternatives can be prescribed, such as a combination of carbamazepine + pipamperone + cyproterone. After hundreds of trials, the therapy that has provided the best results is directed social regression. However, this therapy is sometimes unsuccessful when latent conflicts between the owners lead one or several of them to almost consciously support the dog. Furthermore, the clinician quite frequently encounters situations in which the owners have given up through fatigue or are afraid of their dog and avoid confrontation. In this case, objective therapies with self-evaluation are very effective.

ANXIETY DISORDERS IN ADULTS
Phobias in adults

We shall only mention the non-developmental phobias in this section. This choice is not due to the absence of these phobias in adults, since they are quite often found in subjects aged 12 to 14 months, but because they are disorders that have existed since childhood (stage 1 deprivation syndrome) and have not been treated.

Description: Adult phobias correspond to post-traumatic phobias. They have all the characteristics of phobias and occur after a sensitizing event. From this triggering event, the dog presents phobic responses whenever it is exposed to the stimulus.

Diagnosis: In general, this is the appearance of a state of fear when exposed to a stimulus rendered sensitizing by a traumatic episode. Three stages are identified:

- Stage 1: unique and identifiable stimulus; stream of typical reactions to the state of fear.
- Stage 2: multiple stimuli that have in common their frequent precedence to exposure to the initial sensitizing stimulus; predominance of avoidance responses.
- Stage 3: difficult to identify stimuli because they are very numerous and unrelated to each other; appearance of direct organic manifestations.

Differential diagnosis: This must consider ontogenic phobias, phobic attacks, and dysthymias. The distinction from ontogenic phobias is important both because of the poorer prognosis of these disorders and the possible financial consequences with respect to the breeder. While it may be reasonable to ask breeders to assume responsibility for ontogenic phobias, the same does not go for post-traumatic phobias. Ontogenic phobias appear when the pup arrives at its owners, without there being a traumatizing episode at the start. In the case of phobic attacks, examining the whole clinical picture connected with the hierarchical conflict helps avoid confusion. In the productive phases of dysthymias, changes in reactivity may lead to confusion. However, the existence of other symptoms, noticeably sleep disorders, is sufficient to make the difference.

Prognosis: This is generally favorable, the only limiting factor being the patience and level of motivation of the owners.

Treatment: In drug therapy, the choice is guided by the stage of the phobia. At stage 1, propranolol (5–10 mg/kg divided bid) is useful. At stage 2, we might use antidepressants such as mianserine (5–10 mg/kg divided bid). When panic attacks are common, antiproductive neuroleptics such as fluphenazine (50 mg/m^2 divided bid) can be prescribed. At stage 3, only substituted benzamides such as sulpiride (25 mg/m^2 divided bid), amisulpride (20 mg/m^2 divided bid), or selegiline (0.5 mg/kg) stabilize the animal. As behavior therapies, we use the techniques of systematic desensitization associated with counterconditioning, communication flow control therapies, or even play therapy.

THYMIC DISORDERS IN ADULTS

In this section, we have gathered mood (thymic) altering disorders, i.e., the reactive tendency of individuals. We have divided them into two subsections currently matching the clinical criteria, which could be the expression of different biological mechanisms.

Depressive disorders of adults

The depressive disorders have in common the existence of constant symptoms, which are characterized by a depressive state. They differ however by the existence of associated disorders that usually result from the etiological mechanisms involved.

Reactive depression

Description: This is an acute depressive state, i.e., characterized by the addition of anorexia or hyporexia with hypersomnia. This clinical form of depression appears eight to 10 days after high stress. Reactive depressions result from the loss of reversibility of emotional expression. The clinical presentation is dominated by a loss of voluntary mobility, especially exploratory behavior, but also by anorexia, hypersomnia, and the production of whines without any physical cause. There is also an indifference to all outside stimulation, even those which used to trigger organized behaviors (play, work, etc.).

Diagnosis: The signs include:

- The appearance of the disorder following an identifiable stress.
- The disorder appeared more than 10 days ago.
- Hypersomnia.
- Inhibition of exploratory activity.
- Loss of interest in the environment and the usual activities.
- Production of whines for a substantially long period.

Differential diagnosis: This includes chronic depression and pyrexia. The most obvious criterion for differentiation is the existence of a dysorexia and the development of paradoxical sleeping in chronic depression. With regards to pyrexia, interleukine-1 released during the febrile reaction increases sleeping, inhibits appetite, and may cause a depression-like behavior. For this reason, infectious causes must first be ruled out.

Prognosis: This is generally favorable. However, anorexia can be dangerous in young or debilitated subjects. In these cases, it is especially important to get the treatment to rapidly re-establish eating; otherwise force-feeding may become necessary. These situations are rare in dogs whereas they are quite frequent in cats.

Treatment: Antidepressants can be used for therapy. For reactive depression, noradrenaline or dopamine re-uptake inhibitors seem to be the most useful. We mainly recommend mianserine (2–5 mg/kg divided bid). The primary purpose of drug therapy is to stimulate the resumption of initiative. Play, work, or agility work are also likely to support this resumption.

Chronic depression

Description: Dogs suffering from chronic depression have altered behavioral functions. As in acute depression, a loss of interest in all types of stimulation as well as all usual activities is noticed. But what strikes clinicians is the existence of sudden emotional reactions in the absence of any significant inciting stimulus. These sudden reactions are usually accompanied with cries and excitement. Dietary behavior is profoundly modified with periods of hyporexia following bulimic periods. This sequence has no regularity, changes sometimes occurring within the same day. Sleeping is subjected to profound modifications with qualitative and quantitative disturbances. We also notice a progressive advancement of paradoxical sleep, which may even end up starting the cycle. This inversion in the organization of the cycles is accompanied by a lengthened duration of the phases of paradoxical sleep. During these phases, the dog seems more excited and ends up waking suddenly and frequently by producing howls, and micturition and defecation in its sleeping place (enuresis, encopresis). This dyssomnia rapidly leads to the appearance of a phase of wariness during the period preceding the time before going to sleep. Dogs whimper, pant, try to lie down, and get back up straight away, which the owners interpret (maybe rightly) as being afraid to go to sleep. These pre-sleep anxiety disorders are found in most chronic thymic disorders.

Diagnosis: Chronic depression is associated with the following signs:

- Dyssomnia characterized by an advancement of paradoxical sleep.
- Dysorexia.
- Loss of initiative.
- Loss of control of emotional responses.

Additional signs:

- Pre-hypnotic anxiety.
- Enuresis and/or encopresia.
- 'Dragging their feet' walk.
- Whining while staring at an object or a place.

Hypothyroidism and Cushing's syndrome must be ruled as contributory factors (leading to endogenous depression).

Differential diagnosis: Involutive depression or bipolar dysthymias must be ruled out. The distinction with involutive depression is in the presence of clinical signs of involution. Two characteristics of bipolar dysthymias are distinguishable: first, the bipolar disorders are cyclical in character and develop over several days to several weeks, which is quite different from the sudden and sometimes multiple changes of chronic depression; second, the productive phases of dysthymias are accompanied by a considerable decrease in the duration of sleep, to less than six hours per day.

Prognosis: This is good, although there is an average relapse rate of 11% six months after the end of treatment.

Treatment: This is mainly chemical. Endogenous chronic depression must have a specific drug treatment. Thus, daily thyroxine helps stabilize quite rapidly the mood in hypothyroidism, while recovery of normal cortisol activity in Cushing's syndrome lifts the depression. In addition to treatments based on Op'ddd or ketoconazole, or adrenalectomy, during unilateral hypertrophy, selegiline (0.5 mg/kg) may help to regulate the adrenal corticoid activity by controlling dopaminergic disturbances associated with this illness. Selegiline decreases the resecretion of ACTH. For exogenous depression, the serotonin re-uptake inhibitors are recommended. However, there will be an increase in the frequency of panic attacks, which might accompany the time of increase in 5HT synaptic concentration. This is why it is sometimes useful either to use molecules possessing sedative properties, such as clomipramine, or to combine an anxiolytic with the antidepressant. The 5HT re-uptake inhibitors of interest are fluvoxamine (0.5–4 mg/kg) or even fluoxetine (2 mg/kg). As in reactive depression, the only interest in behavior therapy is supporting the resumption of initiative.

Hyperattachment syndrome in adults

Description: This is a clinical condition which, by its pathophysiological characteristics, is a chronic depressive disorder, but whose symptomatology may sometimes be confusing. The clinical picture resembles at first that of separation anxiety, since there is a hyperattachment. However, in this syndrome the problem was acquired as an adult. Moreover, there is often a great deal of furniture destruction, autonomic disorders are systematically present, and this also occurs outside the separation episodes.

Apart from the above, this syndrome resembles more an anxiety disorder. But a careful semiological approach will pinpoint the existence of clinical signs characteristic of chronic depression. Only proximity to the object of attachment limits the appearance of pre-sleep anxiety in certain patients, as well as sudden awakening. This stabilization by hyperattachment usually has a limited duration, the development of the illness passes through an increasingly characteristic clinical picture. Finally, it must be noted that the phases of excitement during which the dog damages the furniture are limited to certain periods of separation from the object of attachment. These are not periods with a systematic trigger, as is seen in separation anxiety.

Diagnosis: This is based on compulsory symptoms and at least two specific symptoms.

Compulsory symptoms:

- The appearance of a hyperattachment in an adult whose behavioral development is normal.
- Dysorexia.
- An advancement of paradoxical sleep.
- The presence of primary organic manifestations tending to chronicity.

Specific symptoms:

- Destruction of furniture during certain episodes of separation from the attachment figure.
- Vocalization during separation.
- Pre-hypnotic anxiety.
- Sudden awakening with enuresis and/or encopresia.
- The development of a departure and/or welcome ritual.

Differential diagnosis: This has to consider separation anxiety, paroxysmal anxiety, intermittent anxiety, hypocorticalism, and digestive disorders. Regarding separation anxiety, although this is an affection that develops during the pre-pubertal period, it is possible to encounter dogs that have not been treated and thus display a clinical picture that persists into adulthood. The differential diagnosis relies on highlighting the aberrant development when the phase of detachment does not appear, and also on the absence of dyssomnia: here, insomnia is typical of the anxiety (sleep with normal cycles). The issue of paroxysmal anxiety is a concern when the dog belongs to a breed in which this anxiety has a digestive expression (German Shepherds and Mastiffs). But this form of anxiety is characterized by its clinical expression 'by means of crises' only involving the autonomic system with the exclusion of any behavioral disturbance. It is the absence of episodic aggressiveness that allows the distinction from intermittent anxiety. Hypocorticalism usually expresses a clinical picture combining a decrease in reactive dynamism, episodes of diarrhea and insomnia. The differential diagnosis, in addition to adrenal function, relies on the absence of

hyperattachment and the advancement of paradoxical sleep in these patients. The confusion with digestive disturbances can only result from a superficial clinical examination. Moreover, during a somatic illness, neither hyperattachment nor dyssomnia are observed.

Prognosis: Only emotional factors or lack of patience by the owners can render the cure of this disorder difficult, if not impossible.

Treatment: It is important to know how to coordinate chemotherapy and behavior therapy in order to avoid iatrogenic worsening. Chemotherapy uses either clomipramine (1–4 mg/kg) combined with pipamperone (30 g/m^2), or substituted benzamides at an anti-deficient dose. Sulpiride (25 mg/m^2) and amisulpride (20 mg/m^2) are of more use in this indication. Therapy aims to break the hyperattachment and relaunch initiative. But detachment therapy, identical to that used in the treatment of separation anxiety, must not be set up as long as the chronic depressive state is still in place. One must remember that the dogs seeks hyperattachment for 'protection,' and that any misplaced break is likely to aggravate the disorder. This technique is complemented by play, work, or agility exercises. In this case, the owners are unable to assume, sometimes tolerate, detachment therapy.

Dysthymia in Cocker Spaniels

Description: This is an affection whose sociocultural impact is quite powerful. Cocker Spaniels are one of those breeds of dogs whose physical attributes are highly appealing to some people. Fictional characters such as Beauty in Walt Disney's 'The Lady and The Tramp' are illustrations of this affective image and have at the same time done a lot to promote Cocker Spaniels. And yet suddenly, the idyllic relationship is broken. This has been enough for some authors to speak of the 'Jekyll and Hyde' Cocker Spaniel. In fact, Cocker Spaniels suffering from this affection display a clinical picture that is unarguably that of a dysthymia, which develops firstly in a unipolar direction to eventually become bipolar. But this aspect is not sufficient to characterize the dysthymia of Cocker Spaniels. The most spectacular factor is undoubtedly the development of the productive phase. The dog, from the beginning of this phase, grabs a random item. This may be an item belonging to a family member or a toy of the dog, or even a 'neutral' item such as a tea towel or a tissue. This item becomes inseparable from the dog, it takes the item everywhere and the item is always placed where it can watch it. Some dogs can watch their item for hours without moving. They will not tolerate this item being watched or anyone walking past it, and will attack anyone who makes that 'mistake.' However, this aggression has no sequential organization. The bite can be preceded by short growls, but there is no appeasement or renewing of the bite, whatever the reaction of the person attacked. Finally, other aggressions have no relation to the presence of the grabbed item. These incidents are identical to those recognized in the other dysthymias.

Diagnosis: The following symptoms must be met:

- A unipolar or bipolar state.
- Productive phases characterized by the appropriation of an item that is taken everywhere; looking at this item or approaching it triggers aggression.

Differential diagnosis: This must include a sociopathy. This is the affection with which confusion is easiest in Cocker Spaniels. Because of their emotional attachment to Cocker Spaniels, owners frequently have ambivalent hierarchical relationships with their dog. There results from this a sociopathy in which aggression dominates the clinical picture. But, in this case, the aggression contains the characteristic triad of sociopathies. We must however insist on the fact that sociopathies are not mutually exclusive and that any sociopathy in a Cocker Spaniel, in which there are aggressions with no sequential structure and whose triggering is unpredictable, must make clinicians look for a dysthymia. Failing to take this into account, a therapy for sociopathies will prove ineffective.

Prognosis: This is guarded. Only rarely have we obtained a true recovery. The dogs may be efficiently stabilized but it is usually necessary to maintain chemotherapy for life.

Treatment: This requires drug therapy. Two drugs help stabilize the dysthymic disorders of Cocker Spaniels; these are lithium salts (Neurolithium, at 0.05–0.015 mmol/kg; Teralithe ND, at 0.01 mmol/kg) and selegiline (0.5 mg/kg). Lithium carbonate might be used at a dose of 3 mg/kg divided bid to start but then titrated to appropriate serum levels.

Appendix A

Handouts and forms

On the accompanying CD are a set of handouts, most of which have been inserted in the text, to help explain to clients a number of the protocols and behavioral techniques found throughout the text. Handouts that are not found within the chapter text can be viewed in Appendix C and are called C.1, C.2, etc., in the table below.

Handout	Page	Figure
1. Barking – training quiet	318	13.8
2. Training basic commands using food lure training	496	C.4
3. Socialization tips for puppy owners	494	C.2
4. Stereotypic and compulsive disorders	206	10.4
5. Guide to crate/confinement training	54	3.25
6. Destructive chewing and digging	336	15.3
7. Teaching the pet to fetch and drop objects on command	403	19.14
8. Behavior modification for fears and phobias toward noises, locations, and objects in dogs (inanimate stimuli)	232	11.3
9. Behavior modification for fear of people or pets in dogs (animate stimuli)	238	11.8
10. Desensitization and counterconditioning for fear in cats	241	11.9
11. Food bowl exercises	527	C.13
12. Handling and feeding exercises	51	3.23
13. How to use the head halter for training and control of undesirable behavior	67	3.37
14. Canine housetraining	353	17.1
15. Litter training your kitten	367	18.1
16. Infants, children, and cats	523	C.11
17. Infants, children, and dogs	519	C.10
18. Socialization tips for kitten owners	495	C.3
19. Leadership	48	3.20
20. Puppy mouthing, nipping, and biting – bite inhibition and teaching off	417	19.22
21. Products for managing and correcting undesirable behavior	94	5.4
22. Reward-based training	57	3.26
23. Training a dog to settle or relax	113	5.13
24. Dealing with problem behaviors – jumping up, getting on counters and furniture	309	13.3

On the accompanying CD are a number of forms, most of which have been inserted in the text, that may prove useful when offering behavioral services in the clinic. Forms that are not found within the chapter text can be viewed in Appendix C and are called C.1, C.2, etc., in the table below.

Form	Page	Figure
1. Aggression release	526	C.12
2. Canine behavior checklist	8	1.4
3. Canine behavior consultation questionnaire	498	C.5
4. Cognitive dysfunction screening checklist	273	12.4
5. Informed consent for behavior-modifying drug use	518	C.9
6. Feline behavior checklist	10	1.5
7. Feline behavior consultation questionnaire	507	C.6
8. Feline housesoiling therapy worksheet	381	18.12
9. Behavior consultation follow-up	517	C.8
10. Senior pet screening checklist	279	12.11
11. Kitten kindergarten class outline	42	3.13
12. Checklist for new clients	29	3.2
13. Pet selection consultation questionnaire and resource list	491	C.1
14. Puppy class training outline	40	3.12
15. Behavior and temperament evaluation	515	C.7
16. The ARCAD scale – age-related cognitive and affective disorders	298	12.15
17. The EDED scale – evaluation of dog's emotional and cognitive disorders	459	21.3
18. Evaluation grid of aggressiveness in dogs	458	21.1

Appendix B

Behavior resources

USEFUL BEHAVIORAL REFERENCES FOR VETERINARIANS AND BEHAVIOR CONSULTANTS

Askew HR 1996 Treatment of behavior problems in dogs and cats. A guide for small animal veterinarians. Blackwell Science, Oxford, 350 pp

Beaver BV 1994 The veterinarian's encyclopedia of animal behavior. Iowa State University Press, Ames, IA

Dodman NH, Shuster L 1997 Psychopharmacology of animal behavior disorders. Blackwell Science, Malden, MA, 332 pp

Hetts SA 1999 Pet behavior protocols. What to say, what to do, when to refer. AAHA Press, Denver, CO

Horwitz H, Heath S, Mills D 2002 BSAVA manual of canine and feline behavioural medicine. BSAVA, Gloucester, England, 288 pp

Houpt KA (ed) 1997 Progress in companion animal behavior. Veterinary Clinics of North America, Small Animal Practice 27(3):427–697, May 1997, Progress in Companion Animal Behavior

Jackson J, Anderson RK, Line S 2001 Early learning for puppies to socialize and promote good behavior. A program guide for veterinary clinics, canine trainers and humane societies. Premier Pet Products, Richmond, VA

Keltner NL, Folks DG 2001 Psychotropic drugs, 3rd ed. Mosby, St Louis

Lindsay SR 2000 Handbook of applied dog behavior and training. Vol. 1: Adaptation and learning. Iowa State University Press, Ames, IA, 410 pp

Lindsay SR 2001 Handbook of applied dog behavior and training. Vol. 2: Etiology and assessment. Iowa State University Press, Ames, IA, 304 pp

Mills DS, Heath SE, Harrington LJ 1997 Proceedings of the first international conference on veterinary behavioural medicine. Universities Federation for Animal Welfare, Herts, UK

Overall K 1997 Clinical behavioral medicine for small animals. Mosby, St Louis

Overall K, Mills DS, Heath SE et al (eds) 2001 Proceedings of the third international congress on veterinary behavioural medicine. Universities Federation for Animal Welfare, Herts, UK

Pharmacology: For veterinarians using human drugs for behavioral therapy in pets a most recent edition of the human Physicians Desk Reference (PDR-US) or Compendium of Pharmaceuticals and Specialities (CPS-Canada) or equivalent and an updated/recent pharmacology text should be kept for references purposes

Plumb DC 1999 Veterinary drug handbook, 3rd ed. Iowa State University Press, Ames, IA

Reid PJ 1996 Excelerated learning. James and Kenneth, Oakland, CA

Schwartz S 1997 Instructions for veterinary clients: canine and feline behavior problems, 2nd ed. Mosby, St Louis

Veterinary Clinics of North America, Small Animal Practice. A number of previous issues have contained useful behavior information including November 1997, Geriatrics; March 1991, Advances in Companion Animal Behavior; and November 1982, Animal Behavior

Voith VL, Borchelt PL (eds) 1996 Readings in companion animal behavior. Veterinary Learning Systems, Trenton, NJ, 236 pp

REFERENCES ON DOG AND CAT BEHAVIOR

Beaver BV 1992 Feline behavior: a guide for veterinarians. WB Saunders, Philadelphia, PA

Beaver BV 1999 Canine behavior: a guide for veterinarians. WB Saunders, Philadelphia, PA

Bradshaw JWS 1992 The behaviour of the domestic cat. CAB International, Oxon, UK

Coppinger R, Coppinger L 2001 Dogs – a startling new understanding of the origin, behavior and evolution. Scribner, New York

Donaldson J 1996 The culture clash. James and Kenneth, Berkeley, CA

Donaldson J 1998 Dogs are from Neptune. Lasar Multimedia, Montreal

Dunbar I 1999 Dog behavior. Howell Book House, New York

Houpt K 1998 Domestic animal behavior, 3rd ed. Iowa State University Press, Ames, IA

Scott JP, Fuller JL 1965 Dog behavior. The genetic basis. University of Chicago Press, Chicago

Serpell J, Barrett P (eds) 1996 The domestic dog: its evolution, behaviour and interactions with people. Cambridge University Press, Cambridge, 268 pp

Thorne C (ed) 1992 The Waltham book of dog and cat behaviour. Pergamon Press, Oxford, 159 pp

Turner DC, Bateson P (eds) 2000 The domestic cat, the biology of its behaviour, 2nd ed. Cambridge University Press, Cambridge, 244 pp

USEFUL BEHAVIORAL REFERENCES FOR PET OWNERS AND STAFF

*Ackerman L 2001 The contented canine: a guide to pet parenting for dog owners. Iuniverse.com

*Ackerman L, Landsberg G, Hunthausen W (eds) 1996a Cat behaviour and training: veterinary advice for owners. TFH Publications, Neptune, NJ

*Ackerman L, Landsberg G, Hunthausen W (eds) 1996b Dog behavior and training: veterinary advice for owners. TFH Publications, Neptune, NJ

Campbell W 1999 Behavior problems in dogs, 3rd ed. BehaviorRx systems, Grants Pass, OR

Dodman N 1996 The dog who loved too much. Bantam, New York

Dodman N 1997 The cat who cried for help. Bantam, New York

Dodman N 1999 Dogs behaving badly. An A-to-Z guide to understanding and curing behavioral problems in dogs. Bantam, New York

Dunbar I 1987 Sirius puppy training (video). James and Kenneth, Berkeley, CA

Dunbar I 1998 Dog behavior: an owner's guide to a happy healthy pet. Hungry Minds, Inc.

Fisher J (ed) 1993 The behaviour of dogs and cats. Stanley Paul, London

Fogle B 1990 The dog's mind. Viking Penguin, New York

Fogle B 1992 The cat's mind. Howell Book House, New York

Fogle B 1994 ASPCA complete dog training manual. Dorling Kindersley, London, 128 pp

Fox MW 1996 Superdog. Raising the perfect canine companion. Howell Book House, New York

Heath S 1993 Why does my cat …? Souvenir Press, London

*Horwtiz D, Landsberg G Lifelearn CD – client handouts: behavior (62 titles). Lifelearn, Guelph, ON

*Hunthausen W, Landsberg G AAHA client behavior handouts (14 titles). AAHA Press, Denver, CO

Kilcommons B, Wilson S 1994 Child-proofing your dog. Warner Books, New York

Marder A 1994 Your healthy pet: a practical guide to choosing and raising happier, healthier dogs and cats. Rodale Press, Emmaus, PA, 216 pp

Neville P 1991 Do cats need shrinks? Contemporary Books, Chicago

Neville P 1992 Do dogs need shrinks? Citadel Press, New York

Pryor K 1999 Don't shoot the dog: the new art of teaching and training, Bantam Doubleday Dell, 202 pp

Rafe S 1990 Your new baby and Bowser. Denlinger Publications, Fairfax, VA

Ryan T 1990 Puppy primer. Legacy, Pullman, WA

Ryan T 1994 The toolbox for remodeling problem dogs. Legacy, Pullman, WA, 26 pp

Schwartz S 1996 No more myths. Howell Book House, New York

Scidmore B, McConnell P 1996 Puppy primer. Order from Dog's Best Friend Ltd, PO Box 447, Black Earth, WI 53515; 608-767-2435

Wright JC, Lashnits JW 1994 Is your cat crazy? MacMillan, New York

---

*Recommended client handouts authored by Drs Landsberg, Hunthausen, or Ackerman.

USEFUL WEB SITES WITH BEHAVIORAL INFORMATION

Name	URL
American Animal Hospital Association	www.healthypet.com
American Behavior Society	www.animalbehavior.org
American College of Veterinary Behaviorists	www.veterinarybehaviorists.org
American Psychological Association	www.apa.org
American Veterinary Society of Animal Behavior	www.avma.org/avsab/
Animal Behavior Consultant Newsletter	www.mercer.edu/psychology/Certif_Anim_Behave.htm
Applied Ethology Home Page	www.usask.ca/wcvm/herdmed/applied-ethology/
Association of Pet Behaviour Counsellors	www.apbc.or.uk
Association for Pet Loss & Bereavement	www.aplb.org
Association for the Study of Animal Behaviour	www.asab.org
BehaviorRx – Pet Behavior Resources	www.webtrail.com/petbehavior
Cambridge Center for Behavioral Studies	www.behavior.org
Canadian Veterinary Medical Association	www.animalhealthcare.ca
Center for the Integrative Study of Animal Behavior	www.indiana.edu/~animal/index.html
Center for the Interaction of Animals and Society	www.vet.upenn.edu/ResearchCenters/CIAS/
Clicker training	www.clickertraining.com, www.clickandtreat.com
Companion Animal Behaviour Therapy Study Group	www.cabtsg.org
Delta Society	www.deltasociety.org
European Society of Veterinary Clinical Ethology	www.esvce.org
Human Animal Bond Association of Canada	http://home.istar.ca/~habac
Hunthausen WH, Animal Behavior Consultations web site (behavior articles, tips, and resources)	www.westwoodanimalhospital.com
International Society for Adaptive Behavior	www.adaptive-behavior.org
International Society for Applied Ethology	www.sh.plym.ac.uk/isae/home.htm
Landsberg GM	www.doncasteranimalclinic.com
Society of Veterinary Behavior Technicians	www.svbt.org
Society for Behavioral Neuroendocrinology	www.sbne.org
Veterinary Information Network	www.vin.com

PRODUCT MANUFACTURER INFORMATION

Direct interruption devices

Product	Company	Contact
Air horns	L.P.I. Consumer Products	L.P.I. Consumer Products, 2745 E. Atlantic Blvd, Suite 300, Pompano Beach, FL 33062; Tel: (954)-783-5858, Fax: (954)-783-5859
Direct Stop Repellent (citronella spray)	USA: Premier Pet Products Canada: Multivet	www.premier.com www.multivet-inter.com
Handheld Bark Deterrent (audible)	Radio Systems Inc.	www.petsafe.net
Barker Breaker	Amtek Pet Products	www.amtekpet.com
Pet-Agree/Dazzer (ultrasonic)	KII Enterprises	www.kiienterprises.com

Remote-activated collars

Product	Company	Contact
Citronella Spray Remote Trainer Spray commander or Master Plus	USA: Premier Pet Products Canada: Multivet	www.premier.com www.multivet-inter.com
Pet Pager (vibration stimulation remote collar for deaf dogs)	Radio Systems Inc.	www.petsafe.net
Shock collars	Radio Systems Inc., Innotek Pet Products, Tritronics	www.petsafe.net www.innotek.net www.tritronics.com

Booby traps (environmental punishment devices) and containment systems

Product	Company	Contact
Pet Citronella Spray Containment Systems; Indoor – Spray Barrier; Outdoor – Virtual Fence	USA: Premier Pet Products Canada: Multivet	www.premier.com www.multivet-inter.com
Indoor and Outdoor Electronic Containment Systems (electronic stimulation)	Radio Systems Inc. (Pet Safe) Invisible Fencing, Innotek Pet Products	www.petsafe.net www.invisiblefence.com www.innotek.net
Spray motion detector (Ssscat)	Multivet	www.multivet-inter.com
ScareCrow (motion-activated sprinkler)	Contech Electronics	www.scatmat.com
Scat Mat (electronic stimulation mat)	Contech Electronics	www.scatmat.com
Scraminal, Critter Gitter, Scratcher Blaster (motion-activated alarms)	Amtek Pet Behavior Products	www.amtekpet.com
Snappy Trainer	Interplanetary Inc.	www.interplanetarypets.com
SofaSaver	Abbey Enterprises	Abbey Enterprises, 1130 Summerset St, New Brunswick, NJ 08901; 732-873-4242
Tattle Tale, motion (vibration) sensor – audible	KII Enterprises	www.kiienterprises.com

Electronic doors

Product/company/contact

Manufactured or distributed by Staywell, Solo, PetMate, Cat Mate, Johnson, PetSafe: www.catdoor.com, www.dogdoor.com, www.petdoors.com or Hightech Pet Products: http://store.yahoo.com/hightechpet

Bark-activated devices

Product	Company	Contact
Gentle Spray (citronella bark collar) Aboistop (Canada)	USA: Premier Pet Products Canada: Multivet	www.premier.com www.multivet-inter.com
Electronic stimulation bark collars	Radio Systems, Innotek, Tritronics	www.petsafe.net www.tritronics.com www.innotek.net
Sonic Bark (control collar)	Radio Systems Inc.	www.petsafe.net
Silencer Bark Activated Collar (ultrasonic bark-activated collar)	Radio Systems Inc.	www.petsafe.net
Super Barker Breaker, Sure Stop Barker Breaker (audible)	Amtek Pet Behavior Products	www.amtekpet.com

Head halters

Product	Company	Contact
Gentle Leader, USA Gentle Leader, Canada	Premier Pet Products Professional Animal Behavior Associates Inc.	www.premier.com www.gentleleadercanada.com
Halti	Coastal Pet Products	www.coastalpet.com
Snoot Loop	Animal Behavior Consultants Inc.	Animal Behavior Consultants Inc., 102 Canton Court, Brooklyn, NY 11229; 718-891-4200, 800-339-9505

No-pull halters

Product	Company	Contact
K9 Pull Control	Dog Crazy Co.	Dog Crazy Co., 6640 Cobra Way, San Diego, CA 92121; 619-824-0400
Holt	Coastal Pet Products	www.coastalpet.com
No Pull Halter	Four Paws Products Ltd	www.fourpaws.com
Sporn Training Halter	Sporn Company	www.sporn.com

Exercise, play, and chew products

Product	Company	Contact
Activity Ball	Hightower USA	Hightower USA, 4691 Eagle Rock Blvd, Los Angeles, CA 90041; 800-246-6556, 213-255-1112
Bite-A-Bone	Phydeaux Enterprises Inc.	Phydeaux Enterprises Inc., PO Box 36034, Detroit, MI 48236
Buster Cube	Kruuse A/G, Denmark	www.bustercube.com
Goodie Ship, Goodie Bone, Goodie Ball, Kong Toys	Kong Products	www.kongcompany.com
Inflations (black rubber dairy milking devices)	Jeffers	Jeffers, PO Box 948, West Plains, MO 65775-0948; 800-533-3377
Mutt Puck	Mutt Puck Pet Toys	Mutt Puck, 6260 Reber Place, St Louis, MO 63139; 800-274-MUTT, 314-781-MUTT
Nylabone Products, Crazy Ball	TFH Publications	www.nylabone.com
Tricky Treats	Bruin Enterprises	www.trickytreats.com
Pavlov's Cat	Aqualine Innovations	www.mktmkt.com/pavlovscat.html
Play-N-Treat, Push-N-Roll, Zig-N-Zag	Our Pet's	www.petgalaxy.com/ourpets.html
Tennis Bone	Interplanetary Inc.	www.interplanetarypets.com
Laser Mouse	Pet Tech	800-414-3173

Miscellaneous behavior products

Product	Company	Contact
Assess-a-Hand	Rondout Kennels	Rondout Kennels, Sue Sternberg, 4628 Rt. 209, Accord, NY 12404; 914-687-7619
Basket-type muzzles	UPCO Canada (Baskerville Muzzles): B&R Pet Supplies	www.upco.com B&R Pet Supplies; 902-860-3332
Anti-Icky-Poo (AIP)	Bug-A-Boo Chemicals	Bug-A-Boo Chemicals, 11924 NE Sumner, Portland, OR 97220; 503-257-9999, 800-326-3016
Feliway, D.A.P.	Farnam Companies Inc.	www.farnampets.com
Animale	La Ballastiére	La Ballastiére, BP 126, 33501 Libourne Cedex, France
KOE/AOE/Cat Off/Dog Off (odor neutralizers)	Thornell Corp.	www.thornell.com
Moisture urine sensor, Anti-Icky Poo (AIP)	Mister Max	www.mistermax.com
Nature's Miracle/Nature's Miracle Black Light	Pets 'N People Inc.	Pets 'N People Inc., 27520 Hawthorne Blvd, Suite 125, Rolling Hills Estates, CA 90274; 310-544-7125
Outright Stain and Odor Removal Products	The Bramton Company	www.bramton.com
Ropel	Burlington Scientific Corp.	www.burlingtoncorp.com
Soft Paws (plastic nail cap covers)	Soft Paws Inc.	Smart Practice, www.softpaws.com
Sound Desensitization CD	PABA	www.gentleleadercanada.com
Sounds Scary (sound desensitization CD)	John Bowen and Sarah Heath 2001	www.soundsscary.com
Sticky Paws (clear tape to stop scratching furniture)	Fe-Lines Inc.	www.stickypaws.com

Appendix C

This appendix contains the printed versions of forms that are on the accompanying CD but are not found as figures within the chapter text.

PET SELECTION CONSULTATION QUESTIONNAIRE AND RESOURCE LIST

The goal of a selection consultation is to help you choose a pet that is suited to your family, as well as to provide advice that you will need to prepare for the arrival of your pet. If you are interested in a purebred, we ask that you first narrow your selection to a few breeds that appeal to you, since there are now over 400 choices of dog breeds alone (recognized or unrecognized depending on which national or international registry you favor). Once you decide on your preferences, we can then discuss the pros and cons of each breed for your home.

To get some idea as to the size, shape, color, coat type, and other physical characteristics of each breed, you might want to begin by visiting a dog or cat show and interviewing some of the breeders. There are also several web sites, including those operated by most of the major pet food companies, that will help guide you through the selection process. In addition to the Internet there are numerous books available that discuss not only the physical characteristics of the breed, but also a history of how, when, and why the breed was originally developed. This can give you some excellent insight into some of the highly inbred characteristics of that breed. To be completely prepared to deal with a specific breed, it is also worthwhile to be aware of the potential genetic nature of medical conditions seen in that breed.

Even if you are not interested in a purebred pet, the selection consultation can help you decide what age of pet might be best to obtain, the differences between males and females of the breed, as well as where to obtain the pet and what to look for when you get there. It might interest you to note that puppy assessment tests are not a very good way of predicting adult behavior. In fact, you might learn a lot more by assessing the behavior of the parents when you go to visit the kennel. On the other hand, as puppies age, testing may become increasingly more accurate as the puppies emerge into adulthood.

Date of Consult
Name: email:
Address:
City/town: Province/state: Postal/zip code:
Phone: Home   Business   Fax:

1.   Indicate all family members in the household including age and sex:

2.   Indicate any other pets in your household and their age and sex:

3.   Desired pet: _____ Dog   _____ Cat
           Breeds of interest: List up to 5

4.   If you have no specific breeds in mind, list size and coat type that interest you:

5.   For what reason(s) are you interested in obtaining a pet (choose one or more):
       Companionship   Increased family security
       Guarding/Protection   Show/Breeding
       Sport/Hobby   For the kids
       Other: _____

6.   Have you ever owned a pet previously? Y/N If yes, describe the pet(s) and when owned:

7.   Special needs:
       Does any family member have allergies to pets? Y/N If so, what pets and severity:

       Are there any special considerations about your home that might need to be considered (e.g., physical disabilities, illness, infirmities, boarders, etc.):

       Are there any restrictions on pet ownership in your home or building? Describe:

8.   Household (Check one or more that apply)
       Describe the type of home you live in:
       _____ Single family detached – Indicate approximate size:
       _____ Town home or semidetached – Indicate approximate size:
       _____ High rise/apartment – Indicate approximate size:
       _____ Basement flat/room – Indicate approximate size:
       _____ Owned   _____ Rental
       _____ Fenced private yard – Indicate approximate size:
       _____ Unfenced yard – Indicate approximate size:
       _____ No yard   _____ Shared yard
       _____ Nearby park(s)   _____ Nearby dog park
       _____ Busy street   _____ Quiet street   _____ Rural
       _____ Other

9.   Daily schedule/home environment
       Indicate your basic family schedule including how long the pet will be left alone at any one time during the average work or school day?

       What is the longest time your pet will need to be left alone?

       Where do you intend to house your pet when you are out of the home?

Where do you plan for your pet to sleep at nights?

Will you be using a pen or crate confinement/training? Y/N If yes, describe:

10.   Financial (choose one)
        ____ I am concerned about the cost of pet ownership as I will need to watch my expenses
        ____ I have mild concerns about expenses but owning a pet is not likely to significantly affect my budget
        ____ I have no concerns about the cost of owning a pet and this will not have an impact on my budget

Below are a list of financial obligations that responsible pet ownership might entail:
        a) Regular expenses – food, treats, toys, license, cleaning supplies, grooming supplies or regular grooming
            Health care – vaccines, fecal, parasite protection, dentistry, insurance, geriatric care, laboratory tests
        b) One time or infrequent – purchasing the pet, bowls, leash, collar, identification (e.g., microchip), cage
            Health care – spay/castrate, training classes, aging
        c) Occasional recurrent expenses – boarding, medical care for sickness, illness, emergency

Pet Selection References
Breed catalogs:
There are numerous handbooks, field guides, and kennel club publications in this category. For example:
        Alderton D. Cats. Dorling Kindersley, 1995
        Alderton D. DK Handbook Dogs. Dorling Kindersley, 2001
        American Kennel Club Complete Dog Book, 19th ed. Howell House, New York, 1997
        Fogle B. The New Encyclopedia of the Dog. Dorling Kindersley, 2000
        Fogle B. Dogs. Firefly Books/Dorling Kindersley, 2000
        Fogle B. Cats. Firefly Books/Dorling Kindersley, 2000

Breed guides:
In many countries, there are publications that list breeds and breeders; check with breed associations.

Internet sites:
Breeds and pet selection, e.g., waltham.com, purina.com, ckc.ca, akc.org, cfainc.org

Additional books:
1.   Ackerman L. The Genetic Connection. AAHA Press, Lakewood, CO, 1999
2.   Baer N, Duno S. Choosing a Dog. Your Guide to Picking the Perfect Breed. Berkley, New York, 1995
3.   Benjamin CL. The Chosen Puppy: How to Select and Raise a Puppy from an Animal Shelter. Howell Book House, 1990
4.   Clark RD. Medical, Genetic, and Behavioral Aspects of Purebred Cats. Forum Publications, St. Simons, GA, 1992
5.   Coren S. Why We Love the Dogs We Do: How to Find the Dog that Matches Your Personality. Firefly Books, 2000
6.   Hart BL, Hart LA. The Perfect Puppy. WH Freeman, New York, 1988
7.   Kilcommons B, Wilson S. Paws to Consider. Choosing the Right Dog for You and Your Family. Warner Books, New York, 1999
8.   Lowell M. Your Purebred Puppy – A Buyer's Guide. Henry Holt, New York, 1990
9.   Lowell M. Your Purebred Kitten – A Buyer's Guide. Henry Holt, New York, 1995
10.   Tortora D. The Right Dog for You. Simon & Schuster, New York, 1983

Figure C.1   Pet selection consultation questionnaire and resource list (form #13 – printable from the CD).

SOCIALIZATION TIPS FOR PUPPY OWNERS

Even though dogs have been domesticated for thousands of years, each new puppy that comes into our world must learn about humans. Socialization is the process during which puppies develop positive relationships with other living beings. The most sensitive period for successful socialization is during the first three to four months of life. The experiences the pet has during this time will have a major influence on its developing personality and how well it gets along with people and other animals when it grows into adulthood. It is very important for puppies to have frequent, positive social experiences during these early months in order to prevent asocial behavior, fear, and biting. Puppies that are inadequately socialized may develop irreversible fears, leading to timidity or aggression. This is not to say that socialization is complete by four months of age, only that it should begin before that time. Continued exposure to a variety of people and other animals, as the pet grows and develops, is an essential part of maintaining good social skills. It is also extremely important that your new puppy be exposed to new environments and stimuli at this time (e.g., sounds, odors, locations) to reduce the fear of 'the unfamiliar' that might otherwise develop as the pet grows older.

Puppy socialization
Attending puppy classes during this primary socialization period is another excellent way to ensure multiple contacts with a variety of people and other dogs. This relatively new concept in training involves enrolling puppies early, before they pick up 'bad habits,' and at an age when they learn very quickly. Puppy training and socialization classes are now available in many communities where, in some cases, puppies can be admitted as early as their third month. These classes can help puppies get off to a great start with training, and offer an excellent opportunity for important social experiences with other puppies and with a wide variety of people. Eight to ten weeks is an ideal time to begin classes. Since there can be some health risks when exposing young puppies to other dogs and new environments, the best age to begin your puppy in classes should be discussed with your veterinarian.

Socialization biscuits
It is important for every puppy to meet as many new people as possible, in a wide variety of situations. It may be beneficial to ask each person who meets the puppy to give the puppy a biscuit. This will teach the puppy to look forward to meeting people and discourage handshyness, since the puppy will learn to associate new friends and an outstretched hand with something positive. Once the puppy has learned to sit on command, have each new friend ask it to sit before giving the biscuit. This teaches a proper greeting and will make the puppy less likely to jump up on people. You should make certain that the pet has the opportunity to meet and receive biscuits from a wide variety of people of all ages, appearances, and both sexes during the early formative months. Every effort must be made to see that the young pup has plenty of opportunities to learn about children. Kids can seem like a completely different species to dogs since they walk, act, and talk much differently than adults. Puppies that grow up without meeting children when they are young may never feel comfortable around them when they become adults.

And last, but not least, be careful to avoid physical punishment and any interactions with people that might make the puppy anxious. Harshly punishing a young pet will damage its bond with you and weaken its trust in people. Techniques such as swatting the pup, shaking it by the scruff, roughly forcing it onto its back, thumping it on the nose, and rubbing its face in a mess should never be used. Pets that are raised using these methods may grow up to fear the human hand, and are likely candidates to become fear biters. In general, any interactions with people that might make a puppy anxious should particularly be avoided during the early months of its life.

Figure C.2 Socialization tips for puppy owners (handout #3 – printable from the CD).

SOCIALIZATION TIPS FOR KITTEN OWNERS

Even though cats have been domesticated for thousands of years, each new kitten that comes into our world must learn about humans. Socialization is the process during which kittens develop positive relationships with other living beings. The most sensitive period for successful socialization is during the first three months of life, specifically from three to nine weeks. The experiences the pet has during this time will have a major influence on its developing personality and how well it gets along with people and other animals when it grows into adulthood. It is very important for kittens to have frequent, positive social experiences during these early months in order to prevent asocial behavior, fear, and biting. Kittens that are inadequately socialized may develop irreversible fears, leading to timidity or aggression. This is not to say that socialization is complete by three months of age, only that it should begin before that time. Continued exposure to a variety of people and other animals, as the pet grows and develops, is an essential part of maintaining good social skills. It is also extremely important that the kitten be exposed to new environments and stimuli at this time (e.g., sounds, odors, locations) to reduce the fear of 'the unfamiliar' that might otherwise develop as the pet grows and ages.

Kitten socialization
Although kitten socialization classes are not as popular as puppy classes, these may be available in your area. They are an excellent way to ensure multiple contacts with a variety of people and other cats. It may be beneficial to have each family member and each visitor to the home give your kitten a treat each time it is approached or handled. You should make certain that the pet has the opportunity to meet and receive treats from a wide variety of people of all ages, appearances, and both sexes during the early formative months. Every effort must be made to see that your new cat also has plenty of opportunities to learn about children. Kids can seem like a completely different species to kittens since they walk, act, and talk much differently than adults. Cats that grow up without meeting children when they are young may never feel comfortable around them when they become adults.

And last, but not least, be careful to avoid physical punishment or any other interactions with people or experiences in new environments that might make the kitten anxious. Verbally or physically punishing a young pet will damage its bond with you and make it increasingly wary or anxious of being approached or handled by people. Techniques such as tapping the nose, grabbing the scruff of the neck, or hissing at the kitten may only serve to make it more fearful of the owner. In general, any interactions with people that might make a kitten anxious should be avoided.

Best wishes for a long and happy relationship!

Figure C.3   Socialization tips for kitten owners (handout #18 – printable from the CD).

TRAINING BASIC COMMANDS USING FOOD LURE TRAINING

Obedience training is important for all dogs. The best way to get the job done is to start early in the pet's life, use positive motivation, and avoid harsh physical techniques. This will help ensure quick learning and make the training process more fun. If you begin the pet's training when it is a puppy, you'll find that early obedience training can be a big help in establishing leadership, socializing your pet, and controlling unruly behaviors.

An easy, non-force method for teaching obedience commands involves the use of small bits of food for training lures and reinforcements. Most dogs are very motivated to take food, so the best choice for a food lure is the pet's own dry food. If this is not sufficiently appealing, try small, quarter-inch pieces of semi-moist dog treats or freeze-dried liver. An excellent time to train the pet that is picky about treats is just prior to its dinner time, since the dog will be more focused on the food and quicker to respond.

You will use the food to lure the pet into the response you want as you give the command, and then immediately following the response the food will be given as a reward. The food will gradually be phased out as the pet learns the correct response. You'll do this by picking only the best responses (best position, quickest response, etc.) to reward, and withholding food rewards for less exact responses during subsequent training sessions. One of the advantages of food lure training is that your pet will learn two cues for each command. Since hand movements with the food lure accompany the verbal commands, the pet will also be conditioned to respond to hand signals. Learning a double signal (verbal and visual) will make the pet twice as likely to respond to you.

To help ensure that the pet learns with a minimum number of mistakes, avoid training when it seems overly energetic or has a shorter attention span. Work in a quiet area, keep the training sessions short, and stop before the dog begins ignoring commands. When the pet's response to commands becomes dependable, you can gradually take the training to environments with increasingly stronger distractions. Be patient, take your time, and make sure the pet knows one command well before proceeding to the next.

Your tone of voice is important. Use a happy, high-pitched tone of voice when teaching 'come,' 'sit,' and 'down.' An upbeat tone will help motivate the pet to move. Use a deep, commanding tone that is more likely to cause the pet to hold its place when teaching 'stay.' You should avoid repeating a command over and over. If you do this frequently, the pet will learn that it does not have to obey the first time you ask. Whenever you give a food reward, always say 'good dog.' The pet will learn to associate the words with food and the words will eventually become a valuable secondary reinforcer to sustain the response as the food is gradually withdrawn.

Recall on command
This is a fairly straightforward command to teach. Say the dog's name so it turns and makes eye contact with you. Extend your hand toward the pet with a piece of food in it. Wave your hand with the food toward you and say 'come' as the pet runs to you. Give the piece of food to it as you say 'good dog.' Take a few steps back. Show the pet a second piece of food, say its name, and repeat the recall for food. The pet will learn two cues to come on command, a verbal cue and a visual cue.

Sit on command
With the pet in a standing position, hold a small piece of food in front of its nose. In a steady, slow motion, move the food over the dog's head. The pet's nose will point up and the rear end will ease down to the floor taking it into the sit position. Say 'sit' as the rear hits the floor and give the food. Avoid holding the food lure too high over the head or the pet will jump up instead of sit. It won't be long before you'll notice that the dog will go into the sit position when you sweep your hand in an upward movement, even without food. As soon as the pet learns this command, you should ask it to sit before it gets anything it wants. By doing this, you teach the pet that you have control.

Down on command
Begin this lesson with the dog sitting on a smooth surface. Quickly move a piece of food downward from in front of its nose to the floor directly next to its front paws. As the front end of your pet slides down to the floor, say 'down' and give the food. You must make sure that you keep the food on the floor close to the pet's paws.

Otherwise it is likely to stand up and walk toward the food lure. Eventually, a downward sweep of your hand by itself will cause the dog to go into the down position. This command may take a little more patience and time than the first two. Only use the word 'down' when you are teaching this command. If you use the same word to tell the pet to stop jumping on people or to get down off counters and furniture, it may be confused about its meaning.

Stay on command

The 'stay' command is probably the most challenging command to teach a young dog. Don't even attempt to teach this command unless the pet is calm. A helpful strategy is to wear the dog out with a long walk or play session just prior to training.

Ask the pet to 'sit' without using a food lure. The second the pup sits, lean toward it, look it in the eye in an assertive manner, extend the palm of your hand toward it, and say 'stay' in a firm tone. Wait only one second, then approach your dog, calmly praise it while the pet is still sitting, give a release command 'OK,' and hand it a small food reward. Repeat the command, adding a second to the stay following every five or more repetitions. Once the pet can stay for at least 20 seconds, you can begin working on distance. Ask the pet to 'stay' and take one step away from it. Gradually work from a one to a 20-second stay at this position, then move back two steps and repeat the process. In no time at all, you will have the pet staying for longer periods at a significant distance.

Common causes of failure to teach the 'stay' command include attempting to make the dog stay too long or at too far of a distance too quickly, as well as attempting to get the response when the pet is too active or distracted. Try to anticipate when the pet will become bored with training and stop well before then. If the pet's eyes start to wander or it seems like it might move too early, calmly repeat 'stay' in a serious tone of voice, make strong eye contact, and lean toward it. Maintain the stay for just a few more seconds, then quickly release the pet.

Heel on lead

The goal is to teach the pet to walk without pulling on a slack leash. Before training, try to wear the pet out with some aerobic play. The initial training should be short and held inside without distractions. Later, training can be moved to the yard, and then to sidewalks. If the pet is incorrigible about pulling, use a head halter for more control.

Begin the training session by asking the pet to 'sit.' Stand on the pet's right side, facing the same direction. Take the leash in your left hand, holding it about two feet from the pet. Show the pet a treat or toy held in the right hand. Say 'heel' and walk forward, keeping the pet's attention on the object in your right hand. Take a few steps, stop, ask the pet to 'sit,' and reward it with the food or a pat on the head. Repeat, gradually taking more steps between each 'sit' command. Use an upbeat, animated tone to keep the pet's attention. Say 'heel' and reward the pet with praise and/or a treat whenever it walks along at the same speed and the leash is slack. If the pet begins to pull forward, immediately turn and walk in the opposite direction. When the pet catches up, ask it to 'sit' and repeat the above exercise.

Figure C.4   Training basic commands using food lure training (handout #2 – printable from the CD).

CANINE BEHAVIOR CONSULTATION QUESTIONNAIRE

General Information

Date of consultation:

Name: Email:

Address: Postal (zip) code:

Phone: Home: (   )   Business: (   )   Fax: (   )

For referred cases: Veterinarian's name & clinic:

Clinic address: Clinic phone:

How did you hear about our service?

Pet Information

Pet's name: Date of birth: Weight: Sex: M/F   Neutered: Y/N

Age neutered: Any change after neutering?

Breed: Color: Age obtained:

Where did you obtain this pet?   Breeder (if applicable):

Describe previous home/homes (if known):

For what purpose was your pet obtained?

Behavior of parents or littermates (if known):

Briefly describe your dog's personality (e.g., quiet, confident, excitable, unruly, bold, stubborn, etc.)

The Home Environment

Type of food:

How often is your pet fed?   When fed?

Type of treat(s)?

How often do you give treats?   When do you give treats?

List any supplements:

List all other pets, including species, breed, age, and sex:

Describe how your pets get along with each other:

List each family member living in the home (include sex and age of children):

Describe briefly how your pet gets along with each family member including any problems:

Reinforcer Assessment

What is your dog's favorite reward?

If you could give your dog ANY food as a reward, what would be the favorite? List the top five:

Other than food, what rewards (e.g., toy, affection) would be most enticing to your dog? List the top five:

Daily Activities and Routine
Type of exercise/play:
Who exercises/plays?
How often/how long?
Favorite game(s):   Favorite toy(s):
Where is your dog's favored sleeping spot?
Where does the dog sleep at night?
Have you ever used a crate for confinement? Y/N If yes, describe crate and location

Describe the dog's reaction to being crated?
Do you still use a crate? Y/N If no, when and why did you stop?
Briefly describe the usual daily schedule for the family:

Training
Has this pet had obedience training? Y/N Class/Private instructor/I trained my pet at home
Describe training classes your dog has had (including trainer's name if applicable):

Type of training collar used	Dog's response	Success (rate 1–5; 1 = poor, 5 = good)
None, trained off leash		
Neck collar Y/N If yes, indicate type:		
Remote collar Y/N If yes, indicate type, i.e., shock, citronella, etc.		
Head halter Y/N If yes, indicate type:		
Body harness Y/N If yes, indicate type:		

How would you describe the training?
Reward-based Y/N   Assertive/domineering Y/N   Aversive/mostly corrections Y/N   Other: Y/N
Briefly describe the training techniques:

What training was most successful?

What training was least successful?

Describe your dog's learning ability:

Is there any ongoing training? Y/N If yes, describe:

List family member(s) with most control:

List family member(s) with least control:

For each of the following use a scale of 1 (poor) to 5 (excellent) to indicate how your dog responds

1. Sit: Sit-stay 1 minute: Sit-stay 5 minutes: Sit-stay 10 minutes:
2. Down: Down-stay 1 minute: Down-stay 5 minutes: Down-stay 10 minutes:
3. Come (indoors):   Come (in yard):   Come (in park):
4. Heel – with no distractions: Heel – with distractions:
5. Give/drop:

Does your dog know any tricks? Y/N List/explain:

Can you get your dog to settle on command? Y/N If yes, describe:

Punishment

Have you ever used any of the following for punishment or training?

1. Physical punishment: Y/N Dog's reaction:
2. Noise punishment (shaker can/siren): Y/N Dog's reaction:
3. Ultrasonic: Y/N Dog's reaction:
4. Water sprayer: Y/N Dog's reaction:
5. Verbal reprimands: Y/N Dog's reaction:
6. Physical handling: Muzzle grasp: Y/N Dog's reaction:
                   Pinning: Y/N Dog's reaction:
7. Time-out: Dog's reaction: Y/N Dog's reaction:
8. Booby traps/repellants: Y/N Dog's reaction:

What punishment is most effective?

Does any punishment make the problem worse? Y/N If yes, describe:

Has punishment ever led to threatening behavior or aggression? Y/N Explain:

Does your dog respond differently to punishment from different family members? Y/N If yes, describe:

Handling

How does the dog react to the following types of handling:

Nail trimming?   Ear cleaning?
Brushing?   Bathing?
Rubbing belly?   Patting head?
Grabbing collar?   Being lifted?
Rolling over?   Teeth brushing?
Giving pills?   Giving liquid medications?
Hugging/kissing?

Housetraining Screen
Where is your dog's primary location for elimination?
On average, how many times a day does your dog a) urinate _____   b) defecate _____
Is your dog completely housetrained? Y/N
If Yes, please proceed to Medical Screen
If No, please continue to answer the following questions
Does your dog ever eliminate outdoors? Y/N
Do you accompany your dog to its elimination site? Y/N
What is *your dog's* favored location outdoors?
What is *your* preferred location for your dog to eliminate?
What do you do after your dog eliminates in the correct location?
What do you do when you catch your dog soiling in an incorrect location?

Does your dog signal to eliminate? Y/N If yes, describe:

About how often does your dog housesoil?   When is the dog most likely to housesoil?

Does your dog soil in the home by urinating, defecating indoors or both? (circle one)

What are the most likely locations for indoor elimination?

Does your dog housesoil when family members are at home? Y/N If yes, describe:

Does your dog housesoil while you are watching? Y/N If yes, describe:

What do you do when you find urine or stool in the improper location?

Does your dog urine mark? Y/N If yes, describe:

Does your dog ever eliminate in a location where he/she has been sleeping? Y/N
Does your dog ever leak/dribble urine? Y/N
Do you ever confine your dog to a crate? Y/N If-yes, does your dog ever eliminate in the crate? Y/N
Uncontrollable urination when excited? Y/N   Uncontrollable urination when frightened? Y/N
Does urine leak while your dog is
a) sleeping? Y/N   b) walking? Y/N   c) approached by owners? Y/N   d) approached by stranger? Y/N

Medical Screen
Appetite: Normal ___   Voracious ___   Decreased ___   Picky ___   Increased ___   Eats fast ___

Does your pet have any arthritis or other painful conditions? Y/N If yes, describe:

Have you noticed any deficits in your pet's senses? Y/N If yes, describe:

Does your pet drink or urinate excessively? Y/N If yes, describe:

Stools: Normal ___   Constipation ___   Less frequent ___   More frequent ___   Soft/diarrhea ___
Urine: Normal ___   Infrequent ___   More frequent ___   More volume ___

Does your pet have normal eating and bowel movements? Y/N If no, describe:

Does your pet have any other medical problems? Y/N If yes, describe:

Is your pet presently on any medication? Y/N If yes, describe (include name, dosage, duration):

Has your pet had any laboratory tests (blood, urine, X-rays, etc.)? Y/N If yes, indicate any abnormal findings:

If this is a referred case, please have your veterinarian complete the medical section of this questionnaire

Departure Behavior Screening
When you go out is your dog confined or crated? Y/N If yes, indicate if crated or what areas are restricted:

How long is the dog left alone on the average day?
At what time of the day is your dog left alone?
How does your dog react when you prepare to leave?

Has your dog ever been left at a kennel, veterinary office, or with a friend/relative?
If yes, describe your dog's reaction:

Is the dog ever alone outdoors? Y/N How often?   How long (average)?
Where is the dog left when outdoors?
How does your dog react to being left alone outdoors?
Does your dog exhibit any behavior problems when you leave it alone? Y/N
If No, proceed to Reactivity below
If Yes, please continue to answer the following questions
Describe your dog's behavior when left alone at home (list problems and how long after departure they occur):

Does the behavior differ depending on length of time or time of day left alone?

How does your dog react at the time of departure (as the last person prepares to leave)?

Does the behavior differ depending on who is the last to leave?

What is the dog's reaction at homecomings?

Have you ever left the dog alone in the car? Y/N If yes, how does it react?

Reactivity – indicate how your dog reacts to each of the following (check all that apply)

Familiar dogs on property:	Calm ___	Excited ___	Ambivalent ___	Fearful ___	Friendly ___	Aggressive ___
Familiar dogs off property:	Calm ___	Excited ___	Ambivalent ___	Fearful ___	Friendly ___	Aggressive ___
New dogs on property:	Calm ___	Excited ___	Ambivalent ___	Fearful ___	Friendly ___	Aggressive ___
New dogs off property:	Calm ___	Excited ___	Ambivalent ___	Fearful ___	Friendly ___	Aggressive ___
Strangers outside on property:	Calm ___	Excited ___	Ambivalent ___	Fearful ___	Friendly ___	Aggressive ___
Strangers off property:	Calm ___	Excited ___	Ambivalent ___	Fearful ___	Friendly ___	Aggressive ___
Strangers arriving indoors:	Calm ___	Excited ___	Ambivalent ___	Fearful ___	Friendly ___	Aggressive ___
Car rides:	Calm ___	Excited ___	Ambivalent ___	Fearful ___	Friendly ___	Aggressive ___
Thunderstorms/fireworks:	Calm ___	Excited ___	Ambivalent ___	Fearful ___	Friendly ___	Aggressive ___
Other loud noises (e.g., shouting):	Calm ___	Excited ___	Ambivalent ___	Fearful ___	Friendly ___	Aggressive ___

Aggression Screen

Has your pet ever displayed any: Threatening displays? Y/N   Growling? Y/N   Bite attempts? Y/N   Bites? Y/N
When was the most recent attempt to bite or threaten?
If yes, has this problem been entirely resolved? Y/N

Situations causing aggression (please circle)

Petting/handling/restraint:	growled	attempted to bite	bitten	no aggression
If yes, describe:				
Eating food or treats:	growled	attempted to bite	bitten	no aggression
If yes, describe:				
Chewing toys/stolen objects:	growled	attempted to bite	bitten	no aggression
If yes, describe:				
Waking up:	growled	attempted to bite	bitten	no aggression
If yes, describe:				

If there have been no signs of aggression (growl, bite attempts, biting) or if it has been entirely resolved, then proceed to next page

Is aggression the primary reason for today's visit? Y/N
What is the potential for injury: a) none/preventable   b) minimal   c) moderate   d) severe
Is the problem serious enough that you will be unable to keep your pet if it is not improved? Y/N

Is your dog ever aggressive to members of the immediate family? Y/N
If yes, who?
Describe:

Is your dog ever aggressive to visitors to your home? Y/N Were the people known, strangers, or both? (circle one)
Describe:

Is your dog aggressive to people when off property? Y/N Were the people known, strangers, or both? (circle one)
Describe:

Is there a particular person or type (age, sex, uniforms) that your dog is most likely to threaten or bite?

Is there a particular location or situation where aggression is most likely to occur?

Has your dog ever bitten hard enough to break skin or cause injury? Y/N
If yes, describe:

Describe situations where your dog barks, threatens, or growls, but does not bite:

Does your dog ever display aggression to other animals? Y/N If yes, what animals?
Describe aggression:

When your dog threatens or attempts to bite, how do you handle the situation and what is the dog's reaction?

After your dog has bitten how do you handle the situation and what is the dog's reaction?

How would you describe your dog's attitude at the time of the aggression? (bold, protective, outgoing, fearful, etc.)

How would you describe your dog's expression and postures at the time of aggression? (cowering, ears back, tail tucked, hackles raised, retreating, hiding)

Principal Complaint
What is the primary problem? (aggressive, destructive, housesoiling, barking, etc.):

How would you describe the severity of this problem? (circle one)   Mild/Moderate/Severe
Have you considered euthanasia? Y/N Comment:

Please answer all of the following unless they have been entirely covered in another section
When did the problem begin?
What age was your pet when this problem started?
What do you think caused the problem?

Describe the problem, beginning with the most recent incident:

Describe previous incidents:

Describe the first incident:

How often does the problem occur?

Has there been a recent change in frequency or severity? Y/N If yes, describe:

Describe any changes in the home or the pet's health when the problem first started:

What has been done so far to try and correct the problem?

What has been the dog's response?

List any techniques that have been at all successful:

List any techniques that have made the problem worse:

List any drugs (include dosage) tried so far, and the dog's response to medication:

List any other dietary treatments, supplements, or remedies and the dog's response:

Miscellaneous (please answer any of the following that have not been previously discussed)
Disobedient: Jumps up (owners) Y/N   Jumps up (strangers) Y/N
                Won't come when called Y/N   Nips/grabs with mouth Y/N
                Only listens when feels like it Y/N   Pushy/demanding Y/N
                On furniture where not allowed Y/N   In rooms where not permitted Y/N

Exploratory: Normal _____ Infrequent _____ Increased _____ Excessive _____
Activity: Normal _____ Lazy/inactive _____ Restless/won't settle _____ Highly active _____ Overactive _____
Sleep: Normal _____ Increased _____ Less frequent _____ Restless sleep _____ Night waking _____
Stool eating: Y/N   If yes, own stools _____ other dogs ___ cats ___ other:
Garbage raiding: Y/N   Food stealing: Y/N
Eats non-food items (pica) Y/N   Licks objects   Y/N
If yes to any of above, describe:

Destructive chewing Y/N   Digging Y/N   Other:
If yes, describe:

Grooming: Normal grooming ___ Excessive grooming/licking ___ Self-injurious ___
If there is abnormal grooming, describe:

Repetitive/compulsive/unusual activity: Tail chasing Y/N   Sucking Y/N   Star gazing Y/N   Fly chasing Y/N
Light chasing Y/N   Staring Y/N   Other:
If yes to any of above, describe:

Chasing Y/N If yes, describe:
Hunting/predation Y/N If yes, describe:
Sexual habits: Masturbation Y/N   Mounting Y/N   Roaming/running away Y/N
Describe any undesirable sexual habits:

Vocalization: Barking Y/N   Howling Y/N Whining Y/N
If yes, describe:

Anxiety/fear
Noise sensitivity Y/N If yes, describe:

Phobic/excessive fear/panic Y/N If yes, describe:

Shyness/timidity (non-aggressive), e.g., ears back, cowering, tail tucked, shaking, retreating, hiding, etc. Y/N
If yes, describe any situations not discussed previously where your dog is fearful or overly anxious:

How long after exposure to these events is finished does your dog settle down (i.e., back to normal)?

Additional problems or comments:

Veterinary History Form (for referred cases, to be completed by referring DVM prior to consultation)

Clinic: **Phone #:**
Address: **Postal code:**
Doctor's name: **Fax #:**
Client's name: **Pet's name:**

Behavioral History
Describe the pet's behavior in your clinic, including any problems that you have observed:

For what behavior problem is this dog being referred? (i.e., presenting complaint or diagnosis)

Please indicate any advice or counseling that you have given the client thus far (including dates):

Have any medications or products been suggested? If yes, indicate dates, duration, and response:

Medical History
Date of most recent physical/dental examination:

List any abnormal findings:

Vaccination status: Date: Vaccines administered:

List any present medical problems:

Are you aware of any sensory deficits? Y/N If yes, describe:

Are you aware of any painful conditions in this pet? Y/N If yes, describe:

List any recurrent or previous medical problems:

Is the pet presently receiving treatment or medication of any type?

Diagnostic Screening Tests

Attach a copy of all recent diagnostic or screening tests. Alternatively, please complete this section.
Indicate what diagnostic or screening tests have been performed and the date of each:

List any abnormal results:

Figure C.5   Questionnaire for canine behavior consultations (form #3 – printable from the CD).

FELINE BEHAVIOR CONSULTATION QUESTIONNAIRE

General Information
Name:
Address:
Veterinarian/Clinic:
Clinic address:
Clinic phone number:
Referred by (if other than veterinarian):

Date of consultation:
Phone: Home: Business:
Postal/zip code:

Pet Information
Pet's name: Breed: Color:
Date of birth: Weight:
Sex: M/F   Neutered? Y/N   Age neutered: Any change after neutering?
            Declawed? Y/N   Age at declawing: Any change after declawing?
Age obtained: Where did you obtain this pet?
Breeder, if applicable:
Behavior of parents or littermates:

Environment/Lifestyle
Why did you obtain your cat? (companion, breeding, etc.)
Type of food: When is pet fed?
Describe eating habits (e.g., picky, voracious):
List treats or supplements: How often are they given?
Favorite treat:
Do you give catnip? Y/N How often?   Cat's reaction:
Does your cat hunt? Y/N What does your cat hunt?
What does cat do with prey after caught?
Exploratory and self-play. Favored self-play toys:
Favored self-play games: Favored play times:
Does the cat have a play center? Y/N Describe:
Interactive play. List games/activities cat enjoys:
Who plays with cat?   How often?   Favored play times:
How long is the cat home alone on the average day?
Cat's reaction to being alone:
Is cat ever allowed outdoors? Y/N Is cat ever outdoors unsupervised? Y/N
How often and for how long?

Describe where cat stays/sleeps at each of the following times:
Daytime (when owners at home):
Daytime (when owners away):
Night-time:
When guests visit:
How does your cat react to the following: Car rides:
Unusual/loud noises: Strangers in home:
New (non-family) cats: New dogs:

Reinforcer Assessment
If your cat was allowed to have any treat, what would it prefer. List top five:

What other types of rewards would entice your cat (play toys, catnip, attention/affection). List top five:

Family/Relationships

List each family member (include sex and age):

How does your cat get along with each family member?

Who feeds?   Who grooms?   Who gives treats?
Who plays?   Who trains?

Briefly describe the family schedule, including how long the cat is left alone:

List any other pets, including species, breed, age, and sex:

How do the pets get along with each other?

Training

What commands does your cat respond to?
Describe your cat's learning ability:
Who does your cat respond to the best?
List any 'tricks' your cat can perform:
Have you used a body harness on your cat? Y/N   Cat's reaction:

Handling

How does the cat react to the following: Restraining on your lap:
Nail trimming: Grooming/brushing:
Giving pills: Giving liquid medication:
Cleaning/treating ears: Lifting/carrying:
Patting/stroking: Bathing:

Personality

Briefly describe your cat's personality (friendly, bold, active, playful, aloof, independent, fearful, etc.):

Punishment

How does your cat react to each of the following types of punishment:
1. Physical:
2. Noise (siren):
3. Ultrasonic (Pet-Agree™):
4. Water sprayer:
5. Verbal:
What punishment is most effective?

Describe any punishment that has had an adverse effect:

Does the cat respond differently to different family members?

Grooming, Scratching, and Kneading

Does your cat groom itself? Y/N If yes, does the grooming appear to be
a) normal   b) excess   c) less than expected?
When is your cat most likely to groom?
Does your cat lick or groom   a) other cats in the home   b) people in the home   c) objects?
Are there situations/times of year that cause grooming to increase? Y/N If yes, describe:

Does your cat have a scratching post? Y/N If yes, describe:
Does your cat scratch any areas/objects other than its scratching post or play areas? Y/N If yes, describe:
When is your cat most likely to scratch?
Are there any situations/times of year that cause scratching to increase? Y/N If yes, describe:

Does your cat knead? Y/N If yes, describe:
When is your cat most likely to knead?
Are there situations/times of year that cause kneading to increase? Y/N If yes, describe:

Do you feel your cat's scratching, kneading, or grooming is unusual or excessive? Y/N
If yes, describe:

Elimination and Litter Information
Does your cat use a litterbox for stools? Y/N/sometimes   For urine? Y/N/sometimes
Does your cat also eliminate outdoors? Y/N
If yes, what percent of defecation is outdoors?   %   What percent of urination is outdoors?   %
Does your cat dig/bury after eliminating? Y/N
Does your cat housesoil? Y/N If yes, circle all that apply: a) urine horizontal surfaces   b) urine vertical surfaces
c) stools
Where is your cat's preferred elimination location?
How often is the litterbox cleaned/changed?

Litterbox location	Type of litter	Type of box
1.		
2.		
3.		

Indicate which of the above boxes your cat prefers:
If you have more than one cat, do they have different litterboxes? Y/N
Do the cats use each other's litter boxes? Y/N If no, describe where each cat's box is located:

Your cat's home environment
Describe your home: House, apartment, semidetached home, basement, trailer home, etc.
How many stories?   How many rooms?
Please draw a simple diagram of each floor of your home to show all places your cat eliminates:

Use the following keys to indicate the location of each of the following:
Kitty litter: (use numbers **1**, **2**, **3** to correspond to box locations above)
Feeding location: **F**   Play area: **P**
Scratching post: **SP**   Sleeping area (night-time): **SN**
Sleeping spots (daytime): **SD**   Site of inappropriate scratching: **D**
Site of inappropriate elimination/urine: **U**   Site of inappropriate elimination/bowel movements: **BM**

Feline Elimination Problem Questionnaire (please proceed to next page if your cat does not have an elimination problem)

Does your cat defecate outside the litterbox? Y/N
If yes, how often does your cat defecate outside the litterbox? (circle one)
a) Few times a month   b) Few times a week   c) Daily   d) Multiple times daily
When is the cat most likely to defecate outside the litterbox?

What percentage of stools are outside the litterbox?
Where, other than the litterbox, does your cat defecate? List room(s) and type of surface(s):

Does your cat urinate outside the litterbox? Y/N

If yes, is there a preference for urinating on (circle one)
a) Upright surfaces, e.g., walls   b) Horizontal surfaces, e.g., floors   c) Both upright and horizontal
How often does your cat urinate outside the litterbox? (circle one)
a) Few times a month   b) Few times a week   c) Daily   d) Multiple times daily
When is your cat most likely to urinate outside the litterbox?
What percentage of urination is outside the litterbox?
Where, other than the litterbox, does your cat urinate? List room(s) and type of surface(s):

Have you ever observed the cat soil outside the litterbox?
If yes, what did you do?

Does your cat continue to soil outside the box while you are observing?

Does your cat ever use its litterbox while you are observing?

Can you think of any pattern (seasons, days of the week) to the problem?

Was your pet ever completely 'housetrained'? Y/N If yes, at what age was the cat fully trained?
What age was your pet when this problem started?
Describe the first incident:

Were there any changes in the household when the problem began?

Were there any changes associated with the litter or litterbox when the problem began?

What do you think caused the problem?

What has been done so far to try and correct the problem?

What was the cat's response?

List any techniques that have been at all successful:

List any techniques that have made the problem worse:

Is there a particular type of litter or surface your cat seems to prefer?
Are there any surfaces where your cat will not soil?

Have you tried other types of litter? Y/N   Have you ever used litter with a deodorant? Y/N
If yes, describe litter and cat's reaction to each litter type:

Is there a particular type of litterbox your cat seems to prefer?
Have you tried other types of litterbox? Y/N
If yes, describe boxes and cat's reaction:

Is there a particular location your cat seems to prefer for elimination?
Is there a room or location in your house where your cat does not soil? Y/N

Have you tried other litter locations? Y/N
If yes, describe locations and cat's reaction:

Do changes (moving, new furniture, vacations) dramatically affect your cat?

List any drugs tried so far, and the cat's response to medication:

List any medical problems and treatment that your cat has had:

Does any straining or pain accompany urination? Y/N   Or defecation? Y/N
Any blood in the urine or stools? Y/N
Is stool consistency normal? Y/N If no, describe:
Any increase in frequency: Urine Y/N   Stools Y/N
Describe:
Any increase in drinking? Y/N   Is there an increase in appetite? Y/N
How often per day does your cat pass urine? _____ Stools? _____

Feline Skin Disorders

Please answer the following questions if your cat has a problem with overgrooming, behaviorally induced hair loss (psychogenic alopecia), rippling skin (hyperesthesia), or self-traumatic behaviors.

Describe the problem:

When did the problem first begin? (cat's age, time of year, etc.)

Were there any changes in the household, which may have occurred just before the problem began?

Were there any changes in the cat's health or any other physical or behavioral changes when the problem began?

Has the severity, frequency, pattern, or type of hair loss changed since the problem first arose? Y/N
If yes, describe:

Is there a particular event that is most likely to cause or aggravate the problem?

Is there a particular time of month or year that the problem gets worse or begins to improve?

Is the behavior more likely to occur when you are (circle one)
a) at home out of the room   b) at home in the room   c) away from home   d) no difference

What has been done so far to try and correct the problem?

What was the cat's response?

List any techniques that have been at all successful:

List any techniques that have made the problem worse:

List any drugs tried so far, and the cat's response to medication:

Do any pets in your household go outdoors? Y/N If yes, which ones?

Do any other pets in the household have any skin problems? Y/N If yes, describe:

Have any other family members or friends developed skin problems? Y/N If yes, describe:

Principal Complaint (it is not necessary to duplicate previous answers for elimination or skin disorders)
What is the primary problem? (aggressive, destructive, housesoiling, tail chasing, etc.)

How would you describe the severity of this problem? (circle one)   Mild/Moderate/Severe
Have you considered euthanasia? Y/N   Comment:

When did the problem begin?
What age was your pet when this problem started?

Describe the problem, beginning with the most recent incident:

Describe the first incident:

What do you think caused the problem?

Describe any changes in the home or the pet's health when the problem first started:

How often does the problem occur?
Has there been a recent change in frequency or severity? Y/N If yes, describe:

What has been done so far to try and correct the problem?

What has been the cat's response?

List any techniques that have been at all successful:

List any techniques that have made the problem worse:

List any drugs (include dosage, frequency, when started, when stopped), dietary treatments, supplements, or remedies tried so far, and your cat's response to medication:

Aggression
Is your cat aggressive toward family members? Y/N   or other people? Y/N
Describe:

Is your cat aggressive toward other cats? Y/N   or other animals? Y/N
Describe:

What do you do when your cat displays aggression?
What is the cat's response?

Fear
Is your cat fearful? Y/N If yes, would you describe the fear as a) mild, b) moderate, or c) severe?
Describe any situations where your cat is shy, timid, or fearful:

Describe your cat's reaction (retreat, freeze, aggressive, etc.):

For each category circle the answer that best applies
Sleep: a) normal   b) excessive   c) decreased   d) restless/wakes at night
Describe problems:

Eating: a) normal b) overeats c) voracious d) picky e) undereats
Describe problems:
Urine: a) normal b) increased amount c) increased frequency d) decreased
Describe problems:
Stools: a) normal b) increased amount c) increased frequency d) decreased e) soft f) hard/dry
Describe problems:
Activity: a) normal b) overactive – daytime c) overactive – night-time d) decreased e) repetitive (stereotypic)
Describe problems:
Interaction with owners: a) affectionate b) little/minimal affection c) overly affectionate/demanding
Describe problems:

Additional Problems (describe briefly if not previously discussed)
Destructive chewing/eats plants: Y/N
Destructive scratching: Y/N
Scratches people: Y/N
Chews/sucks non-food items: Y/N
Vocalization/howling: Y/N
Hunting: Y/N
Climbing: Y/N
On furniture/counters where not permitted: Y/N
Goes into rooms where not permitted: Y/N
Garbage raiding/food stealing: Y/N
Roaming: Y/N
Additional comments or problems:

Medical: Indicate any ongoing or recurrent health problems and results of any laboratory tests (for referred cases, please have your veterinarian send a review of the medical history and any lab test results)

Veterinary History Form (to be completed for all referred cases prior to consultation)

Clinic: **Phone #:**
Address: **Postal code:**
Doctor's name: **Fax #:**
Client's name: **Pet's name:**

Behavioral History
Describe the pet's behavior in your clinic, including any problems that you have observed:

For what behavior problem is this cat being referred? (i.e., presenting complaint or diagnosis)

Please indicate any advice or counseling that you have given the client thus far (including dates):

Have any medications or products been suggested? If yes, indicate dates, duration, and response:

Medical History
Date of most recent physical/dental examination:

List any abnormal findings:

Vaccination status: Date: Vaccines administered:

List any present medical problems:

Are you aware of any sensory deficits? Y/N If yes, describe:

Are you aware of any painful conditions in this pet? Y/N If yes, describe:

List any recurrent or previous medical problems:

Is the pet presently receiving treatment or medication of any type?

Diagnostic Screening Tests
Attach a copy of all recent diagnostic or screening tests. Alternatively, please complete this section.
Indicate what diagnostic or screening tests have been performed and the date of each:

List any abnormal results:

Figure C.6   Questionnaire for feline behavior consultation (form #7 – printable from the CD).

BEHAVIOR AND TEMPERAMENT EVALUATION

The intent of this form is to provide an organized approach for recording observations made during the behavior consultation.

BEHAVIOR OBSERVATIONS

Consultation location (circle one): Home/Hospital   **Date:**

Pet: **Owner:**   **Attending:**   **Comments:**

Aggressive	0- - - - - - - - - - - - - -10	Friendly	0- - - - - - - - - - - - - -10
Excitable	0- - - - - - - - - - - - - -10	Calm	0- - - - - - - - - - - - - -10
Submissive	0- - - - - - - - - - - - - -10	Assertive	0- - - - - - - - - - - - - -10
Fearful	0- - - - - - - - - - - - - -10	Confident	0- - - - - - - - - - - - - -10
Avoids	0- - - - - - - - - - - - - -10	Seeks contact	0- - - - - - - - - - - - - -10
Shy	0- - - - - - - - - - - - - -10	Outgoing	0- - - - - - - - - - - - - -10
Withdrawn	0- - - - - - - - - - - - - -10	Investigates	0- - - - - - - - - - - - - -10
Hypervigilant	0- - - - - - - - - - - - - -10	Non-reactive	0- - - - - - - - - - - - - -10

Environment

General

Movement

Sound

People

Consultant

   General

   Approach/Greeting

   Physical examination/Handling

   Procedures (e.g., head halter or muzzle application)

Family – Who (indicate which family members were assessed)

   General

   Handling

   Procedures (e.g., head halter or muzzle application)

Others – Who (e.g., strangers/staff)

   General

   Approach/Greeting

   Handling/Procedures

Animals

Family pets

Other dogs

Other animals

Assessment/Comments

Figure C.7   Form to be used for temperament evaluation (form #15 – printable from the CD).

BEHAVIOR CONSULTATION FOLLOW-UP

Please use the following rating scale to answer the questions below:
0   This question is not applicable to my pet's treatment
1   I strongly agree with the statement
2   I agree with the statement
3   I neither agree nor disagree with the statement
4   I disagree with the statement
5   I strongly disagree with the statement

1. ___ The session wasn't too long for the nature of the problem.
2. ___ The session wasn't too short for the nature of the problem.
3. ___ My telephone calls prior to the consultation were handled courteously.
4. ___ The staff were helpful and knowledgeable in setting up the consultation.
5. ___ All telephone calls were returned in a timely manner.
6. ___ The doctor was courteous.
7. ___ The doctor was genuinely concerned with my pet's problem.
8. ___ I was satisfied with the way my pet's care was handled.
9. ___ My pet's behavior problem was diagnosed correctly.
10. ___ The doctor explained the problem clearly.
11. ___ The doctor explained the treatment plan clearly.
12. ___ The doctor was well-informed with respect to this type of problem.
13. ___ The treatment plan for my pet was not too complicated.
14. ___ The treatment plan for my pet was complete enough.
15. ___ I was able to begin the behavioral program.
16. ___ I was able to complete the behavioral program.

17. ___ The program did not require too much of my time.
18. ___ I had sufficient opportunity for follow-up.
19. ___ Medications were recommended for the behavioral problem.
20. ___ I used the medications as directed. If yes, which:
21. ___ I feel that the medications helped my pet.
22. ___ Training products were recommended.
23. ___ I used the training products as directed. If yes, which:
24. ___ Surgery was suggested to help correct the behavior problem.
25. ___ The suggested surgery was performed.
26. ___ I feel that the surgery helped my pet.
27. ___ My pet's behavior improved after treatment.
28. ___ I was satisfied with the outcome of the behavior therapy.
29. ___ The consultation fee was appropriate.
30. ___ I still have my pet (yes or no). If no:
    ___ My pet died from unrelated causes
    ___ I gave my pet away due to its behavior problem
    ___ My pet was put to sleep for its behavior problem

If your pet was improved, please indicate what helped the most:

If your pet was not improved, why do you think treatment was not successful:

Please indicate any comments that might help us to improve our service:

ANY OTHER COMMENTS WOULD BE GREATLY APPRECIATED (commendations, criticism, etc.)

OPTIONAL INFORMATION:
Name and Phone:
Cat ___ Dog ___ Breed _____ Name _____ Sex ___ Neutered ___ Age _____
Pet's problem(s) _____

*Thank you **very** much for your time and cooperation.*

Figure C.8   Form for behavior follow-up and tracking (form #9 – printable from the CD).

INFORMED CONSENT FOR BEHAVIOR-MODIFYING DRUG USE

Pet's name: _____ Sex: _____ Age: _____

Owner name: _____

Owner address: _____

Telephone: _____

I, the undersigned, being the owner or duly authorized agent for the owner of the above animal, understand that the drug

_____

has not been approved for use in dogs and/or cats for the condition being treated. This means that safety, effectiveness, and side effects have not been comprehensively established for the purpose used, although the product is legally available for

_____

I have been advised that the drug is being used in a manner other than that identified on its label, and I accept the consequences of its use. Although I understand that the drug is being prescribed in the hopes that if will be beneficial for my pet, I will not hold the veterinarian responsible for any adverse effects, be they physical or behavioral that might arise out of the use of this drug.

I have been advised of the potential side effects and adverse effects of the medication, which might include:

_____

_____

I have been advised to discontinue the use of the drug and seek veterinary care immediately should any adverse or unexpected effects be exhibited. Since this drug is being used in an attempt to modify or alter behavior, I have also been advised that if there is an undesirable change in my pet's behavior or the problem gets worse, the drug should be discontinued. I also understand that since the product has not been licensed for this use that all potential adverse effects may not be known at this time. I will follow my veterinarian's advice regarding any laboratory or clinical testing that is recommended to safeguard against side effects and to allow adequate patient monitoring as indicated by the condition and the medication used. No other drugs, herbal remedies, or supplements will be used at the same time as this medication, except as discussed with my veterinarian.

I understand it is possible that this drug may not alter the course of the behavior problem, and that my animal may continue with the behavior problem whether or not the medication is administered.

I hereby give my informed consent to the administration of this drug to my animal. I accept full responsibility, legal and financial, for all actions that may occur from the use of this drug.

I have been advised that a follow-up examination or assessment is next due on: _____

_____

Signed: _____ Date: _____

Figure C.9 Form for consent for drug use (form #5 – printable from the CD).

INFANTS, CHILDREN, AND DOGS

New or expectant parents typically have three major concerns: 1) How to prevent pet behavior problems from occurring after the baby arrives; 2) How to introduce the baby to the pet; and 3) How to keep the child safe around the family dog, as well as other animals. Pet owners often assume that jealousy is the cause of problem behaviors associated with the arrival of a new child into the home, but this is not the case. Most problems result from the anxiety caused by significant alterations in the pet's environment and the way the family interacts with the pet. Changes in feeding, exercise, and play schedules; changes in what the pet is allowed to do; changes in how the pet gets attention; and inconsistencies in the way family members interact with the pet can all lead to problems. Preparing the family dog for the new baby includes taking steps to ensure that the changes are gradual and not overwhelming for the pet, and reviewing obedience training and household rules so that the family has the control needed to direct the pet into desired behaviors.

Pets don't innately know how to behave around children, and children need guidance on how to interact with animals. Dogs are most likely to have social problems if they have had little contact or a previous unpleasant experience with babies or children, insufficient handling by humans, or inadequate training. Genetics also plays a role in the dog's sociability, predatory instincts, and temperament, which may have an impact on how the dog interacts with children.

Preparing puppies for children
Preparation for a good relationship between the pet and children begins when the dog is a puppy. To accomplish this, you need to provide frequent opportunities for the young pup to meet children during its early months of life. You should pick times when the pet and children are calm. Having treats available for children to offer to the pup will help the introductions go smoothly. These early interactions help prevent the development of fear, avoidance behavior, and aggression toward children when the pet is older.

Another concept the young pup needs to learn is that being touched can be pleasant and should not be feared. Family members should make a point of gently handling the pet and touching it in all the ways that a child might touch it. Frequently touching the tail, ears, and body, as well as gently tugging on the collar and brushing the hair will make the pet less likely to be upset when a child handles the pet later in life. Any type of physical punishment or threats with a hand should be avoided. If the pet associates hand movement with discomfort, it might bite when the child moves a hand toward it. All pets must learn that the human hand is friendly and not to be feared.

Some dogs show aggression when approached while they eat. This behavior can be avoided by teaching the young pup that it is good to have company when it eats. A family member should occasionally sit on the floor with the puppy while it eats. During this time, the pet can be gently touched all over. Pieces of kibble should be picked from the bowl and hand fed to the pup. The bowl should periodically be picked up for a second and placed back on the floor. If the family member occasionally slips a chunk of canned food into the bowl while the pet is eating its dry food, it will look forward to having humans nearby at dinner time. By doing these exercises, the pup will learn that there is no risk that humans will steal its food, but the meal actually improves when humans are nearby.

Preparing the adult dog for the new baby
The first thing to consider is the pet's temperament. Does your dog growl or snap when touched, disturbed while eating, playing with toys, or resting? If your pet exhibits any type of aggression toward people or animals, seek help from your veterinarian or a qualified pet behavior consultant as soon as possible. Even dogs that get along quite well with children, but exhibit other forms of aggression (such as territorial aggression), can be dangerous for the child that inadvertently gets near the pet when it is aggressive or aroused.

As soon as the mother learns of her pregnancy, some thought should be given to preparing the pet for the inevitable changes that occur when a new baby arrives. Begin by reviewing the dog's obedience training. It is very important to have the pet under reliable verbal control. An unruly, active dog can be as much of a threat to the baby as an aggressive dog. If the pet will readily respond to 'sit,' 'down,' 'stay,' and 'settle,' you will have tools with which to increase desirable behavior and decrease undesirable behavior.

Next, you need to think about the pet's daily schedule, as well as the type and amount of interactions with family members the dog is currently used to getting. Once the baby arrives, this may be dramatically changed. The goal is to make the changes gradual and less noticeable to the pet. Decide on feeding, exercise, and play schedules that can be maintained while providing for the demanding needs of a newborn. Gradually adjust your present schedules until you arrive at ones that will best fit the family's situation once the baby is home. Consideration should also be given to the amount of attention that is given to the dog and how it is given. Tending to the baby's needs is very time consuming and will no doubt reduce the amount of physical attention that can be given to the dog. The amount should be gradually decreased until you arrive at an amount that can be maintained. How the attention is given is also very important. If your pet is used to getting attention whenever he nudges or licks, he will be very confused when he suddenly cannot get what he wants on demand. A good way to handle this is to ignore pushy behaviors and give attention only when the pet is leaving you alone or as a reward for responding to one of your commands ('sit,' 'down'). Other things that will need to be worked on are those behaviors that are permitted now, but won't be permitted when the baby is at home. Jumping up on family members, lying on furniture, climbing onto your lap, or excessive barking are behaviors that often must be changed.

The dog should also be prepared in advance to accept and enjoy the new noises and smells associated with a new baby. If the dog gets upset when it hears strange sounds, a recording can be made of baby noises (cooing, crying, screaming, etc.). Play the recording for the dog so it can barely be heard, and slowly increase the volume until an anxious response is obtained. Then, reduce the volume just below this level and play the tape while jovially requesting obedience commands for tasty food treats. Do at least seven, 15-minute sessions each week. Very gradually increase the volume as the weeks go by until the pet seems comfortable with these noises at high volumes. To prepare the pet for the new smells that will arrive with the baby, take something home from the hospital, such as a towel or blanket with the baby's scent. Ask the dog to sit, then present the object to the pet. While the dog is sniffing, say the baby's name in an upbeat tone and give it lots of praise. On occasion, some dogs will become anxious when the owner carries or nurses the baby. Testing the dog by carrying around and fussing with a doll (especially one that actually moves and makes crying sounds) can be useful. If there is any anxiety, a positive association should be made with this doll using favored food rewards, affection, or a favored play toy (see handouts on desensitization and counterconditioning).

When the baby comes home
Since the pet hasn't seen his mistress for several days, he will probably be very excited and may want to jump up. Therefore, if someone else carries the baby into the home, the mother can greet the dog without worrying that he might accidentally injure the baby. By taking this approach, you avoid scoldings and anxious feelings being associated with the presence of the baby.

Wait until the excitement has died down, the pet is calm, and you are available to supervise before introducing the dog to the baby. That may be later in the same day or could be several weeks afterward. Careful judgment must be exercised in deciding when to allow the dog close enough to sniff. If there is a chance the dog might jump, use a leash, which can be attached to a head halter for even greater control. If there is <u>any</u> likelihood that the dog might bite, consider using a basket wire or plastic muzzle. <u>NEVER</u> (no matter how sweet, trustworthy, or friendly the pet appears) allow an unsupervised dog around the baby. You should be especially vigilant when the baby is crying, kicking, or waving its arms. This could cause a curious dog to jump up and scratch or otherwise injure the infant. During these times, it is wise to either put the pet in a 'down-stay' away from the baby, put it in another room with a very special chew toy, or confine it to the yard. If the pet exhibits any predatory behavior (stalking, strong focus, odd whining, unusual interest) around the baby, take extra precautions and contact your veterinarian or a qualified behavior consultant for advice.

Whenever the dog is in the room with the baby, the family should act very happy and praise all acceptable behaviors (e.g., not jumping, being calm, responding to commands, being relaxed when the baby cries, etc.). The idea is to promote desirable behaviors and to make the dog look forward to the baby's presence because it is associated with a lot of good positive attention. This association can be made more dramatic by reducing the amount of attention or treats the dog gets when the baby is not around. In this way, the dog learns that the presence of the baby is associated with positive events. Similarly avoid punishment or banishing the dog from the room when the baby is present so that a negative association does not develop. The biggest mistake owners make when they try to shape their dog's behavior is to concentrate on telling the dog what is wrong, while neglecting to tell it what is right. A good exercise to bring about the association of good feelings for the baby is for one parent to sit in a room and hold the baby, while the other stands at the opposite end of the room and asks the pet to respond to commands for tasty food treats. Commands should be given in a very happy tone and lots of praise should accompany the food treats. Gradually move the exercises closer and closer to the baby.

Children and dogs

As the baby continues to grow and mature, the dog will be exposed to a variety of new stimuli from crawling to toddling to walking and having things taken away. Even if the dog has adapted nicely to a particular stage in the child's life, owners must always be prepared for a change in the relationship between the child and pet.

Interactions between pups and young children should always be supervised. The spontaneous, active behavior of children is exciting for most dogs, and easily elicits rough play from them. Encouraging the child to give tasty food rewards to the pet for responding to 'sit' commands is a simple way to teach the pup to keep its paws on the ground and expect good things whenever it is around children.

Another important thing to remember is to avoid doing anything to the dog that you don't want your child to do. This includes physical punishment, teasing, and rough play. Set a good example. Children don't innately know how to interact with animals, so they must be taught. You need to teach your child how to play with the pet. For example, fetch is a great game for the child and dog to share with each other. You must also teach the child how to touch the pet. While some dogs will tolerate any type of normal physical contact, the child will be safer if taught to avoid making contact around the eyes, ears, and head, and to pat the dog along its side. Hugging and getting face-to-face are not well tolerated by some dogs and are also best avoided. If the dog is small, you will need to teach the child when and how to comfortably pick it up.

Children should have some control over the pet and this can begin at a relatively early age. Once the child is talking, a family member can hold the child in the lap and teach the pet to sit when the child gives a command. This can be done by coaching the child to say the command word at the same time as the adult. Gradually, the adult can begin whispering the word so the child gives the command alone. This can be repeated with other commands. When the child is old enough, it can request deference from the dog before giving it things that it wants (toys, treats, play) by asking it to respond to a command first. Non-aggressive pets can be taught to look forward to having the child present while they eat by doing a safe, easy exercise. Simply carry the child over to the pet while it eats and hold it a safe distance above the pet. As the pet eats, the child can drop small pieces of meat into the bowl or on the floor next to the bowl.

Children must also learn some rules about other pets. The most important rule is that the child must NEVER pet another family's pet or give it food unless an adult gives permission. Dogs on a leash, by food, by toys, sleeping, acting sick, tied down, or running loose should never be approached. All family members must also follow these rules for them to work. Remember, children are imitators. You must also teach children about avoiding a pet that is exhibiting potentially dangerous behavior. Aggressive behavior is fairly obvious to most children, but few children know that fearful animals should also be avoided. Discuss aggressive postures (growling, loud barking, hair standing on end) and fearful behaviors (trembling, crouching, ears down, tail tucked) and teach the child to avoid animals exhibiting those behaviors. If the child is approached by a dog that is acting aggressive, s/he should stand very still like a tree, say nothing, hold the arms against the body, and avoid eye contact with the dog. If the child is on the ground or knocked down, he should curl into a tight ball, cover the ears with his fists, and remain still and quiet until the animal moves far away. As you might imagine, the necessary responses are contrary to what most children will do when threatened, so it is very important that you actually spend time practicing with them. You should also instruct your children about what to do if a bite occurs. They should try to remember where the bite occurred, what the dog looked like, where it went following the bite, and to report the bite to an adult immediately.

Health concerns

It is rare for a dog to spread disease to humans, but it can occur. The number one health risk is from aggression, so that bite prevention and safety is the overriding concern. With some simple rules most other health problems can be prevented.
1. Have your pet examined and vaccinated at least once a year, and ensure that it is free of parasites.

2. Have a stool sample checked for parasites once or twice a year, and clean all stools from the yard immediately. Ensure that all family members wash hands after cleaning the yard, playing in the yard, or playing with the dog.
3. Have your pet examined immediately if there are any skin conditions or gastrointestinal conditions, as there are fungal infections (ringworm) and parasites (mites, fleas) and some intestinal bacteria that can be contagious to people. Similarly if there are skin conditions or gastrointestinal conditions among family members, have the pet checked.
4. It is also advisable to avoid allowing the dog to lick the face of children (especially around the mouth or eyes) and to teach the children to wash thoroughly after playing sessions with the dog.
5. Any bite or scratch should be thoroughly cleaned and disinfected and wounds that break the skin or appear to become infected should be reported to a medical authority.

Summary
1. Prepare puppies during the early months of life with a variety of people, including young children.
2. Anticipate problems and work on their prevention well before the baby arrives home.
3. ALWAYS supervise pet/child interactions. Prevent access to the child when a responsible adult is not available to supervise.
4. Don't take the relationship between the pet and the baby for granted. Actively take steps to shape it in a positive way.
5. Avoid punishing the pet, banishing it from the room, or ignoring the pet when the child is present.
6. Teach children how to act around their pets, around other animals, and what to do if threatened.

Figure C.10   Client handout on children and dogs (handout #17 – printable from the CD).

INFANTS, CHILDREN, AND CATS

New or expectant parents typically have three major concerns: 1) How to prevent pet behavior problems from occurring after the baby arrives; 2) How to introduce the baby to the family cat; and 3) How to keep the child safe around the family cat as well as other animals. Pet owners often assume that jealousy is the cause of problem behaviors associated with the arrival of a new child into the home, but this is not the case. Most problems result from the anxiety caused by significant alterations in the pet's environment and the way the family interacts with the pet. Changes in feeding, exercise, and play schedules; changes in what the pet is allowed to do; changes in how the pet gets attention; and inconsistencies in the way the owner interacts with the pet can all lead to problems.

Pets don't innately know how to behave around children, and children need to learn how to interact with animals. While most cats accept the new arrival without much fuss, some do not. Cats can be unpredictable around children, varying from avoidance to intense interest. Fortunately, most problems can readily be avoided with some forethought and training.

When the baby comes home
The cat's response to a new baby or to children will be primarily due to previous experiences with babies, children, and strangers, and the cat's genetic temperament. Some cats will adapt quickly to children and new babies by either ignoring them, or eventually seeking them out for investigation or social contact (e.g., cheek rubbing), while others may immediately be inquisitive, playful, and affectionate. While investigation and affection may be desirable, these behaviors must be well supervised since they can still lead to injury to the child, or inappropriate responses from the child toward the pet. On the other hand, some cats may be particularly fearful, which could lead to avoidance or aggression.

There are three basic considerations for helping cats to best adapt to new babies or children. The first is to adapt the cat's schedule, owner interactions, and environment slowly so that it is prepared for the arrival of the new baby. The second is for the owners to supervise all interactions with the cat and the baby to ensure safety and so that positive interactions can be rewarded. The third is to help the child adapt to the needs of the cat.

Adapting the home in advance
Some cats can become stressed and anxious when there are changes to their daily routine, social interactions, or environment. The cat's response may be a change in behavior or attitude with respect to humans or other cats (increased fear and avoidance or increased irritability and aggression), urine or stool marking of the environment, or displacement behaviors such as overgrooming with hair loss (psychogenic alopecia). There may also be an impact on the cat's physical health, such as a change in appetite (whether markedly decreased or increased), activity level (increase or decrease), sleep–wake cycles, or organ dysfunction.

Owners should consider how the daily schedule, social interactions, and household will need to be changed when the new baby arrives and begin to slowly adapt the cat to these changes in advance of the new arrival. Wherever possible the changes should not only be made slowly, but should be associated with positive events and interactions such as food treats, affection, and play. If there are rooms, counters, and areas of the house that will be made out of bounds for the cat when the child arrives, then you should begin in advance to keep the cat out of these areas, and teach the cat where it is allowed to sleep, play, and explore. It may also be advisable to obtain and set up new furniture in advance of the baby's arrival as some cats can be particularly sensitive or reactive to new structures and new odors.

Some cats may be fearful or anxious of strange sounds. For these cats, a recording can be made of baby noises (cooing, crying, screaming, etc.). Play the recording for the cat so it can barely be heard, and slowly increase the volume until an anxious response is obtained, then reduce the volume just below this level and play the tape while offering tasty food treats, play, or catnip toys. Very gradually increase the volume as the weeks go by until the pet seems comfortable with these noises at high volumes. To prepare the pet for the new smells that will arrive with the baby, take something home from the hospital, such as a towel or blanket with the baby's scent. Then teach the cat to associate the object with food or petting. On occasion, some cats may become anxious or overly investigative when the owner carries, changes, or nurses the new baby. Testing the cat by carrying around and fussing with a doll (especially one that actually moves and makes crying sounds) can be useful. If there is any anxiety, a positive association should be made with this doll using favored play toys, treats, or food rewards before the baby arrives (also see our handout on desensitization and counterconditioning). If there is concern that additional safe control will be required to supervise and introduce the cat and baby, then training the cat to wear a body harness can be extremely useful.

When the baby arrives
The simplest rule to help with the arrival is to supervise all interactions with the cat and baby so that any potential problems (whether fearful, overly aggressive, overly affectionate, or overly playful) can be identified. Then, with the aid of a behavior consultant, the particular concerns can be addressed. At all other times, such as when the baby is sleeping or playing in its playpen, access to the baby should be prevented. Even an affectionate cat could choose to lie down next to the young baby, which might be particularly dangerous for babies that cannot yet raise their heads or turn over. When the cat and child are together, be sure to reinforce all positive and appropriate interactions and gradually shape desirable responses. It can be particularly helpful to identify all things positive to the cat (food, affection, play, catnip, treats) and provide them when the baby and cat are together, while reducing their availability when the baby is not around. Conversely do not show anxiety, punish or immediately isolate the cat each time the baby is brought into the room, as this may lead to a negative or unpleasant association. If the cat reacts fearfully, or unpredictably, or there is a potential danger or risk to the new child, then a body harness can be used to help control the introductions.

Also be certain to monitor the cat's general demeanor, health, activity level, feeding, drinking, and elimination, and if there are any changes, report these to your veterinarian. These changes may not pose a risk for your child, but they may indicate that the cat is not coping well with the new arrival. Occasionally, pheromones or even drugs may help the cat to adapt if it is excessively anxious.

Cats and children
As the child grows and becomes more mobile and interactive, the relationship between the cat and child may change. Both fear and anxiety and overexuberant playful behavior could be problematic. As always, supervision to assess the cat's response to the child and the child's interactions with the cat is the best way to ensure that desirable responses are reinforced and any undesirable responses are identified. If problems do arise, preventing interactions may be the safest plan, but a program of careful and entirely positive reintroduction is generally required to improve the relationship (see handout on desensitization and counterconditioning for additional details).

Health concerns
It is rare for a cat to spread disease to humans. The number one health risk is from the physical injury caused by bites or scratches, so that injury prevention is the overriding concern. With some simple rules most other health problems can be prevented.
1. Have your pet examined and vaccinated at least once a year, and ensure that it is free of parasites.
2. Have a stool sample checked for parasites once or twice a year, and clean all stools from the yard immediately. Ensure that all family members wash hands after cleaning the yard, playing in the yard, or playing with the cat.
3. Have your pet examined immediately if there are any skin conditions or gastrointestinal conditions, as there are fungal infections (ringworm) and parasites (mites, fleas) and some intestinal bacteria that can be contagious to people. Similarly if there are skin conditions or gastrointestinal conditions among family members, have the pet checked.
4. It is also advisable to avoid allowing the cat to lick the face of children (especially around the mouth or eyes) and to teach the children to wash thoroughly after playing sessions with the cat.
5. Any bite or scratch should be thoroughly cleaned and disinfected and wounds that break the skin or appear to become infected should be reported to a medical authority.
6. Clean the litter box frequently and keep it out of the reach of children.

Summary
1. Prepare kittens during the early months of life with a variety of people, including young children.
2. Anticipate problems and work on their prevention well before the baby arrives home.
3. ALWAYS supervise pet/child interactions. Prevent access to the child when a responsible adult is not available to supervise.
4. Don't take the relationship between the pet and the baby for granted. Actively take steps to shape it in a positive way.
5. Avoid punishing the pet, banishing it from the room, or ignoring the pet when the child is present.
6. Teach children how to act around their pets, around other animals, and what to do if threatened.

Figure C.11   Client handout on children and cats (handout #16 – printable from the CD).

AGGRESSION RELEASE

Name of animal: _____ Case #: _____

I certify that I am the owner of the above-mentioned animal and that I have sought behavioral counseling for my pet for advice on decreasing its aggressiveness.

I understand that aggression by animals can cause injury, including fatal injury, to other animals, to other people and to me. I understand that treatment for aggressive behavior is not a guarantee that the aggression will be successfully controlled, and that it is impossible to ensure that my pet will not cause harm in the future.

I understand that the only way to **absolutely** ensure that my pet will never cause harm in the future is to euthanize it (end its life). I understand that if I do not euthanize my pet, it will be my responsibility to take appropriate precautions to prevent my pet's causing harm to others. These precautions may include, but are not limited to, informing persons near my pet of its tendency for aggressive behavior, keeping it on a leash, muzzling it, using a head collar, and/or keeping it restrained behind doors, gates, or fencing. I also understand that it is my responsibility to be aware of and comply with all state and local ordinances concerning aggressive animals, as well as any bylaws or acts that specifically apply to my pet. Finally, I understand that, should I choose not to euthanize my pet and it causes harm in the future, I may be held liable for such harm.

I hereby certify that I have read and understood the above and that I am signing this authorization with the full understanding that the treatment given my pet may not eliminate its aggressive behavior.

_____   _____
Signature of Owner   Date

_____
Printed Name

* Original release form courtesy of:
Sharon L. Crowell-Davis DVM, PhD
Diplomate, American College of Veterinary Behaviorists
College of Veterinary Medicine
University of Georgia
Athens, GA 30602

Figure C.12   Sample aggression release form (form #1 – printable from the CD). Modified version of a release form kindly supplied by Dr Sharon Crowell-Davis of the University Georgia College of Veterinary Medicine.

FOOD BOWL EXERCISES

READ THIS FIRST!!

There is <u>ALWAYS</u> a risk of injury when working with an aggressive dog. You may be bitten while performing these exercises. Following the instructions outlined below <u>does not</u> guarantee safety or ensure that a bite or attack will not occur. Never use these exercises or any others designed to change an aggressive dog's behavior unless you fully understand the methods and principles of the exercises and are willing to risk injury.

Preconditioning

1.   Spend at least two to four weeks at this level.
2.   Feeding: Feed two to three times daily. Confine the pet to an area away from feeding room. Place its food in the feeding room. Bring the pet to feeding room, leave and close the door until the pet finishes or 30 minutes pass.
3.   Attend class or review obedience training, occasionally using highly desirable food treats as reinforcers. Practice until the pet will do a very reliable sit/stay.
4.   Perform leadership exercises:
     a)   Make the pet sit or lie down before it gets <u>anything</u> it wants.
     b)   Don't allow the pet to acquire anything by <u>demanding</u> it.
     c)   Make the pet stay and wait for a release to follow you out of a room, up and down stairs, through hallways, and in and out of the home.
     d)   Continue indefinitely as long as the pet is exhibiting any signs of aggression.
5.   Increase the amount of time spent exercising with the pet or engaging in other types of pleasurable, safe activities.
6.   Teach 'fetch' and 'drop it' using only positive reinforcement.
7.   Avoid situations that elicit aggression from the pet.
8.   Avoid punishment.
9.   *Do not begin the following conditioning exercises if*:
     a)   You cannot guarantee complete control of access to food by the dog at <u>all</u> times (a difficult task if young children live in the home).
     b)   The pet will not perform a reliable sit-stay on command.
     c)   The pet lunges toward a person with a highly desirable food treat in the hand.
     d)   You lack confidence, lack control, or feel exceptionally nervous in the presence of the pet.
     e)   You don't completely understand all aspects of the training program.
     f)   You have <u>any</u> reservations about conducting the exercises.

PHASE ONE: Habituation to the owner's presence

- Necessary equipment: 2 bowls, dry food, highly desirable food treats (quarter to half-inch pieces of meat or cheese), 6 feet of rope.
- Optional equipment: leash, head halter.
- The room in which to do the exercises should be at least 10 feet by 10 feet wide. If the pet is more likely to be protective in the room in which it is usually fed, start the exercises in a room other than that room. Later in the program, the exercises can be moved to the original feeding room.

<u>First week of food bowl conditioning</u>

1.   To provide a higher degree of safety, a head halter and leash can be attached to the pet and a second person hold the leash for control. Use a very happy tone of voice during all of the exercises.
2.   Begin the session by requesting several obedience responses that are rewarded with highly desirable food treats.
3.   Place 1/8 of the dog's meal ration in the first bowl.
4.   Request a sit/stay.
5.   Place the bowl on the floor and release the dog to eat.
6.   Place another portion of food in the second bowl, walk a safe distance away (6 to 10 feet), ignore it and wait for the pet to finish eating.

7. When the pet finishes, call it, request a sit/stay, place the food bowl on the floor and release it to eat.
8. Place the third portion of food in first bowl, walk a safe distance away (6 to 10 feet) and wait for the pet to finish eating.
9. When the pet finishes, call it, request a sit/stay, place a bowl of food on floor and release it to eat.
10. Repeat until the meal allotment is finished.
11. Occasionally (every second or third trial, at random) slip a highly desirable food treat into the food bowl before placing it on the floor.
12. Occasionally drop a highly desirable food treat into the bowl just as the pet begins eating.

Second week
1. Repeat the above exercise but decrease the distance between the areas where the bowl is placed by one foot.
2. Gradually request longer stay responses. Vary the duration of the stay.

Following weeks
1. Every one to two weeks, decrease the distance between the areas where the bowl is placed by another six to 12 inches.
2. During the exercises, watch closely for signs of problems, especially during the phases when you remain close during feeding:

- Growling, lifting lip, hackles up
- Slow, stiff tail movement
- Prolonged gaze toward a family member
- Hesitancy approaching food
- Slow, stiff, or cautious behavior
- Nervous glancing
- Eating slower
- Yawning
- Change in carriage of the ears

If you note these behaviors by your pet, stop the session, call the pet to another area of the home, and leave it. Return to the feeding room and place the remaining food in the bowl and return the pet to that room to eat on its own. On the following day, continue the sessions at a previous, less interactive level. If you have any doubt about how to proceed if a problem occurs, be sure to call the behavior therapist before proceeding.

PHASE TWO: Dog and owner together
1. Begin this phase when you have been able to safely stand next to the pet through the whole session of sit/stay, give food bowl, sit/stay, give a second bowl, etc., for at least two weeks.
2. Place 1/8 of the dog's meal ration in the first bowl.
3. Wait until the dog has eaten several allotments of food. While the dog is eating, call its name, show it a highly desirable food treat (meat or cheese), ask it to sit/stay, give it the treat, release it to finish eating.
4. Continue to interrupt the dog at random intervals to sit/stay while it is feeding, gradually increasing the length of the stay.
5. Occasionally slip a highly desirable food treat into the bowl before giving it to the pet.
6. Stay at this level for at least two to four weeks.

PHASE THREE: Bowl in hand
1. Request a sit/stay, release the dog to stand and eat out of the bowl that is being held in your hand.
2. Occasionally slip a highly desirable food treat into the bowl before giving it to the pet.
3. Occasionally interrupt the pet with a sit/stay and hand feed a treat.
4. Stay at this level for at least two to four weeks.

PHASE FOUR: Withdraw bowl while hand feeding
1. Place 1/8 of the dog's meal ration in the first bowl.
2. Request a sit/stay, release the dog to eat out of the bowl that is being held in your hand.
3. Occasionally call the pet's name, ask it to 'stop' in an upbeat tone, give it a highly desirable food treat, and withdraw the bowl at the same time.
4. Ask it to sit/stay, extend the bowl to the dog and release it to eat from the bowl in your hand.
5. Repeat.
6. After seven to 10 days, occasionally say 'good dog' instead of giving a treat.
7. Stay at this level for at least two to four weeks.

PHASE FIVE: Take the bowl on the floor away with a rope
1. Place 1/8 of the dog's meal ration in the first bowl.
2. Attach a rope to the bowl so that it can be pulled away from a distance.
3. Request a sit/stay.
4. Place the bowl on the floor and release the dog to eat.
5. After the pet has eaten about half of its ration, occasionally ask it to 'stop,' sit/stay, and give a highly desirable food treat. Immediately repeat the 'stay' command as you pull the bowl away with the attached rope.
6. Pick up the bowl.
7. Repeat. Gradually use a shorter rope.
8. Stay at this level for at least two to four weeks.

PHASE SIX: Picking up the bowl
1. Place 1/8 of the dog's meal ration in the first bowl.
2. Request a sit/stay.
3. Place the bowl on the floor and release the dog to eat.
4. Occasionally ask the pet to 'stop,' sit/stay, and give it a highly desirable food treat as you pick up the bowl.
5. Give it another treat.
6. Repeat. After seven to 10 days, occasionally say 'good dog' instead of giving a treat.
7. Stay at this level for at least two to four weeks.

PHASE SEVEN: Touching the pet
1. Place 1/8 of the dog's meal ration in the first bowl.
2. Request a sit/stay.
3. Place the bowl on the floor and release the dog to eat.
4. Occasionally ask the pet to 'stop,' sit/stay, and give it a highly desirable food treat or say 'good dog.'
5. As the pet takes the treat from one hand, move the other hand toward its head or shoulder (whichever it is more likely to tolerate), but stop at a safe distance of approximately 24 inches away.
6. As the weeks pass, repeat the above steps. Very, very gradually move the hand toward the pet until it can be lightly touched for one second as it accepts the food. Very, very gradually during following sessions make longer contact with the hand. Work on other areas of the body.

PHASE EIGHT
Repeat the above exercises, starting with phase one, in other rooms of the home.

Figure C.13   Handout for food bowl exercises (handout #11 – printable from the CD).

However, appropriate intro...

Appendix D

Drug dosages

Before using any of the following drugs, please refer to Chapter 6 for treatment suggestions, contraindications, and potential adverse effects. Where more than one dose is listed, it is because a variety of doses have been published, and the lowest effective dose should be utilized. Most of the drugs listed below are not licensed for veterinary use, and few controlled studies have been performed. It is therefore the practitioner's responsibility to know the local regulations regarding off-label dispensing and to have appropriate consent or release forms signed.

The authors have made every effort to ensure the accuracy of the information with regard to drug dosages. However, appropriate information sources should be consulted, especially when new or unfamiliar drugs are first being utilized. It is the responsibility of every veterinarian to evaluate the appropriateness of a particular opinion in the context of actual clinical situations and with due consideration to new developments. For each drug, the authors' recommended dose is listed first followed by dose ranges (DR) that have been published by other authors (where applicable). Doses and descriptions of alternative and herbal remedies can be found in Chapter 7, while drugs used for pain management are discussed in detail in Chapter 8. All drugs are per os unless otherwise indicated.

Class	Drug	Indications/comments	Dosage (dog)	Dosage (cat)
CNS stimulants		• Hyperkinesis • Narcolepsy		
	Methylphenidate	• Paradoxical calming effect in hyperkinesis • Narcolepsy	Hyperkinesis: 2–4 mg/kg bid/tid Narcolepsy: 0.05–0.25 mg/kg bid	
	Dextroamphetamine	• Test for hyperkinesis • Narcolepsy	0.2–1.3 mg/kg prn Narcolepsy: 5–10 mg sid	Narcolepsy: 1.25 mg prn
	Levoamphetamine	• Test for hyperkinesis	1.0–4.0 mg/kg prn	
Anticonvulsants	Phenobarbital	• Psychomotor seizures • Tranquilization • Cats: excessive vocalization • Feline hyperesthesia syndrome	2–4 mg/kg per day divided bid/tid DR: 18–20 mg/kg per day divided bid/tid	2–4 mg/kg sid/bid
	Potassium bromide	• Seizures	70–80 mg/kg divided bid as a sole agent (maintain by monitoring serum levels after 3 months)	20 mg/kg per day divided bid (maintain by monitoring serum levels after 2 months)
	Carbamazepine	• Psychomotor seizures • Fear aggression – cats • Anxiety disorders • May cause vomiting in cats • Chronic/neuropathic pain • Unipolar disorders/mood regulation (Pageat) • Sociopathies (Pageat) • Dyssocialization (Pageat)	4–10 mg/kg divided q8h 20 mg/kg bid for pain management DR: 20–40 mg/kg in divided doses	4–8 mg/kg q12h

	Gabapentin	• Chronic/neuropathic pain • Psychomotor seizures • Anxiety	25–60 mg/kg divided into 3 or 4 doses daily 5 mg/kg tid for pain control	12.5 mg q12h
Benzodiazepines		• Noise phobias • Thunderstorm phobias • Panic attacks associated with separation anxiety • Anxiety disorders • Feline aggression • Urine marking and anxiety-related housesoiling in cats • Night waking • Psychomotor seizures		
	Clorazepate	• See above • Adjunctive seizure control • Complex partial seizures	0.55–2.2 mg/kg sid/tid 1–3 mg/kg bid for seizure control (increase dose with phenobarbital use)	0.2–0.5 mg/kg sid/bid 3.75–7.5 mg/cat bid/tid (seizure control) DR: up to 2.2 mg/kg sid/bid
	Alprazolam	• See above	0.02–0.1 mg/kg prn or bid/qid	0.125–0.25 mg/cat sid/tid
	Lorazepam	• See above (may be safer for liver since no intermediate metabolite)	0.1–0.2 mg/kg prn	0.125–0.25 mg/cat bid
	Diazepam	• See above • Appetite stimulant • Half-life of 2.5 hours in dogs and from 5.5 to 20 hours in cats • Acute, fatal hepatopathy may occur in cats	0.5–2.0 mg/kg, repeat in 4 to 6 hours if necessary for storm phobias 1–2 mg/kg per rectal (used for status epilepticus, may be effective for immediate control of panic/phobic state)	0.2–0.5 mg/kg bid/tid DR: up to 1 mg/kg (for appetite stimulation)
	Flurazepam	• Appetite stimulant • Altered sleep cycles	0.2–0.4 mg/kg for 4–7d	0.2–0.4 mg/kg for 4–7d
	Oxazepam	• Appetite stimulant • Anti-anxiety • Urine marking	0.2–0.5 mg/kg sid/bid DR: up to 1 mg/kg bid	0.2–0.5 mg/kg sid/bid 1–3 mg/cat bid DR: up to 2 mg/kg bid
	Triazolam	• Aggression in cats • Altered sleep cycles	0.01–0.1 mg/kg bid or prn	0.03 mg/cat bid DR: 0.01–0.1 mg/kg bid
	Clonazepam	• Sleep disorders • Seizures • Psychomotor epilepsy	0.1–1.0 mg/kg bid/tid 0.5 mg/kg tid for seizure control (micronized tablets). NB increase dose if concurrent with phenobarbital	0.016 mg/kg sid/qid (sleep disorders) 0.1–0.2 mg/kg sid/bid
	Chlordiazepoxide	• Anxiety • Appetite stimulant • Urine marking	2–20 mg prn DR: 2–6 mg/kg prn	0.2–1.0 mg/kg sid/bid
	Chlordiazepoxide/clinidium	• Stress colitis	1–2 tabs bid	
Neuroleptics/antipsychotics		• Immobilization • Decrease vocalization • Traveling • Noise phobias • Sedation		
	Acepromazine	• Restraint/sedation • Reduce activity • Reduce response to stimuli • Sedation for travel	0.5–1.1 mg/kg sid/qid DR: 0.1–2.2 mg/kg prn	0.5–1.1 mg/kg prn DR: up to 2.2 mg/kg prn
	Chlorpromazine	• Reduce response to stimuli • Reduce activity • Sedation	0.5–3.3 mg/kg sid/qid	0.5–3.3 mg/kg sid/qid
	Promazine	• Reduce activity • Reduce response to stimuli • Sedation	1.0–4.4 mg/kg prn	2.0–4.0 mg/kg prn

	Thoridiazine	• Aggression • Anxiety • Phobias • Compulsive (hallucinatory-type) disorders	1.1–2.2 mg/kg sid/bid 30 mg/m^2 divided bid (Pageat)	
	Perphenazine	• Anxiety • Fears • Phobias	0.88 mg/kg bid/tid	0.88 mg/kg bid/tid
	Pimozide	• Compulsive disorders	1–10 mg sid	
	Haloperidol	• Compulsive disorders • Aggression	1–4 mg bid	
	Risperidone	• Dominance aggression/sociopathies • Dissociative disorders • Hallucinatory-type signs	0.5–1 mg/m^2	
	Sultopride (Pageat)	• For treatment of negative signs. • Hypersensitivity–hyperactivity syndrome (stage 3) • Sociopathies • Stage 3 phobias	200 mg/m^2 divided bid, antideficient dose DR: to 1 g/m^2 divided bid, antiproductive dose	
	Fluphenazine (Pageat)	• Social phobias • Stage 2 phobias	50 mg/m^2 divided bid	
	Sulpiride or amisulpride (Pageat)	• As with sultopride	25–50 mg/m^2 divided bid (antideficient dose)	
	Amisulpride	• As with sultopride	20 mg/m^2 (divided bid)	
	Pipamperone (Pageat)	• Separation anxiety • Primary dyssocialization • Sociopathies	60 mg/m^2 divided bid 30 mg/m^2 divided bid when combined with clomipramine, tiapride, or sultopride	
Tricyclic antidepressants		• Depression • Anxiety • Aggression • Feline urine marking • Narcolepsy • Enuresis • Compulsive behaviors • Mood stabilizing		
	Amitriptyline	• As above • Peak levels 2–12h	2.0–4.0 mg/kg bid DR: 1.0–6 mg/kg bid	0.5–1.0 mg/kg/d DR: up to 2 mg/kg sid
	Doxepin	• Pruritus – self-trauma • Acral lick dermatitis • Compulsive behaviors	3–5 mg/kg bid	0.5–1.0 mg/kg q12–24h
	Clomipramine	• Compulsive behaviors • Anxiety, including separation anxiety • Urine marking	2–4 mg/kg/bid	0.3–0.5 mg/kg sid DR: up to 1 mg/kg sid
	Imipramine	• Separation anxiety • Anxiety disorders • Enuresis • Narcolepsy/cataplexy (peak effects 1–2h)	1–4.4 mg/kg sid/bid Stereotypy: 1.0–2.0 mg/kg bid/tid Narcolepsy or cataplexy: 0.5–1.0 mg/kg tid	0.5–1 mg/kg sid/bid Enuresis: 2.5–5 mg bid
	Protriptyline	• Narcoleptic hypersomnia (e.g., Labrador Retrievers) • Cataplexy	5–10 mg sid/bid (narcolepsy) DR: 0.2–0.5 mg/kg sid/bid	0.5–1 mg/kg sid/bid
	Nortriptyline		0.1–2 mg/kg bid	0.5–2 mg/kg sid/bid
Tetracyclic antidepressant	Mianserine (Pageat)	• Hypersensitivity–hyperactivity syndrome • Stage 2 phobias • Reactive depression	2–5 mg/kg divided bid DR: up to 10 mg/kg daily	

Selective serotonin re-uptake inhibitors (SSRIs)		• Depression • Panic • Compulsive disorders • Aggression • Impulsiveness • Feline urine marking • Mood disorders (Europe) • Overactivity disorders (Europe) • Urine marking		
	Fluoxetine	• See SSRIs above	1.0–2.0 mg/kg sid	0.5–1.0 mg/kg q24h
	Sertraline	• See SSRIs above	1–3 mg/kg sid 2–4 mg/kg divided twice daily (Europe)	0.5 mg/kg sid
	Paroxetine	• See SSRIs above	1 mg/kg sid 2–5 mg/kg sid (Europe)	0.5–1 mg/kg sid
	Fluvoxamine	• See SSRIs above	1–2 mg/kg sid 2–5 mg/kg sid (Europe) DR: up to 7 mg/kg sid	0.25–0.5 mg/kg sid
	Citalopram	• See SSRIs above	1 mg/kg sid	
Hormones		• Aggression • Feline urine marking • Suppress male behavior • Calming effect • Appetite stimulant • Compulsive disorders		
	Megestrol acetate	• As above	1.1–4.4 mg/kg sid, then half dose q2wks to lowest effective dose	2.5–10 mg sid for 1 to 2 weeks then half dose q2wks to lowest effective dose
	Medroxy-progesterone acetate	• As above	5–11 mg/kg sq/im 3X/yr	5–20 mg/kg sq/im 3X/yr
	Diethylstilbestrol	• Estrogen-responsive incontinence	0.1–1.0 mg/dog/day for 3–5 days then reduce to once or twice weekly	
	Testosterone cypionate	• Urinary incontinence in neutered males	2.2 mg/kg im monthly	5–10 mg im
	Cyproterone acetate	• Heterospecific imprints (Pageat) • Sociopathies (Pageat) • Assessing potential effects of castration	1.25–2.5 mg/kg per day DR: 3–5 mg/kg divided bid (Pageat)	
Antihistamines		• Compulsive scratching • Self-trauma • Mild sedation • Sedation for travel • Waking at night		
	Hydroxyzine	• As above	2.2 mg/kg bid/tid	2.2 mg/kg bid/tid
	Chlorpheniramine	• As above	2–8 mg bid/tid 0.2–0.8 mg/kg tid (maximum 1 mg/kg/24h)	1–2 mg bid/tid 0.4–0.7 mg/kg sid/bid
	Diphenhydramine	• As above	2–4 mg/kg bid/tid	2–4 mg/kg bid/tid
	Trimeprazine	• As above	0.5–5.0 mg/dog tid	
	Cyproheptadine	• Serotonin antagonist • Antihistaminic • Appetite stimulant	0.3–2.0 mg/kg bid	2.0–4.0 mg/cat bid/tid
Opiate agonists/antagonists		• Compulsive/stereotypic behaviors • Self-mutilation		
	Hydrocodone	• Compulsive dermatologic disorders	0.22 mg/kg bid/tid	0.25–1.0 mg/kg bid/tid

Beta-blockers		• Decrease somatic components of anxiety		
	Propranolol	• Mild fears and anxiety	0.5–3.0 mg/kg bid or prn DR: 10–20 mg/kg divided twice daily	0.2–1.0 mg/kg tid
	Pindolol	• Mild fears and anxiety	0.125–0.25 mg/kg bid	
Alpha-adrenergics and sympathomimetics		• Urinary incontinence • Excitement urination • Submissive urination		
	Phenyl-propanolamine	• As above	1.1–4.4 mg/kg bid/tid	12.5 mg tid
Alpha-adrenergic antagonists	Nicergoline	• Cognitive dysfunction • Diminished vigor • Sleep disorders • Psychomotor disturbances	0.25–0.50 mg/kg/day 3–30 days. Tablets should not be broken for small dogs. A solution can be concocted with manufacturer's directions	
Antipsychotics	Lithium carbonate	• Unpredictable severe aggression • Ranges for serum therapeutic and toxic levels overlap	3–12 mg/kg q12–24h, titrate dose by blood levels	
Miscellaneous anti-anxiety	Buspirone	• Chronic fears/anxiety • Phobias • Feline urine marking • Aggression • Compulsive disorders • Relatively wide margin of safety	1.0–2.0 mg/kg sid/tid	0.5–1.0 mg/kg sid/tid
	Meprobamate	• Anti-anxiety • Aggression	20–40 mg/kg bid/qid	50 mg/kg prn
	Clonidine	• Anxiety, compulsive disorders, panic, phobia	0.015 mg/kg divided bid (Pageat)	
MAO inhibitors	Selegiline	• Cognitive dysfunction • Neurodegenerative disorders • Hypersensitivity–hyperactivity (Pageat) • Emotional disorders (EDED) • Stage 3 phobias (Pageat) • Dyssocialization (Pageat)	0.5–1 mg/kg sid	0.5–1 mg/kg sid

Key: prn = as needed, sid = once per day, bid = twice per day, tid = three times per day, qid = four times per day.
    DR = dose range published by other authors.

For indications, contraindications, adverse effects, and references, see Chapter 6.

Index

CD-ROM INSTRUCTIONS

This CD-ROM will run on both PCs and Macs. It contains PDF files of the text that can be read using Acrobat Reader 5.0. If you do not already have Acrobat Reader 5.0, and do not have Internet access to obtain it, please install it from the copy supplied on this CD-ROM.

Minimum system requirements

Windows

- Intel® Pentium® processor
- Microsoft® Windows® 95 OSR 2.0, Windows 98 SE, Windows Millennium, Windows NT® 4.0 with Service Pack 5, or Windows 2000
- 64 MB of RAM
- 24 MB of available hard-disk space
- Additional 70 MB of hard-disk space for Asian fonts (optional)

Macintosh

- PowerPC® processor
- Mac OS software version 8.6, 9.0.4, or Mac OS X

- 64 MB of RAM
- 24 MB of available hard-disk space
- Additional 70 MB of hard-disk space for Asian fonts (optional)

Note: No data is transferred to the hard disk, the CD-ROM is self-contained, and the application runs directly from the CD.

Support

Should you have problems with running the disk, please contact us:

In the USA:
- E-mail: technical.support@elsevier.com
- Telephone: +1 800 692 9010

In the UK:
- E-mail: cdrom@eslo.co.uk
- Telephone: +44 (0)20 7611 4202

On initial contact your problem will be logged and passed on to the appropriate technical expert. We will then contact you as quickly as possible with an answer.

MULTIMEDIA CD-ROM
SINGLE USER LICENSE AGREEMENT

1. NOTICE. WE ARE WILLING TO LICENSE THE MULTIMEDIA PROGRAM PRODUCT TITLED *"Handbook of behavior problems of the dog and cat, 2nd edition"* ("MULTIMEDIA PROGRAM") TO YOU ONLY ON THE CONDITION THAT YOU ACCEPT ALL OF THE TERMS CONTAINED IN THIS LICENSE AGREEMENT. PLEASE READ THIS LICENSE AGREEMENT CAREFULLY BEFORE OPENING THE SEALED DISK PACKAGE. BY OPENING THAT PACKAGE YOU AGREE TO BE BOUND BY THE TERMS OF THIS AGREEMENT. IF YOU DO NOT AGREE TO THESE TERMS WE ARE UNWILLING TO LICENSE THE MULTIMEDIA PROGRAM TO YOU, AND YOU SHOULD NOT OPEN THE DISK PACKAGE. IN SUCH CASE, PROMPTLY RETURN THE UNOPENED DISK PACKAGE AND ALL OTHER MATERIAL IN THIS PACKAGE, ALONG WITH PROOF OF PAYMENT, TO THE AUTHORISED DEALER FROM WHOM YOU OBTAINED IT FOR A FULL REFUND OF THE PRICE YOU PAID.

2. **Ownership and License**. This is a license agreement and NOT an agreement for sale. It permits you to use one copy of the MULTIMEDIA PROGRAM on a single computer. The MULTIMEDIA PROGRAM and its contents are owned by us or our licensors, and are protected by U.S. and international copyright laws. Your rights to use the MULTIMEDIA PROGRAM are specified in this Agreement, and we retain all rights not expressly granted to you in this Agreement.

- You may use one copy of the MULTIMEDIA PROGRAM on a single computer.
- After you have installed the MULTIMEDIA PROGRAM on your computer, you may use the MULTIMEDIA PROGRAM on a different computer only if you first delete the files installed by the installation program from the first computer.
- You may not copy any portion of the MULTIMEDIA PROGRAM to your computer hard disk or any other media other than printing out or downloading non-substantial portions of the text and images in the MULTIMEDIA PROGRAM for your own internal informational use.
- You may not copy any of the documentation or other printed materials accompanying the MULTIMEDIA PROGRAM.

Neither concurrent use on two or more computers nor use in a local area network or other network is permitted without separate authorisation and the payment of additional license fees.

3. **Transfer and Other Restrictions**. You may not rent, lend, or lease this MULTIMEDIA PROGRAM. Save as permitted by law, you may not and you may not permit others to (a) disassemble, decompile, or otherwise derive source code from the software included in the MULTIMEDIA PROGRAM (the "Software"), (b) reverse engineer the Software, (c) modify or prepare derivative works of the MULTIMEDIA PROGRAM, (d) use the Software in an on-line system, or (e) use the MULTIMEDIA PROGRAM in any manner that infringes on the intellectual property or other rights of another party.

However, you may transfer this license to use the MULTIMEDIA PROGRAM to another party on a permanent basis by transferring this copy of the License Agreement, the MULTIMEDIA PROGRAM, and all documentation. Such transfer of possession terminates your license from us. Such other party shall be licensed under the terms of this Agreement upon its acceptance of this Agreement by its initial use of the MULTIMEDIA PROGRAM. If you transfer the MULTIMEDIA PROGRAM, you must remove the installation files from your hard disk and you may not retain any copies of those files for your own use.

4. **Limited Warranty and Limitation of Liability**. For a period of sixty (60) days from the date you acquired the MULTIMEDIA PROGRAM from us or our authorised dealer, we warrant that the media containing the MULTIMEDIA PROGRAM will be free from defects that prevent you from installing the MULTIMEDIA PROGRAM on your computer. If the disk fails to conform to this warranty you may, as your sole and exclusive remedy, obtain a replacement free of charge if you return the defective disk to us with a dated proof of purchase. Otherwise the MULTIMEDIA PROGRAM is licensed to you on an "AS IS" basis without any warranty of any nature.

WE DO NOT WARRANT THAT THE MULTIMEDIA PROGRAM WILL MEET YOUR REQUIREMENTS OR THAT ITS OPERATION WILL BE UNINTERRUPTED OR ERROR-FREE. THE EXPRESS TERMS OF THIS AGREEMENT ARE IN LIEU OF ALL WARRANTIES, CONDITIONS, UNDERTAKINGS, TERMS AND OBLIGATIONS IMPLIED BY STATUTE, COMMON LAW, TRADE USAGE, COURSE OF DEALING OR OTHERWISE ALL OF WHICH ARE HEREBY EXCLUDED TO THE FULLEST EXTENT PERMITTED BY LAW, INCLUDING THE IMPLIED WARRANTIES OF SATISFACTORY QUALITY AND FITNESS FOR A PARTICULAR PURPOSE.

WE SHALL NOT BE LIABLE FOR ANY DAMAGE OR LOSS OF ANY KIND (EXCEPT PERSONAL INJURY OR DEATH RESULTING FROM OUR NEGLIGENCE) ARISING OUT OF OR RESULTING FROM YOUR POSSESSION OR USE OF THE MULTIMEDIA PROGRAM (INCLUDING DATA LOSS OR CORRUPTION), REGARDLESS OF WHETHER SUCH LIABILITY IS BASED IN TORT, CONTRACT OR OTHERWISE AND INCLUDING, BUT NOT LIMITED TO, ACTUAL, SPECIAL, INDIRECT, INCIDENTAL OR CONSEQUENTIAL DAMAGES. IF THE FOREGOING LIMITATION IS HELD TO BE UNENFORCEABLE OUR MAXIMUM LIABILITY TO YOU SHALL NOT EXCEED THE AMOUNT OF THE LICENSE FEE PAID BY YOU FOR THE MULTIMEDIA PROGRAM. THE REMEDIES AVAILABLE TO YOU AGAINST US AND THE LICENSORS OF MATERIALS INCLUDED IN THE MULTIMEDIA PROGRAM ARE EXCLUSIVE.

5. **Termination.** This license and your right to use this MULTIMEDIA PROGRAM automatically terminate if you fail to comply with any provisions of this Agreement, destroy the copy of the MULTIMEDIA PROGRAM in your possession, or voluntarily return the MULTIMEDIA PROGRAM to us. Upon termination you will destroy all copies of the MULTIMEDIA PROGRAM and documentation.

6. **Miscellaneous Provisions.** This Agreement will be governed by and construed in accordance with English law and you hereby submit to the non-exclusive jurisdiction of the English Courts. This is the entire agreement between us relating to the MULTIMEDIA PROGRAM, and supersedes any prior purchase order, communications, advertising or representations concerning the contents of this package. No change or modification of this Agreement will be valid unless it is in writing and is signed by us.